ACSM's
Nutrition for
Exercise Science

ACSM's Nutrition for Exercise Science

Second Edition

AUTHOR

Dan Benardot, PhD, DHC, RDN, FACSM

Teaching Professor
Center for Study of Human Health
Emory University
Atlanta, Georgia

Professor of Nutrition, Emeritus
Georgia State University
Atlanta, Georgia

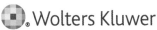

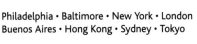
Philadelphia · Baltimore · New York · London
Buenos Aires · Hong Kong · Sydney · Tokyo

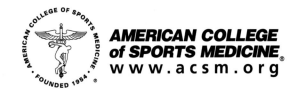

Acquisitions Editor: Lindsey Porambo
Senior Development Editor: Amy Millholen
Editorial Coordinator: Nancy Dickson
Marketing Manager: Danielle Klahr
Production Project Manager: Matthew West
Design Coordinator: Stephen Druding, Leslie Caruso
Manufacturing Coordinator: Margie Orzech
Compositor: Aptara, Inc.
ACSM Publications Committee Chair: Karyn L. Hamilton, PhD, RD, FACSM
ACSM Health-Fitness Content Advisory Committee Chair: M. Allison Murphy, PhD, FACSM, ACSM-EP
ACSM Chief Operating Officer: Katie Feltman
ACSM Assistant Director of Publishing: Angie Chastain

Second Edition

9 8 7 6 5 4 3 2 1

Printed in Mexico

978-1-9751-9716-2
Library of Congress Cataloging-in-Publication Data
available upon request

DISCLAIMER

Care has been taken to confirm the accuracy of the information present and to describe generally accepted practices. However, the authors, editors, and publisher are not responsible for errors or omissions or for any consequences from application of the information in this publication and make no warranty, expressed or implied, with respect to the currency, completeness, or accuracy of the contents of the publication. Application of this information in a particular situation remains the professional responsibility of the practitioner; the clinical treatments described and recommended may not be considered absolute and universal recommendations.

The authors, editors, and publisher have exerted every effort to ensure that drug selection and dosage set forth in this text are in accordance with the current recommendations and practice at the time of publication. However, in view of ongoing research, changes in government regulations, and the constant flow of information relating to drug therapy and drug reactions, the reader is urged to check the package insert for each drug for any change in indications and dosage and for added warnings and precautions. This is particularly important when the recommended agent is a new or infrequently employed drug.

Some drugs and medical devices presented in this publication have Food and Drug Administration (FDA) clearance for limited use in restricted research settings. It is the responsibility of the health care provider to ascertain the FDA status of each drug or device planned for use in their clinical practice.

To purchase additional copies of this book, call our customer service department at (800) 638-3030 or fax orders to (301) 223-2320. International customers should call (301) 223-2300.

For more information concerning the American College of Sports Medicine certification and suggested preparatory materials, call (800) 486-5643 or visit the American College of Sports Medicine Website at www.acsm.org.

shop.lww.com

DEDICATION

To my wonderful children, Jake and Leah, and my incredible grandchildren,
Eva, Nora, Evan, and Jodi, who make my life glow.

Reviewers

Sara C. Campbell, PhD, FACSM
Rutgers University—Douglass Campus
New Brunswick, New Jersey

Nancy Clark, RD, FACSM
Sports Nutrition Counselor
Newton Highlands, Massachusetts

Yvette Figueroa, PhD
Sam Houston State University
Huntsville, Texas

Warren D. Franke, PhD, FACSM
Iowa State University
Ames, Iowa

Jill A. Kanaley, PhD, FACSM
University of Missouri
Columbia, Missouri

Laura J. Kruskall, PhD, RDN, LD, FACSM
University of Nevada, Las Vegas
Las Vegas, Nevada

Foreword

Before the year 2018, there was a great debate in the health fitness world about the extent to which those of us teaching nutrition in classes for exercise science students could go without violating the limitations imposed by state law. The somewhat narrow view was that only Registered Dietitians (RD) or Registered Dietitian Nutritionists (RDN) could provide medical nutrition therapy. The enduring question was whether exercise professionals working in cardiac, pulmonary, or metabolic management programs could discuss ways to change lifestyles including dietary changes with their patients. The problem is compounded by the need of the millions of clients who visit health clubs who also seek help with their diets. The Academy of Nutrition and Dietetics (AND) has recently determined that "medical nutrition therapy and other complex nutrition and dietetics services should only be provided by qualified individuals with the specialized education and training of RDNs or, at a minimum, meet state licensure standards." There are currently 11 states that prohibit any personalized nutrition counseling without a license (and typically require RDN), 3 that provide other pathways besides the RDN and are just as restrictive, but 36 allow for nutrition counseling outside of medical nutrition therapy (https://becomeanutritionist.org/states/).

While versions of the debate continue, many of those initial questions about what could be taught in exercise science classes and what exercise professionals could tell their clients was answered in Dan Benardot's 2018 first edition of this book, *ACSM's Nutrition for Exercise Science*. Filled with case studies and discussion questions, practical advice, in-text learning assists, and other instructor aids made that book an instant hit.

The second edition of *ACSM's Nutrition for Exercise Science* continues the exceptional pathway established by the first edition. Dr. Benardot carefully and skillfully delineates the differences between providing dietary management for a "patient" who has an identified medical condition (which is out of the scope of practice for health fitness professionals who are not RDs or RDNs) and the general guidance given to clients in a health fitness setting. For example, when working as a clinical exercise physiologist (CEP) in a cardiac rehabilitation program, it is fitting for a CEP to conduct a class on general nutrition and would be considered within the scope of practice for that exercise professional. However, trying to answer a question about the resolution (cure) of a disease through specific changes in a diet is beyond the scope of practice and best left to a licensed RD or RDN to answer particularly in those states with restrictive practice guidelines.

Now, on a personal note. I first met Dan Benardot in 1993 when I was interviewing for a new faculty position at Georgia State University. It was Dan who convinced me that moving to the Atlanta area would be a good thing for my career and for my family. He was right. I joined the faculty in 1994 and remained there until retirement in 2020. Dan and I have worked together on countless research projects, traveled the world together as lecturers, and were a writing team for numerous assignments many of them about elite athletes, with and without physical impairments. I am proud to call him my colleague and my friend.

Walt Thompson
Walter R. Thompson, PhD, FACSM
Regents' Professor Emeritus
Former Associate Dean for Graduate Studies and Research
College of Education & Human Development
Georgia State University
Atlanta, Georgia
61st President of the American College of Sports Medicine
(2017–2018)

Preface

Nutrition for Exercise Science, second edition, presents the ever-evolving science of nutrition in an accessible format to enable a high level of understanding of how to best apply the science to athletes in different sports, genders, ages, and environments. The second edition integrates the current science/nutrition guidelines with the ultimate goal of enabling a high level of performance through optimized training and recovery, while reducing health and injury risks. The book has many figures and tables to help facilitate an understanding of the science, and case studies with questions and answers that serve to help the reader understand how different athlete populations have different nutritional risks. In addition, an available test bank and slides serve to help instructors efficiently create an effective classroom environment.

The exponential growth of the field of sports nutrition has provided both science and practical advice that was not readily available until recently. The early guidelines were predictably vague with a low level of agreement among experts on the best strategies to follow to enable a high level of athletic performance while lowering health risks. The scientific knowledge in the field of sports nutrition today, however, is rapidly expanding and increasingly providing science-based and situation-specific recommendations. The information now available is specific to the sport, age, gender, ability, and conditioned capacity of the athlete, and is included in the second edition. As an illustration of how the science of nutrition has changed, in the past we may have recommended the consumption of water or a nondescript sports beverage to help an athlete achieve and/or sustain a desired hydration state. Current recommendations include volume, temperature, electrolyte concentration and composition, and energy substrate concentration and composition for different aspects of the athletic endeavor, including what is recommended before, during, and after training/competition. Importantly these recommendations include a dynamic consideration of sports physiology, nutritional biochemistry, sports medicine, sports psychology, and body composition.

The second edition addresses nutritional problems that impact athletes in different sports, which are often the result of traditions/beliefs on how to eat and drink to optimize performance. It is a common belief that if a small amount of any nutrient is good for you then more must be better. This belief is increasingly being unraveled with scientific findings that have determined that, in most cases, more than enough is not better than enough as excessive intakes fail to support athletic performance while increasing acute and chronic disease risks. To illustrate this point, the heavy consumption of protein, long believed to be the "magic" ingredient in any athlete's diet, is now put into proper perspective with guidelines on how to best consume it for enhanced performance health. To complicate matters further, excessively high consumption of protein invariably results in inadequate carbohydrate consumption, which is a common factor associated with poor athletic performance.

The traditional *calories-in–calories-out* paradigm is now better understood, with a high level of scientific evidence suggesting that energy availability in real time is critically important and that randomly satisfying the energy requirement is not sufficient. We have come to learn that athletes who have satisfied energy needs over a 24-hour period may be at risk for hormonal and body composition struggles if the timing of energy consumption has resulted in periods of significant energy balance deficits. The paradigm for energy intake has shifted to one that should encourage athletes to eat in a way that dynamically satisfies energy expenditure in real time rather than in three daily doses. The endocrine system really does work in real time. Imagine the pancreas waiting until day's end to assess what and how much food was consumed earlier in the day as a way of determining how much insulin it should produce. It just does not happen that way, but the traditional calories-in–calories-out strategy assumes precisely that. A key emphasis for this book, therefore, is to break through our old understandings of how athletes and physically active people should eat and drink to optimize performance by providing an interpretation of the new nutrition science so it can be applied to the athletic endeavor. Included in an enormous body of new scientific literature in sports nutrition are many recent publications that have provided key information for this endeavor, including the joint position statement on *Nutrition and Athletic Performance* from the American College of Sports Medicine, the Academy of Nutrition and Dietetics, and Dietitians of Canada; the recently published International Olympic Committee (IOC) consensus on *Dietary Supplements and the High-Performance Athlete*; the IOC consensus on *Relative Energy Deficiency in Sport (RED-S)*; and numerous publications on the negative impact of within-day energy deficiency in male and female athletes.

Nutrition has an impact on multiple areas, including injury prevention and injury recovery, muscle and skeletal development, exercise recovery, psychological sense of well-being, general health, and resistance to illness. Under ideal circumstances, all members of the sports medicine team, including sports nutritionists, exercise physiologists, sports medicine physicians, sports psychologists, and athletic trainers, should have some understanding of how nutrition will affect their specific areas of expertise. Therefore, while the primary focus of this book is to help exercise science and nutrition students understand the science of sports nutrition, it can also help others on the sports medicine team understand the scientific basis of important nutritional issues that have an impact on athlete health and performance. By doing so, this book will contribute to the cohesiveness and functionality of the sports medicine team and to the ultimate benefit of the athlete. This book is also likely to find other readers who have an interest in athlete health and success, including parents and coaches.

Since an important goal of this book is to make the science accessible, easily understood, and applicable, any reader in a college/university should be capable of reading and understanding the book contents without prerequisite knowledge. A number of courses are taught at the undergraduate and/or beginning graduate level for which this book would be appropriate, including courses with titles such as Nutrition for Physical Activity, Nutrition for Exercise Science, Sports Nutrition, and related titles. Assuming the student is in any field related to applied science and public health, there should be no course prerequisites needed to take a course using this book.

ORGANIZATION AND SPECIAL FEATURES

An important goal of this book is to make it a comprehensive source of nutrition information that relates to athletic needs. All chapters begin with a clear delineation of **Chapter Objectives**, a case study that provides a real-world example of the potential problems an athlete can face, followed by **Case Study Discussion Questions** with **Case Study Considerations** for how to best consider responding to each case study question. Logical and practical solutions are reinforced in each subsequent chapter. Throughout the book, the chapters emphasize the science while making the science accessible and applicable. This is true for each chapter, as follows:

- **Chapter 1** provides an overview of critical issues and terms, common myths, an introduction to nutrients, and information on standards of nutrient intake adequacy. Each topic covered in Chapter 1 is covered in much greater detail in the subsequent chapters.
- **Chapters 2, 3,** and **4** cover the energy substrates (carbohydrate, protein, and fat) with the same goal of breaking through myths by providing the science in a way that demonstrates how to make the right recommendations to athletes seeking to perform at their highest potential.
- **Chapters 5** (vitamins) and **6** (minerals) review the many myths of vitamins and minerals, while providing strategies to assure adequate intakes and avoiding deficiencies and/or toxicities.
- **Chapter 7** addresses the critically important issue of hydration and related problems associated with consuming the wrong fluid in inappropriate volumes, which at times fails to satisfy optimally the nutritional requirement.
- **Chapter 8** focuses on the importance of assessing body composition rather than body weight (mass) to better understand the energy and nutrient needs that help the athlete achieve a physique associated with improved performance.
- **Chapter 9** provides information on how modifications in nutrient intake can alter oxygen transport and utilization to working muscles, and how doing the right things nutritionally can also help to improve muscle recovery and reduce muscle soreness.
- **Chapter 10** emphasizes that athletes of different ages and genders may well have different nutritional needs. A failure to understand these differences may compromise an athlete's potential for optimal performance and could predispose the athlete to nutritional complications that may compromise health.
- **Chapter 11** takes a close look at how athletes involved in different sports (*i.e.*, power, endurance, and team) may well face different nutritional needs that, unless satisfied, may have an impact on athletic performance.
- **Chapter 12** covers how travel and environmental conditions affect nutritional requirements, with strategies that can help to lower nutritional risks.

- **Chapter 13** expands on Chapters 5 and 6 by reviewing more information on dietary supplements and aids that are intended to improve performance. There are many myths uncovered in this chapter, which make it a must-read for anyone working with athletes. Ideally, involvement in sports should be health enhancing, particularly if the correct nutritional strategies are followed.
- **Chapter 14** addresses nutritional issues that relate to athlete health so that those who work with athletes have a better long-term view of how the strategies that are followed today have implications for athlete health tomorrow.
- **Chapter 15** focuses on practical issues related to diet planning by pulling in the information provided earlier in the book that answers this question: Now that I have the science, how should I eat to achieve my goals? The chapter is packed with practical information that includes dietary assessment strategies and practical information for how to satisfy needs in different sports that have different natural breaks (*i.e.*, half-time, intermission, etc.), different training durations (marathoners need different nutrition strategies than do sprinters), and how to eat before, during, and after training. There is also information on issues associated with different "diet" types (*i.e.*, vegan, intermittent fasting, high-fat, gluten-free, etc.), plus a summary overview of the general nutrition strategies that are important for all athletes to follow. The end of the chapter reviews the nutritional considerations for different sports.

Several special features appear frequently throughout the book to enhance the learning experience:

- **Glossary boxes** are placed near the first bolded mention of terms for easy reference.
- **Important Factors to Consider** emphasizes selected key points for the reader to keep in mind.
- **Examples** are used to help the student work through specific applications of the information.
- Plentiful **tables** and **figures** support the content and illustrate complex concepts.

Each chapter ends with the following:

- **Summary** of bulleted points providing chapter highlights
- **Practical Application Activity** providing the reader an opportunity to apply what was learned in the chapter to a real-world situation
- **Chapter Questions** for student review, along with **Answers to Chapter Questions**
- **References** researched and culled from the most up-to-date evidence-based science

Online **Appendices** provide key reference materials (Dietary Reference Intakes, nutrient content of high-risk nutrients, etc.), and a sample health history questionnaire. The appendices also provide a doorway to online resources, which include sample dietary analyses and nutrition problem resolution strategies for both male and female athletes of different ages and in different sports.

A COMPREHENSIVE RESOURCE

From beginning to end, the second edition of *Nutrition for Exercise Science* is intended to provide the reader with a comprehensive resource to help guide the nutritional advice given to athletes and to know when it is appropriate to make a referral to a credentialed health professional (*e.g.*, registered dietitian, physician, certified athletic trainer, etc.) when the athlete's condition warrants a referral.

It is with high hopes that you will find this book to be useful in your professional and sporting activities.

Dan Benardot, PhD, DHC, RDN, FACSM
Teaching Professor, Center for the Study
of Human Health
Emory University
Atlanta, Georgia
Professor of Nutrition, Emeritus
Georgia State University
Atlanta, Georgia

Acknowledgments

My life has been filled with extraordinary friends and colleagues who have enabled the writing of the first and second editions of this book by giving me much needed energy and guidance. There are far too many to name, but there are several individuals who have *always* been available when I needed advice, feedback, and edits, and I want to mention them by name. These people are excessively busy in their own endeavors, but they seem to always be willingly available when assistance is requested. When I need initial advice on whether I'm barking up the right tree, there is nobody better than my dietitian wife Robin, who is always willing and honest with her feedback in the best possible way. My long-time friend and colleague, Dr. Walt Thompson, always finds time to discuss what I'm thinking about writing and is also a superb editor. My new colleagues in the Center for the Study of Human Health at Emory University, Dr. Michelle Lampl, Dr. Jill Welkley, Dr. Myra Woodworth-Hobbs, and Dr. Amanda Freeman have truly been incredibly welcoming and have provided me with an innovative multidisciplinary view of nutrition science. Two of my past graduate students, Dr. Moriah Bellissimo and Dr. Ashley Delk Licata, both now university professors, have been terrific sounding boards with fresh perspectives on how to best communicate ideas to undergraduate students. Anika Jagasia, an undergraduate student in the Center for the Study of Human Health at the time of my writing, provided incredibly useful insights on areas of the book that required more clarity. Zhongyu Li, a PhD student in Nutrition and Health Sciences at Emory University, has been wonderfully creative and tireless in helping me put together the student and instructor test banks. The American College of Sports Medicine assigned Angela Chastain as development editor to work with me on submitting chapters and chapter edits, and Angie has been an absolutely wonderful colleague in this process. The publisher, Wolters Kluwer, assigned Lindsey Porambo as the acquisitions editor, and Amy Millholen as the senior development editor, and I feel truly lucky to have had both of them to work with. All of these people, and many more at Georgia State University, Emory University, and Wolters Kluwer have made this book possible. I gratefully acknowledge their significant contributions to this book and offer my sincere thanks to all of them.

Contents

The Bottom Line—Guiding Nutrition Principles for the Athlete

CHAPTER OBJECTIVES

- Introduce the basic rules of nutrition that can and should be considered for enhancing both athlete health and performance.
- Compare the important ways that nutrition and physical activity interact, demonstrating that a focus on one without the other is likely to result in below-optimal outcomes.
- Discuss the possible factors associated with athletes who are poorly nourished, including issues related to sport tradition, nutrition misinformation, excessive food restriction related to wishing to achieve a desired weight, food allergies, intolerances, and sensitivities.
- Introduce the classes of nutrients that include water, vitamins, minerals, protein, fats, and carbohydrates, and how each is important for health and the athletic endeavor.
- Verify the importance of achieving a balance between nutrients, as overemphasizing a single nutrient over others results in poor health and performance outcomes.
- Assess the differences between essential and nonessential nutrients, showing that these nutrients are all required, but that humans have the capacity to manufacture the nonessential nutrients, provided there has been sufficient consumption of essential nutrients.
- Identify available dietary guidelines and dietary reference intakes (DRIs), and how these are best used with physically active people.

- Examine physical activity guidelines for different age groups and their purpose.
- Identify information on how to read and interpret food labels, and meaning of common terms used on food labels.
- Recall position statements on nutrition and athletic performance that have been jointly published by professional groups, including the American College of Sports Medicine (ACSM), the Academy of Nutrition and Dietetics (AND), and the Dietitians of Canada (DOC).
- Identify position stands published by the ACSM that relate to the athletic endeavor, including positions on bone health, cardiovascular fitness, and the Female Athlete Triad.
- Critique information on common nutritional myths, and how these myths detract from achieving good health and athletic performance.
- Introduce the types of research commonly used to obtain nutritional information, presenting the relative strengths and weaknesses of different types of research studies.
- Explore information on scope of practice, providing basic information on what types of nutrition information can legally be provided to individuals.

Case Study

John, a new college student and former high school athlete, is majoring in exercise science to become a certified athletic trainer. As with many other fellow students, he carries with him many nutrition beliefs. He believes, for instance, that it is a terrible thing to consume too few vitamins and minerals, as the health outcome would be devastating. He also believes that the vitamin supplements he took during his high school days helped his athletic performance. These supplements, depending on the nutrient, had between 200% and 800% of the recommended daily intake amount, but this was no problem because having more vitamins and minerals than tissue requirements can only help—it is having too little that is the problem.

He also did a good deal of dieting during his high school days on the recommendation of his coaches, to help make him a bit lighter and quicker. He is a bit "heavy" now, so he is planning on dieting again to get down to his ideal weight. One of his favorite ways to diet is to skip breakfast, as that is easy and he does not have to think about reducing the size of his meals later in the day. He also makes sure to not eat anything after 7:00 PM, as everyone knows that eating late at night will make you fat. John still tries to exercise most days for about 90 minutes of treadmill running and weight lifting and makes sure to always have water available to drink.

Then John took a class on nutrition and physical activity and came to realize that virtually all of his beliefs about nutrition were wrong. Having excessively large amounts of nutrients on a regular basis could cause problems; not eating something at night may result in a negative energy balance that lowers lean mass and increases fat mass; dieting may make people fatter; drinking water, instead of a fluid that contains carbohydrate and electrolytes, may serve to reduce performance. John has come to learn that nutrition is a *science*, and common beliefs about nutrition often serve to make matters worse rather than better.

CASE STUDY DISCUSSION QUESTIONS

1. What do you think were the errors that John made about his weight?
2. Was it okay for John to take these supplements? If not, what would you change?
3. Is weight a good measure to determine if someone is exercising and eating well?
4. If you were a coach, and you wanted someone to achieve desirable performance fitness, what would you tell this person to do nutritionally?
5. How would you know if they were successful in achieving the fitness goal?

INTRODUCTION TO SPORTS NUTRITION

Nutrition is an applied science integrating the processes by which the components of foods are used to support life through biochemical and physiologic processes. Nutrition guidelines and principles, with many years of scientific evidence, are known to be associated with disease resistance, enhanced injury recovery, better physical performance, and an improved sense of well-being. Nevertheless, there is tremendous pressure from media, acquaintances, and the workplace environment to breach science-based nutrition guidelines and principles with enticements that suggest there are better, easier, faster, and more effective ways to achieve better health and improved performance. In truth, there is no magic bullet that can satisfactorily overcome poor nutritional habits, and believing that there is creates a delusional mindset that does nothing more than make it more difficult to achieve the desired health and performance results. Importantly, the guiding science-based nutrition principles for achieving enhanced health and performance are relatively simple to follow and, if persistently pursued, are likely to create a positive outcome that will be self-motivating so that the right eating patterns continue to be followed. By contrast, unproven quick fixes may achieve what appears to be a sudden positive result, but there is an inevitable outcome failure that eventually makes matters worse. It is clear that following science-based nutrition rules make people feel discernibly better and motivates them to continue doing the right nutritional things. This chapter presents an overview of general guiding nutrition principles that are applicable to all athletes (Box 1.1).

Box 1.1	Basic Guidelines of Nutrition

1. More than enough is not better than enough.
   - If a small amount of nutrient is needed to ensure optimal health, having more than this amount is not necessarily better and may cause problems. For instance, if you need "X" amount of protein, having more than that is not better and creates problems by reducing the intake of other required nutrients.
2. Eating a wide variety of foods is necessary to ensure exposure to needed nutrients.
   - There is no such thing as a perfect food that contains all the nutrients in perfect proportion to cellular needs.

Consumption of a wide variety of foods is necessary to ensure optimal nutrient exposure.
3. Eat enough to satisfy energy and nutrient needs in *real* time.
   - There should be a *dynamic* relationship between the requirement for energy and nutrients, and the consumption of energy and nutrients. Never overfill the tank, and never let it go empty. It is not possible to drive from New York City to San Francisco by providing the car all the fuel it needs for the trip on arrival in San Francisco. The human body cannot do that either.

📖 Nutrition

A biologic science that focuses on the nutrients consumed and how these nutrients are involved in development, tissue metabolism and repair, and health. This term is often misused as follows: "John's nutrition is good." A more appropriate sentence would be: "John's nutrient intake is good" or "John's **nutriture** is good."

📖 Nutriture

The current **nutritional status** of an individual often used in reference to a specific nutrient. Example: Jane's iron nutriture is excellent.

📖 Nutritional Status

The degree to which tissue requirements for nutrients have been met. For instance, someone with poor nutritional status has not adequately satisfied the need for one or more nutrients because of an inadequate intake of the nutrient(s).

📖 Nutrients

Substances that provide needed chemicals to sustain life. The major nutrient categories include vitamins, minerals, carbohydrates, lipids, proteins, dietary fiber, and water (see Table 1.1).

No single food contains all the required nutrients, so consumption of a variety of foods is a critically important component for optimizing nutrient exposure. Eating patterns that have the same few foods being repeatedly consumed (*i.e.,* generally the same breakfasts, and perhaps two or three different lunches and dinners) tend to overexpose cells with some nutrients, while underexposing cells with other nutrients. The result is **malnutrition** and, for the athlete, an inadequate nutrient exposure that may compromise the ability of the athlete to perform up to their conditioned capacity. It is possible that some athletes have come to realize that their food consumption fails to optimally satisfy the need for nutrients, and this may result in them trying to satisfy nutritional requirements by taking nutrient supplements, which carry their own set of potential problems. Surveys have found that many coaches and athletes fail to comprehend how nutrients work and how the human body deals with nutritional mistakes. This chapter will review the essential elements of nutrients, what they do, and how they work.

Food is the carrier of vitamins, minerals, fluids, and energy, and to ensure that people receive all of the **nutrients** required to sustain needs, the right food exposure is required. This basic principle of nutrition demands that people eat a wide variety of foods to ensure that cells are exposed to everything they need. Every cell has a specific need for specific nutrients in specific amounts. Providing too much of any single nutrient may *squeeze* out other nutrients that the cell needs, and providing too little of any nutrient may allow too much of another nutrient to enter the cell. Both scenarios may result in cellular malfunction that has implications for both health and athletic performance.

📖 Malnutrition

A condition of poor health resulting from:

- Inadequate, excessive, or imbalanced intake of one or more nutrients.
- Poor absorption of consumed nutrient(s).
- Abnormal metabolism of consumed and absorbed nutrient(s).

Table 1.1	Understanding the Meaning of "Nutrients"
Classes of Nutrients	■ **Carbohydrates:** A flexible source of energy that can be metabolized oxidatively and anaerobically. Indigestible carbohydrate (fiber) is necessary for normal digestion/absorption of nutrients, and for sustaining a healthy gut microbiome. Digestible carbohydrates provide 4 calories/g. ■ **Proteins:** Necessary for building tissues, hormones, enzymes, and for carrying nutrients. Can also be used as a source of energy by removing the nitrogen and converting the remaining carbon chain to carbohydrate in the liver. Proteins provide 4 calories/g. ■ **Fats:** An important source of energy that can only be metabolized oxidatively. Also serves to protect organs and is a carrier of fat-soluble nutrients. Fats provide 9 calories/g. ■ **Vitamins:** Exist as either water soluble or fat soluble. Involved in energy metabolism, achieving the desired bone mineral density, protecting cells from damage, and important for sustaining the immune system. There are 13 vitamins, 4 of which are fat soluble and 9 of which are water soluble. ■ **Minerals:** Involved in energy production, fluid balance (both blood and cellular), growth, healing, bone mineral density, and the use of vitamins and other nutrients. ■ **Water:** Involved in the regulation of body temperature (sweat), carrying nutrients and oxygen to tissues (blood), removing metabolic by-products from cells (blood), maintaining eye, nose, and mouth moisture, lubricating skeletal joints, removal of waste products via urine and feces, and is necessary for normal digestion and absorption.
Macronutrients	Nutrients required in large amounts (measured in grams) are referred to as "macronutrients". The macronutrients include lipids, carbohydrates, and proteins. All of the macronutrients are a potential source of energy (calories) that is needed to support cellular function and physical activity.
Micronutrients	Nutrients required in smaller amounts (measured in milligrams and micrograms) than macronutrients, but are necessary for using macronutrients and sustaining normal tissue functions. The micronutrients include vitamins and minerals.

INTERACTIONS BETWEEN NUTRITION AND PHYSICAL ACTIVITY

Important Factors to Consider

■ **Physical activity** increases the requirement for energy (calories) per unit of time. Cells require a broad spectrum of other nutrients to enable them to obtain, manufacture, and use the needed energy. Since food is a carrier of both energy and nutrients, anyone performing physical activity should develop an eating strategy *with food* that helps them obtain the needed energy and associated nutrients necessary for metabolizing the energy-providing foods.

■ Metabolizing more energy substrates to create energy is heat creating, and the major means humans have for dissipating this excess heat created from energy metabolism is the evaporation of sweat off the skin. The fluid for sweat comes from the blood volume, which has many functions. It is harder to maintain the sweat rate and these other functions (*i.e.*, oxygen and nutrient delivery to cells) if blood volume drops, so exercisers must have an appropriate strategy for fluid consumption to keep blood volume normal. It is important to consider that this fluid consumption strategy should ideally be one that sustains normalcy, rather than one that attempts to recover from abnormalcy (*i.e.*, dehydration).

The field of sports nutrition represents an interaction between physical activity and nutrition, and the interaction between these two fields can be seen in many ways (Figure 1.1). It is well established that a change in physical activity results in a parallel change in multiple nutrient requirements, including the *rate* of energy (*i.e.*, **calorie**)

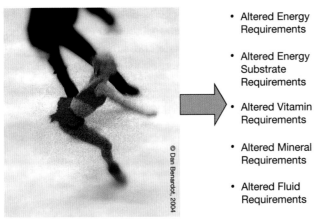

- Altered Energy Requirements
- Altered Energy Substrate Requirements
- Altered Vitamin Requirements
- Altered Mineral Requirements
- Altered Fluid Requirements

© Dan Benardot, 2004

FIGURE 1.1: Interaction between physical activity and nutrition.

utilization. For instance, while you sit reading this sentence you have a relatively low rate of energy utilization for each minute you spend sitting. But if you were to get up from your chair and run outside, the energy consumed by your tissues would be measurably higher for each minute you were running than if you were sitting. In simple terms, higher activity intensity translates into higher energy requirements.

This is only the beginning point, however, for the interaction between physical activity and nutrition. As activity intensity increases, the *type* of nutrients used to satisfy the need for fuel also changes. It is well established that the higher the activity intensity, the greater the utilization of carbohydrate as a fuel. Since humans have relatively low carbohydrate storage, those engaging in relatively high-intensity activity should have a nutrition strategy for assuring the carbohydrate storage "tank" never runs out. Since the rate of utilization of energy substrates also changes with different exercise intensities, it is also important that athletes not mistake "proportion" with "volume." For instance, a higher proportion of fat is used to satisfy energy needs at lower intensity than at higher intensity, but because little energy is used at lower intensity, a relatively small *volume* of fat is metabolized. While a lower proportion of fat is used at higher intensities, the volume of fat utilization is likely to be higher, as shown in the example:

Example: Assume an athlete exercising at low intensity burns 100 calories in 30 minutes, and 80% of the calories are derived from fat. This athlete now increases exercise intensity and burns 200 calories in 30 minutes, and 60% (a lower proportion) of calories are derived from fat. However, 60% of 200 calories is 120 calories from fat, while 80% of 100 calories is 80 calories from fat. Don't mistake proportion with volume.

Physical Activity

Any activity that results in body movement and requires more energy (*i.e.,* calories) above rest is considered physical activity. The greater the energy requirement per unit of time, the more intense the physical activity.

Calorie

The term used in nutrition that is synonymous with **kilocalorie**. Note that the uppercase *C* differentiates this from the lowercase *c* used in **calorie**.

Kilocalorie

The commonly used term in nutrition to refer to the calories in food. *Example:* This bagel has 400 calories actually means 400 kilocalories. This represents the amount of heat energy needed to raise the temperature of 1,000 g (*i.e.,* 1 kg) of water by 1 °C, and is 1,000× greater than a calorie.

Calorie

The heat energy required to elevate the temperature of 1 g of water by 1 °C at sea level. In nutrition, the standard term *calorie, Kcal,* or *Kilocalorie* is 1,000 times this amount, which is why it is more appropriate to refer to Kcal or Calorie when discussing nutritional matters.

We also know that energy substrates (*i.e.,* the nutrients that provide carbon to our cells to produce energy: carbohydrate, protein, and fat) cannot be metabolized (used) by cells to satisfy energy requirements simply because these substrates are present in the cell. Specific vitamins, mainly the B vitamins, are needed to use the energy substrates so that cells can create the energy required to sustain normal body function. The greater the time spent at higher activity intensities, the greater the requirement for energy, and the greater the requirement for specific vitamins to satisfy energy needs. It is important to consider that vitamins do not provide energy, but they are necessary for deriving energy from the energy substrate–containing foods we consume.

Some of the energy that we derive from consumed foods is created with oxygen (aerobic metabolism), whereas other consumed energy can be created without oxygen (anaerobic metabolism). Fat can only be metabolized for energy aerobically, whereas carbohydrate is a flexible fuel that can be metabolized both aerobically and anaerobically. It is important to consider that even the leanest person has plenty of body fat stores to serve as an energy reserve, whereas humans have limited storage of carbohydrate. Therefore, the ability to burn fat via an oxygen metabolic pathway is important for all physical activities, but particularly important for endurance activities. Iron, a mineral, is involved in several ways in aerobic metabolism and is, therefore, a critical nutrient for metabolizing fat for energy. Athletes with poor iron status have poor delivery of oxygen to cells and, as a result, have below-optimal oxidative metabolism that inevitably results in premature fatigue and subpar athletic performance (see Box 1.2 on energy metabolic pathways).

Box 1.2   Quick Check: Energy Metabolic Pathways

Normal breathing suggests that sufficient oxygen is being provided to cells to satisfy energy needs via, primarily, aerobic metabolism. As energy needs increase, as is inevitable with physical activity, the pace and depth of breathing increases to help satisfy the elevated oxygen needs of aerobic metabolism. Fat is the preferred fuel for satisfying energy needs as it is efficiently stored (9 calories/g) and does not produce any negative metabolic byproduct as a result of energy production: Only energy, carbon dioxide, and water are produced. Carbohydrate can also be metabolized aerobically and does not produce any negative byproduct via aerobic metabolism, but carbohydrate stores are limited, making it a less preferred aerobic fuel. In addition, carbohydrate is needed for the complete oxidation of fats for energy, without which ketones are produced. The ketones are acidic and compromise cellular energy metabolism. When the requirement for energy exceeds the individual's capacity to supply sufficient oxygen to metabolize the energy aerobically, then at least a portion of the energy produced is acquired anaerobically (i.e., without oxygen). Carbohydrate is a fuel that can supply energy both aerobically and anaerobically, but as carbohydrate stores are limited, a high reliance on carbohydrate to supply energy is likely to result in early fatigue as carbohydrate stores become depleted. In addition, anaerobic metabolism of carbohydrate is likely to produce lactic acid, which, under certain circumstances, may result in early fatigue. Protein is also a potential source of carbohydrate that can be metabolized either aerobically or anaerobically. Carbohydrate is derived from protein during exercise from body tissues that are broken down when blood sugar is low, so that specific amino acids from the protein can be converted by the liver to carbohydrate to keep the central nervous system functioning. (Blood sugar is the primary fuel for the central nervous system.) In addition, protein is a "dirty" fuel, as nitrogen must be released from the protein carbon chain for energy production. This nitrogen is potentially toxic, so must be excreted via urine, increasing the risk for more urine production and dehydration. Another anaerobic fuel, phosphocreatine (PCr), is capable of supplying an extremely high amount of energy but, because preformed PCr storage is limited, it can only supply energy for a short period of time that typically ranges from 5 to 8 seconds. As an example of fuel utilization, imagine someone running a 100-m sprint. The individual goes so fast there is insufficient time to incorporate oxygen into the cells to satisfy the high energy requirement aerobically. The first 5–8 seconds of energy is derived from PCr, and the remaining energy to finish the ~10-second race is through the anaerobic metabolism of carbohydrate. Now imagine the other end of the exercise intensity spectrum, a marathon runner. The runner runs almost the entire 2+-hour race primarily reliant on fat metabolism but is also using carbohydrate to assure the complete oxidation of fat. Carbohydrates are also used when the marathoner decides the strategic point where they want to pass a fellow competitor, so they must go faster (i.e., burn more energy) to do so. They have fluid stations every 5 kilometers to drink a fluid that will help sustain hydration state and blood sugar. At the end of the race, they may need to sprint to the finish, which is more reliant on PCr and carbohydrate than the fat they were primarily using during the race. In both cases, the sprinter and the marathoner, carbohydrate is likely to be the limiting energy substrate in performance. A sprinter who begins the race with low muscle glycogen (stored carbohydrate) may not be able to finish the race as fast as they would like. A marathoner may not be using a high proportion of carbohydrate during the race, but the limited storage of carbohydrate plus the length of the race clearly requires an effective strategy for keeping blood sugar normal by consuming the right beverage at every 5K opportunity.

Chapters 2, 3, and 4 on the energy substrates cover energy metabolic processes for each energy substrate, and Chapter 11 covers energy metabolism as it relates to power, endurance, and team sports.

Exercise also alters fluid requirements because humans are only 20% to 40% efficient at burning fuel to create muscular movement. Therefore, for every 100 calories burned, 60–80 of these calories create heat. This heat cannot be retained (*i.e.*, body temperature cannot be allowed to increase from the heat created from the metabolism of energy), so we dissipate the heat through the production of sweat. The evaporation of sweat removes this excess heat and lowers body temperature. The greater the intensity of activity, the greater the energy metabolized and the greater the heat produced that must be dissipated through a greater sweat rate.

Exercise

Exercise represents physical activity that is performed for the purpose of improving muscle, heart, skeletal, and lung fitness. Physical activity is typically referred to as *exercise* (*i.e.*, activity requiring physical effort) when it is performed in a planned, structured, and repeated fashion for the purpose of improving health and fitness.

In summary, physical activity alters the total energy requirement, the type of energy required, the vitamins and minerals needed to metabolize the energy, the fluid necessary to dissipate the heat associated with greater energy metabolism, and the electrolytes lost in sweat needing to be replaced (Box 1.3). These interactions are sufficiently important that discussing exercise without also including a related discussion about the nutritional factors that help drive the exercise would be incomplete. In simple terms, these factors constitute the basis of sports nutrition: An increased rate of energy expenditure results in an increased requirement for energy substrates, an increased need for nutrients involved in energy metabolism, and an increased need to replace body fluids lost as a result of energy metabolic heat creation. Although seemingly relatively simple concepts, there is a great deal of science related to what energy substrates are best to consume for different activities, what is the best timing

Box 1.3 Two Major Issues in Sport

Regardless of the sport (power, team, endurance), the big issues revolve around two major factors:

1. Optimally satisfying *energy* needs in terms of amount, type, and timing of intake.
2. Optimally satisfying *fluid* needs in terms of amount, type, and timing of intake.

to consume these substrates, which foods that should be consumed at different times to improve muscle recovery and reduce muscle soreness, the composition of fluids that is best for different events in different environmental conditions, strategies for sustaining an optimal hydration state, and the best eating modalities for assuring that cells have optimal exposure to all the nutrients necessary for the athlete to perform up to their conditioned capacity.

WHY ARE SO MANY ATHLETES POORLY NOURISHED?

Important Factors to Consider

Many factors influence athlete nutritional status, including:

- Whether the athlete has the financial capacity to purchase foods that may be more expensive, such as fresh fruits and vegetables.
- The familiarity an athlete has in consuming certain foods, as eating behaviors established early in life tend to persist.
- Food availability varies by culture and geography that the athlete lives in, and influences the foods consumed.
- The athlete's perception, either real or believed, that consumption of certain foods may negatively impact how they feel, potentially resulting in an inadequate intake of specific nutrients that are associated with the avoided foods.
- The traditions of the sport and the traditions of the organizations that supervise and control the sport may influence how athletes in that sport eat, often with poor outcomes.
- Athletes in sports where weight (*e.g.*, wrestling) or appearance (*e.g.*, synchronized swimming, gymnastics, diving) are important aspects of the sport may place the athlete at nutritional risk because few athletes or those who coach them know about how best to achieve these goals.

Other factors influencing athlete nutritional status include (1):

- The state of hunger and appetite at the time of food availability. This is a particular concern in athletes who overtrain, as this typically lowers appetite and makes it difficult for them to consume the required energy and nutrients.

Sports Organizations and Supplement Use

There are numerous reasons why athletes fail to optimally satisfy nutritional needs. Many athletic event organizers seek sponsors to help defray the costs of the event, and these sponsors provide their nutritional products while inhibiting the use/availability of other products. These products may or may not be appropriate for each competing athlete, but it is safe to say that not all products contain the ideal distribution of nutrients (energy substrates, electrolytes concentrations, etc.) for each athlete in each sponsored event. This leaves athletes with specific nutritional needs that may not be optimally fulfilled with the available products, resulting in a state of poor nutrition that may keep them from performing up to their conditioned capacities (2) (Table 1.2).

National governing bodies are the organizational structures for each sport (i.e., there is a national governing body for track and field, another for gymnastics, another for hockey) and, depending on the organization, may inadvertently perpetuate bad nutritional behaviors because of limited oversight. In addition, coaches certified by the national governing body are often former athletes who tend to encourage nutritional strategies they followed when they were athletes, also resulting in a perpetuation of eating patterns that are not scientifically based. This can result in long-term nutritional difficulties. For instance, athletes in certain sports are often rewarded for having a "thin" appearance desired by judges. However, the drive to achieve this thinness may result in a lifetime of poor eating behaviors that can negatively affect health and could shorten an athlete's competitive life. Ideally, national governing bodies should develop rules that encourage healthy body compositions that would also, ultimately, improve sport-specific performance and competitive longevity.

Many athletes are excessively dependent on supplements, which can be due to a multitude of factors that include convincing advertisements that target athletes, often using sports celebrities as the spokespersons. Some athletes may feel that their eating behaviors are less than

Table 1.2	Factors That Contribute to Poor Nutrition in Athletes
Organization	■ *Event Sponsorships*: Products available to athletes that may not be optimal. ■ *Credentialed Nutritionists/Dietitians Unavailable*: There is often no certified or credentialed nutrition expert at training/competition. ■ *National Governing Body*: There may be a perpetuation of bad nutritional behavior with limited oversight that can result in long-term nutritional difficulties. ■ *Supplements*: Purveyors push supplements with convincing advertisements. ■ *Bad Rules*: Training venues that inhibit easy availability of appropriate foods/beverages.
Knowledge	■ *Inappropriate Modeling*: Copying admired athletes. ■ *Belief vs. Science*: Myths associated with thinking of nutrition as a belief system and not a science. ■ *Misattribution of Perceived Benefit*: Consuming certain foods/beverages may not help for the reasons believed. ■ *Good and Bad Foods*: Oversimplification results in problems. ■ *Magic Bullet*: Looking for the easy fix.
Tradition	■ *Sport Traditions*: Perpetuation of coach/sport-induced nutrition-related problems. ■ *Weight Focus*: Excessive focus on weight, when the focus should be on body composition and strength:weight ratio. ■ *Protein Solves Everything*: High-protein intake will successfully resolve all potential nutrition problems. ■ *Reliance on Supplements*: Lowers food intake and creates World Anti-Doping Agency issues.
Food restriction	■ *Allergies*: Avoidance of foods that cause a potentially life-threatening allergic response. ■ *Intolerances*: Avoidance of foods that cause discomfort, typically related to insufficient digestive enzyme, such as lactose intolerance. ■ *Sensitivities*: Discomfort, bloating, and various other symptoms from foods, often not well identified, that cause gastrointestinal inflammation.

optimal so supplements are used as a nutritional "security blanket." In addition, advertisements for supplements often appear in the official magazine of the sport, giving the supplements a high level of unjustified credibility. Many athletes *believe* that nutrient supplementation will improve their athletic performance but, in truth, supplements taken without evidence of an established biologic weakness may cause more problems than they resolve and, as discussed later in this chapter, supplements may also contain banned substances that are not listed on the label.

Some training venues may have established rules that inhibit easy availability of appropriate foods and beverages. For instance, there may be a rule that prohibits sports beverages in the training room. These rules may make it difficult for the athlete to optimally benefit from the training for multiple reasons, including increasing dehydration risk, limiting energy substrate availability to working muscles, and allowing a low blood sugar state to occur. This failure of satisfying training-associated nutritional needs *in real time*, may result in stress hormone (cortisol) production, with a resultant breakdown of both lean and bone mass. This is certainly not the desired outcome of a training program.

Many of these organizational problems could be overcome with the presence of a credentialed dietitian/nutritionist who specializes in sports nutrition. This void leaves it to others who have an inadequate background in nutrition to provide nutrition information to the athletes. All too often the advice provided is not based on science and may "push" the consumption of products that have a weak scientific basis.

Knowledge

An important contributor to why so many athletes are poorly nourished is because they have poor knowledge of nutritional strategies that could help them achieve their desired athletic goals. The poor understanding of nutrition makes these athletes easy prey to advertisements and also may cause them to inappropriately model what other highly admired athletes are doing. These athletes who are the focus of admiration may have the best coaches in the world and access to superb athletic training facilities, which are both likely to be more important contributors to the athlete's success than the supposed performance-enhancing supplement they consume. However, those who admire them will take the performance-enhancing supplement with the belief that this alone will help. In addition, there may be a misappropriation of benefit with

some supplements that are taken. For instance, a multivitamin supplement that targets athletes may contain banned substances, and any improvement realized may be inappropriately attributed to the vitamins, when in reality it could be due to the banned substance. Related to this is the problem that many athletes perceive nutrition to be a belief system rather than a science. All too often, athletes follow certain inappropriate nutritional strategies because they *believe* those strategies will help them. In fact, there is likely to be good established science that would be a far better guide to the most appropriate nutritional strategies.

Some athletes misattribute the perceived benefit they are receiving from the foods they consume. For instance, a high level of protein consumption is widely believed to be the *critical* nutritional factor in human performance, so many athletes consume extremely high levels of protein from both foods and supplements. Doing this when coupled with an appropriate exercise regimen may result in higher muscle mass, but the benefit may not be from the protein itself but from the higher level of energy the protein has provided to support the larger mass. Protein is certainly important, but using protein as an energy source is not optimal because the nitrogenous waste that is produced must be excreted, resulting in both dehydration and lower bone density. There are clearly better ways to satisfy energy (*i.e.*, calorie) requirements other than through an excessively high consumption of protein.

A common statement made by athletes is, "I eat this because I know it's good for me." The second most common statement athletes say is, "I don't eat that because it's bad for me." This good food versus bad food belief system could create nutritional problems for athletes. Athletes who believe that a particular food is a "good food," may consume it with great frequency and in high amounts. Although the food in question may certainly be a fine food, no single food carries all of the needed nutrients. Therefore, overreliance on this food because of its "good food" label may create its own set of nutritional problems, just as avoidance of a certain food because it is perceived to be a "bad food" may keep the athlete from obtaining a key nutrient present in that food. It is important to remember that there is no magic bullet or perfect food that will help the athlete run faster, jump higher, and move more quickly. All of the nutritional needs must be met in a balanced way for athletic performance to improve and that can only be done through the consumption of a wide variety of foods. Athletes who consume a monotonous diet because they are convinced that a far too limited set of foods is the ticket to crossing the finish line first are badly fooling themselves. Eating a wide variety of foods is critical for exposing tissues to all required nutrients, and also helps to assure that tissues are not overexposed to a substance that may result in toxicity.

Tradition

Sports traditions may also play a role in athlete malnutrition. It is not uncommon for some coaches to apply nutrition strategies that they learned when they were athletes themselves and because it is tradition in the sport. It may be tradition in the sport to keep athletes from consuming fluids during practice because it has never been done (tradition) and because it is wrongly believed that practicing in a dehydrated state will make the athlete more tolerant to dehydration during competition. We know this tradition to be blatantly wrong, as it is well established that there is no adaptation to dehydration, but the tradition continues in many sporting activities.

Making a desired weight is also common in many sports. For instance, linemen in football are often encouraged to get bigger (*i.e.*, have a higher weight), but the focus on weight may be inappropriate from a performance standpoint. Rather, there should be a focus on what constitutes weight (*i.e.*, body composition) because performance is more specifically associated with the strength-to-weight ratio. As an example, try to imagine a football player lineman who went from 250 to 275 lb on the advice of the coach and training staff, but in doing so experienced the weight gain almost entirely from an increase in fat mass. Now this lineman must move a larger mass with the same muscle he had before the weight increase, mandating that the muscle work harder to do the same intensity of work. The likely outcome is that the muscle will fatigue more quickly and with an associated reduction in performance. Also, imagine an athlete in an appearance sport where the coach feels the athlete will have a better competition score with a smaller appearance, so is asked to lose weight through a calorically restricted diet. However, the energy restrictions commonly followed are likely to lower muscle mass more than fat mass, so this athlete becomes weaker because of the weight loss (3). The faster rate of fat recovery relative to muscle recovery following low-calorie diets may also increase health risks that include lower bone density and eating disorders (3). On the other hand, if the focus was to increase muscle while losing only fat, this athlete could maintain the current weight and still look smaller because muscle is more dense than fat, and performance would increase because of more muscle moving less nonmuscle mass. *Weight* is the wrong metric in

both examples, but often remains the common measure in many athletic endeavors. For this reason, body mass index (BMI), a weight-to-height index (kg/m^2), is a poor measure of athlete fitness. BMI was developed as a population index for determining the prevalence of population overweight and obesity, with categories for underweight (16–18.5), normal weight (18.5–25), overweight (25–30), and obesity (30 or higher). By definition, "obesity" represents a condition of having excess body fat. Even though not developed for this purpose, BMI is now commonly used as an obesity measure for individuals, but should not be as it fails to assess the degree to which fat is a contributor to weight. Athletes, because they often carry a high level of muscle for height, can often be mischaracterized as being obese (*i.e.*, BMI >30) when they are not, and some "thin" individuals, who have relatively little muscle mass but a high level of fat mass, can be characterized as "normal" weight with BMI, but because fat contributes significantly to weight, they should more appropriately be characterized as "obese."

The maximal human capacity to use protein anabolically to build and repair tissue, make enzymes and hormones, etc., is ~1.7 g of protein per kg of body mass. But the consumption of protein to derive the optimal anabolic (tissue-building) benefit is far more complicated than the simple consumption of this much protein in a day. Human systems can only process about 30–40 g (120 calories) of protein at a single meal, depending on musculature and, to ensure that this protein can be used anabolically, it must be consumed while in a state of good energy balance (4). It is not unusual for athletes to consume large protein meals containing 80 or more grams of protein, but because only ~20–35 g of this can be used anabolically, athletes are fooling themselves into thinking that this high level of protein at a single meal is contributing to total protein requirements (5–7). The remaining 50 g is either used as a source of calories or stored as fat. It would be far more productive to distribute the required protein throughout the day in amounts that optimize tissue utilization. The frequent distribution of meals (*i.e.*, eating smaller meals more often) also has the added benefit of helping to assure that athletes achieve a better continuous energy balance, which is an important factor in helping to assure that protein can be used the way it is intended (*i.e.*, to make hormones, enzymes, muscle, etc.) rather than using it to satisfy the energy requirement (7).

Another possible reason for why athletes may be at risk for poor nutrition is the excessive reliance on nutrient supplements. The common belief is that "if a little bit is good for me, then taking a lot will make it even better."

Table 1.3	What Consumers Need to Know About Dietary Supplements
Take charge of your health by being an informed consumer	The standards for marketing supplements are very different from the standards for drugs. For example, marketers of a supplement do not have to prove to the Food and Drug Administration that it is safe or that it works before it arrives on grocery store shelves. Find out what the scientific evidence says about the safety of a dietary supplement and whether it works.
"Natural" does not necessarily mean "safe"	For example, the herbs comfrey and kava can cause serious harm to the liver. Also, when you see the term "standardized" (or "verified" or "certified") on the bottle, it does not necessarily guarantee product quality or consistency.
Interactions are possible	Some dietary supplements may interact with medications (prescription or over-the-counter) or other dietary supplements, and some may have side effects on their own. Research has shown that St. John's wort interacts with many medications in ways that can interfere with their intended effects, including antidepressants, birth control pills, antiretrovirals used to treat HIV infection, and others.
Be aware of the potential for contamination	Some supplements have been found to contain hidden prescription drugs or other compounds, particularly in dietary supplements marketed for weight loss, sexual health including erectile dysfunction, and athletic performance or body-building.
Talk to your health care providers	Tell your health care providers about any complementary health products or practices you use, including dietary supplements. This will help give them a full picture of what you are doing to manage your health and will help ensure coordinated and safe care.

Source: National Institutes of Health: National Center for Complementary and Integrative Health. 5 tips: what consumers need to know about dietary supplements. Accessed February 24, 2022. Available from: https://www.nccih.nih.gov/health/tips/tips-what-consumers-need-to-know-about-dietary-supplements

This breaches a key rule of nutrition: *More than enough is not better than enough.* This is based on the Latin saying *Sola dosis facit venenum*, which is attributed to Paracelsus, and translates to "The dose makes the poison." The DRIs published by the National Academy of Sciences are often wrongly viewed as a minimal requirement rather than what they are, which is the average requirement to stay healthy plus two standard deviations above this level (8). Despite this, athletes are the target of advertisements that try to have them consume products containing many multiples, often 300% to 400% or more of the recommended DRI value without any evidence that this intake will enhance health and/or performance. On the contrary, there is an increasing body of evidence suggesting that these excessively high levels of supplemental nutrient intake cause problems (9). There is also evidence that, when taken as supplements, some nutrients may result in the precise opposite of the desired effect. A study assessing vitamin E supplementation (800 IU/day for 2 months) before the Triathlon World Championship in Kona, Hawaii, found that it promoted lipid peroxidation and inflammation during exercise, a finding strongly implying that the triathletes would have been better off without it (10). Studies of dietary supplements have also found the presence of substances banned by the International Olympic Committee (IOC) and the World Anti-Doping Agency, despite these substances not being included on the product label (11). Clearly, consumption of these supplements by an unknowing athlete would put the athlete at risk. (See Table 1.3 for information on what consumers need to know about dietary supplements.)

Food Restriction from Allergies, Intolerances, and Sensitivities

Athletes may be predisposed to poor nutritional status because of issues related to food allergies, food intolerances, and food sensitivities. The symptoms of a **food allergy** are caused by the ingestion of specific antigens that result in an **immunoglobulin E (IgE)**–mediated allergic response that occurs within minutes to 2 hours postingestion. The symptoms involve the gastrointestinal (GI) tract, respiratory system, eyes, and skin, and can be life threatening. The most common food allergies are related to the consumption of peanuts, tree nuts, egg, milk, wheat, soybeans, fish, and crustacean shellfish, with a food-specific protein being the usual offending substance.

Food sensitivities are non–IgE-mediated reactions involving the immune system. Symptoms occur as a result of cytokine and mediator release from granulocytes and T cells, which release mediators, including prostaglandins, histamines, cytokines, and serotonin, that adversely affect gut function through tissue inflammation, smooth muscle contraction, mucus secretion, and pain receptor activation. The food source of symptoms may remain elusive without food sensitivity testing and a personalized elimination diet.

The causes of **food intolerances** involve insufficient or missing digestive substances, such as enzymes or bile salts, causing the rapid onset of distressing GI symptoms. For example, symptoms of lactose intolerance are present in about 10% of the population and occur when the enzyme lactase is not produced in sufficient amounts to adequately break down dairy product lactose. Poor tolerance to dietary fats may occur because of an inadequate production of bile, which is an emulsifying agent that enables removal of the fat from the digestive tract and into the bloodstream.

All of these food-related issues (allergies, sensitivities, and intolerances) have implications for acute and chronic disease states, but they also may cause a dramatic reduction in nutrient exposure by eliminating whole categories of foods. People identified as having any of these conditions require special attention to ensure the diet can deliver the needed nutrients. It is also possible that athletes may unnecessarily restrict foods because they have heard that some foods or food components are "bad" or they believe they have a condition that has not been diagnosed. For instance, athletes may unnecessarily restrict or avoid consuming gluten-containing foods despite have no gluten-related issues; some athletes may unnecessarily restrict dairy foods because they believe they may have lactose intolerance. These unnecessary restrictions may limit the foods they are willing to consume and, therefore, may make it more difficult to consume needed nutrients.

Food Allergy

Food allergy represents an immune response to the consumption of a specific food or an ingredient in a food. An allergic reaction (rash, swelling of tongue, vomiting, diarrhea, etc.) occurs when the body's immune system reacts to the food by binding IgE to the food, resulting in the release of inflammatory chemicals, including histamine. Common food allergies include milk, eggs, shellfish, peanuts, wheat, rice, and fruit.

Immunoglobulin E

These are antibodies produced by the immune system and are involved in allergic reactions. Anyone with an allergy has an excessive immune system response to the allergen, resulting in IgE release. The IgE travels to cells that are the cause of the allergic reaction (*i.e.*, swelling, rash).

Food Sensitivity

Food sensitivities result in non–IgE-localized inflammatory responses in the GI tract. The inflamed GI tract may allow some substances to enter the blood that would otherwise not enter, contributing to inflammatory conditions that include irritable bowel syndrome (IBS), migraine headaches, metabolic syndrome, arthritis, and others. Food sensitivities are more prevalent than food allergies or food intolerances, but they often go undiagnosed because the reaction to the offending food(s)/food substance(s) may take several days.

Food Intolerance

Food intolerance does not affect the body's immune system, and typically occurs because the individual cannot digest a food ingredient because of a missing digestive enzyme, cannot absorb a nutrient because of a missing transport protein, or cannot properly metabolize the consumed food ingredient once it is absorbed because of a missing cellular enzyme. *Example:* One of the common food intolerances is lactose intolerance (affecting ~10% of the adult population), which results from insufficient production of lactase, the digestive enzyme for the sugar lactose.

THE NUTRIENTS

Important Factors to Consider

- People often think that some nutrients are more important than others. This is dangerous thinking, as this may cause them to overconsume these nutrients at the expense of others. Nutrients work together to produce the desired result and having all the nutrients in the right balance is an important key to good nutrition.
- No single food is a good source of all nutrients. Therefore, chronic frequent consumption of the same food(s) fails to expose tissues to a full array of nutrients and phytonutrients, predisposing a person to malnutrition. Consumption of a variety of foods is a key aspect of assuring a good nutritional status.

The six established classes of nutrients include water, vitamins, minerals, proteins, fats, and carbohydrates. Another quasinutrient class is referred to as *phytonutrients*, which are not classically described as nutrients, but which have nutrient-like functions. Phytonutrients are the focus of a great deal of current research, the findings of which are providing useful information on cellular function and repair (Table 1.4). We derive energy (fuel) from foods that contain three of these nutrient classes—carbohydrates, proteins, and fats. We can also derive energy from alcohol, but regular consumption is likely to interfere with normal energy metabolic processes while increasing the potential for dehydration.

There are many people who attribute energy-providing properties to vitamins and minerals, but vitamins and minerals are *not* a source of energy. They are, however, needed to derive energy from carbohydrates, proteins, and fats that are consumed. Athletes who reduce

Table 1.4	The Nutrients	
Nutrient	Subcategories	Functions
Carbohydrates	Sugars Starches Fiber	Muscular fuel to derive energy (from starch, sugars, and glycogen) Cholesterol/fat control (from dietary fiber) Digestion assistance (from dietary fiber) Nutrient/water absorption (from sugars)
Lipids (fats and oils)	Essential fatty acids Nonessential fatty acids Monounsaturated fatty acids Polyunsaturated fatty acids Saturated fatty acids	Delivery of fat-soluble vitamins (vitamins A, D, E, and K) Delivery of essential fatty acids (fatty acids the body needs but cannot make) Energy/muscular fuel (for low-intensity activity) Satiety control (helps make you feel satisfied from eating) Substance in many hormones
Proteins	Essential amino acids Nonessential amino acids	Energy source (if carbohydrates are depleted) Delivery of essential amino acids (amino acids the body needs but cannot make) Essential for developing new tissue (important during growth and injury repair) Essential for maintaining existing tissue (helps control normal wear and tear) Basic substance in the manufacture of enzymes, antibodies, and hormones Fluid balance (helps control water level inside and outside cells) Carrier of substances in the blood (transports vitamins, minerals, and fats to and from cells)
Vitamins	Water soluble Fat soluble	Tissue function and health (e.g., vitamin A helps the eye work correctly) Immune function (e.g., vitamins A and C are well known for this function) Energy metabolism control (e.g., B vitamins, in particular, are involved in helping cells burn energy) Nutrient absorption (e.g., vitamin D helps calcium and phosphorus from the food you eat be absorbed into your bloodstream) Nervous system maintenance (e.g., folic acid and thiamin are important in nerve system development and function) Antioxidants (e.g., help protect cells from oxidative damage)

(continued)

Table 1.4	The Nutrients (*Continued*)	
Nutrient	**Subcategories**	**Functions**
Minerals	Macrominerals Microminerals Ultratrace minerals	Skeletal strength (e.g., calcium, phosphorus, and magnesium are keys to strong bones; fluoride keeps teeth strong by protecting them from bacterial acids) Nerve function (e.g., magnesium and calcium are both involved in nerve communication) Control of the body's pH (acidity level) Oxygen transport (e.g., iron is essential for getting oxygen to cells and removing carbon dioxide from cells) Control of the body's water balance (sodium and potassium play important roles in blood volume)
Water	None	The body's coolant (helps maintain body temperature through sweat production) Carrier of nutrients to cells Remover of waste products from cells Important constituent of muscle Involved in many body reactions (both in digestion of food and in processes inside cells)
Phytonutrients[a]	Phenols Terpenes Polyphenols Sterols	Cell protection agents Cell repair agents Cell longevity agents

[a]Phytonutrients are not officially considered a class of nutrients, but they are receiving a great deal of research attention with findings that they have functions similar to vitamins. They are chemicals naturally found in plants for which there are no current recommended intakes. Plants produce phytonutrients for their own protection against viruses, bacteria, fungi, insects, and the environment, and it is believed they also provide protection for the human body.

food intake because they believe that the reduction in energy consumption will create no difficulty because of their consumption of vitamins are wrong. Many vitamins have very little to work on if there is limited availability of energy. Water, discussed in Chapter 7, is a nutrient that constitutes a high proportion of total body weight and quite literally ties all of the tissues together. Blood, which is mainly water, circulates vitamins, minerals, fats, proteins, carbohydrates, and phytonutrients to tissues and removes the metabolic waste of this tissue utilization. The water in blood is also essential for maintaining body temperature, through sweat production, during exercise.

Nutrient Balance

Each nutrient is uniquely important because each nutrient has specific functions. Athletes cannot eliminate any class of nutrients from the foods they eat and hope to do well athletically, much less survive in good health! Critical to understanding nutrients is the concept that nutrients work together, both within and between nutrient classes. For instance, it becomes more difficult to burn fat for energy without having some carbohydrate present because "fat burns in a carbohydrate flame." It is also impossible to imagine having healthy red blood cells with sufficient iron intake but inadequate vitamin B_{12} and folic acid intake, as these vitamins are essential for forming healthy red blood cells. Having enough total energy intake (from carbohydrate, protein, and fat) is an excellent strategy for optimizing athletic performance. However, doing this with an inadequate fluid intake will impede an athlete's ability to metabolize these energy compounds by limiting their delivery to cells, limiting the removal of metabolic by-products from cells, and limiting the cooling capacity from the heat created when energy compounds are metabolized.

On the other hand, having too much of any one nutrient may damage the opportunity for the normal nutrient absorption and metabolism of other nutrients being consumed at an adequate level. For instance, calcium supplements are commonly taken to help ensure strong and healthy bones that are resistant to stress fractures (an all too common injury in sport) and to reduce the risk of osteoporosis. However, taking too much calcium at the same time as eating foods that contain iron, magnesium, and zinc may inhibit the absorption of these other nutrients, which are equally important in maintaining health and athletic performance. Again, these are issues of nutrient balance. Having one nutrient without the others simply does not work, and having too much of one nutrient may cause difficulties with other nutrients. Therefore, when you review Table 1.2 and see a summary of nutrients and their various functions, it is incorrect to infer that taking a single nutrient will, by itself, encourage that function. Think *balance*.

Essential and Nonessential Nutrients

Nutrients may be referred to as either essential or nonessential, but care should be taken not to misinterpret these terms. An essential nutrient is one that cannot be manufactured by body cells from other nutrients, so it is *essential* that we consume this nutrient from the foods we consume. As an example, we have essential amino acids that we are incapable of making ourselves, so we must consume these amino acids from the foods we eat. The same is true for fatty acids, most of which are considered nonessential because we are fully capable of manufacturing them from other nutrients. However, we still have a small number of fatty acids that are considered essential to consume because we cannot manufacture them.

It is important to *not* think of essential nutrients as more important than nonessential nutrients. We need them *all* (both essential and nonessential nutrients) to function normally, but must purposefully consume the essential nutrients to ensure normal cellular function. Typically, balanced diets that include a variety of foods deliver all of the essential nutrients and also provide the nonessential nutrients. Problems related to essential nutrients are nearly always related to dietary restrictions related to special diets, food allergies, food intolerances, and/or food sensitivities. For instance, people may put themselves on an extremely low-fat diet that eliminates whole categories of foods, such as corn oil, sunflower oil, soybean oil, nuts, and seeds, that are the primary sources of linoleic fatty acid, an essential fatty acid. Over time, this could result in a linoleic acid deficiency, with symptoms ranging from poor growth, fatty liver, skin lesions, and reproductive failure (12). Chapters 2, 3, and 4 on the energy substrates, vitamins, and minerals, respectively, will have a more comprehensive discussion on specific nutrients, their food sources, and the amounts typically required to sustain health. These chapters also cover the impact that physical activity has on specific nutrient requirements, with strategies for athletes on how to ensure they can obtain all of the essential and nonessential nutrients required for health and performance.

NUTRITION GUIDES FOR ATHLETES AND NONATHLETES

Important Factors to Consider

- The U.S. dietary guidelines are general recommendations to help ensure a healthy life. These are generally appropriately used with physically active people, with only a few modifications: (i) sugar-containing sports beverages are appropriate for consumption during bouts of physical activity and (ii) sodium losses through sweat may exceed current intake recommendations, but should be replaced.
- The Dietary Reference Intakes (DRIs) are meant to ensure that 98% of the population will achieve a good nutritional status when daily food intakes of listed nutrients are achieved. However, it is important to consider that the DRI value is two standard deviations *above* the average requirement, suggesting that consumption of DRI level is actually above the level required by most people to sustain a good nutritional status.

The U.S. Department of Health and Human Services and the U.S. Department of Agriculture jointly publish the Dietary Guidelines for Americans (dietary guidelines) every 5 years (13). Each edition of the dietary guidelines reflects the body of nutrition science. The most recent dietary guidelines, 2020–2025 Dietary Guidelines for Americans, provide evidence-based food and beverage recommendations for Americans ages 2 and older (14). These recommendations aim to help people:

- Follow a healthy dietary pattern at every life stage.
- Customize and enjoy food and beverage choices to reflect personal preferences, cultural traditions, and budgetary considerations.

- Focus on meeting food group needs with nutrient-dense foods and beverages, and stay within calorie limits.
- Limit foods and beverages higher in added sugars, saturated fat, and sodium, and limit alcoholic beverages to help prevent chronic disease, and help people reach and maintain a healthy weight.

Public health agencies, health care providers, and educational institutions all rely on dietary guidelines recommendations and strategies. The dietary guidelines also have a significant impact on nutrition in the United States because they:

- Form the basis of federal nutrition policy and programs.
- Help guide local, state, and national health promotion and disease prevention initiatives.
- Inform various organizations and industries (*e.g.*, products developed and marketed by the food and beverage industry).

The intent of the dietary guidelines is to summarize what we know about individual nutrients and food components into an interrelated set of recommendations for healthy eating that can be adopted by the public. Taken together, the dietary guidelines recommendations encompass two overarching concepts: (i) maintain calorie balance over time to achieve and sustain a healthy weight and (ii) focus on consuming nutrient-dense foods and beverages (13).

Maintain Calorie Balance

The first concept is to maintain *calorie balance* over time to achieve and sustain a healthy weight. People who are most successful at achieving and maintaining a healthy weight do so through continued attention to consuming only enough calories from foods and beverages to meet their needs and by being physically active. To curb the obesity epidemic and improve their health, many Americans must decrease the calories they consume and increase the calories they expend through physical activity. As part of this recommendation, there is an emphasis on increasing physical activity and reducing the time spent in sedentary activities to lower the risk of developing obesity or for achieving a better weight if currently overweight or obese. One goal of increasing physical activity is to help achieve a calorically balanced state (*i.e.*, calories consumed equals calories expended) to prevent obesity or to achieve a negative energy balance (*i.e.*, calories consumed is less than calories expended) to lower weight. (More on weight and body composition can be found in Chapter 8.)

Consume Nutrient-Dense Foods and Beverages

The second concept is to focus on consuming nutrient-dense foods and beverages. Americans currently consume too much sodium and too many calories from solid fats, added sugars, and refined grains. Added sugars are considered caloric sweeteners that are added to foods during processing, preparation, or consumed separately. Solid fats are considered fats with a high content of saturated and/or *trans* fatty acids, which are usually solid at room temperature. Refined grains are considered to be grain products missing the bran, germ, and/or endosperm, that is, any grain product that is not a whole grain. These replace nutrient-dense foods and beverages and make it difficult for people to achieve the **recommended nutrient intake** while controlling calorie and sodium intake. A healthy eating pattern limits intake of sodium, solid fats, added sugars, and refined grains and emphasizes nutrient-dense foods and beverages—vegetables, fruits, whole grains, fat-free or low-fat dairy products, seafood, lean meats and poultry, eggs, beans and peas, and nuts and seeds. Care should be taken, however, to not misinterpret *limiting* an intake with *avoiding* an intake. For instance, both low-sodium and high-sodium intakes are associated with higher mortality, so the key is to find an appropriate balance of intake: not too much and not too little (15).

> **Recommended Nutrient Intake**
>
> Nutrient intake guidelines for different ages and genders have been established by various governmental (*e.g.*, National Institutes of Health) and nongovernmental (*e.g.*, World Health Organization) groups. The DRIs (the current U.S. guideline for recommended nutrient intake) provide intake levels for each nutrient that will, statistically, sustain good nutritional status for 98% of the population.

Nutrient-dense foods are foods that, for the calories delivered, have a high concentration of nutrients. An example of a food with low nutrient density is sugar, which is a source of energy but has no other nutrients associated with it. An example of a high nutrient dense food is kale, which is an excellent source of vitamins C, A, K1, and B6, and also an excellent source of the minerals potassium, calcium, magnesium, copper, and manganese. All these nutrients are provided by kale while delivering only 9 calories per cup. Seeking a high nutrient density is logical, as it has been found that the diet of severely obese individuals is unbalanced, with relatively high caloric intakes coupled with inadequate intake of vitamins and minerals (16). There is also an emphasis on consuming alcohol in moderation if it is consumed, by limiting consumption to no more than one drink per day for women and two drinks per day for men, assuming legal drinking age. Alcohol is a source of energy (7 calories/g), but it interferes with the metabolism of a number of nutrients that can increase disease risk. For instance, one of the most common reasons for a thiamin deficiency (Vitamin B1) is alcohol consumption because alcohol interferes with the production of the vitamin's coenzyme (thiamin pyrophosphate) (17). There are also nutrition recommendations for specific populations. As an example, here are some specific eating/nutrient recommendations that are specific to different groups:

- Women of childbearing age who are encouraged to consume sufficient iron and folic acid to reduce pregnancy and fetal complications.
- Women who are pregnant who are encouraged to limit the consumption of certain fish with a high mercury content and to ensure good iron status.
- People who are over 50 years of age who are encouraged to ensure that vitamin B_{12} status is not compromised because of age-related reduced absorption.

Important Factors to Consider

Obesity and overweight have different meanings:

- **Obesity** means having too much body fat
- **Overweight** means weighing too much for your height

  Weight may come from:

- Lean Mass (More = Good)
- Bone Mass (More = Good)
- Fat Mass (More = Bad)
- Body Water (More = Good)

Overweight

Overweight represents someone who is above the desired weight for height, age, and gender. Interpretation of "overweight" is difficult because athletes with a higher level of muscle per unit height may be classified as overweight, but this cannot be considered undesirable. The terms *overweight* and *obese* are often wrongly used interchangeably, as obesity is a condition of excess body fat regardless of weight, whereas overweight represents high weight for height regardless of body fat.

Obese/Obesity

A condition characterized by an excess level of body fat, regardless of body weight. People with a body fat percent (the percent of mass that is fat) that exceeds 25% for men or 32% for women are considered obese. Athletes typically have body fat percent levels that are significantly lower than these values.

DIETARY REFERENCE INTAKES

The DRIs are developed and published by the Institute of Medicine (IOM) and represent the most current scientific knowledge on the nutrient needs of healthy populations (Figure 1.2). The DRIs are composed of the following five components (18):

- *Estimated Average Requirement (EAR):* The average daily nutrient intake level estimated to meet the requirement of half the healthy individuals in a particular life stage and gender group.
- *Recommended Dietary Allowance (RDA):* The average daily dietary nutrient intake level sufficient to meet the nutrient requirement of nearly all (~98%) healthy

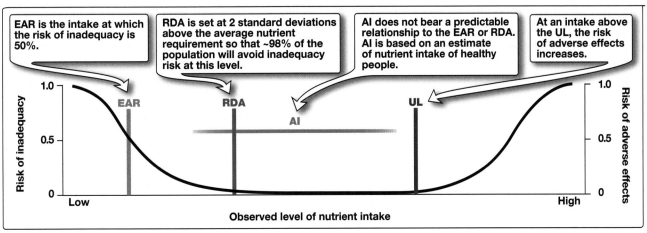

FIGURE 1.2: Dietary reference intakes (DRIs). AI, adequate intake; EAR, estimated average requirement; RDA, recommended dietary allowance; UL, upper intake level. (From Ferrier D. Lippincott illustrated reviews: biochemistry. 7th ed. Philadelphia (PA): LWW (PE); 2017.)

individuals in a particular life stage and gender group. This level amounts to two standard deviations above the average requirement.

- *Adequate Intake (AI):* The recommended average daily intake level based on observed or experimentally determined approximations or estimates of nutrient intake by a group (or groups) of apparently healthy people that are assumed to be adequate—used when an RDA cannot be determined.
- *Tolerable Upper Intake Level (UL):* The highest average daily nutrient intake level that is likely to pose no risk of adverse health effects to almost all individuals in the general population. As intake increases above the UL, the potential risk of adverse effects may increase.
- *Estimated Energy Requirement (EER):* This represents the *average* dietary energy intake predicted to maintain energy balance in a healthy adult of a defined age, gender, weight, and height who has a level of physical activity that is consistent with good health. The EER for children, pregnant women, and lactating women includes the higher energy needs associated with growth and development, pregnancy, or lactation.

As can be seen from Figure 1.2, the DRIs should not be considered a minimum intake level of nutrients to ensure a state of good health. Most healthy people have nutrient requirements that are considerably lower than the RDA (*i.e.*, close to the average requirement and not two standard deviations above the requirement), and a small proportion of people have nutrient requirements higher than the RDA. As indicated in Figure 1.2, having too much of any nutrient above the UL level increases the risk of an adverse effect, and having too little of a nutrient below the EAR level also increases the risk of an adverse health effect. Therefore, the DRI should be considered within the safe range of nutrient intakes that most people should strive for. Given the all-too-common prevalence of nutrient intakes from supplements in athletes, there is reason to be concerned that many physically active people are at greater risk of exceeding the UL than of having an amount below the recommended intake level.

For the individual who exercises regularly, the RDA is an excellent starting point to determine nutrient adequacy. Because exercise results in greater energy utilization than in the average nonexercising person, energy requirements are likely to be higher than those established in the energy RDA, which represents the average requirement. Since burning more energy also requires more nutrients (particularly B vitamins), and performance is closely tied to several minerals (iron and zinc in particular), consuming

the nutrient RDA of these nutrients is important. Serious athletes should periodically have a blood test to determine whether nutrient intakes are adequate and to determine if consuming the RDA level is right for them. In particular, checking adequate iron intake status by evaluating hemoglobin, hematocrit, and ferritin is important and may also be an indicator of the intake adequacy of other nutrients. Periodically assessing vitamin D status, particularly in athletes who train and compete indoors, is also advisable. The DRI tables of EARs, RDAs, AIs, and ULs can be found on the inside cover of this book for easy reference.

Using the DRIs for Planning

The DRI tables are an excellent resource for planning and evaluating nutrient intake adequacy in individuals and groups (Figure 1.3). For individuals, the following guidelines apply:

- **EAR:** Represents the average daily nutrient intake level estimated to meet the requirement for approximately half (*i.e.*, the average) of healthy individuals for each life stage by sex. The EAR should NOT be used as a nutrient intake goal for individuals because of the normal distribution requirements that occur within any population.
- **RDA:** Represents the average daily nutrient intake recommendation plus two standard deviations to satisfy the nutrient need for ~98% of all individuals for each life stage and sex. A typical intake at the RDA level should result in a low risk of nutrient inadequacy.
- **AI:** Represents the observed average daily intake level of nutrient intake by groups of apparently healthy people. As such, it is appropriate to use the AI as a dietary nutrient goal when there is no available RDA for a specific nutrient.
- **UL:** Represents the highest average daily nutrient intake level that is unlikely to pose a health risk for most people. Average intakes above the UL increases the risk for adverse health effects, making it a level inappropriate for dietary planning.

For groups, the following guidelines apply:

- **EAR** is appropriate to use for an acceptably low risk of insufficient nutrient intakes within a group.
- **RDA** should not be used to plan the intakes of groups, as the values represent two standard deviations *above* the average requirement.
- **AI** is appropriate to use for a group, as the average usual intake implies a low prevalence of insufficient nutrient intake.

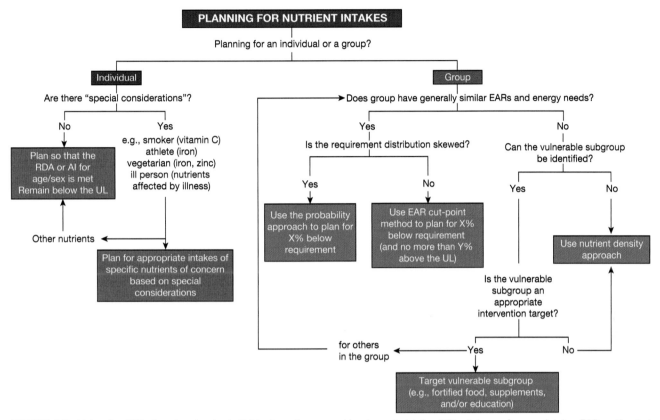

FIGURE 1.3: Using the DRIs for planning for individuals and groups. AI, adequate intake; DRI, dietary reference intake; EAR, estimated average requirement; RDA, recommended dietary allowance; UL, upper intake level (From Institute of Medicine Subcommittee on Interpretation and Uses of Dietary Reference Intakes; Institute of Medicine Standing Committee on the Scientific Evaluation of Dietary Reference Intakes. Using dietary reference intakes in planning diets for individuals. In: Dietary reference intakes: applications in dietary planning. Washington (DC): National Academies Press; 2003. Available from: https://www.ncbi.nlm.nih.gov/books/NBK221374/)

- **UL** can be used in planning to *minimize* the risk that a proportion of the population may receive an excessively high nutrient intake.

PHYSICAL ACTIVITY GUIDELINES

The Office of Disease Prevention and Health Promotion of the U.S. Department of Health and Human Services also publishes *Physical Activity Guidelines for Americans*, last published in 2018 (19). These guidelines are intended to outline the amount and type of physical activity associated with promoting health and reducing the risk of chronic disease. The major health-related research findings that are the basis of the physical activity guidelines include the following:

- Regular physical activity reduces the risk of many adverse health outcomes.

- Some physical activity is better than none.
- For most health outcomes, additional benefits occur as the amount of physical activity increases through higher intensity, greater frequency, and/or longer duration.
- Most health benefits occur with at least 150 minutes (2 hours and 30 minutes) a week of moderate-intensity physical activity, such as brisk walking. Additional benefits occur with more physical activity.
- Both aerobic (endurance) and muscle-strengthening (resistance) physical activities are beneficial.
- Health benefits occur for children and adolescents, young and middle-aged adults, older adults, and those in every studied racial and ethnic group.
- The health benefits of physical activity occur for people with disabilities.
- The benefits of physical activity far outweigh the possibility of adverse outcomes.

The specific key physical activity guidelines for different groups are described as follows:

Preschool-Aged Children

- Preschool-aged children (ages 3 through 5 years) should be physically active throughout the day to enhance growth and development.
- Adult caregivers of preschool-aged children should encourage active play that includes a variety of activity types.

Children and Adolescents

- It is important to provide young people opportunities and encouragement to participate in physical activities that are appropriate for their age, that are enjoyable, and that offer variety.
- Children and adolescents ages 6 through 17 years should do 60 minutes (1 hour) or more of moderate-to-vigorous physical activity daily:
  - **Aerobic:** Most of the 60 minutes or more per day should be either moderate- or vigorous- intensity aerobic physical activity and should include vigorous-intensity physical activity on at least 3 days a week.
  - **Muscle-strengthening:** As part of their 60 minutes or more of daily physical activity, children and adolescents should include muscle-strengthening physical activity on at least 3 days a week.
  - **Bone-strengthening:** As part of their 60 minutes or more of daily physical activity, children and adolescents should include bone-strengthening physical activity on at least 3 days a week.

Adults

- Adults should move more and sit less throughout the day. Some physical activity is better than none. Adults who sit less and do any amount of moderate-to-vigorous physical activity gain some health benefits.
- For substantial health benefits, adults should do at least 150 minutes (2 hours and 30 minutes) to 300 minutes (5 hours) a week of moderate-intensity, or 75 minutes (1 hour and 15 minutes) to 150 minutes (2 hours and 30 minutes) a week of vigorous-intensity aerobic physical activity, or an equivalent combination of moderate- and vigorous-intensity aerobic activity. Preferably, aerobic activity should be spread throughout the week.
- Additional health benefits are gained by engaging in physical activity beyond the equivalent of 300 minutes (5 hours) of moderate-intensity physical activity a week.

- Adults should also do muscle-strengthening activities of moderate or greater intensity and that involve all major muscle groups on 2 or more days a week, as these activities provide additional health benefits.

Older Adults

The key guidelines for adults also apply to older adults. In addition, the following key guidelines are just for older adults:

- As part of their weekly physical activity, older adults should do multicomponent physical activity that includes balance training as well as aerobic and muscle-strengthening activities.
- Older adults should determine their level of effort for physical activity relative to their level of fitness.
- Older adults with chronic conditions should understand whether and how their conditions affect their ability to do regular physical activity safely.
- When older adults cannot do 150 minutes of moderate-intensity aerobic activity a week because of chronic conditions, they should be as physically active as their abilities and conditions allow.

Women during Pregnancy and the Postpartum Period

- Women should do at least 150 minutes (2 hours and 30 minutes) of moderate-intensity aerobic activity a week during pregnancy and the postpartum period. Preferably, aerobic activity should be spread throughout the week.
- Women who habitually engaged in vigorous-intensity aerobic activity or who were physically active before pregnancy can continue these activities during pregnancy and the postpartum period.
- Women who are pregnant should be under the care of a health care provider who can monitor the progress of the pregnancy. Women who are pregnant can consult their health care provider about whether or how to adjust their physical activity during pregnancy and after the baby is born.

Adults with Chronic Health Conditions and Adults with Disabilities

- Adults with chronic conditions or disabilities, who are able, should do at least 150 minutes (2 hours and 30 minutes) to 300 minutes (5 hours) a week of moderate-intensity, or 75 minutes (1 hour and 15 minutes) to 150 minutes (2 hours and 30 minutes) a week of vigorous-intensity aerobic physical activity, or an equivalent combination of moderate- and vigorous-intensity aerobic activity. Preferably, aerobic activity should be spread throughout the week.

- Adults with chronic conditions or disabilities, who are able, should also do muscle-strengthening activities of moderate or greater intensity and that involve all major muscle groups on 2 or more days a week, as these activities provide additional health benefits.
- When adults with chronic conditions or disabilities are not able to meet the above key guidelines, they should engage in regular physical activity according to their abilities and should avoid inactivity.
- Adults with chronic conditions or symptoms should be under the care of a health care provider. People with chronic conditions can consult a health care professional or physical activity specialist about the types and amounts of activity appropriate for their abilities and chronic conditions.

Safe Physical Activity for All Groups

To do physical activity safely and reduce the risk of injuries and other adverse events, people should:

- Understand the risks, yet be confident that physical activity can be safe for almost everyone.
- Choose types of physical activity that are appropriate for their current fitness level and health goals, because some activities are safer than others.
- Increase physical activity gradually over time to meet key guidelines or health goals. Inactive people should "start low and go slow" by starting with lower intensity activities and gradually increasing how often and how long activities are done.
- Protect themselves by using appropriate gear and sports equipment, choosing safe environments, following rules and policies, and making sensible choices about when, where, and how to be active.
- Be under the care of a health care provider if they have chronic conditions or symptoms. People with chronic conditions and symptoms can consult a health care professional or physical activity specialist about the types and amounts of activity appropriate for them.

Although not specifically stated in the dietary and physical activity guidelines, but inherently important is that there should be a dynamic relationship between nutrient and energy intake and energy and nutrient utilization. So, the individual who has increased physical activity should be careful not to achieve a relative energy deficiency (RED) that could create difficulties. For instance, higher energy expenditures associated with physical activity should be closely matched with higher energy intakes to avoid a loss of lean mass and a loss of bone mass, both of which can have short- and long-term negative health effects. Put simply, increasing physical activity without making appropriate changes in the diet may inhibit the potentially positive impact of physical activity from occurring. It is also important to consider that the focus of the DRIs on individual nutrients may detract from the importance of nutrient intake *balance* and that the mix of nutrients consumed from different foods is important. Dietary fiber, for instance, is important for GI health and lowered risk of developing certain cancers. This information may motivate people to consume supplemental pure isolated dietary fiber, such as bran. However, it has pointed out that whole grain cereals, which are also good sources of dietary fiber, may be more important for health than fiber alone because of the other nutrients and phytonutrients that present in whole grains but not in fiber (20). Therefore, the focus should be on delivering a mix of balanced nutrients to improve health and reduce disease risk rather than excessively focusing on single dietary components. More on strategies for dynamically matching energy intake and expenditure are included in Chapter 8.

FOOD LABELS

Important Factors to Consider

- Food labels are important to assess so that there is a good understanding of the level of nutrients contained in a food. However, it is also important to consider that many good foods, such as fresh fruits and vegetables, have no food label. Accessing other sources of the nutrient content of foods is important for fully understanding the nutrient composition of nonlabeled foods.
- Some of the terms used on food labels may be misleading. For instance, the term *Lite* in a label may mean that the food derives less than 50% of its calories from fat, but may still be relatively high in fat, sugar, and/or calories. For instance, "Lite Potato Chips" may only mean that they are a third lower in fat content than a regular potato chip but should still not be considered a low-calorie food.

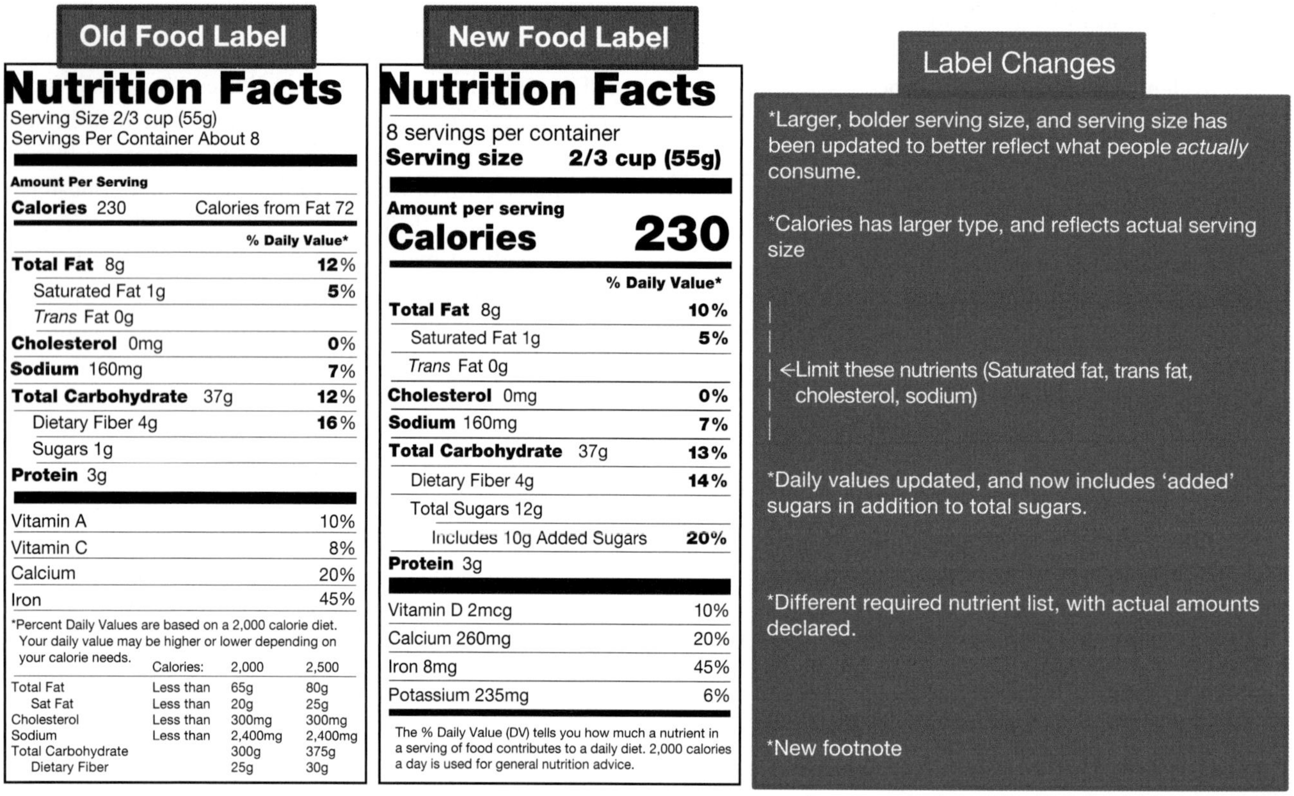

Old Food Label

Nutrition Facts
Serving Size 2/3 cup (55g)
Servings Per Container About 8

Amount Per Serving

Calories 230   Calories from Fat 72

% Daily Value*

Total Fat 8g   **12%**
    Saturated Fat 1g   **5%**
    Trans Fat 0g
Cholesterol 0mg   **0%**
Sodium 160mg   **7%**
Total Carbohydrate 37g   **12%**
    Dietary Fiber 4g   **16%**
    Sugars 1g
Protein 3g

Vitamin A   10%
Vitamin C   8%
Calcium   20%
Iron   45%

*Percent Daily Values are based on a 2,000 calorie diet. Your daily value may be higher or lower depending on your calorie needs.

	Calories:	2,000	2,500
Total Fat	Less than	65g	80g
Sat Fat	Less than	20g	25g
Cholesterol	Less than	300mg	300mg
Sodium	Less than	2,400mg	2,400mg
Total Carbohydrate		300g	375g
Dietary Fiber		25g	30g

New Food Label

Nutrition Facts
8 servings per container
Serving size   2/3 cup (55g)

Amount per serving
Calories   230

% Daily Value*

Total Fat 8g   **10%**
    Saturated Fat 1g   **5%**
    Trans Fat 0g
Cholesterol 0mg   **0%**
Sodium 160mg   **7%**
Total Carbohydrate 37g   **13%**
    Dietary Fiber 4g   **14%**
    Total Sugars 12g
        Includes 10g Added Sugars   **20%**
Protein 3g

Vitamin D 2mcg   10%
Calcium 260mg   20%
Iron 8mg   45%
Potassium 235mg   6%

The % Daily Value (DV) tells you how much a nutrient in a serving of food contributes to a daily diet. 2,000 calories a day is used for general nutrition advice.

Label Changes

*Larger, bolder serving size, and serving size has been updated to better reflect what people *actually* consume.

*Calories has larger type, and reflects actual serving size

|←Limit these nutrients (Saturated fat, trans fat, cholesterol, sodium)

*Daily values updated, and now includes 'added' sugars in addition to total sugars.

*Different required nutrient list, with actual amounts declared.

*New footnote

FIGURE 1.4: Reading *Nutrition Facts* food labels. (From U.S. Food and Drug Administration. Changes to the nutrition facts label [Internet]. 2017. Available from: https://www.fda.gov/food/guidanceregulation/guidancedocumentsregulatoryinformation/labelingnutrition/ucm385663.htm#images)

Learning to read food labels is an excellent strategy for understanding the nutrient contents and caloric content and energy distribution of packaged foods (Figure 1.4). There are some standards for food labels that include the following (21):

■ Every food label must state a common or usual name of the food/product; the name and address of the manufacturer, packer, or distributor; the net contents of the package by weight, measure, and count; and the ingredients in descending order of predominance by weight.

■ Food labels must provide more information if a nutrient is added to it or if a nutrition-related claim is made about the food. (For instance, "This food will lower your cholesterol" or "This food will lower your risk of cancer.") The health message must be truthful and not misleading, must be in general agreement with established medical and nutrition principles, and must have a reference on the label that allows consumers to see a Food and Drug Administration–approved summary of the health claim. Up-to-date labeling requirements can be found at: https://www.fda.gov/downloads/Food/GuidanceRegulation/UCM265446.pdf

■ Information on the food label must include:
  ● *Serving or portion size:* This is how much of the food is considered a serving. Packages may contain multiple servings, so if more is consumed than the serving size listed, the amount of nutrients/calories consumed must be adjusted.
  ● *Servings or portions per container:* Represents the number of servings (based on the servings size listed) in the container.
  ● *Food energy per serving:* The amount of energy (calories) in the food per serving.
  ● *Protein per serving in grams:* This is one of the components in the food that provides energy (*i.e.,* an energy substrate). Protein calories are calculated as grams × 4.
  ● *Carbohydrate per serving in grams:* This is one of the components in the food that provides energy (*i.e.,* an energy substrate). Carbohydrate calories are calculated as grams × 4.
  ● *Fat per serving in grams:* This is one of the components in the food that provides energy (*i.e.,* and energy substrate). Fat calories are calculated as grams × 9.

- *Sodium per serving in milligrams*: Sodium is a component of salt, which is sodium chloride. Most people should consume less than 1,500 mg of sodium/day, which is in a little more than 0.5 tsp of salt.
- *Protein, vitamins, and minerals as a percent of the U.S. RDA*: This lets you know approximately what proportion of the daily requirement is derived by consuming a standard serving of the food.
- *% Daily Value (DV)*: This is intended to help people understand how a food contributes to typical nutrient requirements.
  - ◆ DVs are average nutrient levels for people consuming 2,000 calories/day. Therefore, a food that contains 10% DV of dietary fiber represents 10% of the fiber requirements for an individual consuming 2,000 calories over an entire day.
  - ◆ People consuming more or less than 2,000 calories/day should adjust the DV for the calories consumed to better understand how the individual food serving contributes to the estimated nutrient needs for the day.
  - ◆ One way of interpreting the DV is to assume that 5% or less suggests the food serving has a low concentration of a given nutrient, and 20% or more suggests the food has a high concentration of a given nutrient. It is generally good to seek foods low in saturated fat, trans fat, cholesterol, and sodium and high in vitamins, minerals, and fiber.

It is important for consumers to become fully educated on the meaning of the information on food labels as it has the potential of being misleading and is often used solely for the purpose of marketing. For instance, when an olive oil label has *No Cholesterol* listed on it, the consumer should know that it would be impossible for olive oil to have cholesterol, which can only come from animal products.

As the DRIs are updated with increasing knowledge of health-associated nutrient intakes, the unit of measures for nutrients as they exist on food labels occasionally also change. During the summer of 2019, the FDA released guidance on conversions from the previous measures for folate, niacin, vitamin A, vitamin D, and vitamin E to new units that became required on food nutrition labels. For instance, folate was changed from micrograms (mcg) to mcg of dietary folate equivalents (mcg DFE). For vitamins A and D, food labels stating the Recommended Dietary Intakes (RDI) are now required to use mcg rather than the previously used international units (IU) (22).

An example of the new conversion for folate is provided below. Additional examples for folate and other nutrients can be found at the FDA reference: https://www.fda.gov/foodGuidances:

Folate Conversion to mcg DFE

Example: A serving (30 g) of enriched wheat flour contains a combination of naturally occurring folate (5 mcg) and folic acid (50 mcg)

- Folate Conversion to mcg DFE
  - Folate (mcg DFE) = [Naturally occurring folate (mcg per serving) × 1 (conversion factor for naturally occurring folate)] + [folic acid (mcg per serving) × 1.7 (conversion factor for folic acid)]
  - Folate (mcg DFE) = (5 mcg × 1) + (50 mcg × 1.7) = 90 mcg DFE % DV Calculation
  - % DV = [Folate (mcg DFE) ÷ 2016 RDI for folate (mcg DFE)] × 100% DV = (90 mcg DFE ÷ 400 mcg DFE) × 100 = 23%
- Nutrition Facts Label:
  - Folate. 90 mcg DFE (50 mcg folic acid) = 25% of Daily Value

---

PROFESSIONAL ORGANIZATION POSITION STATEMENTS

Important Factors to Consider

- Position statements by professional organizations represent critically important scientifically based guidelines that bring together the state-of-the-art information on specific health and nutrition-related topics that are important for physically active individuals.
- The 2009 and 2016 position statements on Nutrition and Athletic Performance, published jointly by several professional organizations, present critical scientific summaries of the nutritional strategies that enable both good health and optimal athletic performance (23,24).

The ACSM, AND, and the DOC continue to publish position statements related to nutrition and physical activity. These position statements provide excellent science-based summaries of the state-of-the-art research in the field and provide a good overview of information in a variety of sports nutrition–related areas. The 2009 and 2016 positions on "Nutrition and Athletic Performance," published jointly by the ACSM, AND, and DOC, have come to the following conclusions (23,24):

- Athletes should strive to consume adequate energy during periods of high-intensity and/or long-duration training to maintain body weight and health and maximize training effects. Inadequate energy intakes can result in loss of muscle mass; menstrual dysfunction; loss of bone density or failure to gain bone density in areas of exercise-associated physiologic stress; an increased risk of fatigue, injury, and illness; and a prolonged recovery process.

- Body weight and composition should not be used as the sole criteria for participation in sports; daily weigh-ins are discouraged. Optimal body fat levels are dependent upon the sex, age, and heredity of the athlete and may be sport-specific. Body fat assessment techniques, although currently more accurate than in the past, have inherent variability and limitations. The emphasis should be on the trend of body composition change rather than reliance on a single measure to initiate dietary intervention. Where fat loss is recommended to optimize performance, the best dietary and physical activity strategies to achieve this should, preferably, take place during the off-season or begin before the competitive season and involve a qualified sports dietitian.

- Carbohydrate intake recommendations for athletes range from 6 to 12 g/kg body weight/day, depending on exercise intensity (24). Carbohydrates maintain blood glucose levels during exercise and replace muscle glycogen. The amount required depends on the athlete's total daily energy expenditure, type of sport, gender, and environmental conditions. There should be an emphasis on having a dietary strategy that sustains normal blood glucose during activity.

- Protein recommendations for endurance and strength-trained athletes range from 1.2 to 2.0 g/kg body weight/day, with higher intake levels indicated for short periods during intensified training or when athletes reduce total energy consumption (24). These recommended protein intakes can generally be met through diet alone, without the use of protein or amino acid supplements. Sufficient energy intake is necessary to assure that the consumed protein can be used anabolically rather than to be used to help satisfy the energy requirement.

- Fat intake should range from 20% to 35% of total energy intake. Consuming ≤20% of energy from fat does not benefit performance. Fat, which is a source of energy and a carrier of fat-soluble vitamins and essential fatty acids, is important in the diets of athletes. High-fat diets are not recommended for athletes, and athletes should be cautious about not consuming fats that are potentially inflammatory to tissues, such as trans-fatty acids.

- Athletes who restrict energy intake or use severe weight loss practices, eliminate one or more food groups from their diet, or consume high- or low-carbohydrate diets of low micronutrient density, are at greatest risk of micronutrient deficiencies. Athletes should consume diets that provide at least the RDA for all micronutrients.

- Dehydration (water deficit resulting in an excess of 2% to 3% body mass) decreases exercise performance. Therefore, adequate fluid intake before, during, and after exercise is important for health and optimal performance. The goal of drinking is to prevent dehydration from occurring during exercise, and individuals should not drink in excess of their sweat rate. After exercise, ~16–24 oz (450–675 mL) of fluid for every pound (~0.5 kg) of body weight lost during exercise should be consumed.

- Before exercise, a meal or snack should provide sufficient fluid to maintain/achieve a good hydration state, should be relatively low in fat and fiber to facilitate gastric emptying and minimize GI distress, and should be relatively high in carbohydrate to achieve maintenance of blood glucose, be moderate in protein, be composed of familiar foods, and be well tolerated by the athlete.

- During exercise, primary goals for nutrient consumption are to replace fluid losses and provide carbohydrates (~30–60 g/hr) for maintenance of blood glucose levels. These nutrition guidelines are especially important for endurance events lasting longer than an hour, when the athlete has not consumed adequate food or fluid before exercise, or when the athlete is exercising in an extreme environment (high heat, high humidity, cold, or high altitude).

- After exercise, dietary goals are to provide primarily fluids, electrolytes, energy, and carbohydrates to replace muscle glycogen and ensure rapid recovery. A carbohydrate intake of ~1.0–1.2 g/kg/hr is required for the first 4 hours, followed by resumption of daily fuel needs (24). Proteins providing ~10 g essential

Table 1.5	Negative Impact of Relative Energy Deficiency in Sport (RED-S) on Health and Performance (30)	
Health		**Performance**
■ Impaired immune system		■ Decreased endurance
■ Abnormal menstrual function in females		■ Higher injury risk
■ Lower bone mineral density		■ Poor training response
■ Higher risk of anemia		■ Impaired judgment
■ More psychological issues		■ Lower coordination
■ Elevated cardiac stress		■ Poor concentration
■ Higher risk of gastrointestinal issues		■ Higher irritability
■ Poor growth/development in young athletes		■ Greater depression risk
■ Altered energy metabolism		■ Lower muscle strength

amino acids (or 0.25–0.3 g/kg body weight) should be consumed early in the recovery phase (0–2 hours postexercise) for aiding in muscle recovery and muscle protein synthesis (24).

■ In general, no vitamin and mineral supplements are required if an athlete is consuming adequate energy from a variety of foods to maintain body composition/weight. Supplementation recommendations unrelated to exercise, such as folic acid for women of childbearing potential, should be followed. A multivitamin/mineral supplement may be appropriate if an athlete is dieting, habitually eliminating foods or food groups, is ill or recovering from injury, or has a specific micronutrient deficiency. Single-nutrient supplements may be appropriate for a specific medical or nutritional reason (*e.g.*, iron supplements to correct iron-deficiency anemia). Ideally, nutrient supplementation should only occur if there is a known biologic deficiency, and only under the supervision of a qualified health professional.

■ Athletes should be counseled regarding the appropriate use of ergogenic aids (products advertised as performance enhancers). Such products should only be used after careful evaluation for safety, efficacy, potency, and legality.

■ Vegetarian athletes may be at risk for inadequate intakes of energy, protein, fat, and key micronutrients such as iron, calcium, vitamin D, riboflavin, zinc, and vitamin B_{12}. Educating athletes on how to best obtain these nutrients through consumption of specific foods and food preparation techniques is a desirable strategy for reducing risk.

Consultation with a sports dietitian is recommended to avoid these nutrition problems.

In addition, there are other position stands published by the ACSM that have important nutritional implications. These include positions on the following topics, which will be covered in greater depth later in this book:

■ Exercise and cardiovascular fitness (25)
■ Physical activity and bone health (26)
■ Prevention of heat- and cold-related illnesses during distance running (27)
■ The Female Athlete Triad (28)
■ Weight loss in wrestlers (29)

The IOC and international governing bodies (*e.g.*, Fédération Internationale de Gymnastique, which is the international governing body for gymnastics in sport) also publish nutritionally relevant scientifically based guidelines. Each sporting category, such as swimming, track and field, soccer, has an international governing body. The IOC has published important consensus statements outlining the problems faced by athletes who experience *Relative Energy Deficiency in Sport* (RED-S). These consensus statements outline numerous problems that occur when RED-S occurs (*i.e.*, when a person exercises without sufficient energy availability to support the activity in real time). These problems are wide-ranging and include both performance-related issues and health-related issues (Table 1.5). This consensus is an important scientific statement on the importance of considering both exercise and nutrition as jointly critical for achieving optimal health and performance (30,31).

NUTRITION MYTHS AND MISINFORMATION

Important Factors to Consider

- Nutrition myths are commonly held by many people and often become the standard of understanding for how to achieve desired nutritional goals. This makes it exceedingly difficult to help people achieve desired goals through science-based rather than myth-based strategies. For instance, athletes wishing to reduce weight will follow a standard calorie-restricted weight reduction diet, even though there is scientific evidence that these diets are counterproductive in achieving optimal athletic performance because they tend to lower lean mass, lower bone mass, and increase the proportion body fat mass.

- There are many protein-related myths in athletic environments that fail to produce the desired outcome of more muscle and less body fat. Science-based strategies for how to best consume protein to achieve these goals are far more effective and provide a good way to help athletes believe in the science rather than the myth.

There are many myths associated with nutrition that make it more difficult to help people achieve a good nutritional status. Some of these myths have become so embedded in our culture that they are treated unquestioningly as fact. For instance, there is a common belief that eating anything after 7:00 PM will serve to increase obesity risk. However, some cultures that eat late at night have lower obesity rates than those that do not, and the physiologic reason for this is clear: blood sugar fluctuates in 3-hour units. That is, blood sugar reaches its peak about 1 hour after you eat and is back to premeal levels 2 hours after that. So, if dinner is finished at 7:00 PM and bedtime is 11:00 PM, it is possible that low blood sugar will be achieved before bedtime and will stimulate the production of stress hormone (cortisol), which lowers lean mass and bone mass (32). Although weight may temporarily go down with this strategy, it is possible that the proportion of fat mass (*i.e.*, body fat percent) rises. Here are some of the common myths, which are more fully addressed in subsequent chapters, that are related to nutrition and physical activity:

- *Going on a severe caloric restriction will make you less obese*. In fact, caloric restriction is likely to result in a greater loss of metabolic mass than fat mass, increasing relative body fatness and risk of obesity (3,33,34).

- *3,500 calories equals 1 pound*. This relationship is typically used to demonstrate that if you restrict energy intake by 500 calories every day, you will accrue a 3,500 calorie deficit by the end of the week and will have lost 1 lb. There are no studies showing that this relationship between energy consumption and expenditure is valid for humans (35). Ideally, athletes should consider the importance of dynamically matching energy intake and energy expenditure during the day, rather than simply calculating "energy IN versus energy OUT" over 24 hours as if the endocrine system does not respond to energy balance fluctuations in real time.

- *Eating late at night will make you fat*. Fat loss and fat gain are complex metabolic issues, but it is clear that a failure to sustain normal blood sugar may increase stress hormone production, which may cause a loss of lean tissue and make you relatively fatter. Avoiding severe hunger, including eating a small amount in the evening if that is what it takes, is a good strategy for lowering the risk of developing higher body fat.

- *Eating extra protein will build muscle*. Building muscle is complex and includes having sufficient energy, protein, nutrients, and muscle stimulation (*i.e.*, exercise) to cause the muscle to increase. Simply eating more protein by itself will not build muscle. In fact, there is evidence that an excess intake of high-quality protein in a single dose may lower muscle protein synthesis, while the same level of protein provided in smaller doses will enhance muscle protein synthesis (36,37).

- *Cholesterol-free foods are heart-healthy*. Heart disease may occur from multiple factors, including genetic predisposition, body fat level, and the consumption of fats and sugars. Some cholesterol-containing foods (for instance, eggs) are relatively low in fat and do not contribute significantly to heart disease if consumed without added fats. In general, high-fat diets, even if they are cholesterol free, contribute to heart disease.

- *Athletes do not develop low bone density*. A major factor in higher bone density is putting additional stress on the skeleton, which most athletic events tend to do. However, athletes who fail to eat sufficient energy may also have inadequate calcium intakes, athletes who train and compete indoors may have poor vitamin D status, and amenorrheic female athletes (often the result of insufficient energy consumption) may all develop low bone density and place themselves at increased risk of fracture.

- *Food cravings are a good sign that the foods you crave will provide the nutrients you need.* There is no evidence that food cravings target nutritional need. Most food cravings are the result of multiple factors including, but not limited to, environmental stimuli, coping strategies, past eating habits, or a restrictive eating behavior that may lead to the desire to consume a food that was restricted.
- *Herbal products are natural so, therefore, they are safe.* Herbal products may or may not be safe, depending on whether the contents listed on the label are truly the contents of the supplement. Herbal supplements should contain a secondary label indicating that the contents have been tested by an independent lab to increase confidence that they are safe. In addition, herbal products may be unsafe due to medical conditions, drug–herb interactions, and other medically related issues that should make athletes cautious about their random and unsupervised use.
- *Water is the perfect hydration beverage.* When a person exercises, they lose water and electrolytes, and because of a higher brain and muscle tissue demand, blood sugar may drop rapidly. The ideal hydration beverage should, therefore, contain what is being lost/used (water, electrolytes, carbohydrate), particularly for exercise/activity lasting longer than 1 hour.
- *All fats are bad.* Some fats contain the essential fatty acid(s), so are necessary for sustaining good health, and some fats have anti-inflammatory effects that are desirable. So, not all fats are bad. However, overconsumption of saturated or trans fats increases the risk of obesity and heart disease, so the amounts consumed should be considered a critical factor in both health and performance.
- *Carbohydrates will make you fat.* Not all carbohydrates are the same. Vegetables, fruits, and whole grain cereals are all carbohydrates that are likely to reduce the risk of obesity and contain dietary fiber that is important for glycemic control and gut health. Highly refined carbohydrates, as found in sugars and refined grains, if consumed in excess may stimulate fat production through excess insulin production. There is a difference between learning to sip regularly on a sugar-containing sports beverage to avoid thirst during exercise (good things happen), and waiting to get thirsty and drinking an entire container of a sugar containing sports beverage (bad things happen). So, it's not just what you eat but how you eat it that matters.
- *Periodic fasting helps to cleanse toxins from your body.* The human system, assuming good hydration and nutritional status, has an excellent ongoing strategy for removing toxins that does not require periodic fasting. In fact, if the fasting results in low blood sugar and or RED-S, it could make matters worse.

NUTRITION SCIENCE

Nutrition is a science that draws upon multiple sources of information derived from different types of studies. Nutrition **research** draws upon epidemiological, experimental, and clinical trial evidence to determine the best strategies for people to eat for health and performance.

Research

This represents a systematic and structured investigation to confirm the cause of an existing condition, discover new facts about a condition, or develop new conclusions about a condition. As the name implies, it is a *repeated search* for the truth. Different types of research may provide different levels of understanding about a research question, so care must be taken to not come to conclusions that are not warranted. For instance, some research finds associations between factors, but these associations are not causative. As an example, reading those with cardiovascular disease consume high amounts of decaffeinated coffee should not make you think that consumption of decaffeinated coffee *causes* heart disease. It is more likely, in this example, that this association exists because people with cardiovascular disease are told to consume decaffeinated rather than regular coffee.

Following are three types of research studies:

- *Epidemiological research:* The study of defined populations to assess the patterns of conditions, their causes, and how these conditions may impact health and disease.
- *Experimental research:* A type of study that has an intervention (treatment, program, procedure, etc.) introduced to determine how it affects the studied population. Control groups are often used to see how the intervention group differs from the control group.
- *Clinical trial research:* An experiment conducted on relatively large populations to determine the effectiveness of a treatment, such as a food or a dietary supplement. This is experimental research, but conducted on a larger segment of the population to determine safety and efficacy.

Nutrition studies often assess the impact of food or nutrients, asking this question: Will the person consuming this food or nutrient do better in this outcome? The outcome can be any number of factors, such as lower cholesterol, better iron status, improved endurance, or better exercise recovery. Human studies in the area of nutrition are difficult because the subjects of the studies are typically free-living and, therefore, it is hard to control all aspects of their lives that may influence the outcome of study. Also, the information derived from the subjects is often self-reported, with no capacity to check on the accuracy of the information provided. It is common, for instance, to obtain a 24-hour dietary recall as a research strategy to understand the nutrient and calorie exposure a person has. However, people may forget all the foods they consumed, how the foods were prepared, or how much of a food they consumed, all of which may result in inaccurate results. To counteract this problem, researchers try to obtain information from as many subjects as possible so that a more true population average is obtained. For instance, one subject who overreports intake will be countered by another subject who underreports intake. Also, some nutrients require more days of intake information to fully understand the typical intake, because people do not eat the same thing every day. As an example, typical calorie intake can be estimated from 2 to 3 days of food intake, whereas vitamin C intake may require 20–30 days of intake to obtain a true average consumption pattern (Figure 1.5) (38). To make the interpretation of dietary studies even more complex, few studies go beyond assessing nutrient exposure from diet. We know, however, that it is also important to understand if the consumed nutrients were actually absorbed and used, or if a nutrient is excreted. It is also important to know the frequency of food consumption, as there is likely to be a different outcome in someone who requires 3,000 calories/day and

satisfies their nutrient intake by eating 3 × 1,000 calorie meals vs. 6 × 500 calorie meals. The total energy intake would be the same, but the more frequent consumption is likely to result in a lower total insulin response, lower fat storage, and better muscle maintenance.

Conditions Affecting Nutritional Status

Following are various conditions that have an impact on nutritional status:

- *Inadequate intake:* People may not eat enough for a variety of reasons, including inadequate income, loss of appetite because of a medical or psychological problem, physical incapacity that makes it difficult to eat, food allergies that may limit the intake of whole categories of foods, or drugs that should not be taken with certain foods.
- *Inadequate absorption:* Some individuals may have a GI problem, such as IBS or celiac disease that affects their ability to absorb some of the nutrients they have consumed. Some drug therapies also may produce side effects that inhibit the absorption of specific nutrients. Other issues that may have an impact on nutrient absorption include parasites in the GI tract and surgical removal of a proportion of the small intestine.
- *Defective utilization:* This occurs when nutrients are consumed and absorbed, but a metabolic failure makes it impossible to properly *use* the nutrient. There are numerous reasons that this may occur, including:
  - Inborn errors of metabolism, such as phenylketonuria, which makes it impossible to use the amino acid phenylalanine

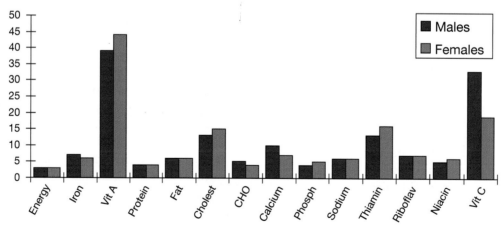

FIGURE 1.5: Days required to estimate average nutrient intake. (Modified from Basiotis PP, Welsh SO, Cronin FJ, Kelsay JL, Mertz W. Number of days of food intake records required to estimate individual and group nutrient intakes with defined confidence. J Nutr. 1987;117:1638–41.)

- Drug–nutrient interference (the drug Dilantin [phenytoin], for instance, interferes with the utilization of vitamin C)
- Alcohol-related liver problems (B-vitamin coenzymes may not be manufactured properly with heavy alcohol consumption)
■ *Increased excretion:* Vomiting and diarrhea cause people to lose nutrients that may otherwise have been absorbed and used. Also, a draining abscess is a common source of nutrient loss.
■ *Increased requirements:* A number of conditions may increase the requirement for energy and/or nutrients, which must be factored into whether a person is consuming an appropriate amount. For instance, an increase in physical activity, an infection, pregnancy, any growth period, a burn, any source of stress, and hyperthyroidism all increase the requirement for both energy and nutrients.

Care should be taken to not assume that an inadequate intake may be best resolved through the intake of a supplement, as the supplement may cause unexpected problems. For instance, a study found that vitamin E supplements, when compared with a placebo and taken prior to a competitive triathlon, promoted lipid peroxidation and inflammation during the triathlon (10). Another study found that there is no convincing evidence that immune-boosting supplements, including high doses of antioxidant vitamins and zinc, prevented exercise-induced immune impairment (39). A study assessing dietary supplements and mortality rate in older women (The Iowa Women's Health Study) found that, with the exception of calcium supplementation, all other vitamin and mineral supplements were associated with higher mortality rates (40). More discussion on specific vitamin and mineral requirements and how best to resolve issues of deficiency and toxicity can be found in Chapters 5 and 6.

SCOPE OF PRACTICE

Important Factors to Consider

■ Many people claim to be nutritionists and provide individuals with information that is intended to enhance health and/or performance. However, most states have laws that restrict the type of nutrition guidance that can be provided, depending on the certification(s) of the individual.

■ Certified fitness professionals without state-mandated certification (often dietetic licensure) typically are considered to be outside their scope of practice if they make recommendations to resolve a clinical condition through nutritional means. For instance, it would be inappropriate for someone without the appropriate state license to recommend a supplement or a diet to someone who has been diagnosed with heart disease or metabolic syndrome.

Currently, 47 of 50 states have laws regulating the practice of nutrition and dietetics, with guidelines clarifying what can or cannot be discussed with clients. As this is a matter of law, people who practice within the field of nutrition and dietetics are subject to prosecution if they exceed the stated boundaries within the law. Importantly, there are guidelines for *all* health professionals who discuss matters related to nutrition with their clients. These guidelines are important because many fitness professionals with inadequate nutrition training, no certifications, or lack of state licensure often exceed their scope of practice by making inappropriate recommendations for special diets that are meant to resolve clinical conditions and/or recommend dietary supplements that are intended to resolve a disease state. It is also inappropriate for fitness professionals to recommend a nutrient supplement to enhance performance if the nutrient content of the supplement exceeds the recommended DRI amount. There are numerous reasons for why these recommendations should not be made, including not knowing the health history of the individuals to whom the recommendation is made, potentially increasing health risks. See Box 1.4 for terms commonly used when discussing the scope of practice.

There are, however, a number of ways that someone who is not a registered dietitian/nutritionist (RD or RDN) can work to help people make better nutritional choices. Importantly, to make these nutritional recommendations people must understand the health implications of the recommendations they are making by knowing the science behind the recommendations. It is also important to understand that recommendations must be limited to nutritional recommendations that are based on the federal dietary guidelines, discussed earlier in this chapter. Noncertified/licensed/registered individuals should not make recommendations that are intended to resolve a clinical condition related to a diagnosed disease, as this is considered to be out of the established scope of practice.

Box 1.4   Common Terms Related to Scope of Practice

Registered Dietitian (RD) or Registered Dietitian Nutritionist (RDN): Individuals who have completed a specific course of study and practice hours are eligible to sit for a national registration examination which, when passed, allows them to have the title RD or RDN. People with this certification have the largest scope of practice in the area of nutrition and dietetic practice.

Licensure: Most states have dietetic/nutrition licensure, where people acting outside their established scope of practice can be prosecuted. Typically, only individuals with the RD or RDN certifications can become licensed.

Certification: Some states have certification where RD or RDN certifications qualify for state certifications. In these states, noncertified people are not allowed to refer to themselves as nutritionists, but they have greater scope of practice in nutrition than in states that have licensure.

Registration: The State of California has registration that makes it possible for RDs and RDNs to practice in the area of nutrition and dietetics, and that makes it illegal for unregistered individuals to refer to themselves as "nutritionists" or "dietitians." However, there is no registration examination and enforcement of registration rules is minimal.

For instance, it is acceptable to discuss with individuals and groups the general principles of good nutrition. But it is *not* acceptable for a noncertified/licensed/registered individual to answer a question from anyone in that group who raises their hand and says: "I have just been diagnosed with hypertension. Can you tell me what I should do nutritionally?" or "I have just been told I have heart disease. Is there something I should be doing nutritionally?" These are complex issues that require the full knowledge of the person's medical background, health history, eating behaviors, prescribed medications, and the recommendations made by the attending physician. It is inappropriate for anyone without this knowledge and without the proper licensure or certifications to make any statement or recommendations regarding these questions. Put simply, noncertified, nonlicensed, and nonregistered individuals may talk about the general nutrition guidelines associated with sustaining a good state of nutritional health, but are considered out of their scope of practice if they discuss nutrition in the context of a disease state.

According to the American Council on Exercise position statement, there are many appropriate avenues for nonlicensed professionals to discuss nutrition for health without exceeding the scope of practice (41). These include:

- Developing cooking classes to show healthy cooking techniques
- Establish recipe exchanges for high–nutrient-density meals
- Creating creative handouts and information packets that motivate people to make appropriate nutritional changes

- Giving nutrition sessions to groups that target key points in the U.S. Dietary Guidelines
- Scheduling individual sessions to discuss strategies for improving nutrient and calorie exposure

Importantly, scope of practice considerations are intended to improve client outcomes. The best outcomes are based on scientific evidence that includes research, national guidelines and policies, professional organization consensus statements, systematic analysis of clinical experience, quality improvement data, and the specialized educational background, knowledge base, and skills of those providing the information and service (42).

SUMMARY

- Nutrition is a science with several established rules that have evolved through many years of cumulative scientific evidence. These basic rules include the following:
  - Consuming more of any nutrient than your body requires does not make you healthier, and it does not improve athletic performance. *Example:* The recommended daily intake for vitamin C is ~60 mg, and there is no evidence that having 500 or 1,000 mg will somehow magically make you healthier or perform better. With some nutrients, having more than you require actually makes matters worse.
  - Consuming a variety of foods is critical to assuring that body tissues are exposed to all the energy substrates, vitamins, minerals, and phytonutrients

your body requires. Thinking that any single food is "perfect" and should, therefore, be consumed with great frequency simply limits exposure to other required foods. No single food is perfect.

- Energy consumption should ideally dynamically match requirement to avoid long periods in the day with excessively high or excessively low energy balance.

■ Physical activity increases the rate of energy utilization that must be matched with energy availability. Just consuming more vitamins, for instance, does nothing to satisfy the requirement for energy, and just consuming more protein fails to provide the vitamins needed to metabolize the protein and fails to satisfy tissue and blood carbohydrate requirements. Increased energy utilization requires the consumption of more foods that contain a variety of energy sources, vitamins, and minerals to satisfy need.

■ Physical activity increases energy metabolism, which is heat creating. Because the heat of exercise cannot be retained, exercise is associated with increased sweat production as the body attempts to dissipate the exercise-associated heat production. Failure to consume sufficient fluids of the right kind and in the right amount to *sustain* blood volume is a sure way to reduce athletic performance, and the resultant dehydration places the athlete at greater risk of heat illness.

■ The higher the intensity of physical activity, the greater the proportionate reliance on carbohydrate as a fuel.

■ Sport traditions often inhibit athletes from pursuing appropriate nutritional strategies to optimally benefit from training and may place athletes at risk of developing nutritionally related disorders.

■ Making "weight" through caloric restriction is now known to be counterproductive, as a failure to satisfy energy needs results in adaptive-thermogenesis (*i.e.*, a metabolic adaptation that excessively lowers the rate of energy metabolism), and is likely to lower more lean mass rather than fat mass.

■ Protein intake often far exceeds requirement, as athletes often believe that protein consumption will, by itself, help to build and maintain musculature. In fact, the recommended protein intake for athletes, ranging from 1.2 to 2.0 g/kg, is easily obtained from food without the need for additional protein supplementation.

■ The manner in which protein is consumed, often as part of large infrequent meals, is not the best way to ensure that the protein can be used to build and repair tissue. Ideally, protein should be consumed in relatively small amounts (~30 g/meal), with enough meal frequency to satisfy need, and at a time when in a good energy balanced state so the protein can be used anabolically rather than used to satisfy the energy requirement.

■ Some nutrients are referred to as essential, whereas others are referred to as nonessential, but this can be misleading as *all* nutrients are needed to sustain health. An *essential* nutrient is a nutrient that our tissues cannot manufacture from other body chemicals, so it is essential that we consume it. A *nonessential* nutrient is one that our tissues can manufacture from other body chemicals, so it is not essential that we consume it. An example is essential and nonessential amino acids. If we consume the essential amino acids, we can manufacture the nonessential amino acids.

■ DRIs have been established to help people understand how much of any nutrient is appropriate to consume on a daily basis (the RDA) and how much of any nutrient is excessive (the safe UL). It is important to understand that these are guidelines and that body tissues can store nutrients, allowing for some daily fluctuation in nutrient intake without compromising health.

■ Dietary guidelines are also available to provide eating guidance by encouraging people to maintain energy balance and by focusing on nutrient-dense foods. Following the dietary guidelines will help people avoid the development of common chronic disorders, including cardiovascular disease and diabetes.

■ Regular physical activity is an important component of maintaining health and fitness. Guidelines for physical activity frequency, time, and type have been developed for children, adults, pregnant women, people with disabilities, and older adults.

■ Food labels should be reviewed carefully, as they provide important information on the nutrient content and energy density of the food. Because food labels contain established terms (*i.e.*, diet or dietetic), it is important to fully understand the meaning of these terms.

■ Professional organizations, including the ACSM, have a variety of science-based position papers on nutrition and athletic performance (the most recent paper on this topic is 2016). These position papers include important information on the best nutrition strategies for achieving optimal performance while sustaining good health.

■ Conditions affecting nutritional status include inadequate nutrient/energy consumption, inadequate absorption of consumed foods, defective utilization of absorbed nutrients, increased excretion of nutrients, and conditions requiring more nutrients.

■ Scope of practice is an important consideration before giving out nutrition information, as most states have nutrition-associated licensure requirements

(*i.e.*, licensed dietitian) for anyone providing clinically based nutrition information. Those without the appropriate nutrition certification(s) have limits on the kind of nutrition information they can provide.

Practical Application Activity

You are likely to find that the nutrients and energy in the foods and beverages you consume are not what you may think. But with an analysis you can begin to see the weaknesses in your diet. Using the *National Nutrient Database for Standard Reference* (available from: https://fdc.nal.usda.gov), analyze a standard day of intake for selected nutrients and compare your intake with the RDA for your age and sex, according to the following directions:

1. Create a spreadsheet organized as follows (select the nutrients listed and any additional nutrients you are interested in for which there is an RDA):

Food (adjusted for consumed amount)	Protein (g)	Calcium (mg)	Iron (mg)	Zinc (mg)	Vit C (mg)	Vit E	Cholesterol (mg)
Food 1~							
Food 2~							
Etc.							
Totals for each nutrient							
RDA (adjusted for age and sex)							
Difference between intake and RDA							

2. When you log into the National Nutrient Database using the preceding link, select the *Food Search* option, enter a description of the food you wish to analyze (*e.g.*, Corn Cob; Broccoli Cooked), and press *Go*.
    a. A list of foods in the database that match your entry will appear. Select the food that comes closest to what you ate. The nutrients associated with the food will appear, with different amount options.
    b. Find a unit of measure (cup, package, etc.) that you can adjust for the amount that you consumed. For instance, if one of the standard units of measure is "Cup" and you had 1.5 cups, put the amount you consumed in the unit of measure you selected.
    c. Select the nutrients under "Cup" (or any other unit of measure you adjusted) to enter into your spreadsheet.
    d. Repeat the above until all the consumed foods have been analyzed.
3. Review the analysis to see the vitamins and minerals that are below the RDAs.
4. Make an adjustment in your food intake by eliminating foods that are poor sources of nutrients and/or adding those foods that can deliver the nutrients that you need more of.
5. Keep adjusting the foods until you can see an approximation of what you would need to eat to expose your tissues to the required nutrients in the spreadsheet.

CHAPTER QUESTIONS

1. Scope of practice represents the legal scope of work based on academic training, knowledge, and experience. Which profession is able, within their scope of practice, to provide dietary information for helping an athlete for a nutritionally related condition?
   a. Nutritionalist
   b. ACSM-Certified Health/Fitness Instructor
   c. ACSM-Registered Clinical Exercise Physiologist
   d. RD
   e. b, c, and d

2. Correlation refers to:
   a. A causal relationship between the same variable between two different groups
   b. A noncausal relationship between different variables
   c. The degree to which two groups of people are the same on any given factor (variable).
   d. A relationship that implies direction (*i.e.,* as weight goes up in one group, weight goes down in another).

3. According to the Dietary Supplement Health and Education Act, the term *dietary supplement* is defined as a "vitamin, mineral, herb, botanical, amino acid, metabolite, constituent, extract, or a combination of any of these ingredients."
   a. True
   b. False

4. The term *macronutrients* typically refers to:
   a. any nutrient that provides energy
   b. the eight key nutrients needed for good health
   c. carbohydrates, proteins, and fats
   d. vitamins and minerals

5. Which of the following best describes the term DRIs?
   a. Minimum amount of nutrients needed by an individual each day
   b. Maximum amount of nutrients that should not be exceeded each day
   c. Current nutrient standard for individuals
   d. Eight key nutrients needed for good health

6. If a food contains 350 calories, how many kilocalories does it contain?
   a. 148
   b. 350
   c. 1,480
   d. 3,250

7. All of the following may negatively affect nutritional status, except:
   a. Inadequate intake
   b. High absorption
   c. Defective utilization
   d. Increased excretion
   e. Increased requirements

8. An effective strategy for lowering obesity is to pursue a calorically restrictive diet.
   a. True
   b. False

9. Following exercise, consumption of _____ carbohydrate for the first 30 minutes following exercise, and again every 2 hours for 4–6 hours is sufficient to replace glycogen stores.
   a. 0.5–0.8 g/kg
   b. 1.0–1.5 g/kg
   c. 2.0–3.0 g/kg
   d. 6.0–7.0 g/kg

10. On food labels, the term *cholesterol-free* means that there is no cholesterol in the food.
    a. True
    b. False

ANSWERS TO CHAPTER QUESTIONS

1. d
2. b
3. a
4. c
5. c

6. b
7. b
8. b
9. b
10. b

Case Study Considerations

1. **Case Study Answer 1:** The big problem is that "weight" is the wrong metric. Ideally, people should assess changes in what constitutes weight (*e.g.*, fat mass vs. fat-free mass). Imagine someone losing 10 lb of fat and gaining 10 lb of muscle. This person would be the same "weight", but their strength:weight ratio would be higher, they would look smaller because lean mass is denser than fat mass, and they would have better endurance because they would have more muscle moving less nonmuscle weight. However, keeping muscle and losing fat requires that individuals sustain a good energy balance all the time. This means that meal skipping or not eating after 7 PM is like to have the opposite of the desired effect, and this strategy is like to result in a severe energy balance deficit.

2. **Case Study Answer 2:** Ideally, vitamins and minerals should be consumed through the appropriate intake of a wide variety of foods. Supplements should only be considered if the individual has been tested and diagnosed as having a specific vitamin or mineral deficiency, and only then if modifying the diet to correct the deficiency is not possible. Importantly, there is an increasing body of evidence to suggest that more than enough is not better than enough, and supplements often provide an amount of nutrient that far exceeds need. This can negatively impact tissue adaptation and health, and may also result in tissue rejection of an overconsumed nutrient, resulting in a deficiency the supplement is intended to avoid.

3. **Case Study Answer 3:** Weight is not a good measure for understanding if someone is exercising and eating well. An individual who has an appropriate energy/nutrient intake to satisfy tissue needs is likely to have a lower body fat level, will have an elevated bone mineral density that is more resistant to fracture, and will at least sustain existing lean mass or increase lean mass as a response to the exercise-associated muscle stress.

4. **Case Study Answer 4:** Ideally, this individual should have an eating plan that avoids large energy deficiencies during the day (typically eating something approximately every 3 hours); drinking an appropriately constituted sports beverage during the physical activity; assuring that the athlete begins the physical activity well hydrated and with muscle glycogen at an appropriate level for the activity; have a recovery plan that includes fluids, carbohydrates, and protein consumed soon after the physical activity ends.

5. **Case Study Answer 5:** Athletes who do the right things nutritionally typically have far lower injury and disease risks, can benefit from the physical activity as evidenced by improved performance, and feel less fatigued as a result of the physical activity they are performing.

REFERENCES

1. Birkenhead KL, Slater G. A review of factors influencing athletes' food choices. Sports Med. 2015 Nov;45:1511–22.
2. Maughan RJ, Burke LM, Dvorak J, Larson-Meyer DE, Peeling P, Phillips SM, Rawson ES, Walsh NP, Garthe I, Geyer H, Meeusen R, van Loon LJC, Shirreffs SM, Spriet LL, Stuart M, Vernec A, Currell K, Ali VM, Budgett RG, Ljungqvist A, Mountjoy M, Pitsiladis YP, Soligard T, Erdener U, Engebretsen L. IOC consensus statement: dietary supplements and the high-performance athlete. Br J Sports Med. 2018 Apr;52(7):439–55.
3. Dulloo AG, Montani JP. Pathways from dieting to weight regain, to obesity and to the metabolic syndrome: an overview. Obes Rev. 2015;16(S1):1–6.
4. Mamerow MM, Mettler JA, English KL, Casperson SL, Arentson-Lantz E, Sheffield-Moore M, Layman DK, Paddon-Jones D. Dietary protein distribution positively influences 24-h muscle protein synthesis in healthy adults. J Nutr. 2014 Jun;44(6):876–80.
5. Paddon-Jones D, Rasmussen BB. Dietary protein recommendations and the prevention of sarcopenia. Curr Opin Clin Nutr Metab Care. 2009;12(1):86–90.
6. Moore DR, Sygo J, Morton JP. Fuelling the female athlete: Carbohydrate and protein recommendations. Eur J Sport Sci. 2022;22(5):684–96.
7. Delk-Licata A, Behrens CE, Benardot D, Bertrand BM, Chandler-Laney PC, Fernandez JR, Plaisance EP. The association between dietary protein intake frequency, amount, and state of energy balance on body composition in a women's collegiate soccer team. Int J Sport Nutr Exerc Metab. 2019;5(123).
8. Institute of Medicine Subcommittee on Interpretation and Uses of Dietary Reference Intakes; Institute of Medicine Standing Committee on the Scientific Evaluation of Dietary Reference Intakes. Using dietary reference intakes in planning diets for individuals. In: Dietary reference intakes: applications in dietary planning. Washington (DC): National Academies Press; 2003. Using dietary reference intakes in planning diets for individuals. Available from: https://www.ncbi.nlm.nih.gov/books/NBK221374
9. Geller AI, Shehab N, Weidle NJ, Lovegrove MC, Wolpert BJ, Timbo BB, Mozersky RP, Budnitz DS. Emergency department visits for adverse events related to dietary supplements. N Engl J Med. 2015 Oct 15;373(16):1531–40.

10. Nieman DC, Henson DA, McAnulty SR. Vitamin E and immunity after the Kona Triathlon World Championship. Med Sci Sports Exerc. 2004;36(8):1328–35.

11. Maughan RJ. Contamination of dietary supplements and positive drug tests in sport. J Sports Sci. 2007;23(9):883–9.

12. Connor WE, Neuringer M, Reisbick S. Essential fatty acids: the importance of n-3 fatty acids in the retina and brain. Nutr Rev. 1992;50:21–9.

13. United States Department of Health and Human Services and U.S. Department of Agriculture. 2015–2020 Dietary guidelines for Americans, appendix 1. 8th ed. 2015. Available from: https://health.gov/dietaryguidelines/2015/guidelines/appendix-1

14. U.S. Department of Agriculture and U.S. Department of Health and Human Services. Dietary guidelines for Americans, 2020–2025. 9th ed. 2020. Available from: DietaryGuidelines.gov

15. Graudal N, Jürgens G, Baslund B, Alderman MH. Compared with usual sodium intake, low- and excessive-sodium diets are associated with increased mortality: a meta-analysis. Am J Hypertens. 2014;27(9):1129–37.

16. Horvath JDC, Dias de Castro ML, Kops N, Malinowski NK, Friedman R. Obesity coexists with malnutrition? Adequacy of food consumption by severely obese patients to dietary reference intake recommendations. Nutr Hosp. 2014;29(2):292–9.

17. Tetsuka S, Hashimoto R. Alcohol-related central nervous system disorders associated with vitamin B deficiency. SN Compr Clin Med. 2021;3:528–37.

18. Ferrier D. Lippincott illustrated reviews: biochemistry. 7th ed. Philadelphia (PA): Lippincott Williams & Wilkins (PE); 2017.

19. United States Department of Health and Human Services. Physical activity guidelines for americans. 2nd ed. The Office of Disease Prevention and Health Promotion, Office of the Assistant Secretary for Health, Office of the Secretary; 2018. Available from: http://health.gov/paguidelines/guidelines/summary.aspx

20. Jacobs DR Jr. Nutrition: the whole cereal grain is more informative than cereal fibre. Nat Rev Endocrinol. 2015;11(7):389–90.

21. United States Food and Drug Administration. Changes to the nutrition facts label [Internet]. 2017. Available from: https://www.fda.gov/food/food-labeling-nutrition/changes-nutrition-facts-label

22. Food and Drug Administration, U.S. Department of Health and Human Services, Center for Food Safety and Applied Nutrition. Converting units of measure for folate, niacin, and vitamins A, D, and E on the nutrition and supplement facts labels: Guidance for Industry. August 2019. https://www.fda.gov/FoodGuidances

23. Rodriguez NR, DiMarco NM, Langley S; American Dietetic Association; Dietitians of Canada. American College of Sports Medicine position stand. Nutrition and athletic performance. Med Sci Sports Exerc. 2009;41(3):709–31.

24. Thomas DT, Erdman KA, Burke LM. American College of Sports Medicine Joint Position Statement. Nutrition and athletic performance. Med Sci Sports Exerc. 2016;48(3):543–68.

25. Garber CE, Blissmer B, Deschenes MR, Franklin BA, Lamonte MJ, Lee IM, Nieman DC, Swain DP; American College of Sports Medicine. American College of Sports Medicine position stand. Quantity and quality of exercise for developing and maintaining cardiorespiratory, musculoskeletal, and neuromotor fitness in apparently healthy adults: guidance for prescribing exercise. Med Sci Sports Exerc. 2011;43(7):1334–59.

26. Kohrt WM, Bloomfield SA, Little KD, Nelson ME, Yingling VR; American College of Sports Medicine. American College of Sports Medicine position stand: physical activity and bone health. Med Sci Sports Exerc. 2004;36(11):1985–96.

27. Armstrong LE, Epstein Y, Greenleaf JE, Haymes EM, Hubbard RW, Roberts WO, Thompson PD. American College of Sports Medicine position stand. Heat and cold illnesses during distance running. Med Sci Sports Exerc. 1996;28(12):i–x.

28. Nattiv A, Loucks AB, Manore MM, Sanborn CF, Sundgot-Borgen J, Warren MP. American College of Sports Medicine position stand. The female athlete triad. Med Sci Sports Exerc. 2007;39(10):1867–82.

29. Oppliger RA, Case HS, Horswill CA, Landry GL, Shelter AC. American College of Sports Medicine Position Stand. Weight loss in wrestlers. Med Sci Sports Exerc. 1996;28(10):135–8.

30. Mountjoy M, Sundgot-Borgen J, Burke L, Carter S, Constantini N, Lebrun C, Meyer N, Sherman R, Steffen K, Budgett R, Ljungqvist A. The IOC consensus statement: beyond the female athlete triad–relative energy deficiency in sport (RED-S). Br J Sports Med. 2014;48:491–7.

31. Mountjoy M, Sundgot-Borgen JK, Burke LM, Ackerman KE, Blauwet C, Constantini N, Lebrun C, Lundy B, Melin AK, Meyer NL, Sherman RT, Tenforde AS, Torstveit MK, Budgett R. IOC consensus statement on relative energy deficiency in sport (RED-S): 2018 update. Br J Sports Med. 2018 Jun;52(11):687–97.

32. Fahrenholtz IL, Sjödin A, Benardot D, Tornberg ÅB, Skouby S, Faber J, Sundgot-Borgen JK, Melin AK. Within-day energy deficiency and reproductive function in female endurance athletes. Scand J Med Sci Sports. 2018;28(3):1139–46.

33. Ochner CN, Tsai AG, Kushner RF, Wadden TA. Treating obesity seriously: when recommendations for lifestyle change confront biological adaptations. Lancet Diabetes Endocrinol. 2015;3(4):232–4.

34. Montani JP, Schutz Y, Dulloo AG. Dieting and weight cycling as risk factors for cardiometabolic diseases: who is really at risk? Obesity Rev. 2015;16(S1):7–18.

35. Hall KD, Heymsfield SB, Kemnitz JW, Klein S, Schoeller DA, Speakman JR. Energy balance and its components: implications for body weight regulation. Am J Clin Nutr. 2012;95:989–94.

36. Elango R, Ball RO, Pencharz PB. Tolerability of leucine in humans. In: Rajendram R, Preedy V, Patel V, editors. Branched chain amino acids in clinical nutrition. Nutrition and health. New York (NY): Humana Press; 2015.

37. Elango R, Chapman K, Rafii M, Ball RO, Pencharz PB. Determination of the tolerable upper intake level of leucine in acute dieetary studies in young men. Am J Clin Nutr. 2012 Oct;96:759–67.

38. Basiotis PP, Welsh SO, Cronin FJ, Kelsay JL, Mertz W. Number of days of food intake records required to estimate individual and group nutrient intakes with defined confidence. J Nutr. 1987;117:1638–41.

39. Gleeson M, Nieman DC, Pedersen BK. Exercise, nutrition and immune function. J Sports Sci. 2004;22:115–25.

40. Mursu J, Robien K, Harnack LJ, Park K, Jacobs DR. Dietary supplements and mortality rate in older women: the Iowa Women's Health Study. Arch Intern Med. 2011;171(18):1625–33.

41. Muth ND. Nutrition coaching: a primer for health and fitness professionals. IDEA Fitness J. 2015. Available from: http://www.ideafit.com/fitness-library/nutrition-coaching-a-primer-for-health-and-fitness-professionals

42. Gibbs L. Evidence-based practice for the helping professions: a practical guide with integrated multimedia. Pacific Grove (CA): Brooks/Cole (Wadsworth Publishers); 2003.

2

Carbohydrates

CHAPTER OBJECTIVES

- Understand the structure of different types of dietary carbohydrates and the foods that are good sources of each type.
- Review the primary functions of dietary carbohydrates.
- Know how to calculate the carbohydrate calories derived from consumed foods and whether the carbohydrate intake will satisfy metabolic requirements.
- Identify the different digestive enzymes that are specific to carbohydrates and the origin of these enzymes.
- Know the energy-producing carbohydrate metabolic pathways.
- Understand the function of insulin, epinephrine, and glucagon, and how these are related to blood sugar.
- Know the difference between glycemic index and glycemic load and how the glycemic effect of foods can affect carbohydrate metabolism.

- Identify human carbohydrate storage systems, the typical maximal storage capacity, and how storage in each storage depot may be affected by diet and activity.
- Review the different possible pathways for blood glucose, and the likely pathway(s) with different blood glucose levels.
- Based on the sugar, starch, and dietary fiber content of foods, explain how different carbohydrate sources are preferred in different circumstances (*i.e.*, pregame, during activity, postactivity, and long-before activity).
- Discuss the preferred carbohydrate composition and concentration in sports beverages.
- Review the possible sources for making carbohydrate from noncarbohydrate sources (gluconeogenesis).

Case Study

Sally was working hard to be a world-class distance runner with the goal of making the marathon team for the next Olympic Games in 3 years. She had moved to train with a well-regarded coach, with whom a plan was developed that included a strict training regimen for daily/weekly mileage and selected competitions to confirm that the training was going as expected. Both Sally and her coach were weight conscious, trying to make sure that Sally ate just enough to support her weight but not so much that her weight would increase. There was some justification for this, as the trend for successful Olympic marathon runners was to be smaller (recent successful male Olympians were typically less than

115 lb, and successful female Olympians were less than 110 lb). However, the "fear of calories" and, especially carbohydrates, that was associated with the "fear of higher weight" resulted in a failure to optimally satisfy energy requirements, particularly as the training progression resulted in longer, harder, faster training mileage. After a year, Sally lost her period, and she started losing some sleep (a common outcome of overtraining). She was losing speed and she felt weaker, so she started eating less carbohydrate and more protein to try to maintain her muscle mass. After 6 months, she developed a stress fracture in her right tibia that stopped the training altogether for 12 weeks. Luckily, the orthopedist

who diagnosed the stress fracture had a Registered Dietitian working with her who was herself a runner and was fully aware of the training demands of elite distance runners. They had long conversations, and the dietitian knew exactly what had happened to Sally. Insufficient energy intake is associated with multiple problems, including low estrogen production that results in a loss of menses, and estrogen is an inhibitor of osteoclasts (the cells that break down bones). Also, inadequate carbohydrate intake resulting in low blood sugar is associated with high **cortisol** (stress hormone) production, which breaks down both muscle mass and bone mass even if extra protein is consumed (1). The extra protein Sally was consuming was mainly being used to satisfy energy requirements (*i.e.,* the protein was being utilized as a source of energy rather than used to sustain or improve the muscle mass). To make matters worse, not eating enough often leads to extra **insulin** being produced when food is eventually consumed, resulting in a greater fat production that may cause the runner to want to eat even less. Therefore, the dietitian showed Sally how to dynamically match energy intake with expenditure on a reasonable diet that included plenty of carbohydrates, some fats, and some proteins. The result was precisely what you would expect when people do the right things nutritionally, and Sally was on the path to making the Olympic team.

CASE STUDY DISCUSSION QUESTIONS

1. If you were working with a distance runner, what would you do to help ensure that energy intake satisfied needs, while lowering the risk of too little energy consumption?
2. Why would cortisol be elevated, and what would you do to help bring cortisol down to normal (nonstress) levels?
3. Would a male distance runner experience the same negative effects of insufficient energy consumption?
4. How often would you need to consume some carbohydrates to help ensure normal blood sugar?
   a. When awake but doing normal daily activity
   b. When asleep
   c. When physically active

Cortisol

A glucocorticoid steroid hormone that is produced by the adrenal gland in response to stress and hypoglycemia (low blood sugar). It functions to increase blood sugar through the breakdown of tissues that are converted to glucose (gluconeogenesis). It is important to note that cortisol breaks down muscle, bone, and fat tissue.

Insulin

A hormone produced by the β-cells of the pancreas that helps to avoid hyperglycemia (high blood sugar) by enabling cells to take blood sugar (glucose). A fast rise in blood sugar from consumption of a large volume of sugar and/or consumption of high glycemic foods results in a high insulin response that enables movement of sugars to tissues. However, this may exceed the tissue requirement for sugar, resulting in tissue conversion of sugar to fat, leading to an increase in body fat levels. A chronically high insulin response may lower tissue sensitivity to insulin, increasing type 2 diabetes risk.

Blood Sugar

The primary fuel for the brain and a source of energy to working muscles that can provide energy aerobically (with oxygen) or anaerobically (without oxygen). Normal blood sugar is in the range of 70–130 mg/dL between meals for adults, and children have slightly higher blood sugar levels between meals. Because blood sugar represents the primary fuel for the brain and the brain is responsible for survival, low blood sugar results in elevated cortisol to break down tissues that can be converted to sugar so that the brain can function. As physical activity increases the rate of blood sugar utilization, it is important for athletes to have a strategy to sustain blood sugar within the normal range to avoid a cortisol response.

INTRODUCTION

Important Factors to Consider

- Humans can derive energy from carbohydrate, protein, and fat, all of which are considered *energy substrates*. Of these, carbohydrate is considered a "flexible" fuel because it is the only energy substrate that can be metabolized for energy both with oxygen (aerobic metabolism) and without oxygen (anaerobic metabolism).
- The human storage capacity for carbohydrates is limited, with only ~300 calories of liver glycogen (which sustains blood glucose) and ~1,500 calories of muscle glycogen. By contrast, even a relatively

lean human can store over 62,000 calories of fat. The limited carbohydrate storage requires that carbohydrates be consumed frequently to ensure that blood glucose and muscle glycogen are sustained.

- While glucogenic amino acids, when converted to glucose, can also be metabolized aerobically and anaerobically, protein breakdown for energy may not be an ideal fuel because the process of converting glucogenic amino acids to glucose requires the release of "nitrogen," the majority of which must be excreted. While this glucose creation from protein may be necessary to satisfy the body's carbohydrate requirement, it takes away from protein's capacity to make other needed substances. Under ideal circumstances, therefore, carbohydrate intake should be sufficient so that protein can perform all its unique functions, including building and repairing tissue, and creating hormones and enzymes, rather than being "burned" as a fuel.

Table 2.1	Tissue Glucose Utilization in the Fasting and Postprandial*a* State	
Tissue/Organ	Fasting (Mainly Insulin Independent) % of Total	Postprandial (Mainly Insulin Dependent) % of Total
Brain	40–45	~30
Muscle	15–20	30–35
Liver	10–15	25–30
GI tract	5–10	10–15
Kidney	5–10	10–15
Other (*e.g.,* skin and blood cells)	5–10	5–10

*a*Period during or immediately after food consumption.

Source: From Gerich JE. Role of the kidney in normal glucose homeostasis and in the hyperglycaemia of diabetes mellitus: therapeutic implications. Diabet Med. 2010;27(2):136–42.

Generations ago, we had culturally appropriate strategies (long since forgotten) for ensuring that basic physiologic needs were satisfied. With the onset of the industrial revolution, however, we forgot why we did what we did, and we have been in trouble ever since. To illustrate this point, consider blood sugar fluctuations. Blood sugar is the primary fuel for the brain, and it fluxes approximately every 3 hours while doing normal casual daily activities (Table 2.1). That is, while you're awake and doing normal

daily activities blood sugar reaches its peak about 1 hour after eating and is back to premeal levels about 2 hours after that (2). When physically active or psychologically stressed, blood sugar may achieve a below-normal level in far less than 3 hours. The intensity of activity influences the rapidity with which blood sugar will drop, with higher intensity causing a faster drop than lower intensity (3–5).

Failing to consume a source of energy that can stabilize blood sugar at that time results in a series of hormonal events that can make a person feel worse and provides a stimulus for the creeping obesity that currently besets many Western cultures. There is such a fear of calories

AEROBIC AND ANAEROBIC METABOLISM

Aerobic Metabolism   Refers to the process of creating energy from the breakdown and combustion (burning) of carbohydrates, proteins, and fats. This process requires oxygen, and thus the reason for it to be called "aerobic metabolism." Fats can *only* be metabolized for energy aerobically, while carbohydrates and modified proteins can be metabolized both with oxygen (aerobically) or without oxygen (anaerobically).

Anaerobic Metabolism   Refers to process of creating energy from the breakdown and combustion (burning) of carbohydrates, modified proteins, and phosphocreatine. This process occurs when there is insufficient oxygen available to satisfy the energy demands of muscles and organs. It is important to note that fats cannot be metabolized for energy anaerobically, resulting in a heavy reliance on carbohydrate and protein when energy demands, as occurs in high-intensity activity, exceed the body's capacity to supply and/or use sufficient oxygen.

See Chapters 8 and 9 for more information on energy metabolism.

that people now migrate toward diet products with caffeine, which stimulates the brain and masks the very real physiologic hunger that is being experienced. In generations past, we had a much more effective strategy, referred to as "morning tea" and "afternoon tea," when a small snack and drink was provided mid-morning and mid-afternoon to ensure that most people had stable blood sugar. There is a cost to pay if hunger is allowed to go unanswered, and the cost gets bigger with each successive day that the same mistakes are repeated.

Physical activity increases the rate at which energy (*i.e.,* calories) is expended, further increasing the risk that energy demands may not be adequately met. It is troubling that surveys of physically active people suggest that they often fail to adequately support their energy needs, detracting from the potential benefits that the activity should impart (6). Specific strategies are required, therefore, to ensure that physically active people obtain the needed extra energy they require.

This chapter discusses carbohydrates, one of the energy substrates, and the natural push and pull between energy delivery and the endocrine system so as to create a balance between the delivered energy and the cellular need for survival (Box 2.1). Understanding this relationship can help physically active people eat in a way that optimizes performance, weight, body composition, and a sense of well-being. There are also common misunderstandings about proteins and fats, with many recommending very high intakes of proteins and/or fats to satisfy energy requirements and enhance performance. The performance issues related to the energy substrates are discussed in this chapter (Box 2.2).

Carbohydrate is one of the energy substrates, meaning that it is a component of food from which we can derive the *energy* needed to support body functions. The other energy substrates, discussed in Chapters 3 and 4, are protein and fat. All carbohydrates are derived from photosynthesis in plants, and the most basic forms of carbohydrate in plants are referred to as **monosaccharides** and **disaccharides**, which are also called *sugars* (Box 2.3). More complex forms of carbohydrates are made by plants through the synthesis of monosaccharides

---

Box 2.2	**Common Questions About Carbohydrates and Physical Activity**

- How much carbohydrates should be consumed immediately before, during, and after physical activity to optimize performance?
- Should the amount of carbohydrates consumed be different for endurance versus power versus team sport athletes?
- If consuming a sports beverage during physical activity, what is the best concentration of carbohydrates?
- Is there any advantage or disadvantage to having different types of carbohydrates in the sports beverage?
- Should physically active people be concerned that consumption of carbohydrates will increase the risk of increasing body fat?
- Are there any types of carbohydrate that should be avoided before exercise? During exercise? After exercise?

---

into **polysaccharides**, which are also referred to as either *starch or fiber*. The older the plants, the greater the proportion of polysaccharides, causing them to taste less sweet and have a less tender consistency. Fruits, however, are initially high in polysaccharides, but as they age, the polysaccharides are broken down into their component monosaccharides and disaccharides, making them taste sweeter as they ripen. Therefore, the age and ripeness of the plant or fruit consumed influence the type of carbohydrate that is ingested. Carbohydrate requirements and sources of carbohydrates in foods are in Box 2.4.

TYPES OF CARBOHYDRATES

Carbohydrates

A class of macronutrients composed of carbon, hydrogen, and oxygen that is a major source of cellular energy provided by foods, including grains, vegetables, fruits, and legumes.

Box 2.1	**Energy Delivery of the Energy Substrates**

Carbohydrates: 4 calories/g
Proteins: 4 calories/g
Fats: 9 calories/g

Box 2.3	**Carbohydrates Come from Photosynthesis**

- Solar energy + carbon dioxide from the atmosphere + water from the ground yield carbohydrate
- Solar energy + CO_2 + H_2O = glucose
- Carbo (carbon) + hydrate (water) = carbohydrate

Monosaccharides

Often referred to as "sugar," the main dietary monosaccharides are the hexoses (6-carbon) glucose, galactose, and fructose, and the pentoses (5-carbon) ribose and xylose. Food sources high in monosaccharides include honey, fresh and dried fruits, jams, and jellies.

Disaccharides

Table sugar is the disaccharide sucrose, which is composed of the monosaccharides glucose and fructose. Other dietary disaccharides are lactose (milk sugar), which is composed of the monosaccharides glucose and galactose; and maltose (grain sugar), which is composed of the monosaccharide glucose. Food sources high in disaccharides include table sugar (and all the foods sugar is added to), milk, cereals, and sweet root vegetables such as carrots and beets.

Polysaccharides

Carbohydrate that is either digestible (starch and glycogen) or indigestible (cellulose, hemicellulose, gums, pectins) depending on the chemical bonds holding the sugar molecules together. Humans have the digestive enzymes to break the α-1,4 and α-1,6 bonds in digestible polysaccharides, but do not have the enzymes to break the β-1,4 bonds in indigestible polysaccharides. These are complex molecules that are composed of many (ten to thousands) monosaccharides bonded together. Food sources high in digestible polysaccharides include cereals (rice, wheat, oats, etc.), potato, corn, and unripe fruits. Food sources high in indigestible polysaccharides (*i.e.*, fiber) include beans, whole grain cereals, nuts, potato skin, and bran.

Monosaccharides

Monosaccharides (mono = single; saccharides = sugars) represent the most elemental form of carbohydrates and require no additional digestion to be absorbed into the blood. The common dietary monosaccharides are the 6-carbon glucose, galactose, and fructose (Box 2.5).

Glucose (also referred to as dextrose) is the principal source of energy for cells and is a moderately sweet sugar derived primarily from fruits and vegetables. Because of its important function in cellular energy metabolism, sustaining blood glucose level is an important strategy for sustaining athletic performance. Sorbitol, the sugar alcohol of glucose, is commonly used as an agent in processed foods to retain moisture (8).

Galactose is found as part of the disaccharide lactose (also called "milk sugar"; see below), which is composed of one molecule of glucose and one molecule of galactose. Galactose is part of several compounds called glycolipids (carbohydrate + fat), and glycoproteins (carbohydrate + protein), and can be manufactured by mammals from glucose so as to enable the production of lactose. While rare, a life-threatening inborn error of metabolism called "galactosemia" is seen in individuals who do not produce the enzymes necessary to metabolize galactose, resulting in an elevation of blood galactose. Elimination of lactose from the diet is necessary for individuals with this condition (9).

Fructose is also referred to as levulose and fruit sugar. It is a component of honey and fruits, and has the sweetest taste of all of the mono- and disaccharides. High levels of fructose may result in gastrointestinal (GI) distress and diarrhea (10). When high levels are absorbed into the blood, the liver capacity to convert the fructose to glucose may be exceeded, with a portion of the fructose being converted to triglycerides (fats) (11). Some excess fructose may also be converted to uric acid, which can result in the symptoms of gout and include joint pain (12). It is important, therefore, to limit the volume of fructose that is consumed at a single time. For instance, beverages sweetened with high-fructose corn syrup may exceed the liver's capacity to convert the fructose to glucose, resulting in an undesired level of blood lipids and/or uric acid (13).

Ribose is a 5-carbon sugar that is part of the genetic compound ribonucleic acid (RNA) and deoxyribonucleic acid (DNA). It can also be converted by cells to provide the carbon chain needed for the synthesis of the amino acids tryptophan and histidine. It is an essential component of respiratory, skeletal, and nervous systems with some evidence that the D-ribose form may enhance athlete potential for performing high-intensity activity (14).

Xylose is a 5-carbon sugar (pentose) that is the main component of hemicellulose, an indigestible dietary fiber component, which is found in many plants/trees. Because it is largely indigestible in the form commonly consumed, the energy concentration of xylose is only 2.4 calories/g (15). The alcohol fermentation product of xylose, xylitol, is sweet tasting but, unlike other sugars, cannot be recognized as a "food" by oral bacteria. Because it is not metabolized by these bacteria, xylitol is noncariogenic (*i.e.,* it does not encourage the development of dental cavities) (Table 2.2) (16). There is also beginning evidence that the addition of D-xylose to processed foods high in other digestible sugars may lower both the insulin response and glucose peak reached by these foods (17).

Disaccharides

The disaccharides sucrose, lactose, and maltose are common constituents of consumed foods and are composed of two monosaccharides joined together with a bond that can be broken with enzymes specific to the disaccharide (Box 2.6).

Sucrose is composed of one molecule of glucose and one molecule of fructose and is a naturally occurring disaccharide of plants. It is found in particularly high levels in sugar cane and beets, from which it is extracted for human consumption and is referred to as "table sugar." The digestive enzyme sucrase, which is present in the human small intestine, can break apart sucrose into its component monosaccharides, and these monosaccharides can then be absorbed rapidly through the intestinal wall into the blood.

Lactose is composed of one molecule of glucose and one molecule of galactose and is a natural component of mammalian milk; hence the common name "milk sugar." The concentration of lactose in human milk (63–70 g/L) is higher than in cow's milk (44–56 g/L) (18). The digestive enzyme *lactase*, which is present in the human small intestine, can break apart sucrose into its component monosaccharides, and these monosaccharides can then be absorbed through the intestinal wall into the blood. Lactase activity is high at birth and through infancy but declines after weaning to solid foods. Because of the gradually reducing lactase production in many populations, an intolerance to milk (lactose intolerance) is often observed (19). The indigested lactose then becomes a readily available "food" for gut bacteria, resulting in

Table 2.2	Acid Production Rate in Mouth in Response to Consumption of Various Carbohydrates
Sugar	Relative Acid Production Rate
Sucrose	100
Glucose	100
Invert sugar[a]	100[a]
Fructose	80–100
Lactose	40–60
Sorbitol	10–30
Xylitol	0

When bacteria (*Streptococcus mutans*) metabolize carbohydrate, acids are produced that have the potential of corroding the tooth enamel and producing cavities.

[a]Invert sugar is an equal mix of glucose and fructose from the breakdown of sucrose. Found naturally in honey and fruits.

Box 2.6	Disaccharides (Di = 2; Saccharide = Sugar. "Disaccharide" Means a Two-molecule Sugar)

Sucrose (glucose + fructose)
- Lactose (glucose + galactose)
- Maltose (glucose + glucose)

bloating, gas, diarrhea, and GI pain. Most adults, however, produce sufficient lactase to consume small amounts of lactose dispersed throughout the day without difficulty, so full avoidance of milk products is not necessary. Some populations have been found to sustain a high-lactase production throughout life, suggesting large population variability in desirable eating patterns. Because milk is an excellent source of calcium, protein, and riboflavin, there is no reason to avoid milk unless an intolerance or allergy is present. Some milk products are fermented (*e.g.,* yogurt, kefir, and cheeses), resulting in a lower lactose content and improved tolerance by people with lactose intolerance. There are also products available that contain the equivalent of lactase, which predigests the lactose in the dairy product and also improves tolerance (20).

Maltose is composed of two molecules of glucose held together in a 1,4 α-glycosidic bond and is the sugar associated with grains and seeds. Often referred to as "malt sugar," it is digested by the enzyme *maltase*, which is present in the human small intestine with the greatest enzyme presence in the duodenum. Because maltose is digested into two molecules of glucose that can readily enter the bloodstream and because the digestive enzyme appears early in the digestive tract, foods that are high in maltose can rapidly elevate blood sugar (*i.e.,* glucose) and may, as a result, produce an excessive insulin response that removes too much sugar from the blood and provides excess sugar to cells. Cells are incapable of utilizing this excess sugar so manufacture it into fat. (Read about the glycemic index and glycemic load later in this chapter.)

Trehalose, a disaccharide of two glucose units linked in a 1,1 α-glycosidic bond, is a naturally occurring nonreducing sugar that is found in several microorganisms, plants, and animals. In nature, trehalose accumulates in fungi, the encrustations of insects, including the underwater insects lobster, shrimp, and crab, and may be directly consumed as such. In all other natural sources, trehalose does not accumulate. In addition, for all other forms of natural trehalose, the plant or organism must be extracted to obtain the trehalose and then the trehalose purified to food grade, a process that makes trehalose both very expensive and available only seasonally. Many cultures commonly consume insects, which are a source of both protein and trehalose. New processes have made commercially available relatively inexpensive trehalose that is approved and suitable for human consumption (21). See Table 2.3 for the relative sweetness of different carbohydrates.

For over 20 years, the ability of trehalose to stabilize proteins has been known (22,23). In addition to the stabilization of proteins, it has been shown that during freeze-drying trehalose enhances the stability of living cells. Recently, the positive effects of trehalose on a variety of cellular processes such as osmotic shock (24), desiccation (25), and temperature tolerance (26) have been demonstrated (27). See Figure 2.1: Disaccharides.

Most disaccharides are disassociated into monosaccharides early in the digestive tract (most disaccharidases are in the proximal duodenum), resulting in fast infusion of monosaccharides into the plasma when a bolus of sugar is consumed. However, the disaccharidase *trehalase* is found throughout the entire length of the small intestine but in relatively small quantities, which results in a relatively low glycemic effect but a prolonged sustained blood glucose with the consumption of trehalose. This characteristic may be the basis for future research related to strategies for recovery or strategies for sustaining blood sugar in physically active people.

Table 2.3	Relative Sweetness of Different Carbohydrates, From Most Sweet to Least Sweet
Sugar	**Relative Sweetness Score**
Sucrose (table sugar, which is the standard against which all other sugars are compared)	100
High-fructose corn syrup	120–180
Fructose (sweeter when cool)	110
Xylitol (sugar alcohol from xylose)	80–110
Glucose	60–70
Mannitol (sugar alcohol from fructose)	60–70
Sorbitol (sugar alcohol from glucose)	60
Maltose	50
Trehalose	40–50
Galactose	35
Lactose	20–30
Dietary fiber	0
Starch	0

Sources: Data from references Dansukker.com. Nordic sugar. Accessed 2018 February 19. Available from: https://www.dansukker.co.uk/uk/about-sugar/sweetness-from-nature; Gwak M-J, Chung S-J, Kim YJ, Lim CS. Relative sweetness and sensory characteristics of bulk and intense sweeteners. Food Sci Biotechnol. 2012;21(3):889–94; Joesten MD, Hogg JL, Castellion ME. The world of chemistry: essentials. 4th ed. Belmont (CA): Thomson Brooks/Cole; 2007. p. 359 (Sweetness Relative to Sucrose, Table 15.1); Noelting J, DiBaise JK. Mechanisms of fructose absorption. Clin Transl Gastroenterol. 2015;6(11):e120.

Chemical Structure of Disaccharides

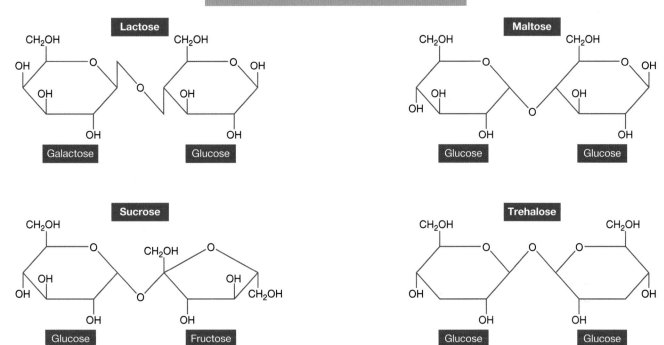

FIGURE 2.1: Disaccharides.

Polysaccharides

Polysaccharides (Box 2.7) are large molecules of at least 10 monosaccharides held together with bonds that humans are capable of breaking apart (*i.e.*, digestible polysaccharides), or not capable of breaking apart (*i.e.*, indigestible polysaccharides). The dietary digestible polysaccharides are commonly referred to as *starch*, which is a storage form of carbohydrate in plants. The storage form of digestible polysaccharides in humans is *glycogen*. Both starch and glycogen combine many molecules of glucose together, but glycogen can be broken down into its component glucose molecules slowly via glucagon, or quickly via adrenalin, making it an important source of energy for humans (28).

Raw starch is difficult to digest because the carbohydrate is stored within thin-walled cells that are difficult for digestive enzymes to penetrate. However, cooking causes the fluid inside the cell wall to expand, causing the starch to swell and burst and making it an easily available source of carbohydrate. Imagine eating raw rice or raw popcorn. Neither could be easily digested. However, using moist heat to cook the rice or corn kernel liberates the starch inside, making the starch available for digestion and absorption. Dextrins are a group of carbohydrates made from the breakdown of either starch or glycogen, with some forms, such as maltodextrin, used as food additives to make solutions thicker or creamier. Dextrins, including maltodextrin, can be easily digested to rapidly provide many molecules of glucose into the blood.

Box 2.7	**Polysaccharides (Poly = Many; Saccharide = Sugar. "Polysaccharide" Means a Many Molecule Sugar)**

- Digestible (α-1,5 and α-1,6 glycosidic bonds). These are polysaccharides that humans can digest and derive energy from.
  - Starch
  - Dextrins
  - Glycogen
- Indigestible (β-1,4 and other bonds). These are polysaccharides that humans cannot digest, so cannot derive energy from, and are often referred to as "fiber."
  - Cellulose
  - Hemicelluloses
  - Pectins
  - Gums
  - Mucilages

Note: Dietary fiber includes indigestible polysaccharides and lignin that cannot be digested by human digestive enzymes but can be partially digested by bacteria in the colon.

The indigestible polysaccharides are commonly referred to as *fiber* or **dietary fiber** and, while they cannot be digested to provide energy, are important for sustaining the health of the GI tract. Different types of dietary fiber, including soluble and insoluble fiber, have different physiologic effects. Foods containing soluble fiber (gums, mucilages, and pectins) include fruits, oats, legumes, and barley, and have the effect of decreasing gastric emptying time (*i.e.,* reduce the amount of time foods are in the stomach), but also decrease the rate at which glucose is absorbed in the small intestine. This is an important health benefit, since lowering the rate of glucose absorption also lowers the insulin response, which would help to sustain normal blood sugar longer and may also lower the rate of fat manufacture by cells (29). Foods containing insoluble fiber (cellulose and hemicellulose) come from foods such as wheat, vegetables, and seeds and have the capacity to absorb many times their own weight in water. This increases stool bulk, which improves peristalsis (the movement of consumed food through the intestines). If consumed with water, insoluble fiber reduces constipation risk. However, insoluble fiber increases gastric emptying time (*i.e.,* foods stay in the stomach longer), which may not be desirable if consumed prepractice or precompetition, when you want *no* foods to be in the stomach during exercise. High-fiber diets, therefore, may intensify GI complaints in physically active people when consumed immediately prior to exercise (30).

It has been noted that fruits and vegetables are both excellent sources of soluble fiber (gums and pectins). While both fruits and vegetables contain oxalic acid, dark green vegetables, such as spinach, are particularly high in *oxalic acid.* The oxalic acid has a high binding affinity for certain minerals (in particular, iron, zinc, calcium, and magnesium). If these minerals become bound to oxalic acid, they are no longer available for absorption (6). The insoluble fibers (cellulose and hemicellulose) that are commonly found in the bran portion of cereal grains are also a good source of *phytic acid.* If these same minerals (iron, zinc, calcium, and magnesium) are bound to phytic acid, they also become unavailable for absorption (31). An easy strategy for removing oxalic acid from vegetables is to quickly blanch them in boiling water, and then prepare the vegetables as desired. The oxalic acid is highly water soluble so it leaches out quickly in boiling water. Since oxalic acid has a bitter flavor and children are especially sensitive to bitter tastes, following this strategy has the double benefit of improving mineral absorption and also making the vegetables more desirable for children to eat. The general strategy for reducing the mineral binding potential of phytic acid is to limit the consumption of foods that are extremely high in it, such as bran, by consuming whole-grain cereals rather than bran-added or bran-only cereals.

FUNCTIONS OF CARBOHYDRATES

Dietary Fiber

Also referred to as *roughage*, is a term used to describe indigestible polysaccharides and includes both soluble dietary fiber and insoluble dietary fiber, both of which have health benefits associated with lower risk of cancer, better blood sugar control, and lower risk of heart disease.

- *Soluble dietary fiber* is found in oats, barley legumes, fruits, and vegetables. It can attach to cholesterol, resulting in reduced cholesterol absorption and lower risk of heart disease. It also reduces rapid blood sugar elevation, lowering the risk of type 2 diabetes. It has a high affinity for water, enabling a greater stool bulk that helps to maintain bowel regularity. This fiber type also improves the good bacteria in the gut (*i.e.,* the gut microbiome), which is associated with lower disease risk.
- *Insoluble dietary fiber* is found in wheat bran, seeds, vegetable stalks, and the skins of fruits. Because of its high binding affinity for water, it improves stool bulk and reduces the risk of constipation and related problems (*e.g.,* hemorrhoids and diverticulitis).

Important Factors to Consider

- Carbohydrates have many functions that are necessary components of good health and athletic performance. Consumption of more protein and/or fat is not a replacement for carbohydrate, and these other energy substrates cannot adequately fulfill carbohydrate functions.
- Low-carbohydrate intakes cause proteins to be broken down to create needed carbohydrate in the liver (gluconeogenesis), but because humans have no storage of protein, this process causes a loss of muscle mass from which the protein is derived. The protein-sparing effect of carbohydrates, therefore, is an important part of why carbohydrates are needed.

Carbohydrates have multiple functions that are critical to both human health and athletic performance. The basic functions include the following: (1) providing a source

Box 2.8	**Functions of Carbohydrates**

- Source of energy that can be used with and without oxygen (4 calories/g)
- Protein sparing
- Complete oxidation of fats
- Instantaneous source of energy
- Part of other body compounds
- Can be converted to and stored as fat for eventual use as energy
- Keeps GI tract healthy

of energy for cellular function, (2) energy storage as glycogen, (3) sparing protein, (4) breaking down fats for energy, (5) normal GI function, (6) being a part of other compounds, and (7) converting carbohydrates to fat. Importantly, carbohydrate in the blood (blood glucose) is the primary source of energy for the brain (Box 2.8).

Source of Energy for Cellular Function and Energy Storage

Carbohydrates provide 4 calories/g and are unique among the energy substrates (carbohydrates, proteins, and fats) in that carbohydrates have the capacity to provide cellular energy both anaerobically (without oxygen) and aerobically (with oxygen). The primary source of energy for cells is glucose, which is a carbohydrate, and some cells are limited in their capacity to derive energy from anything but glucose (Figure 2.2). The primary fuel for the brain and central nervous system is blood glucose, making the

brain sensitive to abnormal fluctuations in blood glucose that can occur from infrequent eating pattern that results in low blood sugar, or excessive consumption of refined or **simple carbohydrates** (*i.e.,* monosaccharides and disaccharides), which can cause a sudden and high rise in blood sugar that results in an excessive insulin response and low blood sugar (32). We can store a limited amount (approximately 306 calories for a 150-lb person) of glucose in the liver as glycogen and a limited amount (approximately 1,530 calories for a 150-lb person) of glucose as glycogen in muscles (33). The amount of carbohydrates stored in muscles may be misleading when calculating time to fatigue as a result of muscle glycogen depletion because specific sports/activities deplete glycogen faster in muscles that are used. For instance, a right-handed pitcher will deplete glycogen faster in the right arm than the left arm, resulting in a more rapid right-arm fatigue (34).

Simple Carbohydrates

Another term for sugars, they are easily and quickly digestible/absorbable disaccharides (sucrose, maltose, and lactose) and monosaccharides (glucose, galactose, fructose, ribose, and xylose).

Sparing Protein

A failure to satisfy the tissue requirements for glucose will initiate a process called **gluconeogenesis**, or the creation of new glucose from nonglucose substances. Protein is a primary gluconeogenic substance, because we have well-established pathways for converting some amino

Common Pathways for Blood Glucose

FIGURE 2.2: What happens to blood glucose.

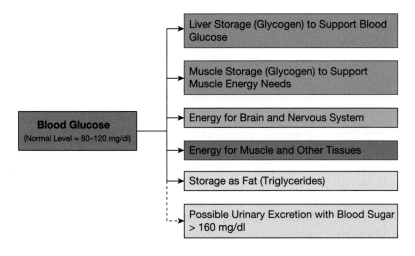

acids (the building blocks of proteins) to glucose. These amino acids are appropriately referred to as glycogenic amino acids. However, we have no storage of extra protein or amino acids for this purpose, so to obtain these amino acids for glucose synthesis, we break down body proteins (muscle, for example) and deliver the amino acids from these proteins to the liver, where they are converted to glucose. Therefore, consuming sufficient carbohydrates spares protein from being broken down to derive glucose. This is an important consideration for athletes because glucose is rapidly utilized during exercise. A failure to maintain sufficient carbohydrates availability in the blood and muscles will break down the very tissues that the exerciser is trying to build through exercise. In body builders, it was found that building muscle could be compromised when on a high-protein, low-carbohydrate diet (35).

Gluconeogenesis

The process of generating glucose from noncarbohydrates. For instance, glycerol, the 3-carbon substance that holds three molecules of fatty acids to make triglycerides (the common storage form of fat), can be converted to glucose by the liver. Glycogenic amino acids, such as alanine and glutamine, also have liver pathways for conversion to glucose. Lactic acid can also be converted to glucose. All of these conversions of taking noncarbohydrate substances and making them into glucose are considered *gluconeogenesis*.

Complete Oxidation of Fats for Energy

When fats are broken down to be metabolized as a source of energy, a small amount of glucose is needed to enable the complete oxidation of fat. Carbohydrates can be synthesized into oxaloacetic acid, which is required for fat metabolism. Insufficient carbohydrate availability causes poor oxaloacetic acid creation, followed by incomplete fat metabolism, which results in the creation of *ketones*. Therefore, ketones are an acidic by-product of incomplete fat metabolism, and when ketone levels become elevated, the condition is referred to as *ketoacidosis* (36). A common ketone is *acetone*, which has a unique odor and can be smelled on the breath of someone who is producing ketones (acetone smells like nail polish remover). Acetone production is common when undergoing a fast because available glucose is depleted, resulting in the incomplete oxidation of fats. The consumption of ketogenic diets (*i.e.*, high-protein, low-carbohydrate diets) as a strategy to lose weight is common (37). These diets

force the metabolism of fats and proteins for energy, but with poor carbohydrate availability, these diets result in ketone formation from the incomplete oxidation of fats (38). There are also potential problems associated with ketogenic diets. An evaluation of the ketogenic diet with male and female exercisers found that reduced aerobic performance and increased risk of developing blood disturbances (39). There is also an increased risk of dehydration in individuals on a ketogenic diet, as the body attempts to excrete ketones, and lower bone mineral density resulting from the kidneys neutralizing ketone acidity via the buffering action of calcium, as ketones are excreted in urine (40).

Helps Normal Gastrointestinal Function

Dietary fiber, derived from fresh fruits, vegetables, legumes, and whole grains, is important for sustaining normal GI function. Inadequate fiber consumption is associated with constipation, hemorrhoids, diverticulitis/diverticulosis, and higher risk of colon cancer. There is also evidence to show that regular consumption of dietary fiber can lower serum lipids, including blood cholesterol, thereby reducing heart disease risk (29).

Being a Part of Other Compounds

Some glucose is converted to ribose and deoxyribose, which are molecular components of our genetic structure (RNA and DNA). Glucose can also be manufactured into nicotinamide adenine dinucleotide phosphate (NADP), which is needed for the synthesis of fats and cholesterol. NADP also lowers the risk of cellular oxidative damage. Carbohydrates are also a part of other compounds, such as glycoproteins and glycolipids. An example of a glycoprotein is *mucin*, which is part of saliva and responsible for making the saliva sticky and more lubricating than water alone. Glycolipids are involved in cellular communication and recognition, as different cell types have different surface glycolipids (41). The blood types A, B, AB, and O are different, for instance, by the type of sugar that is part of the glycolipid in the cell membrane (42).

Conversion of Carbohydrates to Fats

Excess carbohydrates that enter cells can be manufactured into fat for storage and later utilization as a source of energy. Fats are more efficiently stored as energy, containing 9 calories/g versus 4 calories/g for carbohydrates, and we have no upper limit to fat storage. By contrast,

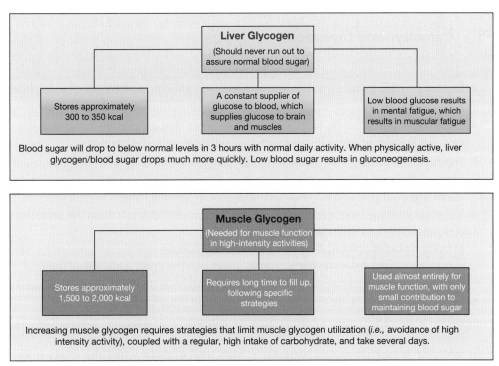

FIGURE 2.3: Two carbohydrate storage systems to consider.

carbohydrate storage as glycogen in the liver and muscles has a finite upper limit. Although we can store excess carbohydrate as fat, it is important to consider that there is no reverse metabolic pathway for converting fats to carbohydrates. Because of the ongoing requirement for carbohydrates, consumption patterns of carbohydrates should dynamically match requirements to avoid excessive use of the limited glycogen stores (Figure 2.3). Chronic over-consumption of highly sweetened beverages and other sugary foods is rapidly absorbed and typically results in a high insulin response that results in excess carbohydrates entering cells with elevated fat creation (43).

DIGESTION, ABSORPTION, AND METABOLISM OF CARBOHYDRATES

Important Factors to Consider

- Starting with saliva in the mouth, there are many components of carbohydrate digestion that involve the mouth, stomach, and small intestine. The more complex the carbohydrate, the greater the time it takes for digestion and absorption to occur, and for some carbohydrates (dietary fiber) we do not have the digestive enzymes needed to digest them and derive energy from them. However, dietary fiber is an important component of GI health and so should be consumed as a regular part of the diet.
- Consuming a high level of sugars at one time, which requires little digestion, causes a large number of sugar molecules to congregate in the GI tract as they await absorption. This results in fluids going from the blood into the GI tract to dilute the sugar. The resulting drop in blood volume that occurs could negatively impact sweat rates, the delivery of nutrients to working muscles, and the ability to remove metabolic byproducts from cells. To sustain physical activity, it is generally better to consume smaller amounts of sugar more often than to consume larger amounts at once.

Digestion

The purpose of digestion is to break down consumed carbohydrates into a form that allows them to be transferred through the intestinal wall and into the blood, where they can be distributed to cells. Digestion of carbohydrate takes place in the mouth and small intestine and involves conversion of more **complex carbohydrates** (starch and glycogen) to less complex carbohydrates (disaccharides)

Table 2.4	Carbohydrate Digestion
Organ	**Role in Digestion of Carbohydrate**
Mouth	▪ Salivary amylase initiates the digestion of starch and glycogen to the disaccharides (maltose, sucrose, lactose).
Stomach	▪ There are no carbohydrate-specific digestive enzymes that are present in the stomach. However, the fluid content and acidity of the stomach may aid in the digestive process.

Small intestine	▪ The pancreas produces a digestive enzyme (pancreatic amylase), which enters early in the small intestine via the common pancreatic/bile duct. Pancreatic amylase is the major digestive enzyme for starch and glycogen, and fully digests the digestible polysaccharides to disaccharides.
	▪ The small intestine produces disaccharidases (enzymes that break down the disaccharides to their component monosaccharides)
	  ● Maltase breaks down maltose to 2 molecules of glucose
	  ● Sucrase breaks down sucrose to 1 molecule of glucose and 1 molecule of fructose
	  ● Lactase breaks down lactose to 1 molecule of glucose and 1 molecule of galactose.
	▪ The monosaccharides are absorbed into the blood in the small intestine.

Note: The digestive enzymes end in *ase*, while the sugar it digests ends in *ose*. Amylose is another word for digestible polysaccharide, or starch.

and then to single-molecule sugars (monosaccharides) to be absorbed (44). A small amount of carbohydrate digestion takes place in the mouth with *salivary amylase,* a digestive enzyme in the saliva. To experience this digestion, put a small amount of starchy carbohydrate (bread, cereal, etc.) into your mouth, and leave it there without swallowing. After a short time, you will sense that the food tastes sweeter as the more complex starch is digested into sugars. The pancreas produces a major carbohydrate digestive enzyme, pancreatic amylase, which enters early in the small intestine via the common duct shared by the pancreas and the gallbladder (45). The pancreatic amylase converts the remaining polysaccharides into disaccharides, which are then further digested by disaccharide-specific enzymes (Table 2.4). The monosaccharides are then absorbed.

📖 **Complex Carbohydrates**

Another term for digestible polysaccharides (starch, dextrin, and glycogen), and indigestible polysaccharides (gums, pectins, cellulose, and hemicellulose). The indigestible polysaccharides are also referred to as *fiber* or *dietary fiber.*

Absorption

The monosaccharides are transported into the intestinal wall for transfer into the blood circulation. Glucose and galactose are absorbed through a specific transporter (SGLT1), while fructose is transported by another transporter (GLUT5). Because GLUT5 availability is limited, a high level of dietary fructose intake may overwhelm the transporter, keeping a significant proportion of the fructose in the intestines rather than getting absorbed (45,46). These molecules of fructose impart a high level of osmolar pressure, causing fluid to move into the intestines, possibly resulting in bloating and diarrhea (Box 2.7). It is for this reason that foods containing added free fructose, as in high-fructose corn syrup, may not be as well absorbed and cause more GI difficulties than foods that contain naturally occurring fructose (46).

Osmolarity and Osmolality

Osmolarity is defined as the concentration of a solution expressed as the total number of solute particles per volume of solution liter (*i.e.,* per liter and per quart). *Osmolality* is osmotic concentration per mass of solvent (*i.e.,* kg solvent/kg solution).

A practical application of this is as follows: 100 calories of sucrose (a disaccharide) has half the number of molecules that 100 calories of glucose does and therefore imparts half the osmotic pressure. Fluid moves in the direction of the highest osmolarity, so for the same caloric load, free glucose will have a greater tendency to "pull" water toward it. Athletic gels are designed to deliver a high level of carbohydrate calories in a relatively low osmolar product. They accomplish this by delivering the carbohydrate in a polysaccharide gel that has many molecules of monosaccharides held together in a single polysaccharide molecule. Only the number of particles per unit volume matters in regard to osmotic pressure, so a single large polysaccharide molecule imparts far lower osmotic pressure than its component individual molecules of carbohydrate.

When delivered to the circulation, the portion of the absorbed monosaccharides that is glucose results in an elevation of blood glucose concentration. The absorbed fructose and galactose must be converted to glucose, mainly in the liver, and do not immediately contribute to the initial elevation in blood glucose. The rise in blood glucose is dependent on the rate of absorption, which is dependent on multiple factors (47,48), including:

- *The complexity of the consumed carbohydrate.* More complex carbohydrates require more digestion and mediate the availability of glucose for absorption.
- *Other substances consumed with the carbohydrate.* Fats and proteins delay the gastric emptying rate, thereby mediating the availability of glucose for absorption.
- *The distribution of monosaccharides in the foods consumed.* Pure glucose causes a slight delay in gastric emptying, but once in the intestines is readily absorbed if the volume of glucose consumed does not exceed transporter (SGLT1) availability. Assuming the same calories, a *mixture* of monosaccharides is more quickly absorbed than any single monosaccharide, as the mixture can capitalize on the availability of transporters and absorption sites.

Insulin is secreted by the β-cells of the pancreas in response to the rise in blood glucose. Insulin is necessary for the update of glucose by body cells. A fast increase in blood sugar, however, may result in a hyperinsulinemic response (*i.e.*, excess insulin production), which takes too much glucose out of the blood and puts too much glucose into cells, exceeding normal cellular requirements and storage capacity. Cells then manufacture the excess glucose into fat and export the fat with the result that body fat mass increases. Insulin production may also be influenced by the protein and fat content of the meal, with higher amounts buffering the speed with which glucose is absorbed, thereby affecting the insulin response.

Unabsorbed Carbohydrate

The indigestible polysaccharides absorb many times their own weight in water, increasing stool bulk and reducing constipation risk. *Prebiotics* are carbohydrates (fiber) that cannot be broken down by digestive enzymes and do not enter the blood circulation but stimulate the growth of "healthy" bacteria by becoming a source of energy/nutrients for the bacteria. The polysaccharides that can be fermented by intestinal bacteria (the gut microflora) do not increase stool bulk to the same degree as nonfermentable

polysaccharides but have the advantage of improving the gut microflora (49,50). The partially digestible polysaccharides, including the oligosaccharides common in beans, encourage the growth of beneficial bacteria, such as *Bifidobacteria*, in the GI tract and are referred to as *probiotics*, live bacteria that are the same as the beneficial bacteria in the human gut, and are consumed as part of dietary supplements or foods, such as "live-culture" yogurt. Probiotic foods help to support good bacteria in the gut. *Synbiotic* refers to a mix of prebiotics and probiotics, which can provide both the bacteria and the nutrients (fiber) that can help encourage the bacteria to flourish. The *Bifidobacteria* that colonize the GI tract help to protect the gut from the potentially damaging effects of pathogenic bacteria (51,52). Recent evidence suggests a strong connection between a healthy GI tract microbiome and exercise, with evidence suggesting a healthy microbiome is associated with improved endurance (53).

After Absorption

The monosaccharides, glucose, fructose, and galactose, are absorbed into the blood, but only glucose is immediately available to cells to satisfy metabolic requirements. The circulating fructose and galactose must be converted by the liver to glucose for these monosaccharides to be available for cellular use. Once converted to glucose, the liver may store the glucose as liver glycogen (used to sustain blood glucose) or may release the glucose directly back into the blood. The amount of glucose that the liver exports to the blood are hormonally controlled by the pancreas, which produces both *insulin* and **glucagon**, and the liver. Having either high or low blood glucose can result in negative health consequences.

> **Glucagon**
>
> A hormone made by the α-cells of the pancreas that helps to avoid hypoglycemia by initiating a slow breakdown of liver glycogen for the resulting glucose to elevate blood sugar.

Blood Sugar Control

Following a meal, insulin is released when blood glucose rises to make the excess blood glucose available to cells. The pancreas monitors the level of blood glucose as the blood flows through it. When it detects that blood glucose is rising above the desired level (~120 mg/dL), it releases the hormone insulin, which affects cell membranes to allow glucose to enter the cell. The effect of insulin is twofold: (1) to lower blood glucose and (2) to make glucose

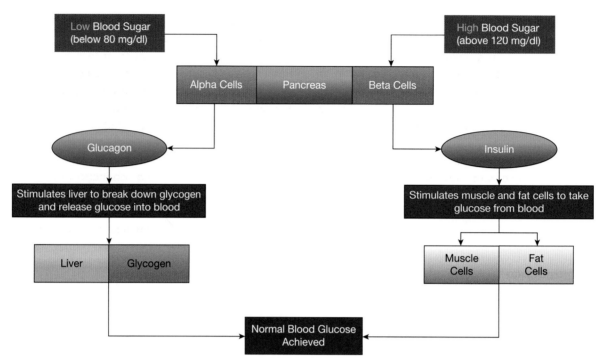

FIGURE 2.4: How the pancreas and liver sustain normal blood sugar.

available to cells. As blood sugar continues to drop and reaches its low threshold (~80 mg/dL), the α-cells of the pancreas release the hormone glucagon (Figure 2.4). Glucagon signals the liver to break down liver glycogen and release the component glucose molecules into the blood. The effect of glucagon is twofold: (1) to raise blood glucose and (2) to lower liver glycogen stores. Up to the limitations of eating frequency and glycogen storage, insulin and glucagon serve to maintain blood sugar within the normal range, while providing needed glucose to the brain and other body cells.

Normal blood glucose maintenance occurs in approximately 3-hour units (2). That is, following a meal, blood sugar reaches its peak 1 hour later and is back to premeal levels about 2 hours after that, suggesting that it is again time to eat. When a person is physically active, however, blood sugar is used at a much faster rate, making it necessary for carbohydrate to be consumed more frequently to sustain blood sugar (Figure 2.5). One of the main functions of carbohydrate-containing sports beverages is precisely to ensure that blood sugar is maintained within desirable limits during exercise. The current recommendation, for

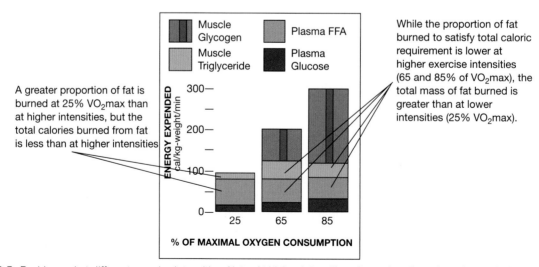

FIGURE 2.5: Fuel burned at different exercise intensities. Note: At higher intensities of exercise, there is an increasingly greater reliance on muscle glycogen to supply the needed fuel. (Modified from Romijn JA, Sidossis LS, Gastaldelli A, Horowitz JF, Wolfe RR. Regulation of endogenous fat and carbohydrate metabolism in relation to exercise intensity and duration. Am J Physiol. 1993;265:E380–91.)

people who exercise 1 hour or longer, is to consume a sports beverage (54–56). Those who exercise at extremely high intensity may require sports beverages to sustain blood glucose even if the exercise duration is less than 1 hour. A failure to sustain normal blood sugar creates difficulties. Low blood sugar (**hypoglycemia**) results in nervousness, dizziness, and faintness. Should hypoglycemia occur during exercise, it will result in mental fatigue, which is associated with muscle fatigue (even if the muscles are full of glycogen). In addition, low blood sugar may result in *gluconeogenesis*, often resulting in a breakdown of lean mass (see more on gluconeogenesis later in this chapter).

Hypoglycemia

An abnormally low blood sugar (blood glucose) level that is commonly the result of excess insulin, either from consuming high glycemic foods or from taking excess insulin if a diabetic. Normal blood sugar is in the range of 80–120 mg/dL, and hypoglycemia is defined as having a blood sugar level of 70 mg/dL or below.

Hyperglycemia

An abnormally high blood sugar (blood glucose) level that is characteristic of metabolic syndrome and diabetes. Normal blood sugar is in the range of 80–120 mg/dL, and high fasting blood sugar (after not eating or drinking for 8 hours) is >130 mg/dL.

Consumption of high glycemic index foods and/or diabetes may result in high blood sugar (**hyperglycemia**), which is associated with dehydration and, if severe, coma. Chronic hyperglycemia resulting from high body fat levels, excess consumption of food, inadequate activity, or consumption of high glycemic foods results in chronic hyperinsulinemia (too much insulin production). This continuous excess insulin production has the effect of reducing cellular sensitivity to insulin and is associated with type 2 diabetes (insulin is produced, but it is ineffective in reducing blood glucose, so blood glucose is elevated). Type 1 diabetes is also associated with high blood sugar but is the result of a failure of the pancreas β-cells to produce insulin. Type 1 diabetes is often seen in children, and may be the result of the body's immune system destroying the body cells or a bacterial infection that targets and destroys the β-cells. Type 2 diabetes is often called adult-onset diabetes because the onset of diabetes is most often seen in adults. However, type 2 diabetes is now being seen with ever-increasing prevalence in obese children. Both type 1 and type 2 diabetes are associated with high blood glucose. Blood glucose that is above the level of 160 mg/dL exceeds the renal threshold and starts

to show up in the urine. Sugar (glucose) in the urine is a sign of uncontrolled diabetes (57).

Another hormone that has an impact on blood glucose is **epinephrine** (adrenaline), which is produced mainly by the adrenal glands. It has the effect of rapidly increasing the breakdown of liver glycogen to infuse a high level of glucose into the blood extremely quickly (58). It also increases muscle blood flow and heart output. It is thought that the main purpose of epinephrine is survival in the "flight-or-fight" response that occurs when in imminent danger. The ready availability of energy (blood glucose) coupled with high cardiac output and improved muscular blood flow serves to help the individual move extremely quickly and with a high level of power. However, the quick depletion of liver glycogen also results in low blood sugar and exhaustion soon after the epinephrine has had its effect. It is because of this later effect that staying calm and being familiar with the surroundings (*i.e., avoiding* an adrenaline production) is helpful for maintaining athletic performance. Epinephrine is also used as a medication to treat a severe allergic response called *anaphylaxis*. People with allergies often carry with them an EpiPen Auto-Injector (filled with epinephrine) to quickly enhance the immune response and avoid the potentially dangerous effects of a serious allergy (59).

Epinephrine

Also referred to as adrenaline, this hormone initiates a quick breakdown of liver glycogen for the resulting glucose to quickly elevate blood sugar. It also increases the insulin-mediated flow of the high-energy (*i.e.,* high-glucose) blood to muscles, enabling fast muscle movement, which is an important component of the fight-or-flight response associated with epinephrine/adrenaline. Note: the depletion of liver glycogen associated with epinephrine is related to exhaustion and signs of hypoglycemia after the initial epinephrine-induced high-energy state.

Glycemic Index and Glycemic Load

The **glycemic index** (Figure 2.6) compares the potential of foods containing the *same* amount of carbohydrate to raise blood glucose. However, the amount of carbohydrate consumed also affects blood glucose and, therefore, the insulin response (32). The **glycemic load** is calculated by multiplying the glycemic index by the amount of carbohydrate (g) provided by a food and dividing the total by 100. Each unit of glycemic load represents the equivalent blood glucose-raising effect of 1 g of pure glucose. The dietary glycemic load equals the sum of the glycemic loads for all the foods consumed in the diet and may be used to describe the relative quality of the diet. In general,

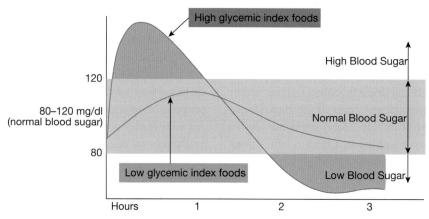

FIGURE 2.6: Glycemic index is a measure of how foods have an impact on blood glucose. Consumption of high glycemic index foods results in a fast high blood glucose, which is responded to with excess insulin. This removes too much glucose out of the blood and puts too much glucose into cells, exceeding cellular requirements. Cells convert the excess glucose into fat (body fat increases). Chronically consuming high glycemic index foods results in high body fat, lower insulin sensitivity, and higher risks of type 2 diabetes. (Data from Granfeldt Y, Björck I, Hagander B. On the importance of processing conditions, product thickness and egg addition for the glycaemic and hormonal responses to pasta: a comparison with bread made from 'pasta ingredients'. Eur J Clin Nutr. 1991;45(10):489–99.)

it is good to be consuming foods with a relatively low glycemic load (Table 2.5).

📖 Glycemic Index

Relative to the standard value of 100 for glucose, the glycemic index indicates a food's effect on blood glucose. High glycemic index foods (*i.e.,* with a value near 100) elevate blood sugar quickly. Low glycemic index foods (*i.e.,* with a value of <55) elevate blood sugar slowly. High glycemic index foods initiate a high insulin response, which puts excess blood glucose in cells, causing cells to create fats from the glucose for storage and later use.

📖 Glycemic Load

Similar to glycemic index, but the glycemic load indicates the impact on blood glucose adjusted for a 100 g serving. A glycemic load of >20 is considered high, while a glycemic load of <10 is considered low. For instance, the glycemic index of watermelon has a relatively high glycemic index value of 72, but a 100 g serving of watermelon has a relatively low glycemic index of 3.6.

As indicated in Table 2.5, one cup of brown rice has a glycemic load (60) below that of cornflakes (28), despite delivering more carbohydrate (33 vs. 26 g). Delivering

Table 2.5	Glycemic Index and Glycemic Load for Selected Foods			
Food	Glycemic Index (Relative to Glucose, Which Equals 100)	Serving	Carbohydrate/ Serving	Glycemic Load/ Serving
Cornflakes	81	1 cup	26	21
Rice cakes	78	3 cakes	21	17
Baked potato	76	1 medium	30	23
White bread	73	1 slice	14	10
Table sugar	68	2 tsp	10	7
White rice (boiled)	64	1 cup	36	23
Brown rice (boiled)	55	1 cup	33	18
Orange, fresh raw	42	1 medium	11	5
Kidney beans, boiled	28	1 cup	25	7
Peanuts, roasted	14	1 oz	6	1

the same amount of carbohydrate as table sugar, a baked potato will exert a higher glycemic load (21 vs. 23). The *type* of carbohydrate consumed, therefore, matters with regard to the expected endocrine response. For instance, table sugar is composed of sucrose, which is 50% glucose and 50% fructose. Baked potatoes are composed of starch, which is mainly a polymer of glucose. The fructose does not immediately contribute to the glycemic load, so baked potatoes have a higher glycemic effect. A lower glycemic load will result in a lower insulin response, a more stable blood sugar, and a lower rate of fat manufacture. The general recommendations for carbohydrate consumption are:

- Consume fiber-rich fruits, vegetables, and whole grains often
- Try to select foods and beverages with little or no added sugars or sweeteners

Metabolism

Humans have ongoing energy requirements, and carbohydrates play an important role in the provision of energy. Ultimately, energy substrates are metabolized into *adenosine triphosphate (ATP)*, which is the fuel for all cellular work, including digestion, muscle contraction, nerve transmission, circulation, tissue synthesis, tissue repair, and hormone production. When the phosphate bond is broken, energy is released, and ATP is formed into *adenosine diphosphate (ADP)*. Humans have a small energy reserve of ATP that must constantly be resynthesized to avoid running out. Some energy for ATP resynthesis is supplied through the anaerobic (without oxygen) splitting of *phosphocreatine (PCr)* into creatine and phosphate, which releases energy. The creatine and phosphate can be joined again into PCr. Carbohydrate is the only nutrient that can provide energy anaerobically to form ATP. Energy released from breakdown of preformed ATP and PCr can sustain high-intensity exercise for approximately 5–8 seconds. For instance, the 100-m world record time of approximately 9.6 seconds exceeds the human capacity to supply the needed ATP from stored ATP and PCr, so the sprinters slow down during the last ~1.5 seconds because the highest-intensity fuel sources are exhausted.

There are four basic energy metabolic systems: phosphocreatine system, anaerobic glycolysis (lactic acid system), aerobic glycolysis system, and aerobic metabolism (oxygen system):

- *Phosphocreatine System (PCr).* This system can produce ATP anaerobically from stored PCr and can be used for maximal-intensity activities that last no

longer than 8 seconds. (After 8 seconds, the PCr is depleted and must be reformed.)
- *Anaerobic Glycolysis (Lactic Acid System).* This system involves the anaerobic production of ATP from the breakdown of glycogen, with lactic acid production as a by-product of this system. This is used for very high–intensity exercise that exceeds the person's ability to consume enough oxygen. Anaerobic glycolysis can typically produce ATP for no more than 2 minutes.
- *Aerobic Glycolysis.* This describes the production of ATP from the breakdown of glycogen through the utilization of oxygen. This system is used for high-intensity activities that require a high level of ATP but remain within the athlete's capacity to supply sufficient oxygen for energy metabolism.
- *Aerobic Metabolism (Oxygen System).* This system (glucose + $6O_2 \rightarrow 6CO_2 + 6H_2O$ + heat) produces ATP from the combined breakdown of carbohydrates and fats and is used for low- to moderate-intensity activities of long duration. This system avoids the production of lactic acid, which allows the energy metabolic process to continue for long periods of time. Fats can *only* be metabolized via this aerobic system. Protein can be metabolized to produce ATP, but only after the nitrogen associated with protein molecules is removed. Once removed, the remaining carbon chain can be converted to carbohydrate and metabolized either aerobically or anaerobically or stored as fat to be metabolized aerobically. As humans have no protein storage for the purpose of supplying energy, using protein as an energy source requires the breakdown of tissue protein (*i.e.*, muscle and organ tissue), to supply the fuel to create ATP, and should not, therefore, be considered a preferred source of energy.

The theoretical yield of ATP molecules from 1 molecule of glucose is 38 ATP: 2 from glycolysis, 2 from Krebs cycle, and 34 from electron transport (61). However, this much ATP production is not normally achieved because of the ATP (energy) cost of moving pyruvate (from glycolysis), phosphate, and ADP (substrates for ATP synthesis) into the mitochondria (62) (Figure 2.7).

Making Carbohydrate From Noncarbohydrate Sources

As noted earlier, gluconeogenesis refers to the process of making glucose from noncarbohydrate substances. Blood glucose is critical for central nervous system function, aids in the metabolism of fat, and supplies fuel to working

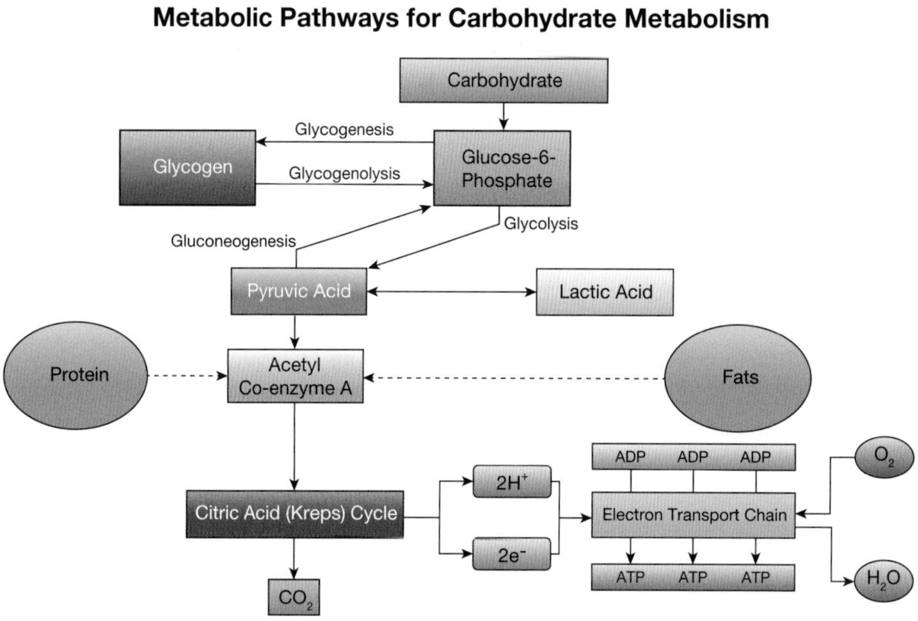

Metabolic Pathways for Carbohydrate Metabolism

FIGURE 2.7: Carbohydrate metabolism.

cells. However, because of its limited storage capacity as liver glycogen, which helps to maintain blood sugar, a minimum level of glucose is always available through the manufacture of glucose from noncarbohydrate substances (see Figure 2.3).

There are three main systems for gluconeogenesis (63–65):

- Triglycerides are the predominant storage form of fat in the human body and consist of three fatty acids attached to a glycerol molecule. The breakdown of triglycerides results in free *glycerol* molecules (a three-carbon substance), and the combination of two glycerol molecules in the liver results in the production of one glucose molecule (a six-carbon substance). The kidney is also capable of manufacturing glucose from glycerol.
- Catabolized muscle protein results in an array of free amino acids that constitute the building blocks of the muscle. One of these amino acids, alanine, can be converted by the liver to form glucose.
- In anaerobic glycolysis, lactic acid is produced. This lactic acid, or *lactate*, can be converted back to pyruvic acid for the aerobic production of ATP, or two lactic acid molecules can combine in the liver to form glucose. The conversion of lactate to glucose is referred to as the Cori cycle (lactate removed from the muscle and glucose returned to the muscle). If blood glucose is low, pyruvic acid can be converted to lactate, and glucose can be produced via the Cori cycle.

CARBOHYDRATE INTAKE RECOMMENDATIONS

Important Factors to Consider

- The recommended intake of carbohydrate for athletes ranges from 5 to 10 g/kg. This level of intake is far higher than that for protein, which has a recommended range of 1.2–1.7 g/kg. Despite this difference, many athletes still wrongly believe that focusing on protein as the primary fuel is beneficial for optimizing athletic performance.
- Regardless of whether an athlete is involved in primarily power or endurance activity, carbohydrate is considered to be that limiting energy substrate in performance. That is, when carbohydrate (glycogen) stores become depleted, performance quickly deteriorates. Because of this, all athletes should have well-developed strategies for ensuring adequate carbohydrate consumption before, during, and following activity to ensure optimal recovery. Consider that, while endurance athletes typically derive a higher proportion of energy from fat than power athletes, endurance athletes exercise for longer periods of time causing a drain on carbohydrate stores. Power athletes typically exercise for shorter periods of time, but a higher proportion of energy is derived from carbohydrate stores. In both cases, carbohydrate is the limiting energy substrate in activity.

Dietary fiber consumption (from indigestible and partially digestible polysaccharides) should be at the level of 38 g/day for adult men and 25 g/day for adult women. Adequate fiber consumption aids in the maintenance of normal blood sugar, reduces heart disease risk, and lowers constipation risk. The difference between genders in recommended fiber consumption is based on the expectation that women typically consume less total energy.

The Institute of Medicine (2002) recommends 130 g (520 calories) of carbohydrate per day, which is the average minimal usage of glucose by the brain. The desirable range of carbohydrate intake is 45% to 65% of total caloric intake (also referred to as the acceptable macronutrient distribution range, or AMDR). The daily value for carbohydrate that is on food labels is based on a recommendation that carbohydrate should constitute 60% of total energy consumed. These recommendations also generally advise that sugar consumption be limited to no more than 25% of the carbohydrate consumed (66,67).

Athlete requirements for carbohydrate are based on several factors, including:

- providing energy to satisfy the majority of needs, particularly for high-intensity activity;
- optimizing glycogen stores;
- allowing for muscle recovery after physical activity;
- providing a well-tolerated source of energy during practice and competition;
- providing a quick and easy source of energy between meals to maintain blood sugar.

Carbohydrate consumption has traditionally been recommended as a proportion of total caloric intake. The recommendation for the general population is that carbohydrate should supply 50% to 55% of total calories, and the dietary reference intake is 130 g/day (520 calories/day) for male and female adults. However, the amount typically recommended for athletes is slightly higher, between 55% and 65% of total calories, assuming an adequate total caloric intake. The current system for recommending carbohydrate requirement is by taking into consideration the amount of carbohydrate to be consumed (in grams) per kilogram of body mass. The current recommendation for athletes ranges from 3 to 12 g/kg body weight per day, depending on the intensity and duration of activity (68). This recommendation is based on a large body of research indicating that carbohydrates maintain blood glucose levels during exercise and replace muscle glycogen, with the range of intake

based on the total energy expended, the type of sport (e.g., high-intensity activity is more reliant on carbohydrate as a fuel), gender, and environmental conditions. Using these values, a 70-kg athlete would be expected to consume between 420 and 700 g/day, a level far greater than that recommended for the general public. The recommended carbohydrate consumption for a large 136-kg (300 lb) football player would be even higher, ranging from 815 to 1,360 g/day, or 3,260 to 5,440 calories/day from carbohydrate alone. However, care should be taken when estimating total carbohydrate requirements, since a diet containing 500–600 g of carbohydrate per day for a 70-kg athlete is likely to adequately support glycogen stores. However, a short athlete consuming 60% of total energy from carbohydrates may not have sufficient carbohydrate to satisfy glycogen stores (69). It is important, therefore, to consider both athlete size and energy expenditure in determining optimal carbohydrate intakes.

Carbohydrate and Human Performance

In virtually all types of physical activity, carbohydrate availability is considered to be the limiting energy substrate in performance. That is, when carbohydrate runs out, the ability to perform physical activity at a high pace is limited, and performance drops. As is evident from the information in Table 2.6, the human system has limited storage of carbohydrate relative to the other energy substrates, fat and protein, and the availability of carbohydrate is worse than it seems. Exercise typically accesses specific muscles that use muscle glycogen at a faster rate than muscles that are not used, and these muscles can deplete muscle glycogen relatively quickly. However, the glycogen present in the nonused muscles is not "shared" by the muscles that use glycogen, so the availability of glycogen is actually lower than it appears to be in Table 2.5.

In actuality, people utilize carbohydrate and fat simultaneously to derive energy, and the more well-conditioned they are, the better able they are to use fat, which uses less carbohydrate and increases the time to exhaustion (i.e., the point at which carbohydrate is depleted). As seen in Figure 2.5, the higher the intensity of activity, the greater the *rate* of carbohydrate utilization to satisfy energy requirements.

The rate of fat utilization still remains significant in high-intensity activity, but the additional energy for activities at and above 65% of maximal oxygen consumption all comes from carbohydrate. Therefore, high-intensity activity will result in a faster depletion of carbohydrate

Table 2.6	Carbohydrate Stores in the Average Weight (154 lb), Lean (10% Body Fat) Male, and Length of Exercise Time If Solely Reliant on the Specific Energy Source		
Source	Mass (kg)	Energy (calories)	Exercise Time (min)
Liver glycogen	0.08	306	16
Muscle glycogen	0.40	1,530	80
Blood glucose	0.01	38	2
Fat	7.0	62,141	3,250
Protein	13.0	52,581	2,750

Source: Adapted from Maughan RJ, editor. Sports nutrition: The encyclopedia of sports medicine. West Sussex: Wiley-Blackwell; 2014.

stores. However, being well conditioned through a good training program can increase the reliance on fat and decrease the reliance on carbohydrate, with the result that time to exhaustion is increased (Figure 2.8).

Maximizing Glycogen Storage

Because stored glycogen is limited and therefore important to maximize prior to a competitive event or exercise,

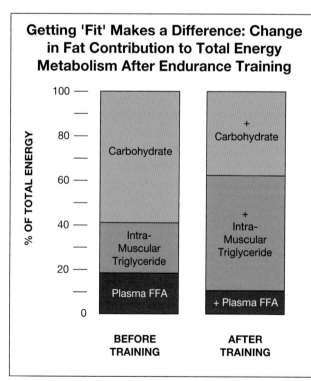

FIGURE 2.8: Getting "fit" makes a difference: Change in fat reliance after endurance training. (Modified from Martin WH III, Dalsky GP, Hurley BF, Matthews DE, Biern DM, Hagberg JM, Rogers MA, King DS, Holloszy JO. Effect of endurance training on plasma free fatty acid turnover and oxidation during exercise. Am J Physiol. 1993;265(5):E708–14).

it is important to consider the dietary strategy needed to optimize its storage. This strategy is often referred to as glycogen loading and was first described by Bergström (70). This glycogen-loading technique involved depleting muscle glycogen storage through hard exercise coupled with a low-carbohydrate diet for 3 days. This was followed by a high-carbohydrate diet and little or no exercise for 3 days. It was believed that muscle depleted of glycogen would behave like a sponge to maximize glycogen storage once carbohydrate was made available. A number of years later, another glycogen-loading strategy was described by Sherman et al. (71). This strategy involved sustaining a high-carbohydrate diet coupled with a tapering of exercise. It was found that the latter technique was equally successful in optimizing glycogen storage, and subsequent studies have confirmed two basic principles for physically active people to follow (60,72):

- Reducing the utilization of glycogen through the tapering off of physical activity is useful for optimizing storage.
- Consuming carbohydrate is necessary for maximizing glycogen storage.

Glycogen synthesis from the consumption of carbohydrates is reliant on the enzyme *glycogen synthase*. This enzyme is highest when glycogen storage is lowest in the period immediately following physical activity. Therefore, carbohydrate should be consumed immediately following physical activity to optimize glycogen synthesis. It has been found that the best glycogen synthesis occurs in the first 4 hours following exercise, when carbohydrate is consumed in frequent small feedings (73–75). It also appears that the form of carbohydrate consumed (liquid vs. solid) may not be an important factor in glycogen resynthesis (76). However, low glycemic index foods (*i.e.,* more complex carbohydrates) are known to be effective in assuring optimal glycogen storage (72). Energy balance is an important factor in glycogen synthesis, as it is known that energy restriction results in lower glycogen storage even when the same amount of carbohydrate is provided (77).

The maximum storage capacity of glycogen in a well-trained male athlete is about 400 g, which equates to around 1,530 calories. As the athlete experiences a decrease in blood glucose and these glycogen stores are depleted, the athlete will experience fatigue, which results in a decrease in athletic performance. Blood glucose is responsible for cognitive brain function, so, as blood glucose levels decline, the brain is not adequately perfused with energy. The decrease in blood glucose causes mental fatigue, which results in muscular fatigue and a reduction in athletic performance (78).

Performance during endurance activities has been shown to heavily rely on carbohydrate availability. Therefore, it is thought that carbohydrate loading and carbohydrate consumption during activity will positively affect athletic performance. Carbohydrate loading is when one consumes high levels of carbohydrate, generally 10–12 g/kg body weight, 2–3 days prior to an athletic event. Another recommendation is to consume carbohydrates during exercise. Carbohydrate consumption during exercise will supplement the body's glycogen stores and prevent blood glucose levels from rapidly declining. This will prevent fatigue and a decrease in performance. The most recent guidelines state that 30–60 g of carbohydrate per hour of exercise is recommended (69). In simple terms, it would be best for athletes to consume a carbohydrate-containing sports beverage in a way that seeks to maintain normalcy rather than waiting until carbohydrate is depleted before carbohydrate is consumed.

It has been found that the intake of glucose plus fructose will allow the human body to utilize more carbohydrates, thus increasing the recommendation of carbohydrate consumption during exercise (79). The reasoning behind why a consumption of mixed carbohydrates is more effective than a single carbohydrate is still unknown. However, it is thought that when mixed carbohydrates are consumed, separate transporter proteins may enhance intestinal carbohydrate absorption (78). It is also important to consume carbohydrates after exercise to replenish the muscle and liver glycogen stores that were utilized during exercise. This is strongly recommended for athletes who compete in multiday competitions or who will compete in two events in 1 day (80).

High-Intensity Sports

In high-intensity sports with a duration between 30 and 60 minutes, there is evidence that carbohydrate consumption during the activity improves performance (81). There is also evidence that the use of a carbohydrate mouth rinse for high-intensity activity lasting between 30 and 60 minutes improves performance, despite no carbohydrate being absorbed. This involves drinking a carbohydrate solution without swallowing and spitting it out after 5 seconds in the mouth (55,82). Care should be taken to not apply these findings to activities that are shorter than 30 minutes or longer than 60 minutes, as longer-duration activities clearly require the actual ingestion of carbohydrate. The likely basis for the improved performance using a carbohydrate mouth rinse is brain stimulation from the taste of carbohydrates in the mouth (83).

Team Sports

Athletes participating in team sports that involve intermittent stop-and-go activities experience a performance benefit when carbohydrate-containing beverages are consumed during the activity (84). The likely benefits from this consumption are from a lower breakdown of muscle glycogen, as a proportion of the required muscular fuel is derived from blood glucose and/or replenishment of muscle glycogen "fuel" during the activity (84). A number of more recent studies have suggested that carbohydrate consumption during intermittent sports improves skill performance either during (85) or at the end of the activity (86,87). A study assessing soccer skills found that consuming a carbohydrate-containing beverage reduced the typical performance deterioration in shooting (kicking) (88).

Endurance Sports

Carbohydrate consumption in sports activities with a duration exceeding 2 hours has been shown to improve time to exhaustion (*i.e.,* improved endurance) (89). It is likely that this consumption reduces the rate of muscle glycogen utilization and also helps to maintain normal blood glucose levels, thereby avoiding the performance deficits associated with mental fatigue. Studies of cyclists competing in the Tour de France have extremely high-carbohydrate consumption patterns of more than 90 g/hr (90). It also appears that carbohydrate polymer (gel) is well tolerated in long-duration events, whether it is composed of glucose or glucose-fructose (91).

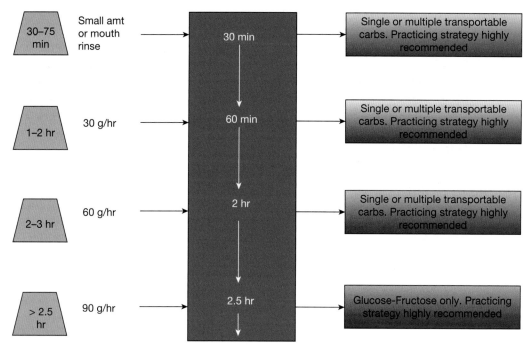

FIGURE 2.9: Recommended carbohydrate intake for different exercise durations in well-conditioned athletes. (Modified from Jeukendrup AE. Carbohydrate ingestion during exercise. In: Maughan RJ, editor. Sports nutrition: The encyclopedia of sports medicine. West Sussex: Wiley-Blackwell; 2014.)

Carbohydrate Consumption in Different Activities

Different durations and intensities of exercise require different carbohydrate intake strategies (Figure 2.9). Total carbohydrate consumption recommendations range from 30–60 g/hr (56) to up to 90 g/hr (92). It is likely that intakes above this level are difficult to achieve and may result in GI upset. One limitation of carbohydrate consumption is absorption capacity. Studies have found that absorption is enhanced when multiple types of carbohydrates are consumed, particularly at the levels of 60–90 g/hr. Therefore, it is recommended that combinations of glucose, maltose, maltodextrin, and fructose be consumed during exercise, particularly at durations >2.5 hours, rather than any single source of carbohydrate (73,79,89).

There is also evidence to suggest that there are wide individual differences in carbohydrate tolerance, but practicing the consumption of carbohydrate during exercise improves tolerance to higher volumes and concentrations of carbohydrate, resulting in lower risk of GI distress. For instance, athletes running the marathon often practice without carbohydrate/electrolyte beverages, but then have the availability of beverages to consume every 5 km during a race. The athletes who practice consuming carbohydrate/electrolyte beverages can consume more during the race with better race outcomes (93,94).

SUMMARY

- Physically active people should consider that only the energy substrates (carbohydrate, protein, and fat) provide the carbon chains needed to produce ATP.
- Vitamins and minerals are necessary to help the process of deriving energy from the energy substrates but do not provide energy themselves.
- Humans have "energy-first" systems, meaning that sufficient energy must be provided to ensure that all normal body processes can take place. A failure to provide sufficient energy in a way that dynamically matches requirements will interfere with performance. Many athletes "postload" energy consumption, that is, they consume the required energy at the end of the day, after they needed it, resulting in poor outcomes.
- Physical activity elevates the rate at which blood glucose is utilized and can result in low blood glucose, which is associated with premature mental muscular fatigue.
- Different carbohydrates are best consumed at different times. When not exercising (pre- and postexercise), starch-based complex carbohydrates are best for ensuring optimal glycogen storage. During and immediately after exercise, a combination of sugars is best to sustain blood glucose to provide energy to working muscles and for replenishing glycogen stores.

Practical Application Activity

Carbohydrate intake can be analyzed as a percentage of total calories consumed (% carb) or as grams of carbohydrate/kg mass (g/kg). The preferred method is g/kg, as this provides an adjustment for the carbohydrate intake based on body mass. Using % carb, it is possible for someone to have what appears to be a desirable carbohydrate consumption (*e.g.*, 55% of total calories), but if insufficient calories are consumed, the carbohydrate consumption will be inadequate. It is also important to know your indigestible carbohydrate consumption (fiber) and how sugar contributes to your total carbohydrate intake. You can assess your food intake for all of these using the procedure described in Chapter 1, accessing the online USDA Food Composition Database (https://fdc.nal.usda.gov); only, this time, focus on carbohydrate, fiber, and sugar with your food search:

1. Create a new spreadsheet analysis of a typical day of intake, creating columns for energy, carbohydrate, fiber (total dietary), and sugars (total).
2. When completed, analyze your dietary intake for these nutrients as follows:
   a. Calculate grams of carbohydrate/kg by dividing carbohydrate by your weight in kilograms. Compare your carbohydrate/kg with the recommended intake.
   b. Calculate percentage (%) of total calories from carbohydrate as follows:
      i. Multiply grams of carbohydrate × 4 to obtain calories from carbohydrate.
      ii. Divide total energy (calories) consumed by calories from carbohydrate to derive the percentage of total calories from carbohydrate.
      iii. Compare this percentage with the recommended intake.
   c. Compare your total dietary fiber intake with the recommended intake (women = 25 g/day; men = 38 g/day)
   d. Calculate percentage of total calories from sugar as follows:
      i. Multiply grams of sugar × 4 to obtain calories from sugar.
      ii. Divide total sugar calories by total calories to derive the percentage of total calories from sugar.
      iii. Calculate "added sugars" by subtracting naturally occurring sugar from total sugar.
      iv. Compare your total sugar intake, as percentage of total calories, with the recommended intake.
3. Review which foods contribute most to your fiber intake and your sugar intake. Make an adjustment, if needed, in your food intake by reducing the foods high in sugar and increasing the foods high in fiber.
4. Keep analyzing and adjusting until the carbohydrate consumption is desirable for g/kg, fiber, and sugar, and to view what type of carbohydrate and how much carbohydrate you would consume to ideally satisfy your needs.

CHAPTER QUESTIONS

1. Why are many people unable to digest milk sugar?
   a. They lack pancreatic amylase
   b. They lack the proper intestinal bacteria
   c. They were not breastfed
   d. They have a lactase deficiency

2. What is gluconeogenesis?
   a. The production of glucose from noncarbohydrate sources
   b. The oxidation of glucose under anaerobic conditions
   c. The maximum amount of glycogen that can be stored
   d. The use of ketone bodies for glucose by the brain

3. Carbohydrate that is consumed during endurance exercise appears to delay fatigue by
   a. Providing a steady supply of glucose that exercising muscle can use
   b. Sparing muscle glycogen
   c. Rapidly resynthesizing muscle glycogen
   d. All of the above

4. Muscle glycogen is a
   a. Monosaccharide
   b. Disaccharide
   c. Polysaccharide
   d. None of the above

5. Sucrose is a
   a. Monosaccharide
   b. Disaccharide
   c. Polysaccharide
   d. None of the above

6. The physiologic response to hyperglycemia resulting from the consumption of carbohydrate-containing foods
   a. Stimulation of α-cells in the pancreas and secretion of insulin
   b. Stimulation of β-cells in the pancreas and the secretion of insulin
   c. Stimulation of α-cells in the pancreas and secretion of glucagon
   d. Stimulation of β-cells in the pancreas and secretion of glucagon

7. Cortisol may be produced when blood sugar is
   a. Normal
   b. Above normal
   c. Below normal
   d. None of the above

8. One difference between epinephrine and glucagon is that glucagon can more rapidly break down liver glycogen to glucose.
   a. True
   b. False

9. Of the following, which is the least sweet tasting?
   a. Sucrose
   b. Maltose
   c. Lactose
   d. Fructose

10. Of the following, which is considered an abnormal (not desired) outcome for glucose?
    a. Conversion to liver glycogen
    b. Utilization as a source of energy (ATP production)
    c. Excretion in the urine
    d. Source of fuel for the central nervous system

ANSWERS TO CHAPTER QUESTIONS

1. d
2. a
3. a
4. c
5. b
6. b
7. c
8. b
9. c
10. c

Case Study Considerations

1. **Case Study Answer 1:** Education is key, so showing Sally what happens when inadequate energy is available, in real time, to satisfy nutrient needs. The information provided should differentiate between *what weight* is being controlled, as the current strategy for maintaining weight resulted in a greater loss of muscle mass than fat mass and caused a deterioration in the strength:weight ratio, which is an important factor for all athletes. The fear of carbohydrate intake is pervasive in many athlete groups, so showing Sally the optimal timing (pre-, during-, and postexercise), source, and volume of carbohydrate consumption to optimize glycogen stores and sustain blood sugar is important for assuring protein can be used anabolically (*i.e.,* to build/repair muscle, make hormones, make enzymes, etc.) while avoiding a decrease in bone density the development of a proportionately greater fat mass. All of this is made easier by visually showing Sally how her current eating pattern fails to satisfy energy/nutrient needs in real time.

2. **Case Study Answer 2:** The stress hormone cortisol becomes elevated when an individual is experiencing stress. This can be psychological stress, which results in a more rapid use of blood sugar (the primary fuel for the brain), or an eating pattern that fails to sustain normal blood sugar. In both cases, low blood sugar is a primary cause of elevated cortisol, which is a catabolic hormone. That is, when cortisol is elevated, the body tries to find a way to normalize blood sugar and it does this by breaking down tissues so that some of the tissue components

can go to the liver to be converted to glucose. A primary pathway is the breakdown of lean tissue so that the glucogenic amino acids (*i.e.*, those amino acids that can be converted to glucose) provide a metabolic source of glucose. While this appears to be desirable, the normalized glucose occurs with the loss of lean tissue, which is not desirable for anyone and especially not desirable for an athlete. It would be far better to have an eating/drinking strategy that assures a reasonably good maintenance of blood sugar so that cortisol is suppressed and there is no loss of lean tissue and bone mass.

3. **Case Study Answer 3:** One of the effects of experiencing elevated cortisol is lower estrogen production in female athletes. Low estrogen results in a cessation of normal menses and is also associated with lower bone mineral density. The lower bone density is the result of a failure to inhibit bone osteoclasts (cells that break down bone), which is a function of estrogen. In male athletes estrogen is not an issue. However, there is now evidence that elevated cortisol in male athletes is associated with lower testosterone production, which would inhibit the repair, recovery, and building of muscle and, thereby, be an inhibitor of achieving optimal performance.

4. **Case Study Answer 4:**
   a. Blood sugar typically fluctuates in 3-hour units when awake and when doing normal daily activity. That is, blood sugar reaches its peak about 1 hour after you eat, and 2 hours after that it is back to the premeal level. This suggest that if eating the typical three meals per day (*i.e.*, breakfast, lunch, and dinner) separated by 5–6 hours between meals, it would be good to have a small snack between meals (*e.g.*, fresh fruit, fruited yogurt, whole grain cereal, etc.) that provides approximately 200–250 calories, primarily from carbohydrate, to restore liver glycogen and assure normal blood sugar until the next meal. Avoidance of highly sweetened beverages and sugary snacks is important, as these will result in a hyperinsulinemic response that quickly lowers blood sugar.

   b. Blood sugar can be maintained for up to 7–8 hours while asleep because of the lower metabolic rate associated with sleeping. This suggests that it would be desirable to have a small snack prior to bedtime to sustain blood sugar while asleep. This snack could be, as in answer "a," fresh fruit, fruited yogurt, whole grain cereal, while highly sweetened foods/beverages are avoided.

   c. Physical activity results in a fast drop in blood sugar, requiring a strategy that can sustain normalcy rather than a strategy that focuses on recovery. That is, far too often athletes do nothing to sustain blood sugar during physical activity but consume a large volume of sports beverage and other high carbohydrate foods after exercise to recover from the low blood sugar that was the result of the exercise. A good strategy is to know that blood sugar is dropping faster than normal when you exercise, so adopting a sports beverage (*i.e.*, carbohydrate- and electrolyte-containing beverage) sipping strategy from the very beginning of exercise is desirable. As an example, low-intensity exercise will use blood sugar more slowly than high-intensity exercise, so an athlete performing low-intensity exercise may take one mouthful of a sports beverage every 15 minutes, while an athlete performing higher-intensity exercise may take two mouthfuls every 10 minutes.

REFERENCES

1. Madave H, Kanawjia P, Chaudhary MJ, Srivastava C, Saxena J. Acute effect of resistance exercise on serum cortisol and its correlation to blood glucose in healthy non obese adults: a pilot study. J Clin Diagn Res. 2021;15(10):OC10–3.
2. American Diabetes Association. Postprandial blood glucose. Diabetes Care. 2001;24(4):775–8.
3. Hargreaves M, Spriet LL. Skeletal muscle energy metabolism during exercise. Nat Metab. 2020;2(9):817–28.
4. Tian D, Meng J. Exercise for prevention and relief of cardiovascular disease: prognoses, mechanism, and approaches. Oxid Med Cell Longev. 2019;2019:3756750.
5. Hearris MA, Hammond KM, Fell JM, Morton JP. Regulation of muscle glycogen metabolism during exercise: Implications for endurance performance and training adaptations. Nutrients. 2018;10(3):298.
6. Bohn T, Davidsson L, Walczyk T, Hurrell RF. Fractional magnesium absorption is significantly lower in human subjects from a meal served with an oxalate-rich vegetable, spinach, as compared with a meal served with kale, a vegetable with a low oxalate content. Br J Nutr. 2004;91(4):601–6.
7. Coy JF, Franz M. The cancer fighting diet. Toronto: Robert Rose Publisher, Inc.; 2013. 41 p.
8. American Chemical Society. Sorbitol provides superior moisture conditioning qualities. Sorbitol provides superior

moisture conditioning qualities. Chem Eng News. 1956;34(48): 5800–1.

9. Demirbas D, Coelho AL, Rubio-Gozalbo ME, Berry GT. Hereditary galactosemia. Metabolism. 2018;83:188–96.

10. Noelting J, DiBaise JK. Mechanisms of fructose absorption. Clin Transl Gastroenterol. 2015;6(11):e120.

11. Ackerman Z, Oron-Herman M, Grozovski M, Rosenthal T, Pappo O, Link G, Sela B-A. Fructose-induced fatty liver disease: hepatic effects of blood pressure and plasma triglyceride reduction. Hypertension. 2005;45(5):1012–8.

12. Lecoultre V, Egli L, Theytaz F, Despland C, Schneiter P, Tappy L. Fructose-induced hyperuricemia is associated with a decreased renal uric acid excretion in humans. Diabetes Care. 2013; 36(9):e149–50.

13. Stanhope KL, Medici V, Bremer AA, Lee V, Lam HD, Nunez MV, Chen GX, Keim NL, Havel PJ. A dose-response study of consuming high-fructose corn syrup-sweetened beverages on lipid/lipoprotein risk factors for cardiovascular disease in young adults. Am J Clin Nutr. 2015;101(6):1144–54.

14. Li S, Wang J, Xiao Y, Zhang L, Fang J, Yang N, Nasser MI, Qin H. D-ribose: potential clinical applications in congestive heart failure and diabetes, and its complications (Review). Exp Ther Med. 2021;21(5):496.

15. Shafer RB, Levine AS, Marlene JM, Morley JE. Do calories, osmolality, or calcium determine gastric emptying? Am J Physiol. 1985;248(4):R479–83.

16. Mussatto SI. Application of xylitol in food formulations and benefits for health. In: da Silva SS, Chandal AK, editors. D-Xylitol. Berlin, Heidelberg: Springer; 2012. p. 309–23.

17. Pol K, Mars M. L-arabinose and d-xylose: sweet pentoses that may reduce postprandial glucose and insulin responses. Food Nutr Res. 2021;65. https://doi.org/10.29219/fnr.v65.6254

18. Claeys WL, Verraes C, Cardoen S, De Block J, Huyghebaert A, Raes K, Dewettinck K, Herman L. Consumption of raw or heated milk from different species: an evaluation of the nutritional and potential health benefits. Food Control. 2014;42:188–201.

19. Swagerty DL, Walling AD, Klein RM. Lactose intolerance. Am Fam Physician. 2002;65(9):1845–50.

20. de Vrese M, Laue C, Offick B, Soeth E, Repenning F, Thob A, Schrezenmeir J. A combination of acid lactase from Aspergillus oryzae and yogurt bacteria improves lactose digestion in lactose maldigesters synergistically: a randomized, controlled, double-blind cross-over trial. Clin Nutr. 2015;34(3):394–9.

21. Yoshizane C, Mizote A, Arai C, Arai N, Ogawa R, Endo S, Mitsuzume H, Ushio S. Daily consumption of one teaspoon of trehalose can help maintain glucose homeostasis: a double-blind, randomized controlled trial conducted in healthy volunteers. Nutr J. 2020;19(1):68.

22. Colaco C, Sen S, Thangavelu M, Pinder S, Roser B. Extraordinary stability of enzymes dried in trehalose: simplified molecular biology. Biotechnology (N Y). 1992;10:1007–11.

23. Roser BJ. Protection of proteins and the like. USP 4,891,319. Issued January 2, 1990. Filed January 15, 1987.

24. Boos W, Ehmann U, Forkl H, Klein W, Rimmele M, Postma P. Trehalose transport and metabolism in *Escherichia coli*. J Bacteriol. 1990;172:3450–61.

25. Tymczyszyn EE, Gomez-Zavaglia A, Disalvo EA. Effect of sugars and growth media on the dehydration of Lactobacillus delbrueckii ssp. bulgaricus. J Appl Microbiol. 2007;102(3):845–51.

26. Hottiger T, DeVirgilio C, Hall MN, Boller T, Wiemken A. The role of trehalose synthesis for the acquisition of thermotolerance in yeast II. Physiological concentrations of trehalose increase the thermal stability of proteins in vitro. Eur J Biochem. 1994;219:187–93.

27. Walsh DT. Ecological significance of compatible solute accumulation by micro-organisms: from single cells to global climate. FEMS Microbiol Rev. 2000;24:263–90.

28. Coyle EF, Coggan AR, Hemmert MK, Ivy JL. Muscle glycogen utilization during prolonged strenuous exercise when fed carbohydrate. J Appl Physiol. 1986;6(1):165–72.

29. Mcintosh M, Miller C. A diet containing food rich in soluble and insoluble fiber improves glycemic control and reduces hyperlipidemia among patients with type 2 diabetes mellitus. Nutr Rev. 2001;59(2):52–5.

30. de Oliveira EP, Burini RC, Jeukendrup A. Gastrointestinal complaints during exercise: prevalence, etiology, and nutritional recommendations. Sports Med. 2014;44(1):79–85.

31. Torre M, Rodriguez AR, Saura-Calixto F. Effects of dietary fiber and phytic acid on mineral availability. Crit Rev Food Sci Nutr. 2009;30(1):1–22.

32. Augustin LSA, Kendall CWC, Jenkins DJA, Willett WC, Astrup A, Barclay AW, I Björck I, Brand-Miller JC, Brighenti F, Buyken AE, Ceriello A, La Vecchia C, Livesey G, Liu S, Riccardi G, Rizkalla SW, Sievenpiper JL, Trichopoulou A, Wolever TMS, Baer-Sinnott S, Poli A. Glycemic index, glycemic load and glycemic response: an International Scientific Consensus Summit from the International Carbohydrate Quality Consortium (ICQC). Nutr Metab Cardiovasc Dis. 2015;25(9):795–815.

33. Maughan RJ, editor. Sports nutrition: The encyclopedia of sports medicine. West Sussex: Wiley-Blackwell; 2014.

34. Vigh-Larsen JF, Ørtenblad N, Spriet LL, Overgaard K, Mohr M. Muscle glycogen metabolism and high-intensity exercise performance: a narrative review. Sports Med. 2021;51:1855–74.

35. Paoli A, Cenci L, Pompei P, Sahin N, Bianco A, Neri M, Caprio M, Moro T. Effects of two months of very low carbohydrate ketogenic diet on body composition, muscle strength, muscle area, and blood parameters in competitive natural body builders. Nutrients. 2021;13(2):374.

36. Hasselbalch SG, Knudsen GM, Jakobsen J, Hageman LP, Holm S, Paulson OB. Blood-brain barrier permeability of glucose and ketone bodies during short-term starvation in humans. Am J Physiol. 1995;268(6):E1161–6.

37. Phinney SD. Ketogenic diets and physical performance. Nutr Metab 2004;1(1):2.

38. Koeslag JH. Post-exercise ketosis and the hormone response to exercise: a review. Med Sci Sports Exerc. 1982;14(5):327–34.

39. Durkalec-Michalski K, Nowaczyk PM, Główka N, Ziobrowska A, Podgórski T. Is a four-week ketogenic diet an effective nutritional strategy in crossfit-trained female and male athletes? Nutrients. 2021;13(3):864.

40. Ashtary-Larky D, Bagheri R, Bavi H, Baker J, Moro T, Mancin L, Paoli A. Ketogenic diets, physical activity, and body composition: a review. Br J Nutr. 2022;127(12):1898–1920.

41. Nature.com. Glycolipids [Internet]. 2015. Accessed 2015 November 30. Available from: http://www.nature.com/subjects/glycolipids

42. Maton A, Hopkins J, McLaughlin CW, Johnson S, Warner MQ, LaHart D, Wright JD. Human biology and health. Englewood Cliffs (NJ): Prentice Hall; 1993. p. 52–9.

43. Faruque S, Tong J, Lacmanovic V, Agbonghae C, Minaya DM, Czaja K. The dose makes the poison: sugar and obesity in the United States-a review. Pol J Food Nutr Sci. 2019;69(3):219–33.

44. Southgate DA. Digestion and metabolism of sugars. Am J Clin Nutr. 1995;62(1):203S–10S.

45. Lentze MJ. Molecular and cellular aspects of hydrolysis and absorption. Am J Clin Nutr. 1995;61(Suppl):946S–51S.

46. Riby JE, Fujisawa T, Kretchmer M. Fructose absorption. Am J Clin Nutr. 1993;58(Suppl):748S–53S.

47. Burkitt DP, Trowell HS. Refined carbohydrate foods and disease: some implication of dietary fibre. London: Academic Press; 2012.

48. Cherbut C. Role of gastrointestinal motility in the delay of absorption by dietary fibre. Eur J Clin Nutr. 1995;49:S74–80.

49. Gibson GR, Beatty ER, Wang X, Cummings JH. Selective stimulation of bifidobacteria in the human colon. Gastroenterology. 1995;108:975–82.

50. Mudgil D, Barak S. Composition, properties and health benefits of indigestible carbohydrate polymers as dietary fiber: a review. Int J Biol Macromol. 2013;61:1–6.

51. Gibson GR, Wang X. Bifidogenic properties of different types of fructo-oligosaccharides. Food Microbiol. 1994;11:491–8.

52. Saez-Lara MJ, Gomez-Llorente C, Plaza-Diaz J, Gil A. The role of probiotic lactic acid bacteria and bifidobacteria in the prevention and treatment of inflammatory bowel disease and other related diseases: a systematic review of randomized human clinical trials. Biomed Res Int. 2015;2015:505878. https://doi.org/10.1155/2015/505878

53. Clauss M, Gérard P, Mosca A, Leclerc M. Interplay between exercise and gut microbiome in the context of human health and performance. Front Nutr. 2021;8:637010. https://doi.org/10.3389/fnut.2021.637010

54. Carter JM, Jeukendrup AE, Jones DA. The effect of carbohydrate mouth rinse on 1-h cycle time trial performance. Med Sci Sports Exerc. 2004;36:2107–11.

55. Carter JM, Jeukendrup AE, Mann CH, Jones DA. The effect of glucose infusion on glucose kinetics during a 1-h time trial. Med Sci Sports Exerc. 2004;36(9):1543–50.

56. Sawka MN, Burke LM, Eichner ER, Maughan RJ, Montain SJ, Stachenfeld NS. American College of Sports Medicine position stand. Exercise and fluid replacement. Med Sci Sports Exerc. 2007;39:377–90.

57. Meyer C, Hanson RL, Tataranni A, Bogardus C, Partly RE. A high fasting plasma insulin concentration predicts type 2 diabetes independent of insulin resistance: evidence for a pathogenic role of relative hyperinsulinemia. Diabetes. 2000; 49(12):2094–101.

58. Stumvoll M, Chintalapudi U, Perriello G, Wells S, Gutierrez O, Gerich J. Uptake and release of glucose by the human kidney. Postabsorptive rates and responses to epinephrine. J Clin Invest. 1995;96(5):2528–33.

59. McIntyre CL, Sheetz AH, Carroll CR, Young MC. Administration of epinephrine for life-threatening allergic reactions in school settings. Pediatrics. 2005;116(5):1134–40. Accessed 2016 December 2. Available from: http://pediatrics.aappublications.org/content/116/5/1134

60. Costill DL, Sherman WM, Fink WJ, Maresh C, Witten M, Miller JM. The role of dietary carbohydrate in muscle glycogen resynthesis after strenuous running. Am J Clin Nutr. 1981; 34:1831–6.

61. Rich PR. The molecular machinery of Keilin's respiratory chain. Biochem Soc Trans. 2003;31(Pt 6):1095–105.

62. Stryer L. Biochemistry. 4th ed. New York (NY): W. H. Freeman and Company; 1995.

63. Gerich JE. Role of the kidney in normal glucose homeostasis and in the hyperglycaemia of diabetes mellitus: therapeutic implications. Diabet Medi. 2010;27(2):136–42.

64. Mithieux G, Rajas F, Gautier-Stein A. A novel role for glucose 6-phosphatase in the small intestine in the control of glucose homeostasis. J Biol Chem. 2004;279(43):44231–8.

65. Widmaier E. Vander's human physiology. New York (NY): McGraw Hill; 2006. p. 96.

66. Institute of Medicine, Food and Nutrition Board. Dietary reference intakes for energy, carbohydrate, fiber, fat, fatty acids, cholesterol, protein, and amino acids. Washington (DC): National Academies Press; 2002.

67. USDA/HHS. Dietary guidelines for Americans. Washington, DC: Government Printing Office; 2005.

68. Thomas DT, Erdman KA, Burke LM, MacKillop M. American College of Sports Medicine Joint position statement. Nutrition and athletic performance. Med Sci Sports Exerc. 2016;48(3):543–68.

69. Rodriguez NR, DiMarco NM, Langley S; American Dietetic Association, Dietitians of Canada. American College of Sports Medicine position stand. Nutrition and athletic performance. Med Sci Sports Exerc. 2009;41;709–31.

70. Bergström J, Hermansen L, Hultman E, Saltin B. Diet, muscle glycogen and physical performance. Acta Physiol Scand. 1967; 71:140–50.

71. Sherman WM, Costill DL, Fink WJ, Miller JM. Effect of exercise-diet manipulation on muscle glycogen and its subsequent utilisation during performance. Int J Sports Med. 1981;2: 114–8.

72. Burke LM. Energy needs of athletes. Can J Appl Physiol. 2001;26(Suppl):S202YS219.

73. Jentjens RL, Moseley L, Waring RH, Harding LK, Jeukendrup AE. Oxidation of combined ingestion of glucose and fructose during exercise. J Appl Physiol. 2004;96(4):1277–84.

74. van Hall G, Shirreffs SM, Caleb JAL. Muscle glycogen synthesis during recovery from cycle exercise: no effect of additional protein ingestion. J Appl Physiol. 2000;88(5):1631–6.

75. van Loon LJC, Saris WHM, Kruijshoop M, Wagenmakers AJM. Maximizing post exercise muscle glycogen synthesis: carbohydrate supplementation and the application of amino acid or protein hydrolysate mixtures. Am J Clin Nutr. 2000; 72(1):106–11.

76. Keizer H, Kuipers H, van Kranenburg G. Influence of liquid and solid meals on muscle glycogen resynthesis, plasma fuel hormone response, and maximal physical working capacity. Int J Sports Med. 1987;8:99–104.

77. Tarnopolsky MA, Zawada C, Richmond LB, et al. Gender differences in carbohydrate loading are related to energy intake. J Appl Physiol. 2001;91(1):225–30.

78. Watters DAK. Does fatigue impair performance? ANZ J Surg. 2014;84(3):102–3.

79. Triplett D, Doyle JA, Rupp JC, Benardot D. An isocaloric glucose-fructose beverage's effect on simulated 100-km cycling performance compared with a glucose-only beverage. Int J Sport Nutr Exerc Metab. 2010;20:122–31.

80. Cermak NM, van Loon LJC. The use of carbohydrates during exercise as an ergogenic aid. Sports Med. 2013;43(11):1139–55.

81. Jeukendrup AE, Brouns F, Wagemakers AJM, Saris WHM. Carbohydrate-electrolyte feedings improve 1 h time trial cycling performance. Int J Sports Med. 1997;18(2):125–9.

82. Rollo I, Williams C, Gant N, Nute M. The influence of carbohydrate mouth rinse on self-selected speeds during a 30-min treadmill run. Int J Sport Nutr Exerc Metabo. 2008;18(6):585–600.

83. Chambers ES, Bridge MW, Jones DA. Carbohydrate sensing in the human mouth: effects on exercise performance and brain activity. J Physiol. 2009;589:1779–94.

84. Nicholas CW, Williams C, Lakomy HKA, Phillips G, Nowitz A. Influence of ingesting a carbohydrate-electrolyte solution on endurance capacity during intermittent, high-intensity shuttle running. J Sports Sci. 1995;13(4):283–90.

85. Currell K, Conway S, Jeukendrup AE. Carbohydrate ingestion improves performance of a new reliable test of soccer performance. Int J Sport Nutr Exerc Metab. 2009;19(1):34–46.

86. Ali A, Williams C, Nicholas CW, Foskett A. The influence of carbohydrate-electrolyte ingestion on soccer skill performance. Med Sci Sports Exerc. 2007;39:1969–76.

87. Winnick JJ, Davis JM, Welsh RS, Carmichael MD, Murphy EA, Blackmon JA. Carbohydrate feedings during team sport exercise preserve physical and CNS function. Med Sci Sports Exerc. 2005;37(2):306–5.

88. Russell M, Benton D, Kingsley M. Influence of carbohydrate supplementation on skill performance during a soccer match simulation. J Sci Med Sport. 2012;15(4):348–54.

89. Jeukendrup AE. Carbohydrate feeding during exercise. Eur J Sport Sci. 2008;8:77–86.

90. Saris WH, van Erp-Baart MA, Browns F, Westerterp KR, ten Hoor F. Study on food intake and energy expenditure during extreme sustained exercise: the Tour de France. Int J Sports Med. 1989;10:S26–31.

91. Pfeiffer B, Cotterill A, Grathwohl D, Stellingwerff T, Jeukendrup AE. The effect of carbohydrate gels on gastrointestinal tolerance during a 16-km run. Int J Sport Nutr Exerc Metab. 2009;19:485–503.

92. Jeukendrup AE. Carbohydrate ingestion during exercise. In: Maughan RJ, editor. Sports nutrition: The encyclopedia of sports medicine. West Sussex: Wiley-Blackwell; 2014.

93. Cox GR, Clark SA, Cox AJ, Halson SL, Hargreaves M, Hawley JA, Jeacocke N, Snow RJ, Yeo WK, Burke LM. Daily training with high carbohydrate availability increases exogenous carbohydrate oxidation during endurance cycling. J Appl Physiol. 2010;109:126–34.

94. Dhiman C, Kapri BC. Optimizing athletic performance and post-exercise recovery: the significance of carbohydrates and nutrition. Monten J Sports Sci Med. 2023;19(2):49–56. https://doi.org/10.26773/mjssm.230907

CHAPTER

3

Protein

CHAPTER OBJECTIVES

- Understand the differences between essential amino acids and nonessential amino acids, and the primary functions of the essential amino acids.
- Be capable of calculating the daily protein requirement for yourself and for others, both athlete and nonathlete, and calculate the optimal distribution of the protein to optimize tissue utilization.
- Know the health risks associated with consumption of too much or too little protein and how other energy substrates help to "spare" protein so that it can be used anabolically (*i.e.*, to build/repair tissues, make hormones and enzymes, help control pH and fluid balance, etc.) rather than being used as a source of energy.
- Explain how proteins are digested and absorbed, including the location and source of the major protein digestive enzymes.
- Understand protein energy metabolic pathways, and the by-products produced when proteins are used as a source of cellular energy.

- Know how supplements of amino acids and other protein-related substances, such as creatine monohydrate, may have an impact on health risks and performance.
- Understand how the presence and distribution of essential amino acids influence protein quality.
- Recognize the primary functions of proteins as they relate to immunity, tissue structure, hormones and enzymes, transportation, and fluid balance.
- Discriminate between food sources that are good sources of high–biologic-value (BV) protein and food sources that are moderate to poor sources of high BV protein.
- Determine foods that, when combined, can improve the protein quality to a level better than if these foods were consumed individually.
- Identify the common methods used for determining the protein quality.
- Describe the factors that are involved in improving muscle mass size and function.

Case Study: Lots of Protein but Poor Delivery Inhibits Benefits

T.J. was a massive freshman defensive guard on his college football team, and he learned from the very beginning, when he was playing football in the Pop Warner league as a 6-year-old, that lots of protein was needed to ensure he could grow and build the muscle needed for a career in football. He was already bigger, heavier, and taller than nearly all of the other players, but he wanted to be bigger still, even as a youngster. So, he ate lots of food and made sure that a high proportion of it was protein. Steak and chicken were his favorite, but he ate fish when his mother made it. He did not care much for veggies, but that did not

matter much to him because he "knew" that protein would get him where he wanted to go.

The massive amount of food T.J. ate did help him get bigger, but as a collegiate athlete, there was a great deal more being asked of him than ever before. His coach also wanted him to be fast and be able to play as hard in the fourth quarter as he did in the first. Right away, the defensive coach saw a problem: T.J. was certainly big, but he was not as quick as he should be and his endurance was terrible. The coach put him on a more severe training regimen to build his strength, quickness, and endurance. Of course,

(continued)

T.J. did what he thought he needed to do, and that was to increase his protein intake, but it did not help. T.J. kept getting fatter from all the extra food he was consuming, but the extra fat he was carrying around made him slower and his endurance kept getting worse. So, they sent him to talk with the sports nutritionist who just started working with the university teams, and the nutritionist immediately found the problem. T.J. was consuming a huge amount of protein, but at the expense of carbohydrates. To make matters worse, his intake of food, including protein, was not spread out well throughout the day. He mainly had two large meals: breakfast and a late dinner, and nearly nothing in-between. This type of eating pattern is associated with many problems that make it difficult to build muscle but easy to store fat. The nutritionist showed him that the typical daily requirement for an athlete is 1.2–2.0 g/kg/day, which is ideally consumed by providing moderate amounts of protein spread out during the day and following a strenuous training session. T.J. was consuming a great deal more protein than the requirement, and he was not distributing it well throughout the day to optimize his body's capacity to use it efficiently for building and repairing muscle. So, the nutritionist showed him how to have seven eating opportunities (breakfast, mid-morning snack, lunch, afternoon snack, dinner, evening snack, and bedtime snack), with about 30 g of protein each time both to provide the recommended level of intake and to optimize protein utilization. Almost immediately T.J. saw the difference. His body fat was decreasing and his muscle mass was increasing. He learned one of the secrets of nutrition: It is not just how much you eat, but how and when you eat it that matters most.

CASE STUDY DISCUSSION QUESTIONS

1. Calculate the protein in your diet to see if you are consuming an amount that satisfies need, and that you are distributing the protein in a way that would optimize protein utilization.
2. Is it likely that active people who eat the standard three meals/day could distribute protein intake in a way that could enable optimal protein utilization?
3. What happens to the excess protein consumed? List the potential problems that may arise from this.
4. How would you set up an athlete environment to help ensure that the athletes could consume foods in a pattern that would be most useful?

INTRODUCTION

Important Factors to Consider

- There is limited evidence that increasing protein consumption above the recommended intake levels as a means of improving musculature is a useful strategy and it may cause problems with kidney health, dehydration, and low bone mineral density (1). In addition, high-protein intake interferes with a balanced intake of other foods/nutrients.
- It is far better to consume the recommended level of protein in amounts that can be efficiently used by tissues, especially when the athlete's energy intake level is satisfied with sufficient intake of carbohydrates and fats.
- Consumption of single amino acids for the purpose of initiating a desired metabolic outcome (*i.e.*, greater muscle acquisition) may be associated with problems that could interfere with the desired outcomes (*i.e.*, muscle protein synthesis [MPS], reduced muscle soreness, improved muscle repair) and is not likely to be a successful strategy.
- Misconceptions about nutrition are commonly held by athletes, resulting in eating and drinking behaviors that may negatively impact athletic performance while increasing injury risk. Protein is commonly thought to be a singularly important nutrient, elevating the potential that athletes consume to much protein, resulting in a diminished intake of other essential nutrients (2).
- It is far better to eat foods that contain a wide array of essential amino acids to ensure an adequate energy intake and to allow tissues to acquire the amino acids they require for metabolic purposes. It is easy to get too much of a single amino acid that may result in the opposite of the desired effect. For instance, the **branched-chain amino acid** (BCAA) leucine is known to be an MPS stimulator, and studies suggest that 20 g of good-quality protein containing leucine has been found to maximally stimulate MPS (3).

Protein Intake Recommendations

Athletes	1.2–2.0 g/day
Per Meal	~30 g/meal
Nonathlete Adults	0.8 g/day
Growing Boys (between ages 3–18)	0.9 g/day
Growing Girls (between ages 3–15)	0.9 g/day

 Branched-Chain Amino Acids

The amino acids isoleucine, valine, and leucine can be metabolized locally in muscle tissue and promote MPS and are involved in glucose metabolism.

Proteins are one of the energy substrates (with carbohydrates and fats), meaning that we are capable of producing adenosine triphosphate (ATP, or energy) from protein molecules, primarily through their conversion to carbohydrates and fat. Besides this energy-producing capacity, however, proteins have many other critical functions that require consideration. Many physically active people consider protein consumption to be the key to athletic performance success, and even a cursory review of the magazines and other literature targeting athletes demonstrates this point, with advertisements for protein supplements and protein-added foods that are intended to, ultimately, enhance winning potential. Often, physically active people consume far more protein than is needed, and an obvious problem with excess protein consumption is that this necessarily translates into consuming too little of other nutrients that are equally important (4). There is evidence that satisfying the total protein requirement by consuming meals containing approximately 30 g protein maximally enhances MPS in both young and elderly subjects, suggesting that higher-protein meals (*i.e.*, those providing more than 30 g protein) may fail to produce greater muscle enlargement (5,6). In addition, high-protein consumption may displace carbohydrates, which is well established as a critically important fuel for all sporting endeavors, ranging from endurance to short-duration, and high-intensity events (4,7,8). In addition, although physically active people often consume far more total protein than body tissues can use to fulfill nonenergy anabolic (*i.e.*, MPS) requirements, the manner in which this protein is consumed (*i.e.*, excess protein in a meal) may inhibit the utilization of the consumed protein for functions that only protein can fulfill (9). Poor protein utilization will result in at least a portion of the protein having the nitrogen removed, with the remaining carbon chain converted to fat and carbohydrates that

can be used or stored as fuel. Although it is clear that athletes have a significantly higher-protein requirement than nonathletes (1.2–2.0 vs. 0.8 g/kg/day), the manner in which the protein is consumed is important, as is satisfying energy balance and seeking a balanced and varied food intake that exposes athletes to all of the nutrients they require. This chapter will review food sources of protein, protein functions, protein requirements, and eating patterns that can help derive the most out of the protein being consumed. There are many questions that this chapter will answer, including:

- Does increasing protein intake beyond a certain level help to increase muscle mass?
- Does supplemental or high-protein intake provide an ergogenic (performance-enhancing) benefit?
- Does supplemental or high-protein intake improve strength and power?
- Is there evidence that, when normalized on a protein/kg basis, athletes tend to overemphasize protein to the detriment of other nutrients?

 Proteins

Molecules consisting of multiple amino acids held together by peptide bonds in a sequence and structure that influence protein function.

STRUCTURE OF PROTEIN

Proteins are made of amino acids, which contain carbon, oxygen, hydrogen, and *nitrogen* (Figure 3.1).

Of the energy substrates, only the amino acids that make up proteins contain nitrogen. The nitrogen content of proteins is an important consideration because when proteins are broken down to be used for energy or stored as fat, this nitrogen must be removed from the protein molecule. This nitrogen waste forms blood urea nitrogen (BUN)

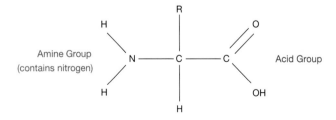

Each amino acid can bond with another amino acid

FIGURE 3.1: Basic structure of an amino acid, the building block of proteins.

FIGURE 3.2: Protein breakdown and nitrogen excretion. ATP, adenosine triphosphate.

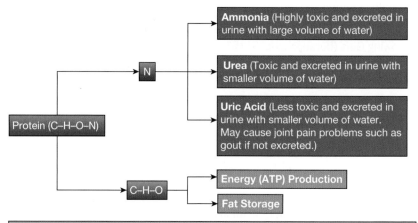

Protein Breakdown and Nitrogen Excretion Resulting from Excess Protein Intake. Possible Outcomes are Energy Production and/or Fat Storage

and, because it is potentially toxic, it must be removed. The primary removal of BUN is via the kidneys, requiring greater urinary volume when the BUN level is high. This higher urine volume may increase dehydration risk, which is a significant problem for athletes because of an already elevated risk of dehydration from sweat loss (Figure 3.2).

Blood Urea Nitrogen

Blood urea nitrogen (BUN) is a measure of the urea nitrogen content in the blood that mainly represents the nitrogen released from the metabolism of protein. It is from the waste product urea. Urea is produced when amino acids are catabolized and the carbon chain is used to supply energy or stored as fat. The nitrogen removed from the amino acid forms urea, which is removed from the body via urine.

Urine

Urine is a liquid produced by the kidneys to excrete the by-products of metabolism. A primary function of urine is to excrete nitrogenous waste (urea) that is a by-product of protein catabolism. High-protein diets that exceed the tissue capacity to use the protein anabolically result in protein catabolism and higher nitrogenous waste that must be excreted via urine.

Amino acids are the building blocks of protein, with several amino acids held together to form **polypeptides** and several polypeptides held together to form a protein.

There are 20 different amino acids, and humans can manufacture 11 amino acids by using the nitrogen discarded by the breakdown of proteins and the carbon, hydrogen, and oxygen available from carbohydrates. The 11 amino acids that we can manufacture are referred to as nonessential or dispensable amino acids, because it is *not essential* that we obtain them from the foods we consume since they can be manufactured. However, do not misinterpret nonessential as meaning unimportant, as these nonessential amino acids are just as metabolically important as the nine **essential amino acids**, which we cannot manufacture and must be obtained from the foods we consume (Table 3.1).

To make proteins, amino acids are held together via peptide bonds, where the acid end of one amino acid connects with the nitrogen of another amino acid and, in the process, water is formed (Figure 3.3). The sequence of how these amino acids are connected determines the function of the protein. So, although a protein may contain the same amino acids, how they are ordered will determine what the protein will do.

Amino Acids

Organic compounds are characterized by an amine group (NH_2) on one end of the molecule and a carboxyl group (COOH) on the other end of the molecule. Amino acids are held together in different sequences to compose polypeptides and proteins.

Table 3.1   Essential and Nonessential Amino Acids

Nonessential Amino Acids (Synthesized by humans from carbohydrates and fragments of other amino acids)			Essential Amino Acids (Cannot be synthesized by humans, so must be consumed from foods)		
Amino Acid	Abbr	Notes	Amino Acid	Abbr	Notes
Alanine (Glucogenic)	Ala	Can be converted to glucose in the liver (gluconeogenesis) via the alanine-glucose cycle.	Histidine (Glucogenic)	His	Unlike the other essential amino acids, does not induce a negative nitrogen balance when removed from the diet. Involved in production of histamine.
Arginine (Glucogenic)	Arg	Conditionally essential amino acid that may become essential under certain metabolic conditions. Used in production of nitric oxide.	Isoleucine (Glucogenic)	Ile	Branched-chain amino acid that may be useful for muscle recovery and the immune system following exercise.
Asparagine (Glucogenic)	Asn	Necessary for the development and function of the brain and plays a role in ammonia synthesis.	Leucine (Ketogenic)	Leu	Branched-chain amino acid that may be useful for muscle recovery and the immune system following exercise. Stimulates muscle protein synthesis
Aspartic Acid (Glucogenic)	Asp	Involved in neurotransmission and may be converted to glucose.	Lysine (Glucogenic)	Lys	Metabolized to form acetyl-CoEnzyme A, the intermediary product in energy metabolism. Also used to help form collagen, a connective tissue protein.
Cysteine (Glucogenic)	Cys	Conditionally essential amino acid that may become essential under certain metabolic conditions.	Methionine (Glucogenic)	Met	Restriction may lower obesity risk and improve longevity in humans, but may also lower production of other amino acids
Glutamic acid (Glucogenic)	Glu	Important neurotransmitter and used as part of the flavor enhancer monosodium glutamate.	Phenylalanine (Glucogenic and Ketogenic)	Phe	Important for production of neurotransmitters norepinephrine, and epinephrine.
Glutamine (Glucogenic)	Gle	Conditionally essential amino acid that may become essential under certain metabolic conditions.	Threonine (Glucogenic and Ketogenic)	The	Used in the synthesis of proteins and glycine.
Glycine (Glucogenic)	Gly	A building block in protein synthesis, and functions as a neurotransmitter.	Tryptophan (Glucogenic and Ketogenic)	Trp	Used to synthesize the neurotransmitters serotonin and melatonin, and the vitamin Niacin
Proline (Glucogenic)	Pro	Conditionally essential amino acid that may become essential under certain metabolic conditions	Valine (Glucogenic)	Val	Branched-chain amino acid that may be useful for muscle recovery and the immune system following exercise.
Serine (Glucogenic)	Ser	Important for normal neurological function.			
Tyrosine (Glucogenic and Ketogenic)	Tyr	Conditionally essential amino acid that may become essential under certain metabolic conditions. Used to manufacture dopamine, norepinephrine, and epinephrine.			
*Glucogenic: May undergo conversion to glucose and stored as carbohydrates (glycogen).					
*Ketogenic: May be degraded directly to acetyl-CoA, a precursor of ketones (common ketones include acetone, methylethyl ketone, and cyclohexanone)					
*Conditionally Essential: Usually not essential except in times of illness and/or stress					

Source: From National Academy of Sciences. Dietary reference intakes for energy, carbohydrates, fiber, fat, fatty acids, cholesterol, protein, and amino acids (macronutrients). National Academies Press; 2005. p. 591, 593; Negro M, Giardina S, Marzani B, Marzatico F. Branched-chain amino acid supplementation does not enhance athletic performance but affects muscle recovery and the immune system. J Sports Med Phys Fitness. 2008;48(3):347–51; Ruzzo EK, Capo-Chichi J-M, Ben-Zeev B, Chitayat D, Mao H, Pappas AL, Hitomi Y, Lu Y-F, Yao X, Hamdan FF, Pelak K, Reznik-Wolf H, Bar-Joseph I, Oz-Levi D, Lev D, Lerman-Sagie T, Leshinsky-Silver E, Anikster Y, Ben-Asher E, Olender T, Colleaux L, Décarie J-C, Blaser S, Banwell B, Joshi RB, He X-P, Patry L, Silver RJ, Dobrzeniecka S, Islam MS, Hasnat A, Samuels ME, Aryal DK, Rodriguiz RM, Jiang Y-H, Wetsel WC, McNamara JO, Rouleau GA, Silver DL, Lancet D, Pras E, Mitchell GA, Michaud JL, Goldstein DB. Deficiency of asparagine synthetase causes congenital microcephaly and a progressive form of encephalopathy. Neuron. 2013;80(2):429–41.

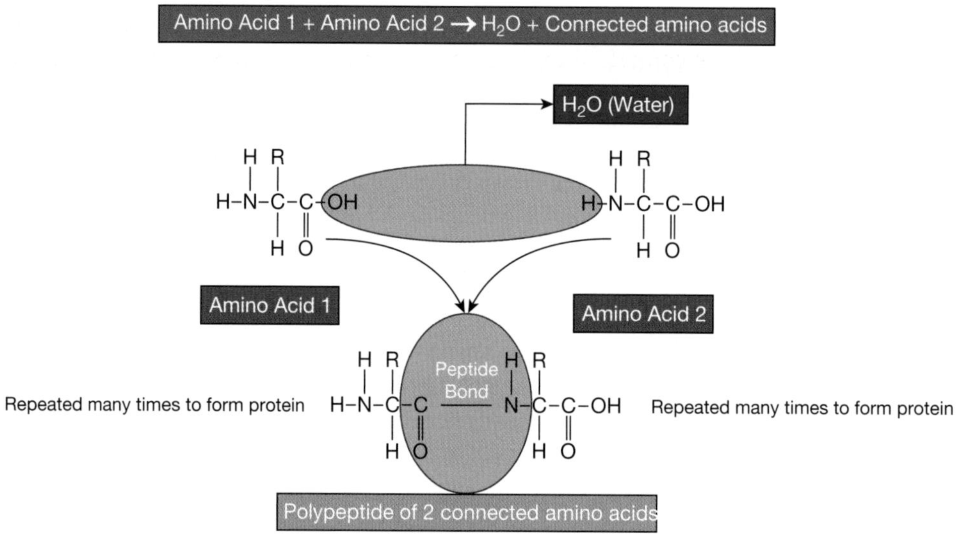

FIGURE 3.3: Proteins formed by connecting individual amino acids via peptide bonds.

Amino Acid 1 + Amino Acid 2 → H₂O + Connected amino acids

H_2O (Water)

Amino Acid 1

Amino Acid 2

Repeated many times to form protein

Peptide Bond

Repeated many times to form protein

Polypeptide of 2 connected amino acids

Polypeptide

A molecule consisting of a chain of amino acids held together by peptide bonds. The molecule is too small to be called a protein.

Essential Amino Acids

Amino acids that humans are incapable of synthesizing from other amino acid skeletons, making it essential that they be in consumed foods. Essential amino acids are also referred to as indispensable amino acids.

Nonessential Amino Acids

Nonessential Amino Acids are those amino acids that humans are capable of synthesizing from other amino acid skeletons, so it is nonessential that they be in consumed foods. Nonessential amino acids are also referred to as dispensable amino acids.

Glucogenic Amino Acids

Glucogenic amino acids are amino acids that can be converted to glucose through the process of gluconeogenesis in the liver. In humans, all amino acids with the exception of leucine and lysine are glucogenic. Alanine is a primary glucogenic amino acid with a robust liver pathway for converting alanine to glucose.

Ketogenic Amino Acids

Ketogenic amino acids are converted to ketones when catabolized. Isoleucine, phenylalanine, threonine, tryptophan, and tyrosine are both glucogenic and ketogenic, whereas leucine and lysine are only ketogenic.

Example:

(AA1+AA3+AA5+AA2+AA1+AA4)

and

(AA3+AA1+AA2+AA5+AA4+AA1)

will have different functions, although they contain the same amino acids, because the amino acids are held together in a different sequence.

All of the necessary amino acids must be present at the same time to build a protein, and as protein synthesis is coded by DNA, amino acid substitutions cannot be made. It is also important to consider that protein synthesis requires energy (calories) and is difficult to accomplish when someone is in a severely energy-deficient state. As the human system is highly adaptive, the synthesis of specific proteins can be stimulated through different actions. For instance, assuming sufficient energy and amino acids are available, an individual lifting weights that are heavier than that person is accustomed to will encourage the synthesis of more muscle protein to enable a more energy-efficient weight lifting.

Proteins have four structural components:

- *Primary structure:* the sequence of the amino acids that compose the protein and is, therefore, the main determinant of the protein's function.
- *Secondary structure:* the hydrogen bonds of the protein, which are connected to the primary structure of the protein.
- *Tertiary structure:* the protein's shape. For instance, the double-helix shape of DNA is part of the DNA protein tertiary structure.

- *Quaternary structure:* the number of polypeptides and proteins that are connected to the protein as side chains.

PROTEIN FUNCTIONS

The proteins we consume are digested into individual amino acids, and these amino acids interact with the amino acids produced by body tissues to make up the total pool of amino acids available to tissues. Tissues have multiple and different amino acid/protein requirements, as they have different functions. For instance, neurologic tissue requires neurotransmitters, which are specialized proteins for carrying nerve impulse messages; muscles require protein to produce and repair muscle; and so on. The main functions of proteins include:

- *Protective:* Proteins help to synthesize antibodies, which attack foreign substances, including bacteria and viruses, to protect the body from invasion and infection. An example of an important antibody is *immunoglobulin G.* Proteins also provide barrier defenses against invasion of bacteria and viruses through skin, tears (to protect the eyes), and mucin (in saliva, to protect the gastrointestinal tract).
- *Tissue structure:* Structural proteins provide the structure to support cell/tissue shape, including organs, muscles, bone, skin, hair, and nails. An example of a structural protein is collagen, which provides strength and resilience to body tissues. The creation of structural proteins is a necessary component of tissue growth and maintenance.
- *Messenger:* Some proteins, including hormones, transmit messages to specific tissues to determine and, literally, control how that tissue will function. For instance, the hormone estrogen provides messages for the creation and function of the uterus.
- *Transport:* Specific proteins are carriers of molecules that are critical to tissue function. As an example, the protein hemoglobin carries oxygen to cells and removes carbon dioxide from cells for normal cellular respiration. Other examples include *lipoproteins,* which carry lipids (fats) in the blood; *transferrin* and *ceruloplasmin,* which carry and transfer iron for the manufacture of hemoglobin; and protein-bound iodine, which is used to make the hormone thyroxine.
- *Enzymes and hormones:* These proteins control the chemical reactions that each cell has and, in doing so, are responsible for the creation of new molecules and tissues. **Enzymes** are the action arm of the genetic

information in each person's DNA. An example of an enzyme is pancreatic amylase, which breaks down large carbohydrate molecules into smaller molecules that can be absorbed. Another example is *phenylalanine hydroxylase*, which converts the amino acid phenylalanine to tyrosine, another amino acid. Examples of protein-based **hormones** include insulin, glucagon, and growth hormone. Amino acids also stimulate secretion of insulin, glucagon, growth hormone, and insulin-like growth factor-1, all of which are related to maintenance, recovery, and enlargement of the muscle mass (10).

- *Fluid balance:* Blood proteins are necessary for controlling fluid inside and outside tissues through osmotic pressure. Protein-deficient states are associated with fluid being lost from tissues and the resulting *edema* (Box 3.1).
- *Acid–base balance:* Proteins are *amphoteric,* as they have the capacity to pick up and release hydrogen, and by doing so they help to control body pH (relative acidity/alkalinity).
- *Nitrogen compound synthesis:* Proteins are involved in the synthesis of other small nitrogen-containing compounds, including creatine, purines, and pyrimidines. Creatine is involved in manufacturing *phosphocreatine,* the compound used for creating a large number of ATPs in extremely high-intensity activity. L-Carnitine is necessary for transporting lipids inside cells to the mitochondria of the cell, where the lipids can be metabolized for energy.
- A good protein intake that is consumed when in a good energy-balanced state helps to assure that amino acids will be available to synthesize these substances, rather than using the available protein to satisfy the energy requirement. It has been found, for instance,

Box 3.1	Edema

Edema refers to swelling resulting from a fluid shift from the blood and/or tissues to the fluid surrounding tissues, most commonly observed in hands, arms, feet, ankles, and legs. There are multiple causes of edema, including excess fluid intake, a compression of the veins in the lower belly from obesity or pregnancy that interferes with fluid flow to the upper body, heart failure, kidney disease, cirrhosis of the liver, and poor protein status. Pitting edema refers to a condition where pressing the swollen area with a finger results in a visible imprint (Figure 3.4).

**Edema, Which Occurs When Excess
Fluid is Trapped in Body Tissues**

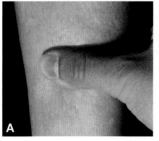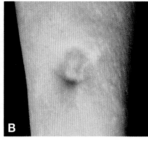

FIGURE 3.4: Pitting edema, a condition where pressing the swollen area with a finger results in a visible imprint. (From Strayer DS, Saffitz JE, Rubin E. Rubin's pathology: mechanisms of human disease. 8th ed. Wolters Kluwer; 2020.)

that female soccer players wishing to achieve a lower fat mass and a higher fat-free mass should consume protein while in a good energy-balanced state, and that those with energy balance deficits exceeding −400 kcal had higher body fat levels (11,12). Satisfying energy needs in real time to diminish the risk of poor energy availability also helps to diminish the risk of developing athlete "burnout" (13). It has also been found that distributing protein throughout the day in 20- to 35-g doses (larger amounts for larger athletes) to satisfy total protein needs is a better strategy for achieving a desired body fat loss than a less frequent protein consumption pattern (14).

In humans, some individual amino acids derived from the consumed proteins also have important biologic roles. Examples of these include the following:

- *Glycine* and *glutamic acid* are neurotransmitters.
- *Tryptophan* is a precursor of the neurotransmitter serotonin.
- *Glycine* is a precursor of heme (part of hemoglobin).
- *Arginine* is a precursor of nitric oxide (part of the process of delivering oxygen to cells).

SOURCES OF PROTEIN

Important Factors to Consider

- Virtually every food we eat has a wide array of amino acids, but not all foods have the essential amino acids in a ratio that allows them to be efficiently used by tissues to fulfill all protein functions. Therefore, athletes should strive to consume regular, small amounts (25–30 g) of good-quality protein from a variety of foods throughout the day to satisfy total tissue needs (1.2–2.0 g/kg/day).
- Although the highest sources of good-quality protein are meats, vegetarians can obtain good-quality protein by mixing foods in a way that improves the distribution of essential amino acids. This strategy of creating complementary proteins to improve protein quality has been practiced for generations by many cultures, including mixing beans with corn (Central and South American) and mixing beans with rice (Mediterranean basin and Asia). Consuming protein in this form also has the advantage of better sustaining a healthy gut microbiome, which is highly reliant on fiber and other nutrients commonly delivered by fruit, vegetables, and whole cereal (15–17). More information on the gut microbiome is covered in the Chapter 2.

Proteins and their component amino acids are found in nearly everything we consume that has not been processed to produce a single substance/chemical (for instance, table sugar). Different foods, however, have different *concentrations* of proteins and amino acids and different *distributions* of amino acids that affect the volume and quality of the protein consumed. The highest sources of protein (*i.e.*, highest volume with the best distribution of amino acids) come from animal-derived foods (*i.e.*, meat, fish, poultry, eggs, dairy), whereas plant-based foods provide the lowest concentrations of protein (*i.e.*, fruits and vegetables) (Table 3.2). This should not suggest, however, that vegetarians are incapable of satisfying protein needs. As indicated in Table 3.3, combining nonmeat foods in a way that improves amino acid distribution can serve to fully satisfy protein requirements. While consuming more plant-based protein would be necessary when compared to animal-based protein to satisfy athlete protein needs, the elevated consumption of these plant-based proteins may have certain benefits, including better meeting the carbohydrates requirement, improving/sustaining the gut microbiome, and helping to satisfy total body fluid needs (18).

MEASURING AND EVALUATING PROTEIN

Besides considering the *volume* of protein delivered from the foods consumed, the distribution of amino

Table 3.2	Selected Food Sources of Protein Based on Volume of Protein/g of Food
High source	▪ Meat • Beef • Lamb • Pork • Etc. ▪ Fish and shellfish ▪ Poultry ▪ Eggs
Moderately high source	▪ Dairy products ▪ Legumes • Beans • Peas • Lentils • Soy
Moderate source	▪ Cereal grains • Corn • Wheat • Rice • Barley • Oats ▪ Seeds and nuts • Cashews • Peanuts/peanut butter • Sesame seeds
Low source	▪ Fruits • Apples • Oranges • Grapes ▪ Vegetables • Broccoli • Leafy greens • Carrots

Table 3.3	Combining Nonmeat Foods to Improve Protein Quality	
Food	**Amino Acids That Are Low (Not Missing)**	**Foods That Can Improve Quality (Complementary Foods)**
Legumes (lentils, peas, beans, peanuts)	▪ Tryptophan ▪ Methionine	▪ Grains ▪ Nuts ▪ Seeds
Grains (wheat, corn, oats, rice, rye, barley)	▪ Lysine ▪ Isoleucine ▪ Threonine	▪ Legumes ▪ Dairy
Nuts and seeds (almonds, sunflower seeds, cashews, etc.)	▪ Lysine ▪ Isoleucine	▪ Legumes

Specific foods have different amino acid profiles. The amino acids listed in this table are based on averages for the food category.

Although it takes some additional planning, it is possible to obtain good-quality protein from nonanimal sources. It should also be considered that pure vegans (*i.e.*, those consuming *no* animal products) must also plan for other nutrients that may more easily be delivered through animal products, including iron, zinc, and vitamin B_{12}. With good planning, however, it is most definitely possible to consume all of the necessary nutrients from a plant-based diet.

Source: Pennington JAT, Douglass JS. Bowes & Church's food values of portions commonly used. 18th ed. Lippincott Williams & Wilkins; 2005. p. 264–314.

acids in the food should also be considered to determine the *quality* of the protein consumed. The higher the **protein quality**, the lower the volume of protein necessary to satisfy our biologic requirements for protein. Animal-based foods have both a high volume and a high quality of protein, whereas nonanimal foods have both lower volume and lower quality of protein. To a large extent, this can be corrected by combining specific plant-based foods to enhance their quality (*i.e.*, the distribution of essential amino acids). Some plant-based foods are low in a specific essential amino acid, whereas other plant-based foods are low in another specific essential amino acid. By combining them (*i.e.*, by eating them at the same time), the essential amino acid mix creates **complementary proteins** that improve the protein quality. Legumes, for instance, have low levels of tryptophan and methionine, whereas grains have low levels of lysine, isoleucine, and threonine. By combining legumes and grains, the distribution of essential amino acids is improved to make a good-quality protein. A common strategy for producing a good-quality protein is to consume peanut butter, which is low in tryptophan and methionine, with wheat bread, which is low in lysine, isoleucine, and threonine. The combination (a peanut butter sandwich) results in a higher-quality protein (Table 3.3). The typical strategy for improving plant protein quality is to consume legumes with grains, or legumes with nuts and seeds.

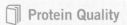 **Protein Quality**

A measure of the net utilization of the dietary protein consumed. There are several methods for determining protein quality, but all are related to the level of nitrogen retained compared with the level of nitrogen consumed. Nitrogen is only derived from protein-related products, and higher nitrogen retention means better tissue utilization and higher-protein quality.

Complementary Proteins

Two or more food sources that individually do not provide high-quality protein, but when combined they complement each other and provide a better distribution of the essential amino acids with higher-protein quality. As an example, combining legumes and cereal in a meal (such as beans and corn tortillas) produces a significantly higher-protein quality than eating either legumes or cereals by themselves.

The *ratio* of amino acids consumed at one time makes a difference in the protein quality (*i.e.*, what proportion of the amino acids consumed can be efficiently used metabolically for one or more of the protein functions listed earlier), and protein quality makes a difference in the proportion of amino acids that are deaminated (*i.e.*, have the nitrogen removed) so the remaining carbon chain can be stored as fat or burned for energy. The lower the quality of the protein consumed, the greater the proportion of nitrogen that is removed and that must be excreted (see Figure 3.1). As a way of visualizing this, Table 3.4 provides a worksheet for estimating how much protein will be retained and used as protein, lost and burned for energy, or stored as fat. The purpose of this table is to help the reader understand that a **complete protein** is determined by both the presence and the *ratio* of essential amino acids, which, together, help to determine protein quality and retention.

Complete Protein

Refers to protein that contains all of the essential amino acids in a concentration/ratio that is capable of supporting growth and preventing deficiency if consumed in appropriate quantities. The ratio of the essential amino acids makes an important difference in the anabolic potential of the protein. Not as much food with a superior amino acid distribution (*i.e.*, higher-quality protein) is required to satisfy the multiple functions of protein (19).

The main considerations for determining protein quality are as follows: (i) the characteristics of the protein and the food matrix in which it is consumed (*i.e.*, how available is the protein from the food that has been consumed) and (ii) the demands of the individual consuming the food, as influenced by age and growth phase (faster growth requires more protein), health status (illness often increases the tissue requirements for protein), physiologic status (activities that increase muscle breakdown require more protein for muscle repair), and energy balance (low energy balance limits protein utilization as humans are energy-first systems). Low energy balance results in the protein being used to satisfy energy requirements rather than being used for the multitude of other functions only proteins can satisfy (20). Clearly, protein status is a much more complicated issue than just how much protein is consumed.

The traditional methods for determining protein quality in humans involve the following:

- The assessment of nitrogen retention, which is referred to as 'Biological Value' (BV).
- The ability of consumed protein to enable tissue growth, which is referred to as 'Protein Efficiency Ratio' (PER).

Table 3.4	Complete Protein Worksheet to Estimate How Much Protein Is Retained or Lost								
	EAA1	EAA2	EAA3	EAA4	EAA5	EAA6	EAA7	EAA8	EAA9
Ideal	20	10	10	20	30	30	40	20	10
Eaten	10	10	10	20	30	30	40	20	10
Used	10	5	5	10	15	15	20	10	5
Lost	0	5	5	10	15	15	20	10	5

How to interpret this table:

1. "Ideal" is the hypothetically perfect distribution of the nine essential amino acids (EAAs) for optimal tissue utilization.
2. "Eaten" is the amino acid distribution in the protein food(s) that was actually consumed. Note that EAA1 is 50% of the ideal, whereas all of the other EAAs are provided in the ideal amounts.
3. "Used" represents the amount of EAA that can actually be used for protein metabolism. Since EAA1 was 50% of the ideal, to keep the ratio of EAA at the ideal ratio, only 50% of the other EAA can be used.
4. "Lost" represents the EAA that cannot be used for protein metabolism, so nitrogen is removed and the remaining carbon chain is stored as fat and/or "burned" to supply energy.

- Satisfying the amino acid requirements and the ability to digest the amino acids, which is referred to as 'Protein Digestibility-Corrected Amino Acid Score (PDCAAS)'.

Biologic Value

The *BV* is a measure of the protein absorbed from consumed foods that is incorporated into total body protein (skin, hair, muscle, organs, hormones, etc.). The proportion that is absorbed but not incorporated into body proteins is excreted. Since only protein contains nitrogen (N), nitrogen is used as an estimate of protein consumption, absorption, and excretion. Therefore, *nitrogen balance* is a measure of nitrogen consumed versus nitrogen excreted. The basic strategy is to have a known nitrogen content in the consumed meal, measure the nitrogen lost in fecal matter, which represents the amount of protein not absorbed, and measure the amount of nitrogen lost in the urine, which represents the amount of protein absorbed but not incorporated into body tissues. Higher quality (*i.e.*, better essential amino acid distribution) proteins have a higher rate of incorporation into body tissues and a lower rate of loss in the urine. The result provides a percent value, with a higher percent equal to a higher BV. The BV can also be compared with a test protein (typically egg albumin, which has a BV of 94%) to determine the quality of a protein compared with a known standard. A comparison of foods with different BV can be found in Table 3.5. The basic formula for BV is as follows (21):

$$BV = (\text{nitrogen retained/nitrogen absorbed}) \times 100$$

$$\text{Nitrogen retained} = \text{nitrogen absorbed} - \text{nitrogen excreted in urine}$$

$$\text{Nitrogen absorbed} = \text{nitrogen consumed} - \text{nitrogen excreted in feces}$$

📖 Nitrogen Balance

Nitrogen balance is a measure of protein adequacy, by providing a measure of the nitrogen consumed versus the nitrogen excreted. (Protein is the only energy substrate containing nitrogen, so measuring nitrogen provides an indirect measure of protein.) Positive nitrogen balance suggests incorporation of protein (which is nitrogen containing) into new tissues/products, whereas negative nitrogen balance suggests a net loss of protein-associated tissues/products. For example, child growth is a prime example of *positive* nitrogen balance and is observed in an athlete who is building muscle. Someone who is consuming insufficient energy will lose tissue weight and will metabolize protein to help satisfy the energy requirements, resulting in a *negative* nitrogen balance.

Table 3.5	Nitrogen and Protein Quality
Proportion of Nitrogen Retained	**Protein Quality Compared With Whole Egg Protein**
■ Whey protein: 96% retained ■ Whole soybean: 96% retained ■ Chicken egg: 94% retained ■ Cow's milk: 90% retained ■ Cheese: 84% retained ■ Rice: 83% retained ■ Fish: 76% retained ■ Beef: 74.3% retained ■ Soybean curd (tofu): 64% retained ■ Whole wheat flour: 64% retained ■ White flour: 41% retained	■ Whey protein: 1.04 ■ Egg protein: 1.00 ■ Cow's milk: 0.91 ■ Beef: 0.80 ■ Casein: 0.77 ■ Soy: 0.74 ■ Wheat protein (gluten): 0.64

Protein Efficiency Ratio

Protein efficiency ratio (PER) is a measure of the weight gained by a test animal (typically a baby rat, chick, or baby mouse) divided by the total protein consumed during a test period. The greater the gain in body mass for any given amount of protein, the higher the PER and, therefore, the better the quality of the protein consumed. In simple terms, if you give 100 g of protein X to a chick and it gains 20 g, and you give 100 g of protein Y to another chick and it gains 10 g, then protein X is a higher-quality protein. It has been observed that the PER may influence food tolerance in individuals who travel to environmental conditions (*i.e.*, high altitude, high humidity, etc.) that they are not well adapted to (22). Food manufacturers are also increasing efforts to elevate the PER of foods commonly consumed, such as high-protein pasta and goat milk whey fortified drink, to enable a way to more easily satisfy the protein requirement (23,24). The basic formula for PER is as follows (25):

$$PER = \text{Increase in body mass (g)/protein intake (g)}$$

Protein Digestibility–Corrected Amino Acid Score

PDCAAS is a method used by the United States Food and Drug Administration (FDA) and the Food and Agricultural Organization of the United Nations/World Health

Organization (FAO/WHO). It involves the determination of protein quality based on both the amino acid requirement and a human's capacity to digest it. The PDCAAS value of "1" is the highest possible value, and a value of "0" is the lowest possible value. It is based on the amino acid requirement of a 2- to 5-year-old child (the most protein-demanding age group per unit of mass) and the amino acid requirements adjusted for digestibility. The PDCAAS provides a protein quality ranking based on the amino acid profile of a specific food protein, compared with a standard amino acid profile with the highest possible score of "1." So, after digesting the protein, it would provide 100% or more of the essential amino acids required. The basic formula for PDCAAS is as follows (26):

PDCAAS = (mg of limiting amino acid in 1 g of test protein/mg of the same amino acid in 1 g of the reference protein) × digestibility percentage

Examples of PDCAAS values include:

- Casein (milk protein) = 1
- Egg white (albumin) = 1
- Whey protein (milk protein) = 1
- Beef = 0.92
- Chickpeas = 0.78
- Vegetables = 0.73
- Other legumes (beans, peas, etc.) = 0.70
- Peanuts = 0.52
- Whole wheat = 0.42

Digestible Indispensable Amino Acid Score

Digestible Indispensable Amino Acid Score (DIAAS) is recommended as a revised score of the PDCAAS by the FDA (27). The purpose of this score is to account for the different digestibilities of individual amino acids that are consumed. It is intended to be a more accurate means of assessing protein quality. DIAAS is defined as (28):

DIAAS % = 100 × [(mg of digestible dietary indispensable amino acid in 1 g of the dietary protein)/(mg of the same dietary indispensable amino acid in 1 g of the reference protein)]

DIAAS can be used as follows (27):

- For calculation of DIAAS in mixed diets for meeting the needs for quality protein, as humans consume proteins from varied protein sources in mixed diets.

- To document the additional benefit of individual protein sources with higher scores in complementing less nutritious proteins.
- For regulatory purposes to classify and monitor the protein adequacy of foods and food products sold to consumers.

An expert panel has concluded that the concept of DIAAS is a method preferable to PDCAAS for the assessment of protein and amino acid quality, but that the usage of DIAAS will be limited until there are good data on the digestibility of commonly consumed foods (29).

Table 3.5 displays protein quality using biologic value (the proportion of nitrogen retained) and the PDCAAS (the degree to which a consumed protein compares with egg albumin) (30,31).

High-quality proteins provide all of the essential amino acids in amounts that tissues can efficiently use. Foods of animal origin (meat, fish, dairy, eggs) deliver high-quality protein with an excellent distribution of the essential amino acids. Foods of plant origin have at least one limiting amino acid that is present in an amount lower than body tissues optimally require. However, different plant foods have different limiting amino acids, so combining different plant foods at the same meal (i.e., legumes with cereals) with different limiting amino acids improves the protein quality of the foods consumed. Lower-quality proteins result in a higher proportion of the amino acids being lost as protein, because the nitrogen is removed and the remaining carbon chain is either stored as fat or burned as a source of energy.

Consumption of too much protein at one time also results in removal of nitrogen from the excess amino acids, with the remaining fragments being stored as fat or burned as a source of energy. Put simply, exceeding the cellular capacity to metabolize protein anabolically will result in removal of nitrogen with the remaining carbon chain burned as fuel, converted to carbohydrates, or stored as fat. The removed nitrogen is potentially toxic and so must be removed, mainly through urine with a concomitant loss of body water. Therefore, low-quality protein consumption or excess protein consumption in conjunction with inadequate fluid intake exacerbates dehydration and kidney damage risk (32,33).

PROTEIN REQUIREMENTS

Important Factors to Consider

- Protein requirements are affected by numerous factors, including the growth phase (fast growth is associated with higher needs), gender, pregnancy/ lactation, and training intensity, duration, and type. A male adolescent athlete in the middle of the adolescent growth spurt will, therefore, have a far higher-protein requirement (g/kg) than a young adult male involved in the same sport.

- It is important to satisfy the total energy requirement with an adequate intake of carbohydrates and fats to ensure that the consumed protein can be used anabolically (*i.e.*, to build tissue and manufacture needed enzymes and hormones) rather than to be used to satisfy the energy requirement. Humans are "energy-first" systems and must satisfy the need for energy before manufacturing other substances needed for optimizing health and performance.

A number of factors influence protein requirements for physically active and inactive people, including the following (31,34):

- *Age (growth phase):* An individual who is growing (childhood, adolescent growth spurt, etc.) has a higher requirement for protein than people who are fully grown.
- *Gender (amount of muscle mass):* There are gender differences in muscle mass that influence protein requirements. Women typically have less muscle mass than men and would, therefore, have a lower protein requirement.
- *Pregnancy/lactation:* Women who are pregnant and/or lactating have a higher requirement for protein to enable fetal growth (pregnancy) and to provide sufficient protein to the breastfeeding infant (lactation).
- *Length of training at time of data collection:* Protein requirements are higher at the initiation of a new training regimen, as there are greater changes in tissues than in people who have adapted to the training.
- *Energy intake and exercise:* Inadequate energy intake and/or exercise that is not adequately supported with sufficient energy may result in protein tissue (muscle, bone, and organ) to help satisfy the requirement for energy. The subsequent necessity to repair these tissues increases protein requirement.
- *Type of exercise:* Some physical activity results in a greater breakdown of protein-based tissue, either to help supply energy or as a result of the nature of the activity, which may be tissue damaging. In either case, more protein would be required to repair the tissue damage.

Skeletal muscle and organ mass represent the major functional deposits of protein and constitute at least 60% of total body protein (35). Body proteins also exist in bone, blood plasma, and skin. There is no active "pool" of protein or amino acids for the body to draw upon when needed, so a failure to provide sufficient energy and protein of adequate quality in a timely fashion will cause a breakdown of existing body proteins to satisfy needs (36). This is an intricate balance that must satisfy current metabolic needs, tissue recovery requirements, and future goals that, for an athlete, may include an enlargement of the muscle mass. It is clear that consuming insufficient protein causes a failure to satisfy metabolic requirements and may compromise the immune system, tissue development, and tissue repair (34,35). However, having protein in excess of 2 g/kg/day may increase dehydration risk, lower bone mineral density, increase the risk for kidney stones, and increase the risk of kidney failure (37–39). To make matters even more complicated, it seems clear that total daily recommendations for protein may be misleading, as they fail to address the following important factors:

- Total daily protein requirement can be estimated based on growth phase, activity, and physiologic goals (40).
- Humans can only process a limited quantity of protein at one time (~20–25 g), suggesting that the amount of protein provided at each meal be considered.
- Maximally stimulating postexercise muscle recovery is best accomplished when protein is consumed in the period immediately postexercise, indicating that timing of intake is an important factor.
- Protein is best used metabolically when individuals are in a state of anabolic energy balance state (*i.e.*, they have not burned more energy than they have consumed), so satisfying energy needs is an important factor in allowing protein to be used anabolically rather than to satisfy the energy requirement (Figure 3.5).
- Consumption of too much total protein over time and too much protein at a single meal can be damaging to both bones and kidneys and may result in a state of dehydration.

DIGESTION, ABSORPTION, AND METABOLISM OF PROTEIN

Digestion

The purpose of protein digestion is to break complex proteins down into their component amino acids. Although the mouth has no protein-digesting enzymes, the saliva (primarily water) helps to denature the consumed proteins (break down some of the bonding structures of the

Possible Pathways for Protein Not Used Anabolically

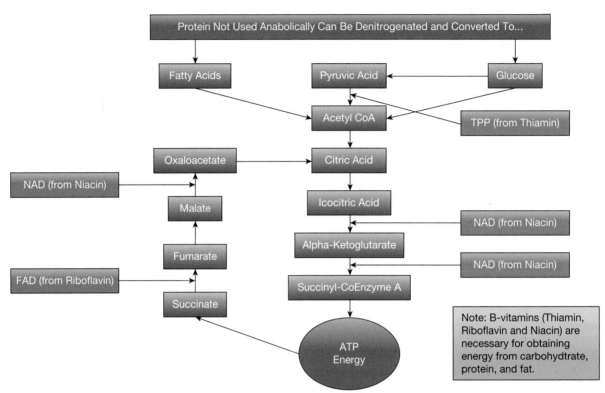

FIGURE 3.5: Citric Acid Cycle (also referred to as "Krebs Cycle" and the "Triacarboxylic Acid Cycle").

protein) and the protein is also "chewed" in the mouth, allowing greater access to protein-digesting enzymes to access protein bonds later in the digestive tract. Once in the stomach, the acidity of the stomach (reaching a pH of 1–2) helps to further denature the protein, and the primary protein-digesting enzyme, pepsin (also referred to as gastric protease), begins the process of breaking down proteins into amino acids. Pepsin breaks down the consumed protein by attacking the peptide bonds that hold amino acids together. This is a step-wise process, with proteins first being broken down into polypeptides (smaller protein) and then eventually into individual amino acids.

Once the stomach contents, including the partially digested proteins (polypeptides and some amino acids), are released into the small intestine, the pancreas releases pancreatic juice and the digestive enzymes trypsin, chymotrypsin, and carboxypeptidase into the small intestine. The pancreatic digestive enzymes are sometimes referred to together as *pancreatic proteases.* The pancreatic juice is highly alkaline and changes the acid pH of the stomach contents to neutral (pH = 7). The shift in pH from highly acidic to neutral further contributes to denaturing of the protein, making the digestive enzymes more effective (Table 3.6).

Absorption

With the digestive process complete, the amino acids are absorbed into the blood through the small intestine. Most protein absorption occurs in the jejunum and ileum. In a healthy individual, protein digestion is highly effective, so only a small proportion of dietary protein is typically lost in the fecal matter. It is important to note that aging commonly results in a reduction in gastric HCl, which makes it more difficult for some older adults to efficiently digest all proteins. Once in the blood, most amino acids are processed by the liver, whereas BCAAs can be processed by the liver, muscle, and other tissues. The metabolism of amino acids involves manufacturing the specific proteins required by the body to function (Figure 3.6).

Important Factors to Consider

■ It is incorrect to think that consumption of a specific protein will result in the manufacture of more of that protein. Once the protein is digested into its individual amino acids and delivered to tissues, the tissues manufacture proteins based on genetic command that are needed for survival and health.

Table 3.6	**Protein-Specific Digestive Enzymes**
Pepsin	Pepsinogen is released by the chief cells of the stomach, and the pepsinogen is converted to pepsin when the pH of the stomach becomes lower (from pH of 7 to 1–2) from the release of hydrochloric acid by the parietal cells of the stomach. The lower pH is a signal that the stomach is in the process of digesting proteins. Pepsin is a primary digestive enzyme, involved in breaking down consumed proteins to polypeptides and amino acids by cleaving the peptide bonds that hold together the amino acids that constitute the protein.
Trypsin	A digestive enzyme produced by the pancreas and enters the small intestine via the common pancreatic bile duct. It breaks down proteins and polypeptides into smaller polypeptides and individual amino acids in the duodenum of the small intestine.
Chymotrypsin	A digestive enzyme produced by the pancreas and enters the small intestine via the common pancreatic bile duct. It has a slower breakdown rate than trypsin, particularly for polypeptides that contain leucine and methionine. Chymotrypsin continues the digestive process initiated by pepsin and trypsin, digesting polypeptides into individual amino acids.
Carboxypeptidase	A digestive enzyme produced by the pancreas and enters the small intestine via the common pancreatic bile duct. It specifically breaks down the acid end of protein and/or polypeptide molecules.

■ As an example, gelatin sold in your local grocery store often advertises itself as being good for making healthy hair and nails. Although gelatin is a relatively low-quality protein that is a major component of hair and nails, eating hair and nails (*i.e.*, gelatin) does not mean that you will have healthy hair and nails!

Metabolism

Proteins are digested into their component amino acids, and these amino acids are absorbed into the blood where they are delivered to tissues to be synthesized into new proteins or metabolized for energy. If the amino acids delivered to tissues exceed current needs, they

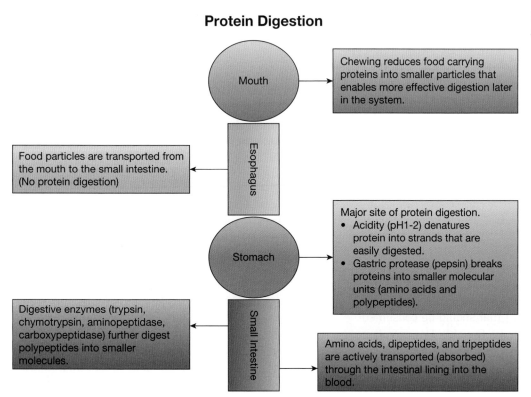

Protein Digestion

FIGURE 3.6: Digestion and absorption of protein.

Mouth → Chewing reduces food carrying proteins into smaller particles that enables more effective digestion later in the system.

Esophagus → Food particles are transported from the mouth to the small intestine. (No protein digestion)

Stomach → Major site of protein digestion.
- Acidity (pH1-2) denatures protein into strands that are easily digested.
- Gastric protease (pepsin) breaks proteins into smaller molecular units (amino acids and polypeptides).

Small Intestine → Digestive enzymes (trypsin, chymotrypsin, aminopeptidase, carboxypeptidase) further digest polypeptides into smaller molecules.

Amino acids, dipeptides, and tripeptides are actively transported (absorbed) through the intestinal lining into the blood.

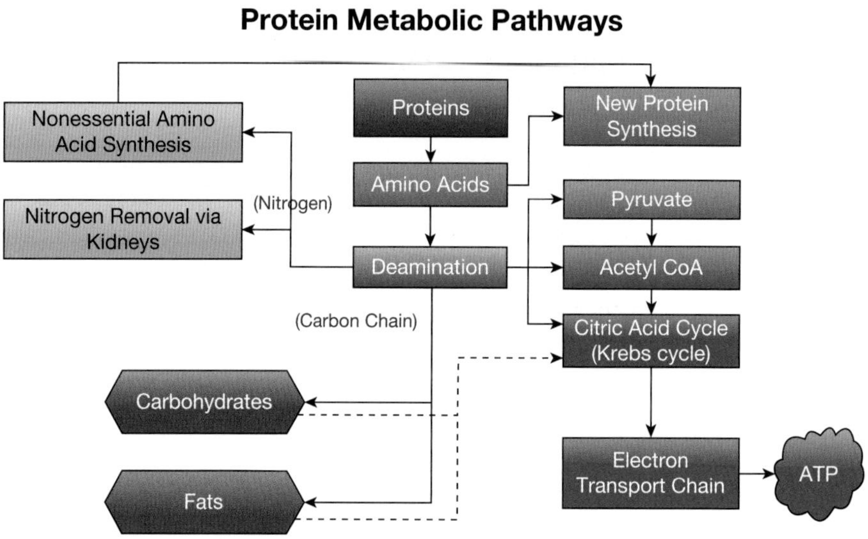

FIGURE 3.7: Protein metabolism. ATP, adenosine triphosphate; CoA, coenzyme A.

Protein Metabolic Pathways

are deaminated (*i.e.*, the nitrogen is removed) and the remaining carbon chain is converted to glucose (gluconeogenesis) or stored as fat (Figure 3.7). The removed nitrogen is either incorporated into a new nonessential amino acid in a process referred to as *transamination* (the transfer of nitrogen from one amino acid, which has had the nitrogen removed, to a newly created nonessential amino acid) or removed via the kidneys. The newly created nonessential amino acids are used to synthesize new proteins.

The deaminated amino acid can also be used to create pyruvic acid, acetyl coenzyme A (the intermediary product in all energy metabolism), or can go directly into the **citric acid cycle**, all of which are products that can go into the electron transport chain for the creation of ATP (energy). Consider, however, that all amino acids used to create ATP must have the nitrogen removed, which has the potential to create kidney stress if the amount of protein consumed is high.

PROTEIN INTAKE RECOMMENDATIONS

Important Factors to Consider

- The recommendations for protein intake are based on age, gender, pregnancy/lactation, and level of activity. In each case, these recommendations are based on the amount that should be consumed per day and per kg mass (weight). However, it is important to remember that the daily requirement cannot be consumed at a single meal, because

that amount of protein would exceed the body's capacity to metabolize it properly. Depending on body size, the total daily protein requirement should be distributed evenly throughout the day in 25–30 g portions to optimize tissue utilization.

- It is relatively easy to consume protein at the level of the established requirement from typically consumed foods. Protein supplements are typically not necessary and may keep athletes from consuming foods that can provide the energy and other nutrients needed to ensure that the consumed protein will be used anabolically rather than to help support the need for energy.

Protein intake recommendations for the general public in the United States are in the range of 10%–35% of total calories for healthy adults, with slightly less for children and adolescents (Table 3.7). This range is based on (41):

- 0.80 g protein/kg weight/day for adults,
- 0.85 g protein/kg weight/day for adolescents,
- 0.95 g protein/kg weight/day for preadolescents aged 4–13 years, and
- 1.10 g protein/kg weight/day for 1- to 3-year-olds.

These values differ from the recommendations of the WHO (42), which suggests an intake of 0.83 g protein/kg weight/day of good-quality protein for all healthy adults of both genders and at all ages. For some groups, this value is considerably less than the upper level of the protein intake recommendation of the U.S. Institute of Medicine (IOM) (41), corresponding to ~8%–10% of total calories consumed. The Nordic Nutrition recommendations are

Table 3.7		Institute of Medicine Protein and Amino Acid Requirements				
Nutrient	Function	Life Stage Group	RDA/AI* g/d[a]	AMDR[b]	Selected Food Sources	Adverse Effects of Excessive Consumption
Protein and amino acids	Serves as the major structural component of all cells in the body and functions as enzymes, in membranes, as transport carriers, and as some hormones. During digestion and absorption, dietary proteins are broken down into amino acids, which become the building blocks of these structural and functional compounds. Nine of the amino acids must be provided in the diet; these are termed indispensable amino acids. The body can make the other amino acids needed to synthesize specific structures from other amino acids.	Infants 0–6 mo 7–12 mo Children 1–3 y 4–8 y Males 9–13 y 14–18 y 19–30 y 31–50 y 50–70 y >70 y Females 9–13 y 14–18 y 19–30 y 31–50 y 50–70 y >70 y Pregnancy ≤18 y 19–30 y 31–50 y Lactation ≤18 y 19–30 y 31–50 y	9.1* 11.0 13 19 34 52 56 56 56 56 34 46 46 46 46 46 71 71 71 71 71 71	ND[c] ND 5–20 10–30 10–30 10–30 10–35 10–35 10–35 10–35 10–30 10–30 10–35 10–35 10–35 10–35 10–35 10–35 10–35 10–35 10–35 10–35	Proteins from animal sources, such as meat, poultry, fish, eggs, milk, cheese, and yogurt provide all nine indispensable amino acids in adequate amounts, and for this reason are considered "complete proteins." Proteins from plants, legumes, grains, nuts, seeds, and vegetables tend to be deficient in one or more of the indispensable amino acids and are called "incomplete proteins." Vegan diets adequate in total protein content can be "complete" by combining sources of incomplete proteins, which lack different indispensable amino acids.	Although no defined intake level at which potential adverse effects of protein were identified, the upper end of AMDR is based on complementing the AMDR for carbohydrates and fat for the various age groups. The lower end of the AMDR is set at approximately the RDA.

The table represents recommended dietary allowances (RDAs) in **bold type**, adequate intakes (AIs) in ordinary type followed by an asterisk (*). RDAs and AIs may both be used as goals for individual intake. RDAs are set to meet the needs of almost all (97%–98%) individuals in a group. For healthy breast-fed infants, the AI is the mean intake. The AI for other life stage and gender groups is believed to cover the needs of all individuals in the group, but lack of data prevent being able to specify with confidence the percentage of individuals covered by this intake.

[a]Based on 1.5 g/kg/d for infants, 1.1 g/kg/d for 1–3 y, 0.95 g/kg/d for 4–13 y, 0.85 g/kg/d for 14–18 y, 0.8 g/kg/d for adults, and 1.1 g/kg/d for pregnant (using prepregnancy weight) and lactating women.

[b]Acceptable macronutrient distribution range (AMDR) is the range of intake for a particular energy source that is associated with reduced risk of chronic disease while providing intakes of essential nutrients. If an individual consumes in excess of the AMDR, there is a potential of increasing the risk of chronic diseases and insufficient intakes of essential nutrients.

[c]ND = Not determinable due to lack of data on adverse effects in this age group and concern with regard to lack of ability to handle excess amounts. Source of intake should be from food only to prevent high levels of intake.

Source: Institute of Medicine. Dietary reference intakes for energy, carbohydrates. fiber, fat, fatty acids, cholesterol, protein, and amino acids (2002/2005). The National Academies Press; 2005. Accessed 2018 April 19. Available from: www.nap.edu

all less than the IOM recommendations, ranging from 10% to 20% of total energy consumed, with an average of 15% of total calories from protein for dietary planning purposes. This translates to 1.1–1.3 g protein/day for healthy adults, and slightly more for those aged over 65 years (1.2–1.5 g protein/kg).

The protein intake recommendations for active people ranges from 1.2 to 1.7 g protein/kg weight/day, depending on type and duration of activity, age, and gender (8,30). Typical recommendations for endurance athletes are 1.2–1.4 g protein/kg weight/day and for strength-trained athletes from 1.6 to 1.7 g protein/kg weight/day (43,44). These higher requirements in athletes are based on higher lean (muscle) mass, a greater exercise-associated loss of protein in the urine, more protein "burned" as a source of energy, and a greater requirement for muscle repair

(30,31,45). However, it should also be considered that endurance athletes may fail to satisfy total energy needs during prolonged activity, creating a higher reliance on protein in these individuals to replace the protein tissue that was lost to satisfy energy needs (46). As demonstrated in Table 3.8, most athletes can easily consume far more protein than the upper level of these ranges from food alone (39).

Most athletes have energy requirements that are considerably higher than same-weight nonathletes, making it far easier to obtain the needed protein if energy requirements are satisfied. Numerous studies have found that athlete protein intake is often in the range of 2–2.5 g/kg/day, and as high as 3 g/kg/day, values that represent nearly double the upper end of the desirable range. Despite the easy access of protein from foods alone, the diets of some

Table 3.8 — Protein Content of Commonly Consumed Foods, Providing ~2,350 Calories

Meal	Food	Amount	Calories	Protein (g)
Breakfast	Orange juice	1 cup (8 oz)	112	1.74
	Whole wheat bread, toasted	2 slices	161	7.97
	Almond butter	1 tbsp	98	3.35
	Whole egg, hard boiled	2 large eggs	156	12.58
Mid-AM snacks	Banana	1 medium	109	1.20
	Peanuts	1 oz	166	4.84
Lunch	Roast beef sandwich			
	▪ Lean roast beef	2 oz	65	10.56
	▪ Whole wheat bread	2 regular slices	161	7.97
	▪ Mustard	1 tsp	3	0.19
	▪ Lettuce	1/3 cup (shred)	2	0.02
	Milk, 1% fat	8 oz (1 cup)	102	8.22
	Strawberries, fresh	1 cup	49	1.02
Mid-PM snacks	Apple, raw	1 medium	95	0.47
	Sports beverage[a]	16 oz	127	0.00
Dinner	Chicken breast (no skin) baked	3 oz	147	26.29
	Broccoli, boiled	1 large stalk	98	6.66
	Potato, baked with melted low-fat cheddar cheese	1 medium potato / 1 oz	145 / 49	3.06 / 6.90
	Multigrain bread	1 slice	69	3.47
	Frozen yogurt (vanilla)	½ cup	114	2.88
Evening snacks	String cheese (low fat)	1 stick (1 oz)	49	6.90
	Fresh orange	1 Orange	69	0.21
	Total Calories and Protein (g)		**2,339**	**126.30**

Based on the maximum recommendation of 2.0 g protein/kg/d a 120 lb (55 kg) athlete consuming these foods would require a maximum of 110 g protein/d, and these foods provide 126.30 g protein.
[a]Consumed as part of physical activity/training.

athlete groups should be carefully assessed to ensure an adequate intake. These groups include (47):

- Athletes who are in a growth phase have a high energy and protein requirement from the combined demands of growth and physical activity. These athletes are often in school settings where getting sufficient food during the day may present difficulties.
- Athletes who restrict food consumption to achieve a lower weight. Food restriction compromises both energy and protein consumption, making it difficult to satisfy protein functions.
- Vegetarian athletes who avoid all animal products, which are the highest sources of protein. Although it is possible for vegetarian athletes to obtain the protein they require, doing so requires planning.

As indicated in Chapter 2, carbohydrates have a protein-sparing effect. That is, if sufficient carbohydrates are consumed to satisfy a sufficient proportion of the energy (calorie) requirement, the consumed protein is not used for energy, therefore making it available to satisfy other functions that are specific to protein. Therefore, protein consumption adequacy can only be viewed in the context of whether sufficient total energy has been consumed. Using the acceptable macronutrient distribution ranges of the IOM, Phillips et al. (39) have predicted the endurance and strength athlete macronutrient ranges (Table 3.9).

Protein and Athletic Performance

Maintaining, Building, and Repairing Muscle

Improving physical performance is a clear goal for athletes and many studies have been conducted to assess how best to achieve this goal through dietary modifications.

It is clear that athletic performance is improved with a lean body mass that enhances the strength-to-weight ratio (48). Studies have found that specific nutritional compounds, when consumed at the right times and in the right amounts, may serve to enhance athletic performance. The essential amino acid *leucine* is known to be a regulator in protein metabolism, including helping to reduce muscle protein breakdown and to stimulate MPS (Tables 3.10 to 3.12).

Muscle protein constantly changes through the breakdown of existing proteins and the synthesis of new proteins (49). This process varies dramatically over the course of a single day, but it is now known that a prolonged period with no food consumption results in a decreased protein synthesis of between 15% and 30% below normal levels, and this catabolic period continues until energy (calories) and amino acids are ingested to stimulate the process of protein synthesis (49). Skeletal muscle is highly responsive to dietary protein and energy intake, and exercise stimulates both MPS and muscle protein breakdown (50–52). Muscle protein acquisition results when there is either increased MPS or decreased muscle protein degradation, so for muscle enlargement to occur, MPS must surpass muscle protein breakdown (53). Consumption of high-quality protein that provides the essential amino acids is essential in encouraging postexercise MPS. Muscle activity and the availability of nutrients strongly influence exercise-induced adaptive changes in muscle (54,55), and a failure to provide sufficient energy and protein soon after an exercise bout will compromise optimal muscle recovery and maintenance (53,56). It has been shown that consumption of protein/amino acids (>15 g) following resistance exercise effectively increases MPS rates (57). It is well established that

Table 3.9	Macronutrient Distribution Ranges for Endurance and Strength Athletes		
Macronutrient	**Dietary Energy (AMDR)[a] (%)**	**AMDR for Endurance Athletes[b] (%)**	**AMDR for Strength Athletes[c] (%)**
Carbohydrates	45–65	55–80	30–65
Fat	20–35	10–25	15–30
Protein	10–35	10–20	20–40

[a]The acceptable macronutrient distribution range (AMDR) of the Institute of Medicine represents "…a range of intakes for a particular energy source that is associated with reduced risk of chronic diseases while providing adequate intakes of essential nutrients."

[b]Derived based on recommendations for carbohydrates intake for optimizing performance.

[c]Derived based on recommendations for protein requirements from retrospective nitrogen balance analysis, and working upward from those estimates to include sufficient nutrients for health, as well as the elevated energy requirements for these athletes to maintain an increased skeletal muscle mass.

Source: Institute of Medicine. Dietary reference intakes for energy, carbohydrates, fiber, fat, fatty acids, cholesterol, protein and amino acids. Food and Nutrition Board. Washington (DC): National Academies Press; 2005; Phillips SM, Moore DR, Tank JE. A critical examination of dietary protein requirements, benefits, and excesses in athletes. Int J Sport Nutr Exerc Metab. 2007;17:S58–76.

Table 3.10 — Summary of Human Studies Related to Dietary Intake of Leucine or Supplementation

Reference	Population	Design	Findings
Alvestrand et al. (89)	12 females	Infusion with intravenous leucine.	Plasma and intracellular levels of AAs decreased, and 40% of excess leucine was oxidized.
Bohé et al. (90)	21 humans	Infusion with mixed AAs at 240% above basal levels.	MPS became saturated at high concentrations of intramuscular EAAs.
Rennie et al. (91)	Humans	Infusion with mixed AAs or leucine.	Leucine stimulated MPS to the same extent as complete meals.
Glynn et al. (92)	14 humans	Consumption of EAAs or EAAs with increased leucine content.	Leucine content in 10 g EAAs is sufficient to maximize MPS.
Casperson et al. (70)	Older humans	Meals supplemented with leucine for 2 wk.	Leucine improved MPS in response to lower protein meals.
Churchward-Venne et al. (63)	24 males	Completion of resistance exercise and consumption of varying doses of whey supplemented with leucine or EAAs without leucine.	Low doses of whey supplemented with leucine or EAAs stimulated MPS to the same degree as larger doses.
Nelson et al. (93)	12 males	Performed high-intensity endurance exercise and subsequently ingested leucine/protein supplement or control.	The high-leucine dose in the supplement saturated BCAA metabolism, increased leucine oxidation, and attenuated MPB.

AAs, amino acids; BCAA, branched-chain amino acid; EAAs, essential amino acids; MPB, muscle protein breakdown; MPS, muscle protein synthesis.

resistance exercise results in greater protein synthesis that continues for up to 48 hours postexercise (58). Therefore, individuals who wish to increase muscle mass must consume protein soon after exercising to gain a positive protein balance and capitalize on the enhanced muscle receptiveness to protein, but should also sustain a good energy balance with well-distributed protein consumption for the days following the resistance activity (59).

Table 3.11 — Summary of Human Studies Related to Timing, Dosing, and Long-Term Effects of Leucine Supplementation

Reference	Population	Design	Findings
Bohé et al. (90)	6 humans	Mixed AAs were infused by IV.	MPS rates declined rapidly after 2 h.
Gaine et al. (94)	7 humans	Consumption of controlled diet and performed aerobic exercise for 4 wk.	Leucine oxidation decreased as protein utilization improved.
Moore et al. (54)	6 young males	Performed resistance exercise then consumed differing amounts of protein.	Leucine oxidation increased after 20 g protein as MPS was maximally stimulated.
Churchward-Venne et al. (63)	24 males	Completed resistance exercise and consumed varying doses of whey supplemented with leucine or EAAs without leucine.	Low doses of whey supplemented with leucine or EAAs stimulated MPS to the same degree as larger doses.
Nelson et al. (93)	12 males	Performed high-intensity endurance exercise and subsequently ingested leucine/protein supplement or control.	The supplemental leucine dose saturated BCAA metabolism, increased leucine oxidation, and attenuated MPB.

AAs, amino acids; BCAAs, branched chain amino acids; EAAs, essential amino acids; MPB, muscle protein breakdown; MPS, muscle protein synthesis.

Table 3.12	Summary of Human Studies Related to the Effect of Leucine Supplementation on Breakdown of Muscle Protein		
Reference	Population	Design	Findings
Schena et al. (95)	16 humans	Trekked 21 day at high altitude and took either BCAA or placebo supplements.	BCAA supplementation decreased muscle loss during chronic hypobaric hypoxia.
Nair et al. (96)	6 healthy males	Leucine or saline infused intravenously.	Leucine decreased MPB across several muscle sites.
Koopman et al. (97)	8 elderly males	Consumed a control diet or one supplemented with leucine after exercise in crossover design.	Coingestion of leucine did not attenuate MPB.
Glynn et al. (92)	14 humans	Consumed EAAs with normal or high-leucine content.	Leucine supplementation showed a modest decrease in MPB.
Stock et al. (98)	20 trained humans	Performed resistance exercise and consumed a leucine-supplemented beverage before and after.	Leucine supplementation did not attenuate MPB.
Kirby et al. (99)	27 males	Performed drop jumps and consumed a placebo, leucine, or nothing.	Leucine supplementation did not attenuate MPB.
Nelson et al. (93)	12 males	Performed high-intensity endurance exercise and subsequently ingested leucine/protein supplement or control.	The high-leucine dose in the supplement saturated BCAA metabolism, increased leucine oxidation, and attenuated MPB.

BCAA, branched chain amino acids; EAAs, essential amino acids; MPB, muscle protein breakdown.

Branched-Chain Amino Acids

The three BCAAs, leucine, valine, and isoleucine, stimulate protein synthesis and inhibit protein breakdown, particularly in skeletal muscle, possibly because BCAAs are the only essential amino acids that are metabolized in muscle and other tissues, but not in the liver (55). Of the three BCAAs, the essential amino acid *leucine* appears to be the most potent stimulator of protein synthesis (60). A number of studies have assessed leucine's role in MPS and its role in reducing muscle protein loss in states of inadequate energy consumption (*i.e.*, in a catabolic state) (49,61). It also appears that leucine regulates protein synthesis in cardiac muscle and adipose (fat) tissue (62).

The value of BCAAs, particularly leucine, in stimulating MPS may be misinterpreted, with athletes sometimes consuming large doses of supplemental protein and/or amino acids with an elevated leucine content. However, there are findings suggesting that metabolic pathway thresholds may be overwhelmed by single bolus doses that exceed ~20–25 g protein and equivalent AA intake, and consuming leucine in large bolus doses greater than these equivalents is not useful (63).

It is also possible that the onset of fatigue during exercise is attributed to changes in concentrations of the neurotransmitters serotonin, dopamine, and noradrenaline, which are dependent on serum amino acids being transported through the blood–brain barrier (64). The amino acids involved in the synthesis of these neurotransmitters use the same blood–brain barrier transporters as the BCAAs, with the possibility that excess leucine and other BCAAs may compete with the transporters and inhibit the production of neurotransmitters, resulting in premature fatigue (65). Supplemental intake of individual amino acids may cause problems, and it is important to remember that amino acids are normally consumed as part of an entire meal consisting of whole proteins, and that the consumed protein is associated with a parallel increase in blood glucose and insulin release, both of which enable leucine's action (60,66). Supplemental amino acids are devoid of carbohydrates, which provide the glucose and subsequent insulin. A good strategy for assuring optimal protein metabolism is to add high-leucine foods, including whey protein, eggs, poultry, fish, and kidney beans, to meals during postexercise recovery to aid MPS by increasing muscle hypertrophy, attenuating muscle breakdown, and maintaining net positive muscle

Distribution of Consumed Protein Makes a Difference in Muscle Development

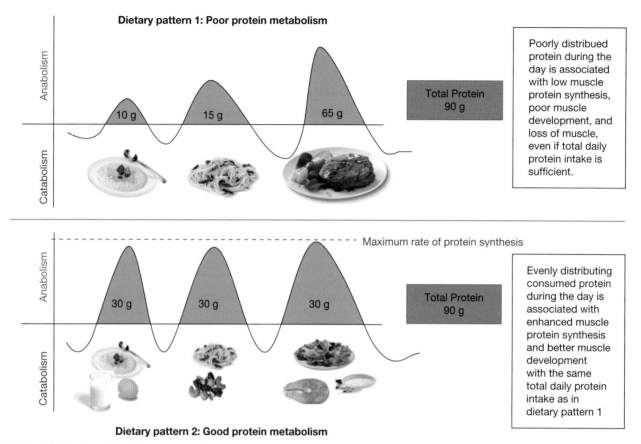

FIGURE 3.8: Protein distribution makes a difference in muscle development. (From Paddon-Jones D, Sheffield-Moore M, Zhang X-J, Volpi E, Wolf SE, Aarsland A, Ferrando AA, Wolfe RR. Amino acid ingestion improves muscle protein synthesis in the young and elderly. Am J Physiol Endocrinol Metab. 2004;286(3):E321–8.)

protein (67). It has also been found that large doses of supplemental leucine are not more effective than doses commonly ingested in a well-balanced healthy diet. Additionally, there are mixed results on whether large doses of leucine may induce detrimental health effects. Some studies have found that large doses are associated with insulin resistance (68,69), whereas other studies have found that increasing dietary leucine has a positive effect on insulin sensitivity (66). Despite the few lingering questions regarding a potentially negative health impact with high-dose intakes, consumption of high-leucine foods and leucine-enhanced foods and supplements (*e.g.*, whey protein food bars) postexercise has been found to enhance MPS across different populations.

The distribution of protein consumption during the day and its intake following exercise and periods of lower activity are also important considerations (see Tables 3.10 and 3.11). Aging is associated with lower MPS following ingestion of essential amino acids, but it has been found that proteins with a slightly elevated leucine content (*e.g.*,

whey protein) when provided in well-distributed intervals throughout the day, increase MPS in both young and older adults (9,70,71) (Figure 3.8).

As noted earlier, the provision of ~25 g of good-quality protein well distributed in daily meals appears sufficient to obtain the desired outcomes, assuming energy balance is sustained (39,72). Studies have determined that large doses of leucine are not more effective than good-quality foods and may negatively impact health (68,69).

From a practical standpoint, consumption of a beverage containing approximately 25 g of protein after heavy resistance training has the potential to improve MPS. Combining this protein with an equal caloric load of carbohydrates also helps to ensure better energy balance, allowing the protein-sparing effect of carbohydrates to manifest itself (so the protein can be used for muscle recovery rather than energy). The carbohydrates provided at this time also aid in glycogen recovery (73). Studies have found that chocolate milk, because of its combination of carbohydrates and high-quality protein that contains

High-Protein Diets May Increase Risk of Kidney Disease

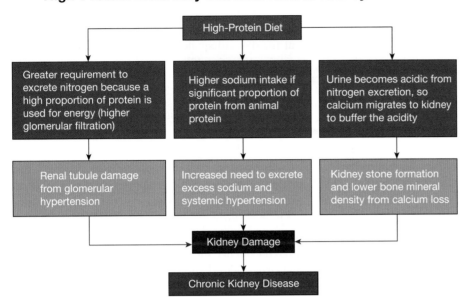

FIGURE 3.9: High-protein diets and increased risk of kidney disease. (Adapted from Marckemann P, Osther P, Pedersen AN, Jespersen B. High-protein diets and renal health. J Ren Nutr. 2015; 25(1):1–5.)

leucine, plus electrolytes (primarily sodium, chloride, and potassium) to help recover a hydrated state, is an effective postexercise replenishment beverage (74,75).

Risks of Too Much Protein

Many physically active people often consume high-protein diets, often at levels exceeding 2.0 g protein/kg or more than 25% of total calories from protein, primarily to enhance muscle mass and strength. There is little scientific support for consuming protein above 2.0 g/day, and there are no long-term data on the potential health effects of this level of regular protein consumption (76). There is an increasing body of evidence to suggest that chronic and excessively high intakes of protein, at levels *exceeding* 2.0 g/kg, may increase the risk of renal damage. A 2-year human intervention study assessing a relatively low-carbohydrate and relatively high-protein meat and dairy-based diet following the basic recommendations of the well-known Atkins Diet found that after 24 months, there were some signs of kidney function loss (77,78). Although this is unlikely to be a major concern for otherwise healthy people, this would be a particular concern for individuals who already have kidney dysfunction (32,79). Animal studies inducing these same high-protein, low-carbohydrate intakes have had similar findings (80). The proposed mechanism for the kidney damage is related to the combination of forced nitrogenous excretion, formation of kidney stones, and hypertension associated with the sodium in animal proteins. This review suggests that protein intakes exceeding 25% of total energy or more than 2–3 g/kg/day are not

recommended (38). Because the excreted urea and uric acid are acidic, blood calcium is used to buffer the acidity in the kidneys. This added calcium increases the risk for uric acid–calcium kidney stones (81,82). Because blood calcium levels cannot change (it is a major pH buffer in the blood), the calcium lost to the kidneys is replaced by calcium from bones, resulting in lower bone mineral density (37) (Figure 3.9).

The IOM has set the protein distribution range at 10%–35% of total calories consumed, with no upper limit on protein intake because of the lack of clearly associated health problems (41). It is common for high-protein intakes, often as much as 300 g/day, to be consumed without any apparent negative health effects. However, the long-term effects of this dietary pattern have not been adequately assessed (32). There is also concern that high-protein intakes above 2.0 g/kg/day negatively affect the consumption of carbohydrates, which could have an impact on performance (32).

SUMMARY

- The recommended protein intake (recommended dietary allowance) for the general adult population is 0.8 g/kg/day, with recommendations for active people in the range of ~1.2–2.0 g/kg/day. The timing of intake and the quality of protein consumed are also important considerations for athletes.
- Resistance activity helps to stimulate the enlargement of muscle mass if coupled with sufficient energy and protein up to 25 g consumed immediately within

2 hours postexercise. Protein intakes above this amount postexercise do not additionally stimulate protein synthesis but merely result in more urea synthesis and nitrogenous excretion (34,83).

■ The protein recommendation, compared with the other energy substrates (carbohydrates and fat), is relatively small for physically active people (~1.2–2.0 g protein/kg/day, compared with the 5.0–12.0 g carbohydrates/kg/day) (8). Ideally, this amount of protein should be evenly distributed during the day in amounts of ~25 g/meal to obtain the greatest benefit. It appears that an average protein intake of 1.25 g/kg/day (assuming sufficient total energy consumption) adequately compensates for muscle protein breakdown during long resistance and endurance exercise sessions (35).

■ The daily requirement of protein should be met with meals that provide a regular distribution of high-quality protein over the course of the day and following strenuous training (8).

■ Current protein recommendations are often expressed in terms of the regular spacing of modest protein intakes (~0.3 g/kg) following physical activity throughout the day. Adequate energy is required to optimize protein utilization (8).

■ High-quality proteins containing the amino acid leucine, particularly when consumed postexercise, are useful for MPS and for sustaining lean mass (8).

■ There is justifiable concern that, despite unanimous recommendations for high-carbohydrates intakes for athletes and recommendations for relatively low intakes of protein, athletes appear to consume far in excess of their need for protein, fail to optimally distribute protein during the day, and consume less than they require from carbohydrates (4,84). In addition, there is limited evidence for whether athletic females having a menstrual period should modify the current recommendations for protein and other energy substrates to better satisfy physiologic needs (85).

Practical Application Activity

Protein intake can be analyzed as a percent of total calories consumed (% protein), or as grams of protein/kg mass (g/kg). The preferred method is g/kg, as this provides an adjustment for the protein consumed based on body mass. Using % protein, it is possible for someone to have what appears to be a desirable protein consumption (*e.g.*, 15% of total calories), but if insufficient calories are consumed, the protein intake will be inadequate. You can assess your protein food intake for both % protein and g/kg following the same instructions provided in Chapter 1, accessing the online USDA Food Composition Database (86), (https://fdc.nal.usda.gov), but this time create a spreadsheet with Energy (calories) and Protein (g) and organize your foods by meal/eating opportunities. Create subtotals for each meal, and totals for the day, as follows:

Food (Adjusted for Consumed Amount)	Energy (Calories)	Protein (g)	Energy from Protein (g × 4)		
Meal 1					
Food 1~					
Food 2~					
Etc.~					
Meal 1 Totals					
Meal 2					
Food 1~					
Food 2~					
Etc.~					
Meal 2 Totals					
All meal Totals				% Energy from protein	Protein g/kg:
Recommended dietary allowance for protein (adjusted for age and sex)					
Difference between intake and recommended dietary allowance					

Note: Repeat meal format (Meal 1, Meal 2, Meal 3, etc.) above for as many eating opportunities that you had.

1. When completed, analyze the diet to view your protein consumption, including protein g/kg, and % energy from protein (calories from protein/total energy).
2. Review the foods that contribute most to your protein intake.
3. Determine if your protein consumption is adequate for a nonathlete (~0.8 g/kg) and for an athlete (~1.2–2.0 g/kg)
4. Assess if the intake of protein per meal is greater than ~30 g at any meal. On average, protein consumed in excess of 30 g/meal may not be efficiently metabolized as protein, with a proportion of the protein being used as energy or stored as fat rather than used anabolically to build and repair tissues, make hormones, etc.
5. If necessary, try to make adjustments to your diet by eating different foods and/or distributing the food consumed so that the consumed protein will be optimally metabolized.

CHAPTER QUESTIONS

1. The chemical composition of proteins differs from carbohydrates or fats because of the presence of:
   a. Sodium
   b. Carbon
   c. Nitrogen
   d. Hydrogen

2. Factors that determine protein quality:
   a. Quantity and rate of intestinal absorption
   b. Rate of utilization as an energy substrate
   c. Amount, type, and distribution of essential amino acids
   d. Digestibility
   e. a and c

3. To have a protein-sparing effect, athletes must consume sufficient:
   a. Nonessential amino acids
   b. Essential amino acids
   c. Carbohydrates
   d. Fluids

4. The anabolic potential of protein is best achieved if it is consumed in a single large dose of between 50 and 60 g.
   a. True
   b. False

5. The daily protein intake recommendation for strength athletes is:
   a. 0.8–1.0 g/kg
   b. 1.2–1.7 g/kg
   c. 2.0–3.8 g/kg
   d. >3.0 g/kg

6. Chronic consumption of excess protein may negatively affect the health of which organ?
   a. Pancreas
   b. Intestines
   c. Kidneys
   d. Brain

7. Because protein is an energy substrate, at least 20% of the total energy requirement should be derived from protein.
   a. True
   b. False

8. Which of the following amino acids is associated with stimulation of MPS?
   a. Leucine
   b. Phenylalanine
   c. Tryptophan
   d. Histidine

9. Protein consumption exceeding 30 g at a single meal may result in an increase in blood urea nitrogen, which is associated with both dehydration and lower bone mineral density.
   a. True
   b. False

10. Consumption of a specific protein will result in better synthesis of that protein. For instance, hair and nails both have a high content of the protein "gelatin," so consuming more gelatin in the diet will result in more healthy hair and nails.
    a. True
    b. False

ANSWERS TO CHAPTER QUESTIONS

1. c
2. c
3. c
4. b
5. b

6. c
7. b
8. a
9. a
10. b

Case Study Considerations

1. **Case Study Answer 1:** Calculate your body mass in kilograms by dividing weight in pounds by 2.2. For instance, if body weight is 140 lb, 140/2.2 = 63.6 kg. Assuming your protein requirement is in the middle of the range of 1.2–2.0 g/kg for an actively exercising person, your protein requirement would be 1.6 g/kg/day. This would make the total daily protein requirement (1.6 × 63.6) a total of ~102 g of protein/day. As this protein should be provided in per-meal amounts of approximately 25–30 g, this person would require about 4 meals/day of about 25 g of protein/meal to satisfy the protein requirement. To calculate the protein you are consuming and how it is distributed during the day, create a spreadsheet that includes the foods consumed, the amounts consumed, and the time it was consumed. Now go to USDA FoodData Central (https://fdc.nal.usda.gov) to find the foods consumed and the protein content of the foods, adjusted for the amount consumed. This is an important step in understanding both whether the total amount of consumed protein is desirable, and whether the distribution of the protein consumed will enable optimal metabolic use of the protein.

2. **Case Study Answer 2:** Using the information obtained in Case Study 1, calculate the protein requirement for three different individuals who weigh 100 lb (requiring about 25 g of protein per meal), 150 lb (requiring about 30 g of protein per meal), and 200 lb (requiring about 30 g of protein per meal). Then calculate the number of meals each person would require to optimally satisfy their protein requirement, assuming the required protein is in the middle of the optimal range (1.6 g/kg). For instance, a 200-lb person would require about 5 meals/day, with each meal providing about 30 g of protein. These calculations will demonstrate the difficulty of satisfying protein needs with 3 meals/day,

particularly if the protein in each meal is not well distributed.

3. **Case Study Answer 3:** Chronic excess protein consumption is associated with multiple disorders, including the following (87,88):
   - Skeletal disorders associated with urinary calcium loss because of a higher excretion of acidic nitrogenous waste (urea). The blood calcium, which is lost to neutralize the acidity in the kidneys, must be replaced to keep blood pH normal and is taken from bones, which lowers bone mineral density and increases fracture risk.
   - Disorders of kidney function because more nitrogenous waste must be excreted, increasing the risk of dehydration. This forces the kidneys to concentrate urine, which over time may result in kidney dysfunction.
   - Increased cancer risk, because high-protein consumers often obtain their protein from red meats, a dietary pattern that is associated with elevated cancer risk of the colon, stomach, rectum, pancreas, bladder, breast, and ovaries.
   - Disorders of liver function, resulting from elevations in amino acid transporters, and elevated blood albumin.
   - High-protein foods are often associated with higher-fat foods, which have been found to elevate cardiovascular disease risk.

4. **Case Study Answer 4:** Nutrition misconceptions are commonly held by athletes, making it difficult for an individual athlete to have food intake behaviors that are different from everyone around them. It is important, therefore, to determine how to best set up an environment that would enable *everyone* to automatically have appropriate food/protein intake behaviors. As an example, athletes who complete a day of training should have a recovery protocol that includes water and electrolytes (to recover from

underhydration), carbohydrates (to replace liver and muscle glycogen and maintain normal blood sugar), and protein (to enable better muscle recovery). Having appropriate foods/beverages available before and after training for everyone, makes it easier to satisfy needs.

REFERENCES

1. Marinaro M, Alexander DS, de Waal D. Do the high-protein recommendations for athletes set some on a path to kidney injury and dialysis? Semin Dial. 2021; Online ahead of print.
2. Eck KM, Byrd-Bredbenner C. Food choice decisions of collegiate division I athletes: a qualitative exploratory study. Nutrients. 2021;13(7):2322.
3. Hall ECR, Semonova EA, Bondareva EA, Hall ECR, Semenova EA, Bondareva EA, Andryushchenko LB, Larin AK, Cięszczyk P, Generozov EV, Ahmetov II. Association of genetically predicted BCAA levels with muscle fiber size in athletes consuming protein. Genes(Basel). 2022;13(3):397. https://doi.org/10.3390/genes13030397
4. Burke LM, Cox GR, Cummings NK, Desbrow B. Guidelines for daily carbohydrate intake: do athletes achieve them? Sports Med. 2001;31(4):267–99.
5. Katsanos CS, Kobayashi H, Sheffield-Moore M, Aarsland A, Wolfe RR. A high proportion of leucine is required for optimal stimulation of the rate of muscle protein synthesis by essential amino acids in the elderly. Am J Physiol Endocrino Metab. 2006;291(2):E381–87.
6. Symons TB, Sheffield-Moore M, Wolfe RR, Paddon-Jones D. A moderate serving of high-quality protein maximally stimulates skeletal muscle protein synthesis in young and elderly subjects. J Am Diet Assoc. 2009;109(9):1582–86.
7. Phillips SM. Defining optimum protein intakes in athletes. In: Maughan RJ, editor. Sports nutrition: the encyclopaedia of sports medicine-an IOC medical commission publication. Wiley Blackwell; 2014. p. 136–46.
8. Thomas DT, Erdman KA, Burke LM. American College of Sports Medicine Joint Position Statement. Nutrition and athletic performance. Med Sci Sports Exerc. 2016;48(3):543–68.
9. Paddon-Jones D, Sheffield-Moore M, Zhang X-J, Volpi E, Wolf SE, Aarsland A, Ferrando AA, Wolfe RR. Amino acid ingestion improves muscle protein synthesis in the young and elderly. Am J Physiol Endocrinol Metab. 2004;286(3):E321–28.
10. Wilcox G. Insulin and insulin resistance. Clin Biochem Rev. 2005;26(2):19–39.
11. Delk-Licata A, Behrens CE, Benardot D, Bertrand BM, Chandler-Laney PC, Fernandez JR, Plaisance EP. The association between dietary protein intake frequency, amount, and state of energy balance on body composition in a women's collegiate soccer team. Int J Sports Med. 2019;5(3).
12. Behrens CE, Delk-Licata A, Benardot D, Bertrand BM, Chandler-Laney PC, Plaisance EP, Fernández JR. The relationship between hourly energy balance and fat mass in female collegiate soccer players. J Hum Sport Exerc. 2020;15(4):735–46.
13. Becker L, Dupke A, Rohleder N. Associations between C-reactive protein levels, exercise addition, and athlete burnout in endurance athletes. Front Psychol. 2021;12:615715.
14. Ruiz-Castellano C, Espinar S, Contreras C, Mata F, Aragon AA, Martínez-Sanz JM. Achieving an optimal fat loss phase in resistance-trained athletes: a narrative review. Nutrients. 2021; 13(9):3255.
15. Hughes RL, Holscher HD. Fueling gut microbes: a review of the interaction between diet, exercise, and the gut microbiota in athletes. Adv Nutr. 2021;12(6):2190–15.
16. Cai J, Chen Z, Wu W, Lin Q, Liang Y. High animal protein diet and gut microbiota in human health. Crit Rev Food Sci Nutr. 2022;62(22):6225–37.
17. Mancin L, Rollo I, Mota JF, Piccini F, Carletti M, Susto GA, Valle G, Paoli A. Optimizing microbiota profiles for athletes. Exerc Sport Sci Rev. 2021;49(1):42–9.
18. Pinackaers PJM, Trommelen J, Snijders T, van Loon LJC. The anabolic response to plant-based protein ingestion. Sports Med. 2021;51(Suppl 1):S59–S74. https://doi.org/10.1007/s40279-021-01540-8
19. Park S, Church DD, Schutzherr SE, Azhar G, Kim I-Y, Ferrando AA, Wolfe RR. Metabolic evaluation of the dietary guidelines' ounce equivalents of protein food sources in young adults: a randomized controlled trial. J Nutr. 2021;151(5):1190–96.
20. Millward DJ, Layman DK, Tomé D, Schaafsma G. Protein quality assessment: impact of expanding understanding of protein and amino acid needs for optimal health. Am J Clin Nutr. 2008;87(5):1576S–81S.
21. Moore DR, Soeters PB. The biological value of protein. In: Meier RF, Reddy BR, Sorters PB, editors. The importance of nutrition as an integral part of disease management. Vol. 82. Nestec Ltd., Vevey/S. Karger; 2015. p. 39–51.
22. Anusha MB, Shivanna N, Kumar GP, Anilakumar KR. Efficiency of selected food ingredients on protein efficiency ratio, glycemic index and in vitro digestive properties. J Food Sci Technol. 2018;55(5):1913–21.
23. Messia MC, Cuomo F, Falasca L, Trivisonno MC, Arcangeli ED, Marcone E. Nutritional and technological quality of high protein pasta. Foods. 2021;10(3):589.
24. Garay PA, Villalva FJ, Paz NF, de Oliveira EG, Ibarguren C, Alcocer JC, Curti CA, Ramón AN. Formulation of a protein fortified drink based on goat milk whey for athletes. Small Rumin Res. 2021; 201:106418. https://doi.org/10.1016/j.smallrumres.2021.106418
25. Chapman DG, Castillo R, Campbell JA. Evaluation of protein in foods. I. A method for the determination of protein efficiency ratios. Can J Biochem Physiol. 1959;37(5):679–86.
26. Schaafsma G. The protein digestibility-corrected amino acid score. J Nutr. 2000;130(7):1865S–67S.
27. Food and Agriculture Organization of the United Nations. Dietary protein quality evaluation in human nutrition: report of an FAO expert consultation. FAO food and nutrition paper. FAO; 2013. ISBN 978-92-5-107417-6.
28. Mathal JK, Liu Y, Stein HH. Values for digestible indispensable amino acid scores (DIAAS) for some dairy and plant proteins may better describe protein quality than values calculated using the concept for protein digestibility-corrected amino acid scores (PDCAAS). Br J Nutr. 2017;117(4):490–99.
29. Lee WTK, Weisell R, Albert J, Tomé D, Kurpad AV, Uauy R. Research approaches and methods for evaluating the protein

quality of human foods proposed by an FAO expert working group in 2014. J Nutr. 2016;146(5):929–32.

30. Rodriguez NR, DiMarco NM, Langley S; American Dietetic Association; Dietitians of Canada; American College of Sports Medicine. American College of Sports Medicine position stand. Nutrition and athletic performance. Med Sci Sports Exerc. 2009;41(3):709–31.

31. Tarnopolsky MA, MacDougall JD, Atkinson SA. Influence of protein intake and training status on nitrogen balance and lean body mass. J Appl Physiol(1985). 1988;64(1):187–93.

32. Tipton KD. Efficacy and consequences of very-high-protein diets for athletes and exercisers. Proc Nutr Soc. 2011;70(02):205–14.

33. Marinaro M, Alexander DS, de Waal D. Do the high-protein recommendations for athletes set some on a path to kidney injury and dialysis? Semin Dial. 2021:1–6.

34. Phillips SM. Dietary protein requirements and adaptive advantages athletes. Br J Nutr. 2012;108(S2):S158–67.

35. Poortmans JR, Carpentier A, Pereira-Lancha LO, Lancha A Jr. Protein turnover, amino acid requirements and recommendations for athletes and active populations. Braz J Med Biol Res. 2012;45(10):875–90.

36. Liu Z, Barrett EJ. Human protein metabolism: its measurement and regulation. Am J Physiol Endocrinol Metab. 2002;283(6): E1105–12.

37. Barzel US, Massey LK. Excess dietary protein can adversely affect bone. J Nutr. 1998;128(6):1051–53.

38. Marckemann P, Osther P, Pedersen AN, Jespersen B. High-protein diets and renal health. J Ren Nutr. 2015;25(1):1–5.

39. Phillips SM, Moore DR, Tang JE. A critical examination of dietary protein requirements, benefits, and excesses in athletes. Int J Sport Nutr Exerc Metab. 2007;17:S58–S76.

40. Butterfield GE, Calloway DH. Physical activity improves protein utilization in young men. Br J Nutr. 1984;51(2):171–84.

41. Institute of Medicine. Dietary reference intakes for energy, carbohydrate, fiber, fat, fatty acids, cholesterol, protein and amino acids. food and nutrition board. National Academies Press; 2005.

42. Joint WHO/FAO/UNU Expert Consultation. Protein and amino acid requirements in human nutrition. World Health Organ Tech Rep Ser. 2007;935:1–265.

43. Gibala MJ. Dietary protein, amino acid supplements, and recovery from exercise sports. GSSI Sports Sci Exchange. 2002; 15(4):1–4.

44. Meredith CN, Zackin MJ, Frontera WR, Evans WJ. Dietary protein requirements and body protein metabolism in endurance-trained men. J Appl Physiol. 1989;66(6):2850–56.

45. Gibala MJ. Regulation of skeletal muscle amino acid metabolism during exercise. Int J Sport Nutr Exerc Metab. 2001;11(1): 87–108.

46. Röhling M, McCarthy D, Berg A. Continuous protein supplementation reduces acute exercise-induced stress markers in athletes performing marathon. Nutrients. 2021;13(9):2929. https://doi.org/10.3390/nu13092929

47. Holwerda AM, van Vliet S, Trommelen J. Refining dietary protein recommendations for the athlete. J Physiol. 2013;591(12): 2967–68.

48. Reid KF, Naumova EN, Carabello RJ, Phillips EM, Fielding RA. Lower extremity muscle mass predicts functional performance in mobility-limited elders. J Nutr Health Aging. 2008;12(7):493–98.

49. Norton LE, Layman DK. Leucine regulates translation initiation of protein synthesis in skeletal muscle after exercise. J Nutr. 2006;136(2):533S–37S.

50. Koopman R, Verdijk L, Manders RJF, Gijsen AP, Gorselink M, Pijpers E, Wagenmakers AJM, van Loon LJC. Co-ingestion of protein and leucine stimulates muscle protein synthesis rates to the same extent in young and elderly lean men. Am J Clin Nutr. 2006;84(3):623–32.

51. Tipton KD, Elliott TA, Ferrando AA, Aarsland AA, Wolfe RR. Stimulation of muscle anabolism by resistance exercise and ingestion of leucine plus protein. Appl Physiol Nutr Metab. 2009;34(2):151–61.

52. Tipton KD, Wolfe RR. Protein and amino acids for athletes. J Sports Sci. 2004;22(1):65–79.

53. Coburn JW, Housh DJ, Housh TJ, Malek MH, Beck TW, Cramer JT, Johnson GO, Donlin PE. Effects of leucine and whey protein supplementation during eight weeks of unilateral resistance training. J Strength Cond Res. 2006;20(2):284–91.

54. Moore D, Robinson MJ, Fry JL, Tang JE, Glover EI, Wilkinson SB, Prior T, Tarnopolsky MA, Phillips SM. Ingested protein dose response of muscle and albumin protein synthesis after resistance exercise in young men. Am J Clin Nutr. 2009; 89(1):161–68.

55. Wilkinson DJ, Hossain T, Hill DS, Phillips BE, Crossland H, Williams J, Loughna P, Churchward-Venne TA, Breen L, Phillips SM, Etheridge T, Rathmacher JA, Smith K, Szewczyk NL, Atherton PJ. Effects of leucine and its metabolite B-hydroxy-B-methylbutyrate on human skeletal muscle protein metabolism. J Physiol. 2013;591(11):2911–23.

56. Adechian S, Rémond D, Gaudichon C, Pouyet C, Dardevet D, Mosoni L. Spreading intake of a leucine-rich fast protein in energy-restricted overweight rats does not improve protein mass. Nutrition. 2012;28(5):566–71.

57. Koopman R, Saris WHM, Wagenmakers AJM, van Loon LJ. Nutritional interventions to promote post-exercise muscle protein synthesis. Sports Med. 2007;37(10):895–6.

58. Phillips SM. Protein requirements and supplementation in strength sports. Nutrition. 2004;20(7-8):689–95.

59. Helms ER, Zinn C, Rowlands DS, Brown SR. A systematic review of dietary protein during caloric restriction in resistance trained lean athletes: a case for higher intakes. Int J Sport Nutr Exerc Metab. 2014;24(2):127–38.

60. Garlick PJ, Grant I. Amino acid infusion increases the sensitivity of muscle protein synthesis in vivo to insulin. Effect of branched-chain amino acids. Biochem J. 1988;254(2):579–84.

61. Garlick PJ. The role of leucine in the regulation of protein metabolism. J Nutr. 2005;135(6):1553S–56S.

62. Suryawan A, Torrazza RM, Gazzaneo MC, Orellana RA, Fiorotto ML, El-Kadi SW, Srivastava N, Nguyen HV, Davis TA. Enteral leucine supplementation increases protein synthesis in skeletal and cardiac muscles and visceral tissues of neonatal pigs through mTORC1-dependent pathways. Pediatr Res. 2012;71:324–31.

63. Churchward-Venne TA, Burd NA, Mitchell CJ, West DWD, Philp A, Marcotte GR, Baker SK, Baar K, Phillips SM. Supplementation of a suboptimal protein dose with leucine or essential amino acids: effects on myofibrillar protein synthesis at rest and following resistance exercise in men. J Physiol. 2012;590(Pt 11):2751–65.

64. Portier H, Chatard JC, Filaire E, Jaunet-Devienne MF, Robert A, Guezennec CY. Effects of branched-chain amino acids supplementation on physiological and psychological performance during an offshore sailing race. Eur J Appl Physiol. 2008;104(5):787–94.

65. Meeusen R, Watson P. Amino acids and the brain: do they play a role in "central fatigue"? Int J Sport Nutr Exerc Metab. 2007;17(Suppl):S37–46.

66. Li F, Yin Y, Tan B, Kong X, Wu G. Leucine nutrition in animals and humans: mTOR signaling and beyond. Amino Acids. 2011;41(5):1185–93.

67. Cockburn E, Hayes PR, French DN, Stevenson E, Gibson ASC. Acute milk-based protein-CHO supplementation attenuates exercise-induced muscle damage. Appl Physiol Nutr Metab. 2008;33(4):775–83.

68. McCormack SE, Shaham O, McCarthy MA, Deik AA, Wang TJ, Gerszten RE, Clish CB, Mootha VK, Grinspoon SK, Fleischman A. Circulating branched-chain amino acid concentrations are associated with obesity and future insulin resistance in children and adolescents. Pediatr Obes. 2013;8(1):52–61.

69. Zanchi NE, Guimarães-Ferreira L, de Siqueira-Filho MA, Felitti V, Nicastro H, Bueno C, Lira FS, Naimo MA, Campos-Ferraz P, Nunes MT, Seelaender M, Carvalho CRO, Blachier F, Lancha AH. Dose and latency effects of leucine supplementation in modulating glucose homeostasis: opposite effects in healthy and glucocorticoid-induced insulin-resistance States. Nutrients. 2012;4(12):1851–67.

70. Casperson SL, Sheffield-Moore M, Hewlings SJ, Paddon-Jones D. Leucine supplementation chronically improves muscle protein synthesis in older adults consuming the RDA for protein. Clin Nutr. 2012;31(4):512–9.

71. Cuthbertson D, Smith K, Babraj J, Leese G, Waddell T, Atherton P, Wackerhage H, Taylor PM, Rennie MJ. Anabolic signaling deficits underlie amino acid resistance of wasting, aging muscle. FASEB J. 2005;19(3):422–4.

72. Paddon-Jones D, Rasmussen BB. Dietary protein recommendations and the prevention of sarcopenia. Curr Opin Clin Nutr Metab Care. 2009;12(1):86–90.

73. Zawadzki KM, Yaspelkis BB III, Ivy JL. Carbohydrate-protein complex increases the rate of muscle glycogen storage after exercise. J Appl Physiol. 1992;72(5):1854–9.

74. Hartman JW, Tang JE, Wilkinson SB, Tarnopolsky MA, Lawrence RL, Fullerton AV, Phillips SM. Consumption of fat-free fluid milk after resistance exercise promotes greater lean mass accretion than does consumption of soy or carbohydrate in young, novice, male weightlifters. Am J Clin Nutr. 2007;86(2):373–81.

75. Thomas K, Morris P, Stevenson E. Improved endurance capacity following chocolate milk consumption compared with 2 commercially available sports drinks. Appl Physiol Nutr Metab. 2009;34(1):78–82.

76. Santesso N, Aki EA, Bianchi M, Mustafa R, Heels-Ansdell D, Schünemann HJ. Effects of higher- versus lower-protein diets on health outcomes: a systematic review and meta-analysis. Eur J Clin Nutr. 2012;66(7):780–8.

77. Friedman AN, Ogden LG, Foster GD, Klein S, Stein R, Miller B, Hill JO, Brill C, Bailer B, Rosenbaum DR, Wyatt HR. Comparative effects of low-carbohydrate high-protein versus low-fat diets on the kidney. Clin J Am Soc Nephrol. 2012;7(7):1103–11.

78. Skov AR, Toubro S, Bülow J, Krabbe K, Parving HH, Astrup A. Changes in renal function during weight loss induced by high vs low-protein low-fat diets in overweight subjects. Int J Obes Relat Metab Disord. 1999;23(11):1170–7.

79. Martin WF, Armstrong LE, Rodriguez NR. Dietary protein intake and renal function. Nutr Metab(Lond). 2005;2:25.

80. Jia Y, Hwang SY, House JD, Ogborn MR, Weiler HA, Karmin O, Aukema HA. Long-term high intake of whole proteins results in renal damage in pigs. J Nutr. 2010;140(9):1646–52.

81. Hiatt RA, Ettinger B, Caan B, Quesenberry CP, Duncan D, Citron JT. Randomized controlled trial of low animal protein, high-fiber diet in the prevention of recurrent calcium oxalate kidney stones. Am J Epidemiol. 1996;144(1):25–33.

82. Romero V, Akpinar H, Assimos DG. Kidney stones: a global picture of prevalence, incidence, and associated risk factors. Rev Urol. 2010;12(2–3):e86–96.

83. Burd NA, West DWD, Staples AW, Atherton PJ, Baker JM, Moore DR, Holwerda AM, Parise G, Rennie MJ, Baker SK, Phillips SM. Low-load high volume resistance exercise stimulates muscle protein synthesis more than high-load low volume resistance exercise in young men. PLoS One. 2010;5(8): e12033.

84. Burke LM, Loucks AB, Broad N. Energy and carbohydrate for training and recovery. J Sports Sci. 2006;24(7):675–85.

85. Moore DR, Sygo J, Morton JP. Fuelling the female athlete: carbohydrate and protein recommendations. Eur J Sport Sci. 2022;22(5):684–96. https://doi.org/10.1080/17461391.2021.1922508

86. USDA/HHS. Dietary guidelines for Americans. Government Printing Office; 2005.

87. Delimaris I. Adverse effects associated with protein intake above the recommended dietary allowance for adults. ISRN Nutrition. 2013;2013:126929.

88. Schutz Y, Montani J-P, Dulloo AG. Low-carbohydrate ketogenic diets in body weight control: a recurrent plaguing issue of fad diets? Obes Rev. 2021;22(S2):e13195.

89. Alvestrand A, Hagenfeldt L, Merli M, Oureshi A, Eriksson LS. Influence of leucine infusion on intracellular amino acids in humans. Eur J Clin Invest. 1990;20(3):293–8.

90. Bohé J, Low A, Wolfe RR, Rennie MJ. Human muscle protein synthesis is modulated by extracellular, not intramuscular amino acid availability: a dose-response study. J Physiol. 2003;552(1): 315–24.

91. Rennie MJ, Bohé J, Smith K, Wackerhage H, Greenhaff P. Branched-chain amino acids as fuels and anabolic signals in human muscle. J Nutr. 2006;136(1 Suppl):264S–8S.

92. Glynn EL, Fry CS, Drummond MJ, Timmerman KL, Dhanani S, Volpi E, Rasmussen BB. Excess leucine intake enhances muscle anabolic signaling but not net protein anabolism in young men and women. J Nutr. 2010;140(11):1970–6.

93. Nelson AR, Phillips SM, Stellingwerff T, Rezzi S, Bruce SJ, Breton I, Thorimbert A, Guy PA, Clarke J, Broadbent S, Rowlands DS. A protein-leucine supplement increases branched-chain amino acid and nitrogen turnover but not performance. Med Sci Sports Exerc. 2012;44(1):57–68.

94. Gaine PC, Pikosky MA, Bolster DR, Martin WF, Maresh CM, Rodriguez NR. Postexercise whole-body protein turnover response to three levels of protein intake. Med Sci Sports Exerc. 2007;39(3):480–6.

95. Schena F, Guerrini F, Tregnaghi P, Kayser B. Branched-chain amino acid supplementation during trekking at high altitude. The effects on loss of body mass, body composition, and muscle power. Eur J Appl Physiol Occup Physiol. 1992;65(5): 394–8.

96. Nair KS, Schwartz RG, Welle S. Leucine as a regulator of whole body and skeletal muscle protein metabolism in humans. Am J Physiol. 1992;263(5 Pt 1):E928–34.

97. Koopman R, Verdijk LB, Beelen M, Gorselink M, Kruseman AN, Wagenmakers AJM, Kuipers H, van Loon LJC. Co-ingestion of leucine with protein does not further augment post-exercise muscle protein synthesis rates in elderly men. Br J Nutr. 2008;99(3):571–80.

98. Stock MS, Young JC, Golding LA, Kruskall LJ, Tandy RD, Conway-Klaassen JM, Beck TW. The effects of adding leucine to pre and postexercise carbohydrate beverages on acute muscle recovery from resistance training. J Strength Cond Res. 2010;24(8):2211–9.

99. Kirby TJ, Triplett NT, Haines TL, Skinner JW, Fairbrother KR, McBride JM. Effect of leucine supplementation on indices of muscle damage following drop jumps and resistance exercise. Amino Acids. 2012;42(5):1987–96.

CHAPTER OBJECTIVES

- Recognize the different types of fatty acids and the primary food sources of these fatty acids.
- Describe the recommended intakes of lipids for athlete and nonathlete populations and the best dietary sources of these lipids.
- Identify the major lipid-digesting enzymes and associated substances and their sources in the gastrointestinal (GI) tract.
- Demonstrate an understanding of the major blood lipoproteins, their sources, and how they are metabolized.
- Explain the association between lipids and atherosclerosis and heart disease, and the exercise and dietary strategies that can be followed to lower atherosclerosis and heart disease risks.

- Discuss how trans fats are made, the foods most likely to be high in trans-fatty acids, and the health problems these pose.
- Describe how fats are metabolized to provide adenosine triphosphate (ATP) energy to tissues, and the dietary, hormonal, and exercise factors associated with increasing fat metabolism.
- Recognize the major functions of lipids in helping to sustain good health.
- Understand the major reactions that take place with dietary lipids.
- Know the essential fatty acids and the processes for making nonessential fatty acids.

Case Study

John was a talented defensive lineman on his high school football team, getting a lot of pressure from his coach to "put on some weight"! He was not given any guidance on how to best do this, so he maintained the same training regimen as before but started eating more—a lot more. More bacon, more sausage, and five fried eggs in the morning instead of his usual two. Sure enough, his weight was going up. The problem was that the weight increase was nearly all body fat, so he had the same amount of muscle trying to move more nonmuscle weight, and everyone noticed he was slower off the line with his endurance getting worse. To make matters even more terrible, he had a great deal of muscle soreness that slowed him down even more and made it difficult for

him to recover from football practice. By the end of each week, he literally felt lame and had terrible performances at Saturday games. So his coach said the inevitable: "You need to lose some weight"! So John went on a self-prescribed low-calorie "diet" that was near starvation, because he was desperate to lose that weight. Yes, he lost weight, but almost all the weight he lost was muscle, which made his strength-to-weight ratio even worse (he had relatively less muscle mass and more nonmuscle mass). His endurance was terrible, and he was pretty sure he would have to give up football.

Out of desperation for what they were witnessing, John's parents made an appointment with a Registered Dietitian who specialized in sports nutrition. The dietitian

(continued)

showed John how to dynamically match energy intake with expenditure, and showed him how all those saturated and trans fats he was consuming added to his muscle soreness. He also spoke to a certified athletic trainer and a strength and conditioning coach who worked together with the dietitian to work up a coordinated diet and exercise plan that would help John benefit from the exercise to enhance muscle mass and lower fat mass. It worked, and John learned some important lessons. Caloric intake needs to be distributed dynamically with calorie expenditure, and consuming a high-fat diet with three meals/day makes it inevitable that too much energy will be consumed at one time. He also learned that not all fats are the same. Some fats, such as omega-3 fatty acids (from fish and vegetables) can reduce muscular inflammation, while some fats, such as n-6 saturated fatty acids and trans fats (mainly from fried foods, meats, and margarine), can add to inflammation. He also found out the hard way that too much fat will most definitely make it easy to get too many calories and will, inevitably, make it easy to become fatter.

CASE STUDY DISCUSSION QUESTIONS

1. If you were working with John, what kind of diet would you recommend for him to help ensure he gets the energy he needs to support his perceived need to put on weight?

2. How would you explain to John that the kind of weight he wants to increase is an important factor in his performance? How would you get John to think about increasing muscle weight rather than just weight?

INTRODUCTION

Important Factors to Consider

■ Dietary lipids (*i.e.*, dietary fats) have many important functions, but the majority of populations in industrialized nations eat too much fat, particularly of the wrong kinds that are high in saturated fatty acids, placing them at risk for obesity and early development of cardiovascular disease. Not all fats are the same in terms of their atherogenic potential, but excess fat intake, regardless of the source, is likely to cause problems. While reading this chapter, think about ways to (i) improve the kinds of fats consumed and (ii) eat to lower total fat consumption. See Table 4.1 for common fatty acids in foods.

■ There is a common misunderstanding that consumption of foods high in **cholesterol** (a waxy, fat-like substance that occurs naturally in all parts of the body) is dangerous as these foods increase **heart disease** risk. For instance, eggs are high in cholesterol but relatively low in fat, but they are often avoided because people fear that the cholesterol will increase heart disease risk. However, consumption of fatty foods, even if they contain *no* cholesterol will also elevate blood cholesterol because the bile used to emulsify these dietary fats is 50% cholesterol. Therefore, the key to lowering heart disease risk is to consume better fats (*i.e.*, mono- and polyunsaturated fats associated with vegetables, nuts, and seeds) and to lower total fat intake. Just lowering cholesterol intake will not achieve the desired goal.

■ Athletes are sometimes encouraged to consume a high-fat diet with the aim of forcing the body to adapt to this elevated fat intake by increasing the proportion of fat metabolized to satisfy energy needs. This higher fat metabolism will theoretically lower the carbohydrate contribution to satisfying energy needs and, because carbohydrate stores are limited, will have the effect of improving endurance performance. A recent study found that a short-term high-fat diet did slightly improve fat metabolism when compared to a high-carbohydrate diet but did not improve time-trial performance on a 5-km run (1). A similar result was found when elite athletes were placed on a low-carbohydrate, high-fat diet with a relatively rapid adaptation to the diet but with impaired endurance capacity. Importantly, acute restoration of carbohydrate after the fat adaptation failed to improve the impairment of high-intensity endurance performance (2). These findings suggest that the body does its best to adapt to the nutrients provided, but this does not necessarily translate into improved performance following the adaptation.

Table 4.1	Common Fatty Acids in Foods		
Fatty Acids	**Carbons: Double Bonds (First Double Bond)**	**Foods High in Fatty Acid**	**Primary Functions**
▪ Palmitic acid	16:0	▪ Dairy/dairy products ▪ Red meat/red products and red meat products ▪ Foods made with palm oil (crackers, potato chips, etc.) ▪ Coconut oil ▪ Avocado/avocado oil ▪ Poultry/poultry products ▪ Eggs/egg-containing products ▪ Macadamia and other nuts and nut oils. ▪ Wheat/wheat products	▪ Fuel source ▪ Component of cell membranes ▪ Component of signaling molecules
▪ Stearic acid	18:0	▪ Dairy and dairy products ▪ Red meat and red meat products (sausage, etc.) ▪ Egg and products using eggs	▪ Component mineral salts (calcium stearate, magnesium stearate, sodium stearate, etc.) ▪ Major component of stored body fat (~30%) ▪ Enables solubility in organic solvents
▪ Oleic acid	18:1 (Omega-9)	▪ Olive oil ▪ Canola oil ▪ Almonds/almond oil ▪ Sesame oil ▪ Cocoa butter	▪ Improves autoimmunity ▪ Facilitates wound healing ▪ Lowers heart disease risk ▪ Lowers inflammation
▪ Linoleic acid (Essential)	18:2 (Omega-6)	▪ Safflower oil ▪ Sunflower seeds and oil ▪ Safflower oil ▪ Pine nuts ▪ Corn oil ▪ Pecans ▪ Brazil nuts ▪ Sesame oil	▪ Involved in transdermal water barrier of epidermis ▪ Inadequate intake in infants may result in growth retardation and scaly skin lesions.
▪ Arachidonic acid	20:4 (Omega-6)	▪ Egg ▪ Poultry ▪ Sardines ▪ Salmon ▪ Red meat	▪ Synthesis of prostaglandins (involved in repair of injury and illness) ▪ Synthesis of leukotrienes (chemicals released when in contact with allergic substances) ▪ Cellular signaling for nerve impulses, muscle contraction, and hormone secretion.
▪ Eicosopentaenoic acid (EPA)	20:5 (Omega-3)	▪ Cold water fish (salmon, tuna, mackerel, sardines, herring)	▪ Protects from unwanted blood clot ▪ Pain reduction ▪ Improved wound healing ▪ Lower muscle soreness ▪ Improved cognitive function

(continued)

Table 4.1	Common Fatty Acids in Foods (Continued)		
Fatty Acids	Carbons: Double Bonds (First Double Bond)	Foods High in Fatty Acid	Primary Functions
■ Docosapentaenoic acid (DPA)	22:5 (Omega-3)	■ Cold water fish (salmon, tuna, mackerel, sardines, herring) ■ Grass-fed beef	■ Protects from unwanted blood clot ■ Improves lipid metabolism ■ Improves neural health
■ Alpha-Linolenic acid (Essential)	18:3 (Omega-3)	■ Flaxseeds and flaxseed oil ■ Chia seeds ■ Walnuts and walnut oil ■ Canola oil	■ Normal growth and development ■ Maintains normal heart function ■ Protects from unwanted blood clot

Note: Most foods contain a variety of different fatty acids. This table provides a summary of the foods that are relatively high in the fatty acid listed.

Note: Not included in this table are short-chain fatty acids (acetate, propionate, and butyrate), which are not typically consumed but are manufactured with the assistance of the gut microbiome. More information on the ergogenic importance of short-chain fatty acids can be found in Chapter 15: Diet Planning for Optimal Performance.

Cholesterol

A sterol molecule manufactured by animal cells with protective cell membrane functions. (It is not found in foods of nonanimal origin.) Bile, made by the liver to aid in dietary fat absorption, is 50% cholesterol. High blood cholesterol may occur, therefore, from either a high level of animal food consumption or a high level of fat consumption. High blood cholesterol is associated with higher risk of atherosclerosis and heart disease deaths.

Heart Disease

Cardiovascular disease involves reduced blood flow to the heart and other tissues from an atherosclerotic narrowing of the arteries, dramatically increasing the risk of a heart attack (myocardial infarction) and stroke. High-fat diets and inadequate exercise are associated with higher risk of cardiovascular disease because of the atherosclerotic vascular tissue damage they cause. The high blood lipids associated with high-fat diets result in inflammation of the vessel wall, and the constant repair of the damaged area results in thickened vessel walls that are both narrower and less flexible. Saturated fats and trans-fatty acids have a greater atherogenic potential than polyunsaturated and monounsaturated fatty acids (MUFAs). Once the vessel walls become repeatedly damaged from chronically high-fat intake and other factors (e.g., cigarette smoking), the repair response becomes dysfunctional resulting in high risk of cardiovascular disease.

The term **lipid** is the scientific term for organic molecules that are not soluble in water but are soluble in organic solvents (soaps, chloroform, benzene, etc.). Lipids are commonly referred to as *fats*, but traditionally the word *fat* refers to a lipid that is solid at room temperature (*e.g.*, butter), while the word *oil* refers to a lipid that is liquid at room temperature (*e.g.*, corn oil). Fats and oils are typically also different in composition, and this can have an impact on the health or disease potential when different fats or oils are consumed. Some lipids, such as cholesterol, are a common part of health assessments because the amount of cholesterol in the blood is associated with cardiovascular disease risk. There are many other lipids as well, including the lipid–protein molecules that are created when dietary fats are digested and absorbed. The degree to which these molecules are present in the blood is also an indicator of cardiovascular disease risk, and it provides an indication of whether more lipids are being removed from storage to supply energy than being delivered to storage.

Lipids

Molecules that include fats, waxes, sterols, monoglycerides, diglycerides, triglycerides, phospholipids, and fat-soluble vitamins.

Virtually every food we consume contains lipids, including fruits, vegetables, cereals, meats, and fish. However, different foods contain different types and concentrations of lipids that may either increase or decrease disease risk. For the purpose of this book, the term *lipid* is used to refer to all lipids in general, and specific fats or oils will be identified where the difference is important for health, disease risk, or athletic performance.

In humans, lipids have a wide range of functions that are critically important to sustaining good health. These include:

- *Concentrated source of energy:* Lipids are an extraordinarily efficient storage form for energy (i.e., calories). One gram of lipid (fat or oil) provides 9 calories, while 1 g of either carbohydrate or protein provides 4 calories. One way of thinking about the difference in caloric density is that, for every gram of fat removed from the diet, you can consume twice as many grams of carbohydrate and protein and still consume less total energy. Another way of considering the caloric density of lipids is that eating high-fat foods (e.g., fried foods, fatty meats) is an easy way to obtain too many calories in a single meal.

- *Insulation from environmental temperature:* Body fat is evenly distributed between the fat stored subcutaneously (under the skin) and visceral fat (the fat stored around the organs). This fat plays dual roles that are both important, acting as a source of energy that can be delivered to tissues in a time of need and also acting as an insulation blanket to help sustain body and organ temperature when exposed to extreme environmental temperatures (3).

- *Cushion against jarring:* The subcutaneous fat layer protects the underlying muscle, which is far more vascular (has more blood running through it), from being bruised when struck. Athletes of all kinds, but particularly athletes in concussive sports (boxing, football, etc.), must be cautious of being too lean as the direct "hits" on muscle would be damaging and require more repair.

- *Prolong satiety:* Consumed lipids have a delayed gastric emptying time, and while food remains in the stomach, the desire to eat again is delayed. This feeling of satiety, or the feeling of fullness after eating, is considered desirable because it helps to avoid overeating. Importantly, the delayed gastric emptying helps to ensure that the consumed foods/nutrients are better absorbed and enter the blood more gradually. This graduated absorption enhances tissue utilization of the nutrients.

- *Improve the flavor and palatability of foods:* For anyone who has tasted fried chicken and boiled chicken at the same meal, it is easy to understand how higher-fat foods improve food flavor and palatability (having a more pleasant taste). Traditionally, higher-fat foods were consumed mainly on special occasions, but many foods that are high in fat are easily available and at low cost. The high palatability, coupled with the low cost and easy availability, increases the risk that excess lipids will be consumed with related higher health risks. This feature of lipids is difficult to overcome, as it would require major dietary changes that involve a dramatic reduction in consumed fried foods and elimination of visible fats (i.e., added butter/margarine, the fat surrounding a steak, etc.).

- *Carry the fat-soluble vitamins A, D, E, and K:* Some vitamins require a lipid environment, so some lipids must be consumed to be assured of obtaining these fat-soluble vitamins. Vitamin E, for instance, is a vitamin commonly found in cereal oils (i.e., corn oil), while vitamin A is found in animal sources (i.e., eggs, meat, dairy, liver). Avoiding high-fat foods of animal does not dramatically increase the risk of deficiency for these vitamins, as beta-carotene (a precursor of vitamin A) is a common component of vegetables, and vitamin E and vitamin K (phylloquinone) are also found in green leafy vegetables. Vitamin D can be obtained through ultraviolet irradiation of the skin from the sun. More information on these vitamins is available in Chapter 5.

- *Provide the essential fatty acids:* While humans can manufacture most of the lipids required to ensure health, we are unable to manufacture the **essential fatty acids**, *linoleic acid* (LA) and *alpha-linolenic acid*. Therefore, it is *essential* that we consume these fatty acids from the foods we eat. These fatty acids are available in a wide range of foods, including fish, shellfish, leafy vegetables, walnuts, flax, and more. Failure to consume foods with essential fatty acids is associated with central nervous system and cardiac problems.

Essential Fatty Acids

The essential fatty acids, linoleic acid (*LA*) and alpha-linolenic acid (*ALA*), are referred to as essential because humans are unable to manufacture them. Therefore, it is *essential* that we obtain these fatty acids from consumed foods.

- *LA* is an unsaturated omega-6 fatty acid (i.e., the double bond is at the sixth carbon atom) and is required for normal neurologic function, the growth and maintenance of hair and skin, and the maintenance of good bone mineral density. There is evidence that diets relatively high in LA also lower heart disease risk (4). Food sources of LA include plant seed oils, including corn, sunflower, and soybean oils. Certain nuts, including pecans, Brazil nuts, and pine nuts, are relatively high in LA. Humans convert consumed LA into γ-linolenic acid (GLA) and arachidonic acid, both of which have important physiologic functions. GLA inhibits the tissue inflammation associated with rheumatoid arthritis, diabetes, and allergies (5). Arachidonic acid not only supports brain and muscle function but also promotes inflammation (6).

■ *ALA* is an unsaturated omega-3 fatty acid (*i.e.*, the double bond is at the third carbon atom) and is necessary for healthy cell membranes and cardiovascular function because of its cholesterol-lowering and inflammation-lowering properties (7). The consumed form of linolenic acid is in the form of the omega-3 fatty acid ALA, the omega-3 fatty acid eicosapentaenoic acid (EPA), and the omega-3 fatty acid docosahexaenoic acid (DHA). Common food sources of ALA include flaxseed, soybeans, pumpkin seeds, walnuts, and canola oil; common food sources of EPA include fatty fish, fish oils, and marine foods (*i.e.*, marine algae, seaweed); common food sources of DHA include marine foods, fatty fish, and DHA-enriched eggs (8,9).

TYPES OF LIPIDS

Important Factors to Consider

■ Different types of lipids have different metabolic outcomes when consumed. Saturated lipids tend to maintain serum lipids and cholesterol longer and are therefore more atherogenic. Monounsaturated lipids tend to be well tolerated and are cleared relatively quickly from the serum. Polyunsaturated lipids tend to be cleared from the serum quickly and have the effect of lowering blood lipids and cholesterol. However, excess intake of all lipids may have an atherogenic effect, so the amount consumed at a single meal should be relatively low.

■ Saturated fatty acids are often used in food processing because they are less likely to interact with the environment and undergo oxidative reactions that cause them to become rancid. Saturated fatty acids that are liquid, such as those found in palm oil, tend to be even more popular with food manufacturers because liquids are more easily mixed with other food ingredients. Therefore, athletes should be cautious about consuming too many processed/packaged foods, which tend to be higher in saturated fat. Recommendation: Read the label!

Fatty Acids

Most **fatty acids** consist of an even-numbered carbon chain of 12–28 carbon atoms, with hydrogen atoms attached to the carbons, but there are also less common fatty acids with 8 and 10 carbon atoms. At one end of the carbon chain, there is a carboxylic acid (hence the name "fatty acid"). When not attached to other molecules, fatty acids are referred to as free fatty acids. Typically, dietary fatty acids are attached to a glycerol molecule in the form of a triglyceride. Some fatty acids are *saturated*, others *monounsaturated*, and still others *polyunsaturated*. These different types of lipids have different types of bonds that hold together the carbon atoms, which make up the skeleton of the fatty acids.

Fatty Acids

A fat molecule with a carbon chain that has a carboxylic acid (COOH) at the terminal end. In the diet, they are typically part of triglycerides. Fatty acids have variable carbon chain lengths, from short chain (fewer than six carbons such as butyric acid), medium chain (between 6 and 12 carbons), and long chain (longer than 12 carbons). The carbon chains may be saturated, monounsaturated, or polyunsaturated.

Saturated fatty acids have carbon atoms that are held together entirely with single bonds, meaning that the carbon atoms are *saturated* with hydrogen atoms. Single bonds are stronger, more stable, and less chemically reactive than double bonds. **Monounsaturated fatty acids** have a single (*i.e.*, *mono*) double bond in the carbon chain, meaning that the two adjoining carbon atoms are each missing a hydrogen atom and are held together with a weaker bonding structure, a double bond. **Polyunsaturated fatty acids (PUFAs)** contain two or more double bonds in the carbon chain. Do not be confused by the terminology, as double bonds are weaker and less stable than single bonds. Because of that, greater the number of double bonds, greater the opportunity for the chemical environment to react with the fatty acid. It is this ability to react with the fatty acid that makes the difference when it is consumed. In general, saturated fatty acids are commonly found in the highest concentration in fats of animal origin, but they are also high in other dietary lipids, including palm kernel oil and coconut oil (Figure 4.1).

Saturated Fatty Acids

These fatty acids have no double bonds between the carbon atoms and tend to stay elevated in the blood longer, increasing their potential for creating atherosclerosis.

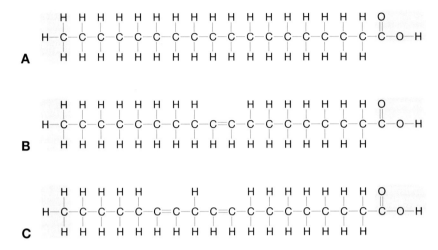

FIGURE 4.1: (**A**) Saturated, (**B**) monounsaturated, and (**C**) polyunsaturated fatty acids. (From Kraemer WJ, Fleck SJ, Deschenes MR. Exercise physiology. 2nd ed. Philadelphia (PA): Lippincott Williams & Wilkins; 2015.)

Common saturated fatty acids are found not only in animal fats (*i.e.*, stearic acid) but also in palm oil (*i.e.*, palmitic acid).

Monounsaturated Fatty Acids

These fatty acids have a single double bond between the carbon atoms and are well tolerated by humans. The most common monounsaturated fatty acid consumed is oleic fatty acid, which is high in olive oil and canola oil.

Polyunsaturated Fatty Acids

These fatty acids have two or more double bonds between the carbon atoms, making them easy to digest and interact with, enabling faster clearance from the blood and reducing atherosclerosis potential. The omega-3 fatty acids, in particular, are polyunsaturated fatty acids from seafood that have been shown to lower heart disease risk.

The most common form of lipid in the human diet, whether from fat or oil, is in the form of **triglycerides**, which is the primary form of lipid (*i.e.*, fat) storage in humans and other mammals. Nearly all dietary lipids (~95%) are in the form of triglycerides. The triglyceride molecule, as the name suggests, is composed of one glycerol molecule with three fatty acids connected to it (Figure 4.2). Triglycerides are extremely efficient forms of energy storage, providing 9 calories/g, compared with 4 calories/g from either proteins or carbohydrates. It takes less than half the dietary fat to deliver the same calories as carbohydrates and proteins, so it is easier to consume excess calories if the foods consumed have a high proportion of fat.

Connecting 3 Fatty Acids to Glycerol Creates a Triglyceride Molecule Plus 3 Molecules of Water

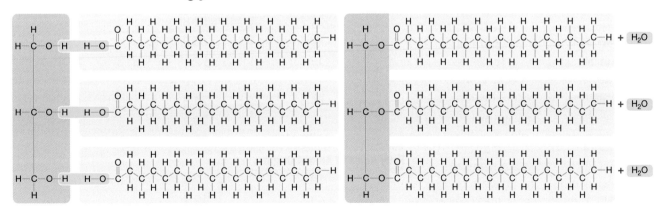

Glycerol + 3 fatty acids ⟶ 1 Triglyceride + 3 water molecules

FIGURE 4.2: Triglyceride molecule. (From Kraemer WJ, Fleck SJ, Deschenes MR. Exercise physiology. 2nd ed. Philadelphia (PA): Lippincott Williams & Wilkins; 2015.)

Triglycerides

A fat molecule composed of glycerol plus three fatty acids, which is the most common form of dietary lipids consumed by humans. Triglycerides are also the main storage form of lipids (*i.e.*, body fat) in humans.

The triglycerides in each food we consume can have some saturated, monounsaturated, and PUFAs. The PUFAs, which are highly prevalent in sunflower oil, corn oil, and safflower oil, have a tendency to *decrease* serum cholesterol, which is associated with lower cardiovascular disease risk. The MUFAs, which are highly prevalent in olive oil, and canola oil, also tend to *decrease* serum cholesterol. The saturated fatty acids, commonly found in high proportions not only in animal fats, but also in coconut oil, palm kernel oil, and cocoa butter, tend to *increase* serum cholesterol, which is associated with higher cardiovascular

disease risk. Table 4.2 shows the distribution of saturated, monounsaturated, and PUFAs in dietary lipids.

Long-chain fatty acids are the most common dietary lipids, but other lipids also exist in nature or are manufactured and used in the food supply. These include:

- *Diglycerides:* 1 glycerol and 2 fatty acids
- *Monoglycerides:* 1 glycerol and 1 fatty acid
- *Short-chain fatty acids:* 4 or 6 carbon atoms
- *Medium-chain fatty acids:* 8, 10, or 12 carbon atoms
- *Long-chain fatty acids:* 14 or more carbon atoms (these are the most common in the diet)

As indicated in Table 4.2, not all oils are high in polyunsaturated fats (*e.g.*, coconut oil and palm kernel oil). The characteristics of these lipids often determine how they are used. As an example, palm kernel oil is often used in processed foods because it is highly saturated and therefore stable. In addition, the fact that it is an oil that

Table 4.2   Distribution of Saturated, Monounsaturated, Polyunsaturated, and Trans-Fatty Acids in Commonly Consumed Dietary Lipids of Plant and Animal Origin

Food	% Saturated	% Monounsaturated	% Polyunsaturated	% Trans-Fatty Acids
Fatty Acids of Plant Origin				
Coconut oil	85.2	6.6	1.7	0.0
Cocoa butter	60.0	32.9	3.0	0.0
Palm kernel oil	81.5	11.4	1.6	0.0
Palm oil	45.3	41.6	8.3	0.0
Cottonseed oil	25.5	21.3	48.1	0.0
Wheat germ oil	18.8	15.9	60.7	0.0
Soybean oil	14.5	23.2	56.5	0.0
Olive oil	14.0	69.7	11.2	0.0
Corn oil	12.7	24.7	57.8	0.0
Sunflower oil	11.9	20.2	63.0	0.0
Safflower oil	10.2	12.6	72.1	0.0
Hemp oil	10.0	15.0	75.0	0.0
Canola oil	5.3	64.3	24.8	0.0
Mixed vegetable oil—stick margarine	13.6	33.5	20.2	14.8
Mixed vegetable oil—tub margarine	16.7	24.7	23.8	3.3
Fatty Acids of Animal Origin				
Butter	54.0	19.8	2.6	0.04
Duck fat	33.2	49.3	12.9	0.0
Lard	40.8	43.8	9.6	0.0

Source: From Pennington JAT, Douglass JS. Bowes & Church's food values of portions commonly used. 18th ed. Baltimore (MD): Lippincott Williams & Wilkins; 2005; U.S. Department of Agriculture, FoodData Central, Accessed May 2024. https://fdc.nal.usda.gov/

Table 4.3	Common Terminology for Lipids
Term	**Meaning**
Essential fatty acids	Fatty acids that we are incapable of synthesizing, so they are *essential* that we consume them in the diet. These include: ■ Linoleic acid ■ α-Linolenic acid
Most prevalent fatty acid	The fatty acid that is most commonly found in the food supply: ■ Oleic fatty acid (monounsaturated)
Simple lipids	Lipids that exist in nature include: ■ Fatty acids ■ Glycerol ■ Triglycerides ■ Diglycerides ■ Monoglycerides ■ Sterols ■ Waxes
Compound lipids	Lipids attached to nonlipid compounds include: ■ Phospholipids ■ Glycolipids ■ Lipoproteins
Structured lipids	Lipids manufactured from simple and/or compound lipids include: ■ Medium-chain triglyceride oil
Short-chain fatty acids	Fewer than six carbons
Medium-chain fatty acids	6–12 carbons
Long-chain fatty acids	Greater than 12 carbons

makes it easier to mix with other ingredients (Table 4.3). The common fatty acid reactions can help in understanding how fats are used or why they behave as they do.

Common Lipid Reactions

Peroxidation

Peroxidation is defined as oxidation reactions of fatty acids and cholesterol that contain one or more double bonds in the carbon chain. The oxidized lipids may create free-radical peroxides that, in foods, make the food taste rancid (spoiled). Meat fats that have at least one double bond (see Table 4.2) are not associated with high levels of antioxidants (vitamins E and C), so they can easily undergo this oxidation rancidity reaction. For example, imagine leaving raw bacon uncovered and unrefrigerated on the kitchen counter for several hours. The fats in the bacon will become oxidized and smell rancid. By contrast, vegetable oils, such as olive oil and safflower oil, are high in mono- and polyunsaturated fats, but they also have a high level of vitamin E, a powerful antioxidant that captures oxygen and keeps the fatty acids from becoming oxidized and rancid. Because of this, vegetable and cereal oils have a high shelf life without becoming rancid. In humans, antioxidant vitamins protect the fatty membranes of cells from becoming oxidized and creating peroxide *free radicals*, which can destroy the cell or can alter the DNA structure of the cell and initiate a disease process (Example 4.1).

Example 4.1: Free Radicals

Free radicals are unstable and react in unpredictable ways as they attempt to gain a missing electron. As a free radical, such as peroxide, steals an electron from a compound it has come in contact with, the compound with the stolen electron itself becomes unstable, causing a chain reaction. When free radicals enter a cell, they move around the cell in an unpredictable and damaging pattern, destroying the cell or nicking the nucleus of the cell. The nucleus contains the DNA of the cell, which can get damaged, and if this cell reproduces, the reproduced cell will not be normal, initiating a disease process such as cancer. Antioxidants, such as vitamin E, help to protect cells by capturing oxygen and avoiding the creation of peroxide and other free radicals that can be made from oxidized fatty acids. One of the reasons consumption of fresh fruits and vegetables is associated with good health is that these foods are high in protective antioxidants.

Iodination

Iodination reactions are performed in a laboratory to determine the number of double bonds (*i.e.*, its relative saturation/unsaturation) that are present in a lipid (10,11). For instance, to determine if there is a difference in saturation/unsaturation between olive oil from Greece and olive oil from Italy, a laboratory could perform an iodination test. The oils are bathed in a solution containing iodine, which has a distinct dark brown color. The iodine attaches itself to the carbon atoms that have double bonds, and the color of the oil is checked in a machine (spectrophotometer) that can determine the degree of color (Table 4.4). The darker the color, the higher the

Table 4.4	Iodination Values of Selected Lipids
Corn oil	109–133
Grape-seed oil	124–143
Olive oil	80–88
Palm oil	44–51
Peanut oil	84–105
Soybean oil	120–136
Walnut oil	120–140

Note: Iodination values are a laboratory marker of the total number of double bonds in the fatty acids of the oils listed. Higher iodination values indicate a greater number of double bonds.

iodine value (the more the molecule has attached iodine) and therefore the greater the number of double bonds (12).

Hydrogenation

Hydrogenation reactions involve treating lipids with hydrogen, which attaches itself to carbon atoms with double bonds, thereby reducing the relative saturation level of the lipid (*i.e.*, it makes the lipid more saturated). These are common reactions for converting oils into semisolids or solids. For instance, hydrogenation reactions convert corn oil into corn oil *margarine*. Because hydrogenation reactions reduce the number of double bonds, the fatty acids become more saturated and therefore have a greater disease risk potential than the oil equivalent. In addition, some hydrogenation reactions may result in the formation of **trans-fatty acids**, which are strongly implicated in increasing heart disease risk (13). It is for this reason that many states are passing laws that ban providing fats that contain trans fats to customers in restaurants and shoppers in grocery stores. Trans fats are banned for use in human food products sold in restaurants and public kitchens in New York City and in California. In Europe, trans fats are banned in Denmark and Switzerland. In 2015, the United States Food and Drug Administration gave the food industry 3 years to phase trans fats out of the food supply (Figure 4.3).

Trans-Fatty Acids

Unsaturated fatty acids that have been hydrogenated to make them more solid (*i.e.*, conversion of corn oil into corn oil margarine) may result in 'cis' or 'trans' fatty acids. Cis fatty acids have the added hydrogen atoms attached on the same side of the carbon atom, while 'trans' fatty acids have hydrogen atoms attached on opposite sides of the carbon atom. Trans fatty acids have been shown to be highly inflammatory, causing increased risk of heart disease and heart disease deaths.

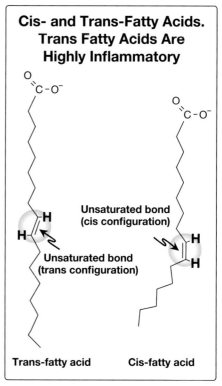

FIGURE 4.3: Cis- and trans-fatty acids. (From Ferrier DR. Biochemistry. 7th ed. Philadelphia (PA): Lippincott Williams & Wilkins; 2017.)

LIPID DIGESTION AND ABSORPTION

Important Factors to Consider

- Fats have the effect of slowing gastric emptying, delaying the speed with which consumed foods leave the stomach and enter the intestines for further digestion and absorption.
- Athletes typically feel uncomfortable exercising with food still in the stomach, as it makes them feel uncomfortable, and the delayed gastric emptying is likely to also inhibit appropriate fluid consumption during exercise. Therefore, the pregame meal should be relatively low in fats and should be consumed early enough prior to exercise to ensure that there is no longer food in the stomach.

Dietary lipids, mainly in the form of triglycerides, are physically broken up into smaller particles through chewing, which do not chemically digest the lipids into smaller

Table 4.5	Lipid Digestion and Absorption	
Site	**Chemical Action**	**Outcome**
Mouth	None	▪ There is no chemical breakdown in the mouth, but chewing food physically breaks down the food into a smaller size that enables more effective digestion later in the digestive tract.
Esophagus	None	▪ No additional action.
Stomach	Acidity	▪ The stomach acid initiates some breakdown of triglycerides into diglycerides and fatty acids. ▪ The stomach contents that enter the small intestine are referred to as "chyme."
Small intestine	Pancreatic lipase (pancreas) Bile salt (liver)	▪ Pancreatic lipase enters the small intestine via the pancreatic duct and effectively breaks down diglycerides and triglycerides into component glycerol and fatty acids. ▪ Bile salt enters the small intestine via the common bile duct and emulsifies the glycerol and fatty acids into small and water-soluble compounds. One end of an emulsifying agent is fat soluble, so can attach itself to the lipid, while the other end of the emulsifying agent is water soluble and wraps itself around the lipid to make it water soluble. ▪ Bile is 50% cholesterol that is manufactured by the liver, so high-fat intakes require more bile, and this bile-related cholesterol is absorbed into the blood with the consumed lipids. Therefore, high-fat intakes, even if no cholesterol is consumed, are associated with high blood cholesterol.
Intestinal lining	None	▪ The water-soluble "micelle" (emulsified fat) is transported into the lining of the small intestine, where it is reformed into a triglyceride and formed into the lipoprotein "chylomicron." The chylomicron enters the blood.
Blood	Lipoprotein lipase	▪ Chylomicrons are converted into low-density lipoproteins (LDL) via lipoprotein lipase (LPL) and the LDL leaves the blood and is taken up by tissues for utilization.

molecular substances (*i.e.*, fatty acids and glycerol) but does enable more effective digestion later in the GI tract. When the lipids enter the stomach, the acidity of the stomach and fluids create still smaller lipid droplets referred to as *chyme*. When this chyme enters the small intestine, a chemical in the small intestine, cholecystokinin, travels up the common bile/pancreatic duct and causes the gall bladder to release bile into the small intestine. At the same time, the pancreas releases its lipid-digesting enzyme, pancreatic lipase, which breaks the lipids into individual fatty acids and glycerol, monoglycerides, and diglycerides. Bile, an effective emulsifying agent, converts these smaller lipid molecules into water-soluble micelles, which are then absorbed into the blood. Once in the blood, the micelles are attached to a protein carrier to create *chylomicrons*, which are relatively large lipid molecules with a relatively small protein carrier. There are no receptors for chylomicrons that allow the lipids to leave the blood, so the enzyme lipoprotein lipase converts

the chylomicrons into low-density lipoproteins (LDLs), for which we do have receptors that allow the lipids to be cleared from the blood and taken up by tissues (Table 4.5).

Lipoproteins

There are four major types of lipid carriers in the blood. These lipoproteins (lipid and protein combinations) have different origins and actions. These are chylomicrons, very–low-density lipoproteins (VLDLs), LDLs, and high-density lipoproteins (HDLs).

Chylomicrons

Chylomicrons are the least dense of the lipoproteins, meaning that they have the highest amount of fat attached to the protein carrier. These molecules have a high atherogenic potential (*i.e.*, may increase **atherosclerosis** risk, a factor in heart disease and which is a hardening of the arteries from fatty streak formation) because they are so high in lipid and because they must stay in the blood until they are converted by lipoprotein lipase to LDL. Chylomicrons are synthesized in the intestinal wall from dietary fat, so the greater the amount of dietary fat consumed at a single meal, the higher the level of circulating chylomicrons. Since conversion of chylomicrons to LDL takes time, a high-fat meal will have a higher sustained level of chylomicrons than a meal that delivers the same calories but is lower in fat (14).

Atherosclerosis

A vascular disease characterized by a thickening and narrowing of the artery wall, making it less able to adjust to fluctuations in blood pressure. The narrowed artery also increases the risk of blood clot formation, leading to a heart attack or stroke. Maintaining high blood lipids, typically from high dietary consumption of saturated and trans-fatty acids, increases atherosclerosis risk. Some diets popular with athletes, such as high-protein, low-carbohydrate, high-fat ketogenic diets have been found to result in elevated LDL that elevates cardiovascular disease risk (15).

Very–Low-Density Lipoproteins

VLDLs are made by the liver from triglycerides and cholesterol and are converted by lipoprotein lipase to LDLs. Lowering the liver's production of VLDL requires a reduction in triglycerides, which requires a loss of body fat, lower consumption of sugary foods, lower consumption of fructose (*i.e.*, foods with high levels of high-fructose corn syrup are a particular problem), and a reduction in alcohol consumption. High levels of VLDL are associated with a higher risk of atherosclerosis and associated higher heart disease risk.

Low-Density Lipoproteins

High levels of LDLs are a known risk factor in heart disease, as LDLs have a high potential for creating fatty streaks in the arteries, where they can cause blockage and a **myocardial infarct** (heart attack) and/or stroke. Clearing LDLs from the blood for delivery to tissues is time related, as the receptors for LDL are limited, and the longer they remain at a high level in the blood, the greater their disease potential. It is for this reason that LDL is often referred to as the "bad" cholesterol. Lowering LDL cholesterol requires lowering the consumption of fat (both total and per meal) and lowering body fat levels (Figure 4.4).

Myocardial Infarct

Literally meaning heart muscle death, it is another name for a *heart attack*, which is a sudden failure of blood supply (*i.e.*, failure to supply oxygen and nutrients) to the heart as a result of an arterial blockage. The blockage results in damage to the portion of the heart that is no longer receiving blood and is associated with chest pain or radiating pain in the arm, neck, and jaw. Heart attacks are typically the result of atherosclerosis.

High-Density Lipoproteins

HDLs are the smallest and densest of the lipoprotein particles, carrying the smallest proportion of lipid to a protein carrier. HDLs are manufactured by the liver, and they are involved in removal of lipid and cholesterol from tissues and blood. Therefore, these molecules are often referred to as "good" cholesterol. Ideally, it is best to have a relatively *low* amount of LDL and a relatively *high* amount of HDL. Moderate alcohol consumption (*i.e.*, one glass of wine with dinner for a female; two glasses of wine

Progression of Arterial Atherosclerosis

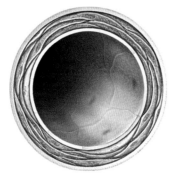 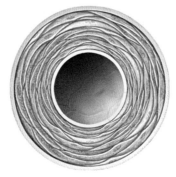 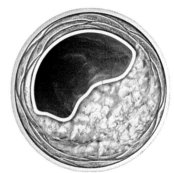

FIGURE 4.4: Atherosclerotic artery. (From Anatomical Chart Company. Hypertension anatomical chart. 2nd ed. Philadelphia (PA): LWW (PE); 2005.)

with dinner for a male) has been found to elevate HDL cholesterol, as does a lowering of body fat through an appropriate exercise and diet program (16).

Sources of Different Lipid Types in the Human Diet

The following are examples of lipid types that occur in the human diet:

- *Monounsaturated fatty acids (MUFAs):* Fatty acids that have a single double bond and are typically liquid at room temperature. Foods rich in MUFAs include vegetable oils (*e.g.*, olive, canola, sunflower, high oleic safflower) and nuts. MUFAs tend to lower bad blood cholesterol (LDL), while maintaining good cholesterol (HDL).

- *Polyunsaturated fatty acids (PUFAs):* Fatty acids that have two or more double bonds and are typically liquid at room temperature. The main food sources of PUFAs are vegetable oils and some nuts and seeds. PUFAs provide the essential fatty acids, which are n-3 (ALA, where the first double bond occurs at the third carbon) and n-6 (LA, where the first double bond occurs at the sixth carbon). Hydrogenating PUFAs to make margarine (*e.g.*, hydrogenating corn oil to make corn oil margarine) reduces the number of double bonds in the hydrogenated fatty acids.

- *n-3 PUFAs:* Include an essential fatty acid (ALA) with an 18-carbon chain and three cis double bonds. Primary sources include soybean oil, canola oil, walnuts, and flaxseed. Other n-3 fatty acids include EPA and DHA, which have very long carbon chains and are found in fish and shellfish. EPA and DHA are also referred to as "omega-3" fatty acids.

- *n-6 PUFAs:* Include an essential fatty acid (LA) with an 18-carbon chain and two cis double bonds. Primary food sources include nuts and liquid vegetable oils, including soybean, corn, and safflower oils. These are also referred to as "omega-6" fatty acids.

- *Saturated fatty acids:* These are fatty acids with no double bonds and are typically solid at room temperature. Common food sources of saturated fatty acids include meats and dairy products. Some tropical oils (liquid at room temperature) are also high in saturated fatty acids, including coconut and palm oils.

- *Trans-fatty acids:* These are derived from partially hydrogenated vegetable oils and are used in desserts, microwave popcorn, frozen pizza, some margarines, and coffee creamer. While not as prevalent, trans fats also occur in fats from ruminant animals, including cattle and sheep. Trans fats are highly inflammatory and are strongly associated with increased risk of heart disease and cancer.

LIPID METABOLISM

Deriving Energy from Lipids

Triglyceride catabolism produces more than double the ATP energy produced from either protein or carbohydrate, but lipids can be metabolized only aerobically (with oxygen). The by-product of lipid catabolism through the citric acid cycle (Krebs cycle) is carbon dioxide, water, and energy. However, the complete oxidation of fats, via a metabolic pathway called *β-oxidation,* requires carbohydrates and the vitamins B_1, B_2, niacin, and pantothenic acid. It is referred to as "β" oxidation because two carbon atoms at a time enter the metabolic sequence to produce energy.

Without sufficient carbohydrates, ketones may be produced when lipids are catabolized (17). Ketones are typically produced in the liver mitochondria when blood glucose level is low and after glycogen stores are exhausted. Blood glucose is the primary fuel for the brain/central nervous system, but with inadequate blood glucose, ketones are produced from fatty acids as a means of supplying ketones to the central nervous system for energy. Fatty acids are normally broken down via β-oxidation to form acetyl-coenzyme A (acetyl-CoA), and this acetyl-CoA is further oxidized in the citric acid cycle to produce energy. However, if the acetyl-CoA generated in β-oxidation exceeds the capacity of the citric acid cycle because of insufficient intermediates, such as oxaloacetate, then the acetyl-CoA is used to make ketones, such as acetone, rather than ATP (energy). Insufficient intermediate products in the citric acid cycle are more likely with insufficient carbohydrate availability (Figure 4.5). High levels of ketones may result in *ketoacidosis*, which is a dangerous state that can be damaging to tissues, including the kidneys. Ketoacidosis occurs in diabetics who are not controlling blood sugar well, people who are fasting, and people on high-protein, high-fat, low-carbohydrate diets that are referred to as ketogenic diets. People making high levels of ketones typically have acetone breath (acetone is a ketone that smells like nail polish remover), suggesting that blood sugar is low.

Making New Lipids

Humans are effective manufacturers of lipids and are capable of making and storing lipids from excess protein,

FIGURE 4.5: Oxidation of lipids for energy.

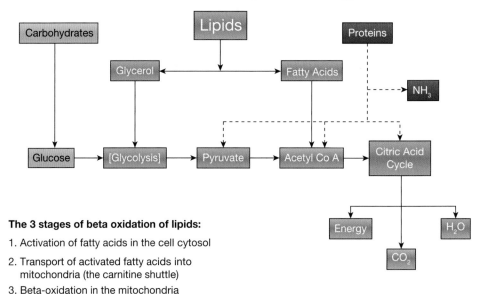

Beta Oxidation of Lipids for Energy

The 3 stages of beta oxidation of lipids:

1. Activation of fatty acids in the cell cytosol
2. Transport of activated fatty acids into mitochondria (the carnitine shuttle)
3. Beta-oxidation in the mitochondria

excess carbohydrate, and excess lipids. The ability to manufacture lipids is important for a number of critical cellular processes, including cell membranes and internal structure, production of lipid-based hormones, and storage of excess energy. The fatty acids that we can manufacture for these processes are referred to as nonessential fatty acids (*i.e.*, it is not essential that we consume them because we can make them), and they are synthesized in body cells from acetyl-CoA via an enzyme referred to as *fatty acid synthase*. Following the formation of the fatty acid, the enzymes called *acetyltransferases* attach three fatty acids to a glycerol molecule to create triglycerides. Also important to this process are insulin and the vitamins biotin, B_2, niacin, and pantothenic acid. Insulin aids new fatty acid synthesis by making glucose and fatty acids available to cells, and any amount of glucose that exceeds cellular requirements can be made into triglycerides and placed in storage (*i.e.*, the fat mass) (18,19).

LIPID RECOMMENDATIONS AND FOOD SOURCES

One of the key principles of the U.S. 2015–2020 Dietary Recommendations is to limit energy consumption from saturated fats because they tend to increase blood cholesterol and cardiovascular disease risk. As can be seen from Table 4.6, it is good to have a *high* amount of HDLs and a *low* amount of LDLs (Figure 4.6).

The current intake of saturated fat in most people is excessive, primarily from the consumption of animal fats (20). The Institute of Medicine recommendation for healthy people is to have a fat intake that constitutes between 25% and 35% of total calories consumed. Of this, less than 10% should come from saturated fats. This level of intake is ~1.0 g/kg, but may be greater than this amount depending on fitness and energy needs. For instance, endurance athletes may require up to 2.0 g/kg satisfying energy requirements, but endurance athletes typically have a high capacity to metabolize fats as a source of energy (21). Some athletes with extraordinarily high energy requirements may have even higher fat requirements as the only reasonable means of satisfying the need for energy.

Lipids also deliver the essential fatty acids, with recommendations for **linoleic acid** that range from 7 to 17 g/day (depending on age) and for linolenic acid that range from 0.7 to 1.6 g/day (Table 4.6).

Linoleic Acid

An *essential* polyunsaturated fatty acid (*i.e.*, it must be consumed as humans cannot manufacture it) with the first double bond at the sixth carbon (n-6). It is found in cell membranes and is involved in the production of other fatty acids and protective substances. Common dietary sources are vegetable oils, and it is particularly high in safflower, sunflower, corn, and soybean oils.

When required for energy, the stored subcutaneous and visceral triglycerides are broken apart into their component fatty acids and glycerol and transported to the tissues in the blood plasma. The glycerol is metabolized like

Table 4.6 Daily Nutritional Goals for Age–Sex Groups Based on Dietary Reference Intakes and Dietary Guidelines Recommendations

Value	Source	1–3 y	F 4–8	M 4–8	F 9–13	M 9–13	F 14–18	M 14–18	F 19–30	M 19–30	F 31–50	M 31–50	F 51+	M 51+
Total fat, % kcal	AMDR	30–40	25–35	25–35	25–35	25–35	25–35	25–35	20–35	20–35	20–35	20–35	20–35	20–35
Saturated fat, % kcal	DGA	<10%	<10%	<10%	<10%	<10%	<10%	<10%	<10%	<10%	<10%	<10%	<10%	<10%
Linoleic acid, g/day	AI	7	10	10	10	12	11	16	12	17	12	17	11	14
Linolenic acid, g/day	AI	0.7	0.9	0.9	1	1.2	1.1	1.6	1.1	1.6	1.1	1.6	1.1	1.6

AI, adequate intake; AMDR, acceptable macronutrient distribution range; DGA, Dietary Guidelines for Americans.

Source: United States Department of Agriculture and United States Department of Health and Human Services. 2015–2020 Dietary Guidelines for Americans. 8th ed. December 2015. Accessed 2018 April 20. Available from: http://health.gov/dietaryguidelines/2015/guidelines/; Institute of Medicine. Dietary Reference Intakes for Energy, Carbohydrate, Fiber, Fat, Fatty Acids, Cholesterol, Protein, and Amino Acids 2005. Washington (DC). The National Academies press: https://doi.org/10.17226/10490

FIGURE 4.6: Reference ranges for blood lipids. (From Reference Ranges for Blood Lipids. Understanding what your cholesterol level means [Internet]. Accessed 2017 September. Available from: http://www.cholesterolmenu. com/cholesterol-levels-chart/).

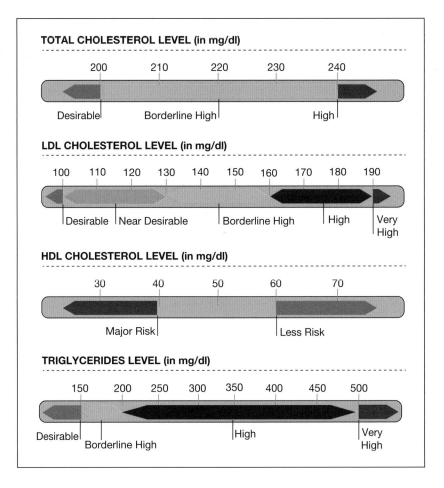

a carbohydrate and is available to all tissues for energy created via aerobic or anaerobic metabolism. Glycerol also has gluconeogenic potential, where it can be converted into glucose and stored as liver glycogen or used to satisfy central nervous system, organ, and muscular energy needs as blood glucose. The fatty acids are transported to muscle and organ tissue, where they are oxidized to create ATP energy.

LIPIDS AND HEALTH

Monounsaturated and Polyunsaturated Fatty Acids

Both MUFAs and PUFAs have been found to be protective against the development of cardiovascular disease by lowering blood cholesterol, but PUFAs are more vulnerable to peroxide formation (rancidity) than are MUFAs. There is also some evidence that MUFAs may help to sustain good cholesterol (HDL) (22). The most commonly consumed MUFA is oleic fatty acid, which is highly prevalent in olive oil and, possibly, one of the reasons (along with higher fish and vegetable consumption) why the Mediterranean Diet is recommended for reducing disease risks. As an example, the food intake of Crete, a Greek Island, has a typical fat intake that is high, providing about 40% of total calories, but a large proportion of the fat consumed is from olive oil. The population of Crete has relatively low coronary heart disease and colon cancer prevalence (23). The Mediterranean Diet also has a balance of omega-3 and omega-6 fatty acids, which is important because some omega-6 fatty acids tend to be inflammatory to tissues, while omega-3 fatty acids tend to be anti-inflammatory. By contrast with the Mediterranean Diet, the typical diet in the United States may contain 14–25 times more omega-6 than omega-3 fatty acids. These differences are important, as MUFA intake has been found to be inversely associated with risk of all-cause mortality (24). It has also been found that elevating the intake of omega-3 fatty acids for 1 month results in a lowering of postexercise fatigue and reduced delayed onset muscle soreness (DOMS) in trained male athletes (25). There is also evidence that a diet replacing omega-6 fatty acids with omega-3 fatty acids results in a cardioprotective and neuroprotective effect in football players (26).

Because saturated fats are associated with an increase in harmful LDL cholesterol, which increases cardiovascular disease risk, the intake of saturated fatty acids should be less than 10% of total calories. There is evidence that maintaining a relatively low total fat consumption while replacing saturated fats with polyunsaturated fats from vegetable oils is an effective strategy for reducing heart disease risk.

Trans Fats

As potentially harmful as a high intake of saturated fats may be, consumption of trans fats places individuals at even higher risk of cardiovascular disease (27). Trans fats are typically found in margarine and shortening which were partially hydrogenated to make the original oil more solid. Margarine and shortening were commonly used in commercial cooking as deep-fat frying oil for French fries and are used in commercial pastries (cookies, cakes, etc.). Trans fats increase harmful LDL cholesterol and are inflammatory to tissues, both of which are associated with stroke, heart disease, diabetes, and cancer. Some studies have found that even very small amounts of trans fats, as little as 2% of consumed fat, may increase heart disease risk by over 20% (13).

Omega-3 Fatty Acids

There are three different omega-3 fatty acids, all of which are polyunsaturated:

- ALA
- EPA
- DHA

They are referred to as omega-3 fatty acids because the first double bond, counting from the nonacid end of the fatty acid, occurs at the third carbon atom. EPA and DHA are derived from fish, and ALA (one of the essential fatty acids) is derived from vegetables, seeds, and nuts. Flax seed is a commonly used nonfish food used to enhance the dietary intake of ALA, which we can use to synthesize the other omega-3 fatty acids. They have been found in a number of studies to be profoundly important for health:

- DHA is highly concentrated in the cell membranes of the retina of the eye, and animal studies have

determined that DHA is necessary for the development and function of the retina (28). In several studies assessing visual function in preterm infants, DHA added to the formula resulted in significant improvement of visual function (29).

- A study that assessed 1,822 males for 30 years found that death from coronary heart disease was 38% lower in men who consumed an average of 1.2 oz/day of fish than in men who ate no fish. In addition, the men who ate fish had a mortality rate from heart attack that was 67% lower. Fish is a primary source of the omega-3 fatty acids ALA and EPA (30). Studies have found that women consuming more ALA from foods have a 54% lower risk of death from coronary heart disease than women consuming less food-based ALA (31). Based on these and other studies, the American Heart Association recommends the consumption of 1 g/day of an EPA and DHA combination, either from food or through supplemental intake (32).
- Fish oils (EPA and DHA) have been found to significantly lower serum triglyceride in diabetics. High circulating triglycerides are a common serious health risk in type 2 diabetics (33). In addition, fish oils have the potential to enable healthier aging in master athletes by beneficially altering the membranes of mitochondria and other cellular membranes (34)
- Consumption of omega-3 fatty acids has been shown to reduce the debilitating inflammatory effects of rheumatoid arthritis after 12 weeks of increased consumption (35).
- Several studies have found that increased consumption of EPA and DHA reduced the inflammation associated with ulcerative colitis, which is an inflammatory disease of the large intestine (36).
- In studies of people with psychological disorders (schizophrenia, depression, and bipolar disorder), consumption of EPA and DHA resulted in less depression than in those taking a placebo (37).

However, it has also been suggested that *excess* intake of omega-3 fatty acids may have adverse effects, including higher risks of prostate cancer, reduced immunity, and atrial fibrillation that could result in stroke (38). Taken together, these studies suggest that increasing the food consumption of omega-3 fatty acids from more regular (~2/wk) fish consumption may result in improved health without risking the health problems that could occur from regular excess intakes through supplementation. In simple terms, getting enough is important, but regular exposure to too much may create health problems.

LIPIDS AND EXERCISE

Stored lipids are sufficient to satisfy, theoretically, the energy needs of even healthy and lean athletes who participate in multiday ultramarathons without having the need to refuel. Of course, other nutrient limitations would cause the exercise to stop before fat was exhausted, but this point is to demonstrate that lipid availability is not likely to be the limiting substrate in exercise. Typical lipid storage is between 5,500 and 11,100 g or between 50,000 and 100,000 calories. In an average 70 kg (154 lb) man with a relatively low body fat of 15%, fat storage is about 10,311 g or 92,800 calories (39). Since the average cost of going 1.6 km (1 mile) is about 100 calories, this represents enough fuel to go between 800 and 1,660 km (500–1,000 miles). In addition to the caloric potential of subcutaneous and visceral-stored lipid, muscle tissues also store 2,000–3,000 calories of triglycerides, which can become quickly available to cells as a fuel under the right oxidative conditions.

Oxygen is required to derive energy from lipids, and lower-intensity exercise makes it easier to satisfy the oxygen requirement for fat metabolism. As a result, lower-intensity activities are associated with a high proportion of fat metabolism to satisfy the need for energy. As the intensity of exercise increases, more carbohydrate is metabolized to satisfy the energy requirement, and a lower *proportion* of fat is metabolized (Figure 4.7). It is also important to remember that carbohydrate is required for the complete oxidation of fat for energy, without which ketones are produced. Ketones are acidic and may compromise exercise endurance (40).

Many people perform low-intensity exercise (often referred to as *cardio*) in the desire to burn fat as an energy substrate and therefore lower the body fat level. However, the *proportion* of fat metabolized should not be confused with the *volume* of fat metabolized, because as exercise intensity increases, more energy is burned per unit of time than in lower-intensity activity (see Example 4.2).

Example 4.2: Burning Fats for Energy

The following scenarios illustrate the potential for confusing proportion with volume:

■ *Scenario 1:* A person is exercising for 1 hour and doing low-intensity activity that burns about 100 calories every 15 minutes, for a total of 400 calories burned during the hour. Of this, ~80% of the energy is supplied by fat (320 calories from fat), and 20% is supplied by carbohydrate (80 calories from carbohydrate).

■ *Scenario 2:* A person is exercising for 1 hour, and doing higher intensity activity that burns about 150 calories every 15 minutes, for a total of 600 calories burned during the hours. Of this, ~60% of the energy is supplied by fat (360 calories from fat), and 40% is supplied by carbohydrate (240 calories from carbohydrate).

While lower-intensity exercise burned a higher *proportion* of calories from fat (80%; 320 calories from fat), the higher-intensity exercise burned a higher *volume* of calories from fat but at a lower proportion of fat burned for energy (60%; 360 calories from fat). When calculating the metabolism of energy substrates to supply energy, both proportion and volume should be considered.

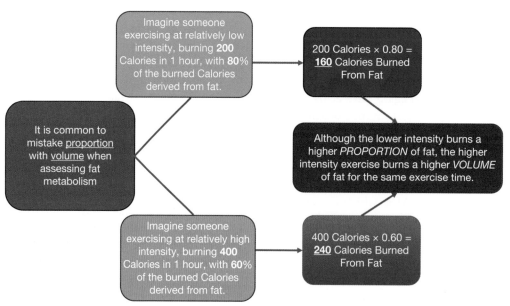

FIGURE 4.7: Fat burned at different intensities. (See Figure 2.4 in Chapter 2.)

Other factors in addition to exercise intensity also play a role in terminating the use of fat during exercise. These include the following:

- *Available fat reserves in muscle:* Some muscle fiber cells have a higher capacity to store triglycerides than other cells. Type I slow-twitch aerobic fibers have a high capacity for cellular lipids, while Type II fast-twitch anaerobic fibers have a lower capacity for cellular lipids. Most people have an even distribution of Type I and Type II fibers, but some people have a higher proportion of Type I fibers, enabling them to use more fat to satisfy the energy requirement.

- *Ability to mobilize and transport lipids from adipose tissue to working muscle:* An exercise-associated increase in sympathetic nerve activity stimulates the production of epinephrine (*i.e.*, adrenalin), which binds to adipose tissue and begins the process of transporting fats to muscle cells. Glycerol is transported to the liver for gluconeogenesis or directly to the muscle cell for metabolism. Fatty acids are bound to albumin to form HDL, which is actively transported into the muscle cell for metabolism. There are several hormones, besides adrenalin, that either stimulate or inhibit the utilization of fat (Table 4.7).

- *Availability of stored glycogen:* Higher carbohydrate intakes are associated with higher glycogen storage, and the better carbohydrate availability during exercise enhances the capacity to completely metabolize fats as an energy substrate. Insufficient carbohydrate availability inhibits β-oxidation, creating incompletely burned fats (ketones), and compromising total energy and fat expenditure.

- *Amount of carbohydrate consumed during exercise:* Sustaining a normal blood glucose level helps to sustain carbohydrate availability and enhances fat metabolism in aerobic activities.

- *Effect of training on fat utilization:* Exercise training has multiple effects on fat utilization, with studies indicating that both endurance and resistance training increase intermuscular triglyceride utilization, resulting in a lower requirement for glycogen at the same exercise intensity. Since glycogen storage is limited, using more fat to satisfy energy needs "spares" glycogen, resulting in improved endurance. In physically fit individuals who are training regularly, peak fat oxidation occurs at a higher $\dot{V}O_{2max}$ (59%–65%) than in untrained individuals (47%–52%) (20,41). (See Chapter 2, Figure 2.8.)

- *Postexercise period:* In the period immediately after exercise, there is a high metabolic priority to resynthesize muscle glycogen that limits carbohydrate utilization for energy. This results in a sustained high fatty acid oxidation following an exercise bout (42).

A good deal of attention is being given to whether increasing total fat consumption, coupled with an exercise program, results in an adaptation toward greater fat utilization that warrants an increase in fat consumption. Regular endurance training does cause skeletal muscle to adapt by enhancing the utilization of all energy substrates, including a particularly high improvement in the utilization of lipids (43). This is an important adaptation, because greater lipid utilization to satisfy the energy requirement reduces the utilization of glycogen, which has limited storage, with the result that it takes longer to deplete glycogen and endurance performance is enhanced.

Some have hypothesized that increased fat consumption will greatly enhance the lipid metabolism adaptation and improve endurance performance still further. However, the effect of consuming a high-fat (60%–65% of energy consumed) diet that is relatively low in carbohydrate (less than 20% of energy consumed) for even short durations of less than 3 days has the effect of lowering muscle and liver glycogen storage. The outcome of these short-term high-fat/low-carbohydrate diets is to reduce endurance, likely because of an insufficient amount of time for adaptation to occur (44). Indeed, there are studies suggesting that high-fat/low-carbohydrate diets that

Table 4.7	Hormonal and Nutritional Factors That Influence the Utilization of Lipids for Energy (Lipolysis)	
Stimulators of Lipolysis	**Inhibitors of Lipolysis**
Epinephrine	Insulin
Norepinephrine	Leptin
Dopamine	Niacin/nicotinic acid
Cortisol	
Growth hormone	
Thyroid-stimulating hormone	
Calcium	
Caffeine	

Source: From Duncan RE, Ahmadian M, Jaworski K, Sarkadi-Nagy E, Sul HS. Regulation of lipolysis in adipocytes. Annu Rev Nutr. 2007; 27:79–101.

are coupled with endurance activity for longer periods may improve fat oxidation in both lower- and moderate-intensity activities, suggesting an adaptation to the lower glycogen availability (45). Should this strategy be followed, endurance athletes should carefully monitor the impact of this dietary change to balance the risk of reduced performance in higher-intensity activity as a result of reduced carbohydrate stores (2,46). Ideally, athletes should plan to enhance lipid metabolism while also maximizing glycogen storage, enabling more high-intensity bursts of activity, even during endurance events/training. Studies have found that a single day of high-carbohydrate intake coupled with avoidance of any activity that would utilize glycogen (typically complete rest) is enough to maximize stored glycogen in athletes who are endurance trained (47,48). Therefore, a higher fat consumption, to enhance fat metabolism in endurance training, coupled with a high-carbohydrate intake and rest on the day prior to competition may be an important strategy for improving endurance performance (49,50). A word of caution, however, since these findings appear relevant only to *endurance* athletes. For those who require frequent bursts of speed (*i.e.*, team sports) or are performing at the top intensity possible (*i.e.*, sprinters, gymnasts), the training protocols they follow would not allow for the appropriate adaptations, suggesting that a higher-fat/lower-carbohydrate diet would not be appropriate for them. High body fat levels are inversely associated with the amount of time people spend in exercise training. It is possible that higher-intensity activity, because it lowers glycogen stores, can force a higher reliance on fat oxidation for fuel and therefore compensate for the excessively high-fat intakes of most Western cultures. However, those wishing to lower body fat should be cautious of consuming a higher-fat diet, regardless of the exercise protocol, because the higher energy density of fat could more easily contribute to greater fat storage, obesity, and associated health risks (51).

SUMMARY

- Lipids are a highly concentrated source of energy, providing more than double the calories per gram (9 calories/g) than either carbohydrate or protein (4 calories/g).
- Lipids have many functions other than the provision of energy—providing the essential fatty acids, providing a carrier for the fat-soluble vitamins, improving food flavor and meal satiety, and serving as a protective blanket to help control body temperature in environmental extremes.
- The essential fatty acids are alpha-linolenic acid and linoleic acid, which must be consumed from foods as humans are unable to synthesize these fatty acids.
- There are many different kinds of lipids, and triglycerides make up the majority of fats in the human diet and in the human body. These triglycerides have one glycerol and three fatty acids linked together in a single molecule.
- There are different kinds of fatty acids. Some fatty acids are saturated, some are monounsaturated, and some are polyunsaturated. Each type of fatty acid has a different function, and different kinds of fatty acids pose different health risks or health benefits.
- The general recommendation for fat intake for adults is between 20% and 35% of total calories consumed. Of this amount, it is generally considered more healthful to have a higher proportion of mono- and polyunsaturated fats than saturated fats.
- When fats are consumed, they are absorbed into the blood as chylomicrons, a very LDL that must be converted by lipoprotein lipase into LDL to be taken up by tissues and cleared from the blood.
- Chylomicrons and LDLs are considered "bad" lipids/cholesterol because they can increase atherosclerosis and heart disease risks. Avoiding large meals that are high in fats helps to reduce circulating chylomicrons and LDLs.
- When lipids are removed from storage (*i.e.*, removed from adipose tissue) to be metabolized for energy, HDLs are formed. HDLs are considered "good" lipids/cholesterol because they suggest that lipids are being metabolized for energy.
- The physical activity/training associated with sport and exercise increases the requirement for energy. Because lipids are highly concentrated in energy, they can help athletes satisfy their energy requirements.

Physically active people are better able to metabolize lipids for energy and, in doing so, are less likely to have high body fat levels. Lipid metabolism for energy requires oxygen, and one of the adaptations that occur in people who exercise is to improve the oxygen delivery system to muscle cells so they can more efficiently burn fats for energy.

Practical Application Activity

Lipid intake can be analyzed as a percentage of total calories consumed (% fat) or as grams of fat/kg mass (g/kg). The usual method is to calculate the proportion of calories derived from fats, which should be ~25% to 35% of total calories. Cholesterol intake should be less than 300 mg/day to help ensure that LDL cholesterol is below 100 mg/dL. You can assess your fat and cholesterol content of consumed foods using the same strategy followed in earlier chapters, accessing the online USDA Food Composition Database (https://fdc.nal.usda.gov/), but this time create a spreadsheet with Energy (calories), Total Lipid (g), Total Saturated Fatty Acids (g), Total Monounsaturated Fatty Acids (g), Total Trans-Fatty Acids (g), and Cholesterol (mg).

1. Enter the foods/beverages with amounts consumed for an entire day, and create totals for Energy (calories) and each lipid component.
2. Calculate percentage of total calories from fat (Total Fat Grams × 9/Total Energy).
3. Calculate grams of fat/kg mass (Total Fat Grams/Your Weight in kg).
4. Determine if total fat intake as percentage of total calories is within the acceptable range (20%–35% of total calories). If above 35% of total calories, what dietary changes would you make to lower total fat consumption?
5. Determine if your cholesterol is above the dietary guidelines recommended limit of 100–300 mg/day for various calorie levels. If above 300 mg/day, what dietary changes would you make to lower dietary cholesterol intake?
6. Determine if your saturated fat intake is below the recommended intake limit (<10% of total calories/day). If so, what changes would you make to replace saturated fat with healthier monounsaturated and polyunsaturated fats?
7. It is generally recommended that trans fats be avoided because they are highly inflammatory and may significantly increase the risk of heart disease. Assess your trans-fat intake, and determine what dietary changes would be needed to avoid trans-fat consumption.

CHAPTER QUESTIONS

1. The fat that contains only one double bond between carbons is:
   a. Saturated fat
   b. Monounsaturated fat
   c. Polyunsaturated fat
   d. Cholesterol

2. An example of a food containing predominantly saturated fat is:
   a. Skim milk
   b. Corn oil
   c. Margarine
   d. Butter

3. An example of a food containing predominantly monounsaturated fat is:
   a. Olive oil
   b. Corn oil
   c. Hamburger
   d. Butter

4. Cholesterol is found in which food categories?
   a. Fruits, vegetables, and grains
   b. Meats and poultry
   c. Fish and shellfish
   d. All the above
   e. b and c only

5. The type of fat that is inflammatory and has the highest risk of increasing the risk of heart disease is:
   a. Monounsaturated fat
   b. Omega-3 fatty acids
   c. Omega-6 fatty acids
   d. Trans-fatty acids

6. What happens to vegetable and cereal oils when they are hydrogenated?
   a. The carbon chains become longer
   b. The fatty acids become solid and more saturated
   c. They taste less rancid but can spoil more quickly
   d. They are more easily digested

7. With the onset of moderate-intensity, steady-state exercise, about how long does it take for the oxidation of fat to reach its maximal rate?
   a. 1.5 minutes
   b. 10–20 minutes
   c. 30–45 minutes
   d. A minimum of 60 minutes, with 90 minutes being the average

8. Good food sources of omega-3 fatty acids include:
   a. Whole wheat bread and corn oil
   b. Olive oil and fish
   c. Fresh vegetables and fresh fruits
   d. Rice and rice oil

9. Trans-fatty acids are created when:
   a. Saturated fatty acids are hydrogenated
   b. Unsaturated fatty acids are hydrogenated
   c. Soft margarine is heated during normal cooking
   d. The solid fatty acids in margarine and butter are turned to liquid oil during cooking

10. Good lipoproteins are _____, and bad lipoproteins are _____.
    a. Chylomicrons and HDL
    b. LDL and HDL
    c. VLDL and HDL
    d. HDL and LDL

ANSWERS TO CHAPTER QUESTIONS

1. b
2. d
3. a
4. e
5. d
6. b
7. c
8. b
9. b
10. d

Case Study Considerations

1. **Case Study Answer 1:** The kind of high-intensity work that is required of football linemen is highly dependent on carbohydrate, making the distribution of energy substrates (carbohydrate, protein, and fat) a critically important consideration. John's early focus on simply increasing total energy intake, much of it coming from fat, fails to consider this issue. For instance, the calories of carbohydrate consumed should be approximately double that of calories from fat. In addition, there should be a dynamic link between energy consumed and energy expended, so that John can maintain a reasonably good energy balanced state throughout the day. This will require a snacking/drinking pattern that can sustain both energy balance and blood sugar to avoid production of cortisol, a catabolic hormone that will negatively impact the muscle mass John is seeking to increase. Increasing muscle weight requires that the physical activity is slightly elevated beyond what John is accustomed to so that the muscle will adapt to the elevated stress. Because muscle mass changes slowly, the elevation in energy intake should also be relatively small so that excess energy consumption is not stored as fat. A proportion if this increased energy consumption should be derived from protein to both increase and support the elevation in musculature. However, providing a high level of protein via a typical three meals/day meal pattern may exceed the body's capacity to use it as intended (*i.e.*, to elevate and sustain muscle mass). Therefore, a greater meal frequency that could help to sustain energy balance is also more likely to provide protein in the smaller more frequent doses that could help enlarge and sustain musculature. In addition, a greater meal frequency that has more carbohydrates (*i.e.*, whole grains, fresh vegetables, fresh fruits, etc.) should help to lower the intake of fats, many of which are inflammatory and make the athletic endeavor more difficult. Athletes should be cautious of satisfying elevated carbohydrate requirements via the consumption of refined grain products, as the elevated insulin response to these foods is likely to increase total body fat storage and detract from the strength-to-weight ratio. However, consumption of less refined carbohydrate foods does not have this same negative effect (52).

2. **Case Study Answer 2**: It is important for John to understand that "weight" is not the right metric for what he wishes to achieve. While the coach encouraged him to put on some "weight," what he really should have encouraged John to do is to put on some "muscle." Elevating musculature relative to total weight increases the strength-to-weight ratio, making it easier for the athlete to move more quickly. In addition, because more muscle is moving less nonmuscle weight, endurance is also enhanced because muscle doesn't have to work as hard to

achieve the desired outcome. To do this a body composition assessment that is taken twice monthly to track changes in muscle mass and fat mass is a desirable strategy to determine if the diet and exercise protocol being followed is achieving the desired result (*i.e.*, more muscle mass and the same or less fat mass). Following this body composition assessment strategy would have quickly found that John's weight increase was predominantly from fat, and that his strength-to-weight ratio was moving in the wrong direction.

REFERENCES

1. Che K, Qiu J, Yi L, Zou M, Li Z, Carr A, Snipe RMJ, Benardot D. Effects of a short-term "fat adaptation with carbohydrate restoration" diet on metabolic responses and exercise performance in well-trained runners. Nutrients. 2021;13:1033.
2. Burke LM, Whitfield J, Heikura IA, Ross MLR, Tee N, Forbes SF, Hall R, McKay AKA, Wallett AM, Sharma AP. Adaptation to a low carbohydrate high fat diet is rapid but impairs endurance exercise metabolism and performance despite enhanced glycogen availability. J Physiol. 2021;599(3):771–90.
3. Anderson GS. Human morphology and temperature regulation. Int J Biometreorol. 1999;43(3):99–109.
4. Farvid MS, Ding M, Pan A, Sun Q, Chiuve SE, Steffen LM, Willett WC, Hu FB. Dietary linoleic acid and risk of coronary heart disease: a systematic review and meta-analysis of prospective cohort studies. Circulation. 2014;130:1568–78.
5. Horrobin DF. Nutrition and medical importance of gamma-linolenic acid. Prog Lipid Res. 1992;31(2):163–94.
6. Ivanov I, Kuhn H, Heydeck D. Structural and functional biology of arachidonic acid 15-lipoxygenase-1 (ALOX15). Gene. 2015;573(1):1–32.
7. Calder PC. Functional roles of fatty acids and their effects on human health. J Parenter Enteral Nutr. 2015;39(1 Suppl):18S–32S.
8. Raper NR, Cronin FJ, Exler J. Omega-3 fatty acid content of the US food supply. J Am Coll Nutr. 1992;11(3):304–8.
9. Williams CM, Burdge G. Long-chain n-3 PUFA: plant v. marine sources. Proc Nutr Soc. 2006;65(1):42–50.
10. Li H, van de Voort FR, Ismail AA, .Sedman J, Cox R, Simard C, Buijs H. Discrimination of edible oil products and quantitative determination of their iodine value by Fourier transform near-infrared spectroscopy. J Am Oil Chem Soc. 2000;77(1):29–36.
11. Mattson FH, Lutton ES. The specific distribution of fatty acids in the glycerides of animal and vegetable fats. J Biol Chem. 1958;233(4):868–71.
12. Firestone D. Determination of the iodine value of oils and fats: summary of collaborative study. J AOAC Int. 1994;77(3):674–6.
13. Brownell KD, Pomeranz JL. The trans-fat ban—food regulation and long-term health. N Engl J Med. 2014;370:1773–5.
14. Tomkin GH, Owens D. The chylomicron: relationship to atherosclerosis. Int J Vasc Med. 2012;2012.
15. Burén J, Ericsson M, Damasceno NRT, Sjödin A. A ketogenic low-carbohydrate high-fat diet increases LDL cholesterol in healthy, young, normal-weight women: a randomized controlled feeding trial. Nutrients. 2021;13(3):814.
16. Ruidavets J-B, Ducimetiére P, Arveller D, Amouyel P, Bingham A, Wagner A, Cottel D, Perret B, Ferrières J. Types of alcoholic beverages and blood lipids in a French population. J Epidemiol Community Health. 2002;56:24–8.
17. Cox PJ, Kirk T, Ashmore T, Willerton K, Evans R, Smith A, Murray AJ, Stubbs B, West J, McLure SW, King MT, Dodd MS, Holloway C, Neubauer S, Drawer S, Veech RL, Griffin JL, Clarke K. Nutritional ketosis alters fuel preference and thereby endurance performance in athletes. Cell Metab. 2016;24(2):256–68.
18. Kulkarni SS, Salehzadeh F, Fritz T, Zierath JR, Krook A, Osler ME. Mitochondrial regulators of fatty acid metabolism reflect metabolic dysfunction in type 2 diabetes mellitus. Metabolism. 2012;61(2):175–85.
19. Wakil SJ, editor. Lipid metabolism. New York (NY): Academic Press, Inc; 1970.
20. United States Department of Agriculture and United States Department of Health and Human Services. 2015–2020 Dietary Guidelines for Americans. 8th ed. 2015 December. Accessed 2018 April 20. Available from: http://health.gov/dietaryguidelines/2015/guidelines/
21. Horvath PJ, Eagen CK, Fisher NM, Leddy JJ, Pendergast DR. The effects of varying dietary fat on performance and metabolism in trained male and female runners. J Am Coll Nutr. 2000;19(1):52–60.
22. Mensink RP, Katan M. Effect of monounsaturated fatty acids versus complex carbohydrates on high-density lipoproteins in healthy men and women. Lancet. 1987;329(8525):122–5.
23. Simopoulos AP. The Mediterranean diets: what is so special about the diet of Greece? The scientific evidence. J Nutr. 2001;131(11):30655–735.
24. Lotfi K, Salari-Moghaddam A, Yousefinia M, Larijani B, Esmaillzadeh A. Dietary intakes of monounsaturated fatty acids and risk of mortality from all causes, cardiovascular disease and cancer: a systematic review and dose-response meta-analysis of prospective cohort studies. Ageing Res Rev. 2021;72:101467.
25. Benson L, Mushtaq S. Dietary supplementation with n-3 fatty acids (n-3 FA) for 4 weeks reduces post-exercise fatigue and delayed onset muscle soreness (DOMS) in trained male athletes. Proc Nutr Soc. 2015;74(OCE5):E280.

26. Heileson JL, Anzalone AJ, Carbon AF, Askow AT, Stone JD, Turner SM, Hillyer LM, Ma DWL, Luedke JA, Jagim AR, Oliver JM. The effect of omega-3 fatty acids on a biomarker of head trauma in NCAA football athletes: a multi-site, non-randomized study. J Int Soc Sports Nutr. 2021;18(1):65.

27. Kim Y, Je Y, Giovannucci EL. Association between dietary fat intake and mortality from all-causes, cardiovascular disease, and cancer: a systematic review and meta-analysis of prospective cohort studies. Clin Nutr. 2021;40(3):1060–70.

28. Bazan NG. Neuroprotectin D1 (NPD1): a DHA-derived mediator that protects brain and retina against cell injury-induced oxidative stress. Brain Pathol. 2005;15(2):159–66.

29. Makrides M, Neumann MA, Byard RW, Simmer K, Gibson RA. Fatty acid composition of brain, retina, and erythrocytes in breast- and formula-fed infants. Am J Clin Nutr. 1994;60(2):189–94.

30. Leaf A. Prevention of sudden cardiac death by n-3 polyunsaturated fatty acids. J Cardiovasc Med. 2007;8(1):S27–9.

31. Willet WC. The role of dietary n-6 fatty acids in the prevention of cardiovascular disease. J Cardiovasc Med. 2007;8:S42–5.

32. Chiuve SE, Cook NR, Vandenburgh MJ, Rimm EB, Manson JE, Albert CM. Abstract 15888: N-3 polyunsaturated fatty acids in erythrocyte membranes and risk of sudden cardiac death in primary and secondary prevention. Circulation. 2015;132:A15888.

33. Cormier H, Rudkowska I, Lemieux S, Couture P, Julien P, Vohl MC. Changes in plasma phospholipid fatty acid patterns and their impact on plasma triglyceride levels following fish oil supplementation. Int J Food Sci, Nutr Diet. 2015;S2:001:1–10. http://dx.doi.org/10.19070/2326-3350-SI02001

34. Murphy CH, McGlory C. Fish oil for healthy aging: Potential application to master athletes. Sports Med. 2021;51(Supplement 1):S31–41.

35. Leitzmann MF, Stampfer MJ, Michaud DS, Augustsson K, Colditz GC, Willett WC, Giovannucci EL. Dietary intake of n-3 and n-6 fatty acids and the risk of prostate cancer. Am J Clin Nutr. 2004;80:204–16.

36. Middleton SJ, Naylor S, Woolner J, Hunter JO. A double-blind, randomized, placebo-controlled trial of essential fatty acid supplementation in the maintenance of remission of ulcerative colitis. Aliment Pharmacol Ther. 2002;16(6):1131–5.

37. Morgan AJ, Jorm AF. Self-help interventions for depressive disorders and depressive symptoms: a systematic review. Ann Gen Psychiatry. 2008;7:13.

38. Fenton JI, Hord NG, Ghosh S, Gurzell EA. Immunomodulation by dietary long chain omega-3 fatty acids and the potential for adverse health outcomes. Prostaglandins Leukot Essent Fatty Acids. 2013;89(6):379–90.

39. Maughan R. IOC encyclopedia of sports medicine: nutrition and exercise. Chichester: Wiley Blackwell; 2000.

40. Whitfield J, Burke LM, McKay AKA, Heikura IA, Hall R, Fensham N, Sharma AP. Acute ketogenic diet and ketone ester supplementation impairs race walk performance. Med Sci Sports Exerc. 2021;53(4):776–84.

41. Saltin B, Astrand PO. Free fatty acids and exercise. Am J Clin Nutr. 1993;57(5):752S–75.

42. Kimber NE, Heigenhauser GJ, Spriet LL, Dyck DJ. Skeletal muscle fat and carbohydrate metabolism during recovery from glycogen-depleting exercise in humans. J Physiol. 2003;548(3):919–27.

43. Brooks GA, Mercier J. Balance of carbohydrate and lipid utilization during exercise: the "crossover" concept. J Appl Physiol. 1994;76:2253–61.

44. Burke LM, Hawley JA. Effects of short-term fat adaptation on metabolism and performance of prolonged exercise. Med Sci Sports Exerc. 2002;34:1492–8.

45. Stepto NK, Carey AL, Staudacher HM, Cummins NK, Burke LM, Hawley JA. Effect of short-term fat adaptation on high-intensity training. Med Sci Sports Exerc. 2002;34:449–55.

46. Burke LM. Ketogenic low-CHO, high-fat diet: the future of elite endurance sport? J Physiol. 2020;599(3):819–43.

47. Stellingwerff T, Spriet LL, Watt MJ, Kimber NE, Hargreaves M, Hawley JA, Burke LM. Decreased PDH activation and glycogenolysis during exercise following fat adaptation with carbohydrate restoration. Am J Physiol Endocrinol Metabol. 2006;290:E380–8.

48. Yeo WK, Carey AL, Burke L, Spriet LL, Hawley JA. Fat adaptation in well-trained athletes: effects on cell metabolism. Appl Physiol Nutr Metabol. 2011;36:12–22.

49. Hawley JA, Yeo WK. Metabolic adaptations to a high-fat diet. In: Maughan RJ, editor. Sports nutrition. Chichester: Wiley Blackwell; 2014:166–73.

50. Martin WH, Dalsky GP, Hurley BF, Matthews DE, Bier DM, Hagberg JM, Rogers MA, King DS, Holloszy JO. Effect of endurance training on plasma free fatty acid turnover and oxidation during exercise. Am J Physiol Endocrinol Metab. 1993;265(5):E708–14.

51. Schrauwen P, Westerterp KR. The role of high-fat diets and physical activity in the regulation of body weight. Br J Nutr. 2000;84(4):417–27.

52. Swaminathan S, Dehghan M, Raj JM, Thomas T, Rangarajan S, Jenkins D, Mony P, Mohan V, Lear SA, Avezum A, Lopez-Jaramillo P, Rosengren A, Lanas F, AlHabib KF, Dans A, Keskinler MV, Puoane T, Soman B, Wei L, Zatonska K, Diaz R, Ismail N, Chifamba J, Kelishadi R, Yusufali A, Khatib R, Xiaoyun L, Bo H, Iqbal R, Yusuf R, Yeates K, Teo K, Yusuf S. Associations of cereal grains intake with cardiovascular disease and mortality across 21 countries in Prospective Urban and Rural Epidemiology Study: prospective cohort study. Br Med J (Clin Res Ed). 2021;372:m4948.

53. Anatomical Chart Company. Hypertension anatomical chart. 2nd ed. Philadelphia (PA): LWW (PE); 2005.

54. Duncan RE, Ahmadian M, Jaworski K, Sarkadi-Nagy E, Sul HS. Regulation of lipolysis in adipocytes. Annu Rev Nutr. 2007;27:79–101.

55. Ferrier DR. Biochemistry. 6th ed. Philadelphia (PA): LWW (PE); 2014.

56. Kraemer WJ, Fleck SJ, Deschenes MR. Exercise physiology. Philadelphia (PA): LWW (PE); 2011.

57. Pennington JAT, Douglass JS. Bowes & Church's Food Values of Portions Commonly Used. 18th ed. Baltimore (MD): Lippincott Williams & Wilkins; 2005.

58. Reference Ranges for Blood Lipids. Understanding what your cholesterol level means [Internet]. Accessed 2017 September. Available from: http://www.cholesterolmenu.com/cholesterol-levels-chart/

59. U.S. Department of Agriculture, FoodData Central, Accessed May 2024. https://fdc.nal.usda.gov/

5

Vitamins: Good Foods Give You What You Need

CHAPTER OBJECTIVES

- Identify the established guidelines for recommended daily intakes of vitamins and how to best interpret these guides.
- Recall the common name(s) for each vitamin, the common foods that are good sources for each vitamin, and the primary functions for each vitamin.
- Analyze the vitamins that athletes may be at highest risk of deficiency for, based on the sport, common training protocols, and traditional eating behaviors.

- Discuss the theories behind why there are common beliefs that higher intake levels of specific vitamins may improve athletic performance.
- Identify the specific water- and fat-soluble vitamins and the potential risks of deficiency and toxicity for each.
- Explain the potential health risks and benefits associated with vitamin supplementation.

Case Study

Leah finally made it big. She got an invitation to the trials to compete for a spot on the national team as a 200-m freestyle swimmer, and she was finally going to the Olympic Training Center for a meeting before the trials with the national team coaches and sports medicine staff. Getting to this point was definitely not easy, with before-school drives to the pool at 5:00 AM, after-school practices, always feeling hungry and thirsty but somehow managing to stay healthy—all with the hard work of her parents who saw to it that she got plenty of good food to eat and enough rest to keep from getting overly tired and sick. But now, just 6 months after graduating from high school as an 18-year-old and starting her new life as a college student, she has a chance to make the national swim team. Life was exciting and good, but also more complicated than ever.

Leah often found herself wondering where she was going to get her next meal. Although her mother always made sure she had something to eat before her early morning practices, her life in college was too hectic to figure out where and what to eat before practice. She noticed she was getting fatigued

a bit earlier than before, but no problem—she figured that she could get some vitamin and mineral supplements to keep her going. That was her first big mistake. Contrary to the advertisements, vitamin supplements do not give you energy. Rather, specific vitamins participate in reactions that derive energy from the energy substrates (carbohydrate, protein fat) consumed. Some vitamin supplements might be useful for someone on a low-quality diet and who has a specific nutrient deficiency, but broad-spectrum nutrient supplements do not help give an athlete who is not eating enough at the right time more energy. Leah became convinced that taking supplements was an important key to success, and started taking a huge array of vitamin supplements before practice with the hope that this would be an easy meal substitute to make sure she had the energy to swim fast. The supplements cost a huge amount, but she did not care because, she believed, it was a logical solution to giving her body what she needed. She was wrong.

Leah was now at the National Training Center and it was her turn to meet with the sports medicine staff. The

(continued)

first question they asked was about her eating pattern. She indicated that it was fine while she was at home, but that when she went to live at college it was difficult—but no problem because she found these amazing supplements. The look of disbelief on the faces of the sports medicine staff made Leah think she had said something wrong and then when the head of sports medicine spoke she began to realize that she did. He said, "Look, Leah; we are not about to invest in an athlete who is going to make herself sick from not eating enough and who is taking supplements that may contain banned substances (a large number of supplements targeting athletes have been found to contain banned substances that are not listed on the label), so even if you do swim well, we are not going to invest in you until we are sure that you are *eating food.*" He also asked Leah three questions:

- What are these vitamins supposed to work on if you are not eating enough food?
- Are you concerned that having 1,000 times the recommended intake level on a daily basis is a bit much?
- What will you do if you are found to have consumed banned substances?

She could not answer any of these questions, and realized all too quickly that she was playing a bad chemistry game with her body. But, she was not about to give up on having

a chance to make it on the team, so she asked an important question: "Can someone guide me on what and when to eat to optimize my performance?" The dietitian looked at Leah and said, "OK, you have just asked the right question. Let us see if we can get you ready for next week's competition. You are too good a swimmer to not have a shot at this."

After some time, Leah was back to form and was doing well, eating properly, and realizing that there is no easy alternative to eating. For many reasons, good food is the best way to get what you need. It gives you the vitamins, minerals, and energy to keep you healthy and performing at your best.

CASE STUDY DISCUSSION QUESTIONS

1. Look at a magazine that targets athletes and look at the nutrition-related advertisements in the magazine to see what vitamin supplements the advertisements are encouraging athletes to consume. Describe the weaknesses in the advertisements.
2. Make a list of the recommended supplements, then look up each supplement in the National Institutes of Health Office of Dietary Supplements Web site for a state-of-the-art listing of what the potential benefits or problems are with each of the supplements (Go to Dietary Supplement Fact Sheets Web site—https://ods.od.nih.gov) (1).

INTRODUCTION

Important Factors to Consider

- There is a common belief that the recommended intake of vitamins represents the *minimum* level needed to sustain good health and that having more than this level is always better. It is also believed that if too much of any given vitamin is consumed, then the excess will simply be urinated away without difficulty.
- In fact, the recommended intake level (the dietary reference intakes [DRI]) is two standard deviations higher than the average amount needed to sustain good health. Also, even water-soluble vitamins are potentially toxic when too much is consumed chronically.
- The simple rule in nutrition, including for vitamins, that should be followed is: *More than enough is not better than enough* (Figure 5.1).

Vitamins are substances needed by cells to encourage specific chemical reactions that take place in the cell. Some vitamins (particularly B-vitamins) are involved in energy reactions that enable cells to derive energy from carbohydrate, protein, and fat. Because athletes require a higher level of energy than nonathletes, these vitamins are of particular interest here. Other vitamins are involved in maintaining mineral balance and are also important for athletes to ensure adequate iron and calcium status. Female athletes of child-bearing age, for instance, are at relatively high risk of iron deficiency because of the menstrual blood loss. Vitamin C has a unique characteristic that can improve the bioavailability of iron in vegetables, which enhances iron absorption from these foods and may help to diminish the risk of iron deficiency. Vitamin D, which we can derive from both sunlight and food, encourages the cells in a specific part of the small intestine to allow more calcium and phosphorus to be absorbed from food into the blood, helping to sustain and/or improve bone mineral density. Importantly, vitamins work together, making food consumption, which

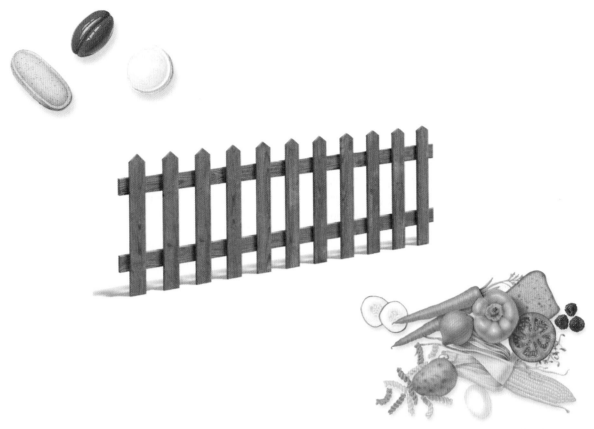

FIGURE 5.1: Belief-based versus science-based nutrition. Nutrient supplements are often viewed as the ultimate "back-up system" for athletes, but when taken without cause, not only do they not work, they often make matters worse. Real foods are the best way to obtain needed nutrients. (From Anatomical Chart Company. Keys to healthy eating. Philadelphia [PA]: Lippincott Williams & Wilkins; 2011.)

simultaneously delivers a wide array of vitamins, a far better strategy for good health than single-vitamin supplementation. For instance, both vitamin E and vitamin C have antioxidant properties, with vitamin E in the cell membrane and vitamin C in the blood. When vitamin E captures a potentially damaging oxidative free radical and protects the cell, it can hand off the free radical to vitamin C so that it is free to capture another free radical and continue its cell membrane–protective function.

Vitamin

An organic compound/nutrient that is necessary for sustaining human health and that cannot be synthesized by tissues, therefore mandating that it be consumed. Vitamins have a variety of functions, including tissue growth, tissue development, tissue repair, tissue protection, red blood cell (RBC) development, energy metabolism, immune function, and bone development.

Vitamins are organized into fat- and water-soluble categories. The **fat-soluble vitamins** literally require a

fat-based environment (*i.e.*, commonly found in food higher in oils/fats, such as whole grain cereals, nuts, and animal fats) in which to be transported and function, whereas the **water-soluble vitamins** require a water-based environment (*i.e.*, commonly found in foods with a higher water content, such as fruits and vegetables). Contrary to popular belief, we have the capacity to store all vitamins and, therefore, have a backup supply of all vitamins. That is to say, if a meal were consumed 2 days ago that had a large amount of vitamin C and the foods consumed the following 2 days had no vitamin C, we would not expect to suffer from symptoms of vitamin C deficiency today. Cells that require or deliver vitamin C have a capacity to store slightly more than they need. However, in the case of water-soluble vitamins such as vitamin C, there are no clear storage depots where large amounts of the vitamin can be stored. Fat-soluble vitamins, however, do have a large storage capacity, allowing for high-level seasonal consumption of certain vitamins. As an example, β-carotene (the precursor of retinol, the active form of vitamin A) is particularly highly concentrated in orange- and yellow-colored vegetables that are harvested in autumn. It appears the storage capacity for vitamins is associated to traditional seasonally based food availability. For instance, eating the pumpkin or squash that provides high levels of β-carotene when seasonally available, typically only during a short period during the Fall, results in a high-level storage that has the potential of preventing a deficiency for the remainder of the year.

Fat-Soluble Vitamins

These are vitamins that are soluble in fat and are in the fat-based portion of the foods we consume. They include vitamins A, D, E, and K.

Water-Soluble Vitamins

These are vitamins that are soluble in water and are in the water-based portion of the foods we consume. They include the B-vitamins and vitamin C.

Doing the math will help illustrate this. A typical body can hold onto about 1,500 mg of vitamin C at a time. The typical rate of utilization of vitamin C in a healthy person is ~15 mg/day. So, the typical healthy person has about a 100-day supply of the vitamin before the vitamin C deficiency disease would occur (1,500/15 = 100). In the 1850s, it was discovered that British sailors who were on long voyages and eating foods not containing vitamin C would start to show signs of scurvy, the deficiency disease of vitamin C, after about 3 months (~90 days) at sea. It was discovered, however, that if these sailors were given lime juice periodically during these long voyages, no scurvy would occur. A British sailor is still now called "limey" because of the common introduction of lime juice in the diet.

Important Factors to Consider

- There are many risks to health that can be found all around our environment. For instance, a person with *pink eye* who rubs his eyes and then touches a table surface places everyone who touches that surface at risk of contracting pink eye, which is highly contagious. The public is now well informed that smoking increases the risk of developing cancer. A smoker is not assured of getting cancer, and the person touching a table surface that had been touched by someone with pink eye is not assured of getting pink eye, but exposure to smoking or a contagious disease increases the risk of getting sick.

- In simple terms, *health risk* represents the likelihood that something (an act, an exposure, no exercise, poor eating habits, etc.) may have a negative impact on a person's health. A 20% increase in health risk means that if five people are equally exposed to a factor that can affect health, one in five (20%) are actually likely to get sick from exposure to that factor. The higher the health risk, the greater the likelihood that a higher proportion of those exposed to the risk will actually get sick. *Mortality risk* is similar to health risk, except the risk of exposure is expressed as the risk of dying (*i.e.*, mortality) from the exposure.

- Typically, an individual's health/mortality risk is comprised of multiple factors that include age, gender, disease history of close family members, activity patterns, food intake, and genetic predisposition to disease. Some factors are within an individual's control (*e.g.*, diet, physical activity), whereas other health/mortality risk factors are not within an individual's control (*e.g.*, the level of air pollution, genes, sex).

Source: United States Department of Health and Human Services, National Institutes of Health. NIH news in health. understanding health risks. Bethesda (MD): USDHHS; 2016. Accessed 2018 April 23. https://newsinhealth.nih.gov/2016/10/understanding-health-risks

It is a myth to believe that consumption of excessively high levels of any vitamin, including the water-soluble vitamins, is without problems. Many people wrongly believe that the excess vitamin consumption will simply and benignly be excreted in the urine. Excess intake of some vitamins, particularly preformed vitamin A (retinol), can produce severe **vitamin toxicity**, and even taking excess water-soluble vitamins creates difficulties. An example of this is the neurologic problem (peripheral neuropathy—loss of feeling in the fingers) created with excess intake of vitamin B_6 (500 mg/day over time) that will create permanent damage (2). The problem of having too many vitamins at once, typically with high-dose supplements, is clearly illustrated in Table 5.1. In this study, it was found that older women ($N = 38,772$) who regularly consumed commonly available dietary vitamin and mineral supplements were at increased mortality risk. Calcium supplementation was the only supplement associated with decreased risk. It was noted that in 1986, 66% of women studied took supplements; and in 2004 that increased to 85% of women (3).

Table 5.1	Dietary Supplements and Mortality Rate in Older Women
Dietary Supplement	**Mortality Rate in Older Women**
Multivitamins	2.4% increased risk
Vitamin B$_6$	4.1% increased risk
Folic acid	5.9% increased risk
Iron	3.9% increased risk
Magnesium	3.6% increased risk
Zinc	3.0% increased risk
Copper	18.0% increased risk
Calcium	3.8% decreased risk

Source: Data from Mursu J, Robien K, Harnack LJ, Park K, Jacobs DR. Dietary supplements and mortality rate in older women: The Iowa Women's Health Study. *Arch Intern Med.* 2011;171(18):1625–33.

Vitamin Toxicity

Also referred to as *hypervitaminosis*, is the result of consuming a vitamin in amounts that exceed the body's capacity to store, neutralize, or excrete the excess. Typically, vitamin toxicities occur when individuals chronically take a high-dose supplement of a vitamin. Some vitamins are more potentially toxic than others, with vitamin A (retinol) known to have high potential toxicity with excess consumption. Water-soluble vitamins are also potentially toxic. As an example, vitamin B$_6$ is known to cause permanent peripheral neuropathy (loss of feeling in fingers and toes) with chronically high-intake doses. The likelihood of developing vitamin toxicity from the consumption of food alone, however, is highly unlikely unless a food that is chronically consumed has a particularly high concentration of a vitamin. For instance, there is evidence that early explorers of the arctic regions resorted to consuming polar bear and seal liver, as they knew that the liver is a storage depot for fat-soluble vitamins and would help diminish the risk of deficiency when consuming a diet with limited variety. However, because cold-weather animals store a far higher concentration of vitamin A than warmer-weather animals, these arctic explorers experienced severe vitamin A toxicity and, in some cases, death because of this exceedingly high intake (4,5).

Consumption of vitamin supplements by athletes is high, with studies finding that up to 81% of studied athletes are regular supplement users (6). The primary reason provided by the athletes for taking supplements was to gain a competitive edge or a desire to prevent possible nutritional deficiencies, with some athletes saying that they consumed supplements to enhance recovery from exercise (7). However, only a small proportion of supplement-taking athletes consulted with health professionals, indicating that these supplements were self-prescribed (8,9). As noted earlier, the supplement consumption by athletes carries risk, as many supplements have been found to contain banned substances not listed on the label, and chronic supplementation may create a risk of toxicity (10,11). Athletes are, of course, the target of marketing efforts by supplement companies, but there is scant evidence that nutrient supplements trump the regular consumption of good food in getting the desired performance outcomes. To illustrate this point, a study of competitive triathletes found that providing 800 IU of vitamin E for 2 months prior to a triathlon, compared with taking a placebo, promoted more lipid peroxidation and inflammation during the race (12). This is precisely the opposite effect that would have been expected from the consumption of an antioxidant vitamin (vitamin E). But if amounts consumed are chronically too high, the tissues develop a resistance to the vitamin and the opposite of the desired effect occurs. Strenuous physical activity is known to be associated with depressed immune cell function, making athletes at higher risk of illness. This is made worse in athletes who have poor intakes of certain nutrients, including protein, iron, zinc, and vitamins A, E, B$_6$, and B$_{12}$. However, it has been found that excess consumption of these nutrients, often through supplements, also impairs the immune function, and there is no evidence suggesting that so-called immune-boosting supplements actually work (13). Other studies have also found that multivitamin and mineral supplementation resulted in no performance enhancement, suggesting that supplementation was not needed in athletes consuming a normal diet (14). Clearly, the best way to obtain the needed nutrients, including vitamins, is to have a regular consumption of good foods that meet the requirements for energy.

Vitamin Enrichment and Fortification

Many vitamins and minerals are added to foods in processes referred to as food **enrichment** and food **fortification**. The process of enrichment is to return vitamins and minerals to foods that were lost during food processing, and the process of fortification is to add selected vitamins and minerals to foods for the purpose of reducing the risk of developing a nutrient and/or **vitamin deficiency** and associated health problems.

Enrichment

This represents the addition of nutrients that were originally present in the food, but were removed during food processing. For example, the processing of wheat grain has the effect of removing many of the B-vitamins that are present in the bran and germ of the grain, and enrichment puts back these same vitamins as a means of restoring the original nutrient composition of the grain.

Fortification

Food fortification adds key vitamins and minerals to commonly consumed foods to enhance the food's nutritional content and reduce the potential of specific nutrient deficiencies in a population. Iodine added to salt (*i.e.*, iodized salt) is an early example of food fortification for the purpose of reducing the chance of developing goiter (enlarged thyroid gland). Vitamins A and D have been fortified in milk for many years to lower the risk of rickets, and more recently in the United States folic acid has been added to grains to ensure that women who become pregnant have a normal folic acid status to reduce the risk that their offspring will have spina bifida or anencephaly.

Vitamin Deficiency

Also referred to as *avitaminosis* or *hypovitaminosis*, a vitamin deficiency results when the tissues have become depleted of a needed vitamin. For example, a vitamin D deficiency may result in rickets or osteoporosis, a vitamin C deficiency may result in scurvy, and a riboflavin (vitamin B_2) deficiency may result in glossitis and photophobia and poor energy metabolism. The deficiency may be the result of poor diet, or a diet that does not adequately satisfy lifestyle-related needs. For instance, smokers require more vitamin C than nonsmokers. It is also important to consider that vitamin deficiencies may also negatively impact mental health, which could adversely impact interactions with friends, teammates and coaches, all of which would negatively impact athletic performance (15,16).

Important Factors to Consider

Enrichment

- Nutrients that were lost during food processing have been added back. For example, refining wheat to make white flour removes several B-complex vitamins and iron that are contained in the part of the grain that is removed during processing. Flour can be called enriched when the removed nutrients are added back to the food before packaging.
- The US Food and Drug Administration (FDA) has rules that food manufacturers must follow to claim that a food is enriched. According to the FDA, a food can claim to be enriched if it contains at least 10% more of a specified lost nutrient than a food of the same type that has not been enriched (17).
- In addition, foods can be labeled as enriched when they meet the FDA's definition for a type of food with a name that includes that term, including

enriched bread or enriched rice. Processed flour can only be labeled as enriched flour if it contains specified amounts of vitamins B_1, B_2, niacin, and iron. Examples of enriched foods include:
- Bread
- Pasta
- Breakfast cereal
- Rice products
- Corn products
- Wheat products

Fortification

- Nutrients have been added to a food that were not originally in the food. The World Health Organization (WHO) and the Food and Agriculture Organization of the United Nations (FAO) define fortification as "the practice of deliberately increasing the content of an essential micronutrient, that is, vitamins and minerals (including trace elements) in a food irrespective of whether the nutrients were originally in the food before processing or not, so as to improve the nutritional quality of the food supply and *to provide a public health benefit with minimal risk to health.*" The primary goal of fortification, therefore, is to identify nutrients that are not easily obtained in foods commonly consumed, and adding those nutrients with the hope of reducing disease associated with specific nutrient deficiency.
- A prime example of fortification that has been practiced for a long time is fortifying milk products with vitamins A and D, and more recently adding (*i.e.*, fortifying) vitamin D to orange juice. Folic acid has been more recently added to (*i.e.*, fortified) cereal grains to lower the risk of women having babies with spina bifida and anencephaly.
- Examples of foods that have been fortified include:
- Cereals and cereal-based products
- Milk and milk products
- Fats and oils
- Beverages
- Infant formulas

Sources: Academy of Nutrition and Dietetics. Enriched, fortified: what's the difference? Accessed 2008 February 12. Available from: Olson, R.; Gavin-Smith, B.; Ferraboschi, C.; Kraemer, K. Food Fortification: The Advantages, Disadvantages and Lessons from *Sight and Life* Programs. *Nutrients* **2021**,13,1118. https://doi.org/ 10.3390/nu13041118; United States Department of Agriculture, Food and Drug Administration. Are foods that contain added nutrients considered "enriched"? Accessed 2018 June 4. Available from: https://www.fda.gov/Food/GuidanceRegulation/GuidanceDocumentsRegulatoryInformation/ucm470756.htm

WATER-SOLUBLE VITAMINS

Vitamin B$_1$ (Thiamin)

Vitamin B$_1$, also referred to as thiamin, is present in a variety of foods, including whole grains, nuts, beans, dried peas, and pork. It works together with other B-vitamins in metabolic processes involving conversion of the potential energy in consumed foods to muscular energy (Box 5.1). Thiamin does this through its involvement in the removal of carbon dioxide in energy reactions with its active **coenzyme**, called *thiamine pyrophosphate (TPP)*. TPP is particularly important in deriving energy from carbohydrates. Thiamin consumption has been reported to be below the recommended daily intake level in certain athlete populations, but thiamin deficiency in athletes has not been reported in the literature (18). In groups of people consuming a low-quality diet of *unenriched* polished rice or other processed and unenriched grains, thiamin deficiency has been reported. It has also been reported in clients with anorexia nervosa, as a result of a severe underconsumption of all foods, including foods containing thiamin (19). There is evidence that having a thiamin intake above the recommended dietary intake level may have some positive effect on exercise performance and reduced fatigue. However, athletes who consume a diet that satisfies their higher energy needs are likely to also satisfy their elevated thiamin level needs (20).

Coenzyme

Coenzymes are small organic molecules that are often the active result of vitamin consumption and are involved in encouraging enzymes to fulfill their chemical functions. For instance, the active coenzyme for thiamin (vitamin B$_1$) is TPP; and the active coenzymes for niacin are nicotinamide adenine dinucleotide (NAD) and nicotinamide adenine dinucleotide phosphate (NADP). TPP, NAD, and NADP are all involved in energy metabolic processes that would not occur without the presence and encouragement of these coenzymes.

The primary thiamin-deficiency disease, called *beriberi*, involves nervous system malfunction (especially in the hands and legs, as well as in balance) and heart failure. A study has found that up to one-third of hospitalized congestive heart failure patients were diagnosed with thiamin deficiency and that, in this population, increasing thiamin availability through food and/or thiamin supplementation improved thiamin status (21). One form of beriberi is referred to as "dry" beriberi, and while another form of beriberi causes edema (water retention), which would be a contributor to congestive heart failure. See Box 5.2. Both dry and wet beriberi are most often seen in individuals with compromised gastrointestinal (GI) absorption, as seen in celiac disease, HIV/AIDs, and individuals who have had GI surgery (22–24).

As expected for a vitamin involved in energy reactions, early thiamin deficiency is characterized by muscle fatigue, which progresses to muscular weakness as the deficiency becomes more severe. Other symptoms of thiamin deficiency include loss of appetite, nausea, constipation, irritability, depression, loss of coordination, and confusion. A deficiency of thiamin is not likely to occur in US athletes. However, because alcohol inhibits normal thiamin metabolism, it is possible that thiamin-deficiency symptoms may occur in athletes who frequently consume alcoholic

---

Box 5.1   Vitamin B$_1$ (Thiamin) Basic Information

- **DRI**
  - Adult males: 1.2 mg/day
  - Adult females: 1.1 mg/day
  - Recommended intake for athletes: 1.5–3.0 mg/day, depending on total calories consumed (high calories = more)
- **Functions:** (active coenzyme: thiamine pyrophosphate [TPP])
  - Carbohydrate, fat, and branched-chain amino acid metabolism
  - Nervous system function
- **Good food sources**
  - Whole-grain cereals
  - Beans
  - Pork
  - Enriched grains
- **Deficiency**
  - Confusion
  - Anorexia
  - Weakness
  - Calf pain
  - Heart disease
  - Deficiency disease: Beriberi
- **Toxicity:** None known (no safe upper limit [UL] established)

Box 5.2	Dry and Wet Beriberi Caused by Thiamin Deficiency

Dry Beriberi

- Loss of muscle/tendon reflexes
- Tender, sore, and tingling muscles
- Imbalanced gait
- Loss of memory
- Loss of feeling in hands and feet
- Emaciated appearance
- Confusion

Wet Beriberi

- Cardiac failure
- Irregular breathing
- Irregular heartbeat
- Enlarged (swollen) heart
- Edema (water retention) in the lower extremities
- Lactic acidosis
- Confusion

beverages. Athletes have a high requirement for energy, but because the thiamin requirement is based on 0.5 mg of thiamin for each 1,000 calories consumed, this level of intake should satisfy athlete needs when energy needs are met.

Adequate intake (AI) of thiamin is important for energy metabolism, muscle protein synthesis, and muscle repair (25,26). Athletes commonly consume high-carbohydrate foods that, because of enrichment, are good sources of thiamin that help to ensure that athletes who meet energy requirements also satisfy the physiologic needs for thiamin. A study of collegiate swimmers found that higher-intensity training was associated with lower circulating thiamin levels in the blood than lower-intensity training, suggesting that dietary intakes should be adjusted to dynamically match the energy requirements of the activity (27). Consumption of more food with higher-intensity activity should adequately provide the thiamin needed for the additional energy metabolic needs.

Thiamin is present in a variety of food sources, including whole grains, nuts, legumes (beans and dried peas), fish, sunflower seeds, and pork. It works in unison with other B-vitamins to convert the energy in the foods we consume to muscular energy and heat. It is naturally found in fish, meat, and whole grain cereals, and is fortified (in the United States and many other countries) in breads, cereals, and baby formulas.

Vitamin B$_2$ (Riboflavin)

Riboflavin is involved in energy production and normal cellular function through its coenzymes *flavin adenine dinucleotide* (FAD) and *flavin mononucleotide* (FMN), both of which are involved in producing energy from consumed carbohydrates, proteins, and fats (Box 5.3). Food sources of riboflavin include dairy products (*e.g.*, milk, yogurt, cottage cheese), dark leafy green vegetables

Box 5.3	Vitamin B$_2$ (Riboflavin) Basic Information

- **DRI**
  - Adult males: 1.3 mg/day
  - Adult females: 1.1 mg/day
  - Recommended intake for athletes: 1.1 mg/1,000 calories
- **Functions:** (active coenzymes: FMN and FAD)
  - Energy metabolism (electron transfer reactions)
  - Protein metabolism
  - Hormone production
  - Skin health
  - Eye health
- **Good food sources**
  - Fresh milk and other dairy products
  - Organ meats (kidney and liver)
  - Lean meats
  - Eggs
  - Dark green leafy vegetables
  - Whole-grain cereals
  - Enriched grains
- **Deficiency**
  - Inflamed tongue
  - Cracked, dry skin at corners of mouth, nose, and eyes
  - Bright light sensitivity
  - Weakness
  - Fatigue
  - Deficiency diseases: cheilosis and photophobia
- **Toxicity: None known** (no safe UL established)

(*e.g.,* spinach, chard, mustard greens, broccoli, green peppers), whole-grain foods, and enriched grain foods. While riboflavin is present in a wide variety of foods, consider that dairy products are high in riboflavin, grains that have undergone enrichment are good sources of riboflavin, and some fruits and vegetables contain riboflavin. There is also a difference in the riboflavin content of animal foods: Beef is high in riboflavin, while chicken, fish, and eggs contain riboflavin but have lower concentrations than beef (28).

No studies suggest that riboflavin-deficiency symptoms commonly occur in athletes, possibly because riboflavin is reabsorbed by the kidneys when blood levels are low (14,27,29). Also, no apparent toxicity symptoms occur from consuming more than the DRI. Several studies have suggested that athletes may have higher requirements than the DRI, which is based on consumption of 0.6 mg riboflavin per 1,000 calories. In a series of studies performed on exercising women and women seeking to lose weight, the riboflavin requirement was found to range between 0.63 and 1.40 mg/1,000 calories (30–32). There is some evidence that physical activity increases the requirement to a level slightly higher than 0.6 mg/1,000 calories, but not more than 1.6 mg/1,000 calories (33). However, even with this apparently higher requirement for athletes, no studies clearly demonstrate an improvement in athletic performance with dietary intakes that exceed the established DRI (34,35). Vegetarian athletes may be at higher risk of riboflavin deficiency, particularly if they avoid consuming foods high in riboflavin, including soy and dairy products (36–38). Vegetarian athletes who increase exercise intensity would also be considered at higher risk, particularly if the regular food intake does not provide the needed energy with greater consumption of plant sources of riboflavin, which includes whole grain and enriched cereals, soy products, almonds, asparagus, bananas, sweet potatoes, and wheat germ (39).

It is never easy to make a determination about what level of intake is appropriate for athletes because there are many factors to consider. For riboflavin, understanding the requirement is made even more complex because riboflavin is easily destroyed by ultraviolet light (the reason behind opaque milk bottles in the grocery store, which serve to inhibit ultraviolet insertion through the milk). The delivered riboflavin content in fresh dairy products is not the same, therefore, as older products have more opportunities for multiple light exposures. This makes it difficult to understand the actual amount of riboflavin that is commonly delivered by food, and whether any earlier risks that may have been found are no longer present.

Niacin (Niacinamide, Nicotinic Acid, Nicotinamide, or Vitamin B₃)

Niacin is involved in energy production from carbohydrate, protein, and fat, glycogen synthesis, and normal cellular metabolism through its active coenzymes (Box 5.4). These enzymes, *nicotinamide adenine dinucleotide (NAD)* and *nicotinamide adenine dinucleotide phosphate (NADP)*, are produced by body tissues and are essential for normal muscle function. Although niacin deficiency is well documented in human populations suffering from famine or monotonous intakes of unenriched grain products, there is no evidence that athletes are at risk of niacin deficiency.

Niacin is found in meat, whole or enriched grains, seeds, nuts, and legumes, and body cells have the capacity to synthesize niacin from the amino acid tryptophan (60 mg of tryptophan yields 1 mg of niacin), which is found in all high-quality protein foods (*e.g.,* meat, fish, poultry). Given the broad spectrum of foods that contain niacin, it is relatively easy for people to consume the DRI of 12–14 mg/day, or 6.6 niacin equivalents (NEs) per 1,000 calories. NEs are equal to 1 mg of niacin or 60 mg of dietary tryptophan. Niacin can be obtained directly from food or indirectly by consuming the amino acid tryptophan. The NE unit of measure takes both sources into account.

Niacin deficiency results in muscular weakness, loss of appetite, indigestion, and skin rash, with an extreme deficiency leading to the deficiency disease *pellagra*. Symptoms of pellagra include diarrhea, dementia, dermatitis, and, if left untreated, results in death. An excess intake of niacin may result in toxicity symptoms, including GI distress and feeling hot (becoming red faced or flushed). It may also result in a tingling feeling around the neck, face, and fingers. These symptoms are commonly reported in people taking large doses of niacin to lower blood lipids, suggesting that niacin supplementation should only occur with medical supervision. There is also beginning evidence that excess niacin consumption may negatively impact exercise performance by resulting in premature fatigue (20). Excess niacin consumption is unlikely to occur from food intake but may occur from supplemental niacin intake. Animal studies have found that supplementation with niacin may increase muscle mitochondrial biogenesis, resulting in an increased potential for fat metabolism. However, there are no studies on humans that have assessed the impact of supplemental niacin on mitochondrial adaptation (40). In fact, early studies that have evaluated the performance effects of niacin supplementation found that endurance was *reduced* because the

Box 5.4   Vitamin B₃ (Niacin) Basic Information

■ **DRI**
- Adult males: 16 mg/day
- Adult females: 14 mg/day
- Recommended intake for athletes: 14–20 mg/day (higher levels based on expected higher energy intakes)

■ **Functions:** (active coenzymes: NAD, which is phosphorylated to NADP and reduced to nicotinamide adenine dinucleotide hydride)
- Energy metabolism
- Glycolysis
- Fat synthesis

■ **Good food sources**
- *Foods high in tryptophan* (an amino acid that can be converted to niacin):
    - Milk
    - Eggs
    - Turkey
    - Chicken
- *Foods high in niacin:*
    - Whole grains

- Lean meat
- Fish
- Poultry
- Enriched grains

■ **Deficiency**
- Anorexia
- Skin rash
- Dementia
- Weakness
- Lethargy
- Deficiency disease: Pellagra

■ **Toxicity**
- Tolerable ULs:
    - 10–15 mg/day for young children (age 1–8 y)
    - 20–35 mg/day for children and adults (age 9–70+ y)
- Toxicity symptoms:
    - Flushing
    - Burning and tingling sensations of extremities
    - Hepatitis
    - Gastric ulcers

excess niacin resulted in lowered fat metabolism (41–43). Lower fat metabolism leads to a greater reliance on carbohydrate fuels (glucose and glycogen) to support physical activity, but glycogen storage is limited, resulting in lower endurance. To date, there is no evidence that the requirement for niacin is increased beyond the DRI with physical activity.

Vitamin B₆ (Pyridoxine, Pyridoxal, and Pyridoxamine)

Vitamin B₆ refers to six compounds (pyridoxine, pyridoxal, pyridoxamine, pyridoxine-5-phosphate, pyridoxal-5-phosphate [PLP], and pyridoxamine-5-phosphate [PMP]) that display similar metabolic activity (Box 5.5). It is found in highest quantity in meats (especially liver) and is also available in wheat germ, fish, poultry, legumes, bananas, brown rice, whole-grain cereals, and vegetables. The function of this vitamin is closely linked to protein and amino acid metabolism, and so the requirements are also linked to protein intake (higher protein intakes require higher vitamin intakes). Because high-protein foods are also typically high in vitamin B₆, those consuming protein from food are most likely to have adequate B₆

levels as well. However, many athletes consume additional protein in purified, supplemental forms (protein powders, amino acid powders, etc.) that are devoid of vitamin B₆, suggesting that it is conceivable that athletes with high supplemental protein intakes will have an inadequate B₆ intake. The adult requirement is based on 0.016 mg of B₆ per gram of protein consumed each day and is adequate for those consuming typical protein intakes (44). Except in alcoholism, which affects B₆ intake and impairs B₆ metabolism, severe deficiency of B₆ is uncommon. The estimated deficiency prevalence of vitamin B₆ in the general population is 10.6% (45). When deficiency occurs, it is most associated with neurologic symptoms (irritability, depression, and confusion) and inflammation of the tongue and mouth (46,47).

Vitamin B₆ functions in reactions related to protein synthesis by aiding in the creation of amino acids and proteins (transamination reactions) and is also involved in protein catabolism through involvement in reactions that break down amino acids and proteins (deamination reactions). It is involved, therefore, in manufacturing muscle, hemoglobin, and other proteins critical to athletic performance. The major enzyme of vitamin B₆, pyridoxal phosphate, is also involved in the breakdown of

---

Box 5.5	Vitamin B$_6$ (Pyridoxine, Pyridoxal, and Pyridoxamine) Basic Information

- **DRI**
  - Adult males: 1.3–1.7 mg/day
  - Adult females: 1.3–1.5 mg/day
  - Recommended intake for athletes: 1.5–2.0 mg/day
- **Functions:** (active coenzymes: PLP and PMP)
  - Metabolism of protein, including protein synthesis
  - Metabolism of fat
  - Metabolism of carbohydrate
  - Neurotransmitter formation
  - Glycolysis
  - Antioxidant
- **Good food sources**
  - Meats
  - Whole grain and enriched cereals
  - Eggs
- **Deficiency**
  - Nausea
  - Mouth sores
  - Muscle weakness
  - Depression
  - Convulsions
  - Impaired immune system
- **Toxicity**
  - Tolerable ULs:
    - 30–40 mg/day for young children (age 1–8 y)
    - 60–100 mg/day for children and adults (age 9–70+ y)
  - Toxicity symptoms:
    - Loss of limb sensation and loss of coordination

---

muscle glycogen for energy through the enzyme glycogen phosphorylase.

A deficiency of vitamin B$_6$ will lead to symptoms of peripheral neuritis (loss of nerve function in the hands, feet, arms, and legs), ataxia (loss of balance), irritability, depression, and convulsions. An excess intake of vitamin B$_6$ does lead to toxic symptoms that have been documented in humans. These symptoms are similar to those seen in B$_6$ deficiency and include ataxia and severe sensory neuropathy (loss of sensation in the fingers). The toxicity symptoms were found in women taking doses that, on average, equal 119 mg/day for the purpose of treating premenstrual syndrome and several types of mental disorders (2,48).

There is a theoretical basis for investigating vitamin B$_6$ and athletic performance. B$_6$ is involved in the breakdown of amino acids in muscle as a means of obtaining needed energy and in converting lactic acid to glucose in the liver (49). Vitamin B$_6$ is also involved in the breakdown of muscle glycogen to derive energy. Other functions of vitamin B$_6$ that may be related to athletic performance include the formation of serotonin and the synthesis of carnitine from lysine. There is evidence that some athletes may be at risk for inadequate vitamin B$_6$ status (50–52). Poor B$_6$ status also reduces athletic performance (53). It has also been proposed that lower antioxidant capacity in athletes may result from vitamin B$_6$ deficiency (54).

Because many athletes are always looking for that extra edge, there is an understandable attractiveness to the consumption of natural substances that are legal. Vitamin B$_6$ is sometimes marketed as one of those natural (and legal)

substances because, besides its importance in energy metabolism, it is linked with the production of growth hormone, which can help to increase muscle mass (55). It appears as if the combined effect of exercise and vitamin B$_6$ on growth hormone production is greater than either of these factors individually (56,57). Given the importance of this vitamin to athletic performance, it is easy to see why athletes may rush to obtain more. However, these factors should be considered (49,58):

- Most athletes have adequate vitamin B$_6$ intakes and adequate vitamin B$_6$ status.
- Those athletes with poor vitamin B$_6$ status are generally those with inadequate energy intakes.
- A greater proportion of female athletes and athletes participating in sports that emphasize low weights (gymnastics, wrestling, skating, etc.) are likely to have inadequate energy intakes and, therefore, inadequate vitamin B$_6$ intakes.
- High doses of vitamin B$_6$ have been shown to have toxic effects, including damage to the nervous system.
- There is no good evidence that having more than the recommended intake has a beneficial effect on athletic performance (59).
- Vitamin B$_6$ supplementation does not appear necessary to enhance athletic performance if a balanced diet, with adequate energy intake, is consumed (60).

Taken together, these factors should encourage athletes to consume an AI of energy before they consider taking supplements of vitamin B$_6$.

> ## Box 5.6 Vitamin B₁₂ (Cobalamin) Basic Information
>
> - **DRI**
>   - Adult males: 2.4 mcg/day
>   - Adult females: 2.4 mcg/day
>   - Recommended intake for athletes: 2.4–2.5 mcg/day
> - **Functions**
>   - Protein metabolism, including protein synthesis
>   - Metabolism of fat
>   - Metabolism of carbohydrate
>   - Neurotransmitter formation
>   - Glycolysis
>   - RBC formation
>
> - **Good food sources**
>   - Foods of animal origin (meat, fish, poultry, eggs, milk, cheese)
>   - Fortified cereals
> - **Deficiency**
>   - *Disease:* Pernicious anemia (more likely caused by malabsorption of the vitamin than by dietary inadequacy, although vegans are at higher risk of deficient intakes)
>   - *Deficiency disease symptoms*: Weakness, easy fatigue, neurologic disorders
> - **Toxicity:** Tolerable ULs not established; the daily value (DV) is 6 mcg/day

Vitamin B₁₂ (Cobalamin)

Vitamin B_{12} is perhaps the most chemically complex of all the vitamins. It contains the mineral cobalt (hence the name cobalamin) and has a major involvement in RBC formation, folic acid metabolism, deoxyribonucleic acid (DNA) synthesis, synthesis of succinyl-coenzyme A (CoA; an intermediary product of the citric acid cycle), and nerve development, but it is essential for the function of all cells (Box 5.6).

Dietary sources of this vitamin are mainly foods of animal origin (meats, eggs, dairy products), and it is essentially absent from plant foods. While there may also be some very small amount of absorbable vitamin B_{12} that is produced by gut bacteria and from fermented foods (*e.g.*, tofu), vegetarian athletes who avoid all foods of animal origin are at risk of vitamin B_{12} deficiency (61). Vegan sources of vitamin B_{12} include fortified and fermented foods, including:

- B_{12}-fortified almond milk
- B_{12}-fortified coconut milk
- Nutritional yeast
- B_{12}-fortified soymilk
- Tempeh or tofu
- B_{12}-fortified cereal

The primary disease associated with vitamin B_{12} deficiency is *pernicious anemia*, but inadequate intake is also associated with higher risk of neural tube defects (*i.e.*, spina bifida and anencephaly), lower synthesis of neurotransmitters, reduced mental function, and elevated levels of homocysteine (a risk factor in heart disease). Pernicious anemia most commonly occurs in older adults who have experienced a reduction in normal stomach function. The stomach produces a substance called *intrinsic factor* that is required for vitamin B_{12} absorption. Without intrinsic factor, a person can consume an adequate level of B_{12} but still develop a deficiency because of poor absorption. Symptoms of deficiency include fatigue, poor muscular coordination (possibly leading to paralysis), and dementia.

There is a long history of vitamin B_{12} abuse by athletes. It was (and continues to be) common for many athletes to be injected with large amounts of vitamin B_{12} (often 1,000 mg) before competitions (62,63). However, the athletic performance benefits of vitamin B_{12} injections and supplementation have not been established for athletes consuming unrestricted diets (39,64–66). While the risk of toxicity is very small, there is some risk of toxicity with the consumption of frequent high doses of vitamin B_{12}, resulting in skin problems, anxiety, headache, and other symptoms (67,68).

It certainly makes sense that athletes consume foods that will avoid deficiencies of any kind, including the avoidance of B_{12} deficiency. The resulting anemia would clearly have an impact on performance by producing a reduction in endurance and, potentially, a lowering of muscular coordination. However, there is no logical basis or proven benefits for consumption or injections of such large doses as has been reported in the literature for vitamin B_{12}. Without a genetic predisposition to B_{12} malabsorption (typically because of an inadequate production of intrinsic factor), there is no basis for taking supplements if a balanced mixed-food diet is consumed. Pure vegetarian athletes (*i.e.*, those who avoid the consumption of all foods of animal origin), on the other hand, may have a good reason to be concerned about vitamin B_{12} status. A supplement that provides, on average, the daily requirement (2.4 mcg) makes good sense, as does the consumption of foods that are fortified with vitamin B_{12} (such as some soy milk products).

Folic Acid (Folate)

Folic acid, also referred to as vitamin B_9, is widespread in the food supply, but is present in the highest concentrations in liver, yeast, leafy vegetables, fruits, and legumes. "Folate" is the form naturally found in foods, and "Folic Acid" is the form found in fortified foods and dietary supplements. It is a water-soluble vitamin that naturally occurs in some foods (*e.g.*, dark green leafy vegetables, legumes, and fruits), and is fortified in other foods (*e.g.*, grains and cereals). Because folate comes in different forms, the common unit of measure is micrograms of Dietary Folate Equivalents (mcg DFE) (69):

- 1 mcg DFE = 1 mcg food folate
- 1 mcg DFE = 0.6 mcg folic acid from fortified foods or dietary supplements consumed with foods
- 1 mcg DFE = 0.5 mcg folic acid from dietary supplements consumed without foods

(Note: Approximately 85% of supplemental folic acid is bioavailable when consumed with foods, and approximately 100% bioavailable when consumed without foods.)

Folate is easily destroyed through common household food preparation techniques and long storage times, so AIs are most associated with the intake of fresh foods. Folate functions in amino acid metabolism and nucleic acid synthesis (ribonucleic acid and DNA), so a deficiency leads to alterations in protein synthesis (Box 5.7) (44). Tissues that have a rapid turnover are particularly sensitive to folic acid. This includes RBC and white blood cells, as well as tissues of the GI tract and the uterus. More recently, adequate folate intake during pregnancy has been associated with the elimination of fetal neural tube defects (most notably spina bifida) (70). The average US folate intake exceeds the requirement of between 180 and 200 mcg/day by between 25% and 50%, but its importance in RBC formation and in preventing neural tube defects has led to the supplementation with folic acid during pregnancy. The recommended intake of folate during pregnancy (400 mcg) is double that of the adult requirement. A deficiency of folate leads to anemia, GI problems (diarrhea, malabsorption, pain), and a swollen, red tongue. Because folate works with vitamin B_{12} in forming healthy new RBCs, a chronic deficiency leads to megaloblastic anemia. Excess folic acid intake may mask vitamin B_{12} deficiency and may also increase cancer risk (71–73).

A primary function of folic acid is in the creation of red blood cells, which is a critical element in oxygen delivery to cells. Folic acid also participates in the production of nitric oxide through involvement in the production

Box 5.7	Folic Acid (Folate) Basic Information

- **DRI**
  - Adult males: 400 mcg/day
  - Adult females: 400 mcg/day
  - Recommended intake for athletes: 400 mcg/day
- **Functions**
  - Methionine (essential amino acid) metabolism
  - Formation of DNA
  - Formation of RBCs
  - Normal fetal development
- **Good food sources**
  - Dark green leafy vegetables
  - Enriched and fortified grains and cereals
  - Beans
  - Whole-grain cereals
  - Oranges
  - Bananas

- **Deficiency**
  - Megaloblastic (macrocytic) anemia
  - Neural tube defects (as a result of poor folate status at initiation of pregnancy)
- **Symptoms**
  - Weakness
  - Easy fatigue
  - Neurologic disorders
- **Toxicity**
  - Tolerable ULs:
    - 300–400 mcg/day for young children (age 1–8 y)
    - 600–1,000 mcg/day for children and adults (age 9–70+ y)

Folate naturally occurs in foods; *folic acid* is the synthetic form of folate.

of nitric oxide synthase. Nitric oxide is an important vasodilator that enables better oxygen and nutrient delivery to tissues and, therefore, is an important factor in athletic performance (74). Therefore, there is a clear relationship between a satisfactory folic acid status and athletic performance. However, no studies have reported that supplementing with additional folic acid above the established requirement has an added benefit on athletic performance (75). However, because athletes have an above-normal tissue turnover because of the pounding the body takes in various sports, and with evidence that RBC turnover is faster in athletes than in nonathletes, there is a good reason for athletes to be certain that adequate folic acid intake is satisfied (14,76). The prudent approach is through the regular consumption of folate/folic acid containing foods, including whole grains (fortified with folic acid), fresh fruits, and vegetables.

Biotin (Vitamin H, Vitamin B₇)

Biotin works with magnesium and adenosine triphosphate (ATP) in carbon dioxide metabolism, new glucose production (gluconeogenesis), carbohydrate metabolism, and fatty acid synthesis (Box 5.8) (44). Biotin is a cofactor for five carboxylases involved in the metabolism of glucose, amino acids, and fatty acids, these metabolic reactions are involved in new glucose production (gluconeogenesis), carbohydrate metabolism, and fatty acid synthesis (Box 5.8) (44). Recent data suggest that biotin is also involved in protecting brain metabolism during periods of malnutrition and starvation, with a deficiency linked to neurologic disorders (77). Biotin is found in a wide spectrum of food sources that include egg yolk, soy flour, liver, sardines, walnuts, pecans, peanuts, and yeast. Fruits and meats are, however, poor dietary sources

of the vitamin. Biotin is also synthesized by bacteria in the intestines. A deficiency of this vitamin is rare but can be induced through the intake of large amounts of raw egg whites (from about 20 eggs), which contain the protein *avidin* (78). This protein binds to biotin, making it unavailable for absorption. When a deficiency of biotin occurs, symptoms include hair loss; scaly red rash around eyes, nose, and mouth; loss of appetite; vomiting; and depression. However, because there are not many people who consume large quantities of raw egg white, deficiencies of this vitamin are rare. While athletes should be cautious of consuming large amount of raw egg whites as a strategy for increasing protein intake, there is no evidence that athletes are at risk for biotin deficiency. Clearly, anyone with a biotin deficiency would have compromised athletic performance because of its involvement in energy metabolism, but there are no findings suggesting that, as a group, athletes are at risk for biotin deficiency (79).

Pantothenic Acid (Vitamin B₅)

Pantothenic acid is a structural component of acetyl-CoA, which is the intermediary product of all energy metabolic processes (Box 5.9). Through CoA, pantothenic acid is involved in carbohydrate, protein, and fat metabolism. Because pantothenic acid is widely distributed in the food supply, it is unlikely that an athlete would suffer from a deficiency, particularly if sufficient total energy is consumed. The highest concentrations of pantothenic acid are found in meat, whole-grain foods, beans, and peas, but it should be considered that food processing can cause a significant reduction in pantothenic acid availability (80). Nevertheless, even with this potential reduced availability, a pantothenic acid deficiency is rare. If a deficiency does occur, symptoms include easy fatigue, weakness,

| Box 5.8 | Biotin (Vitamin H) Basic Information |

- **DRI**
  - Adult males: 30 mcg/day
  - Adult females: 30 mcg/day
  - Recommended intake for athletes: 30 mcg/day
- **Functions**
  - Glucose synthesis (gluconeogenesis)
  - Fatty acid synthesis
  - Gene expression regulator
- **Good food sources**
  - Egg yolks
  - Legumes, dark
  - Green leafy vegetables
  - Note: Also produced by intestinal bacteria
- **Deficiency**
  - Rare; if it occurs, due to high egg white intake
  - *Deficiency symptoms:* anorexia, depression, muscle pain, dermatitis
- **Toxicity:** Tolerable ULs not established

Box 5.9	Pantothenic Acid (Vitamin B$_5$) Basic Information

- **DRI**
  - Adult males: 5 mg/day
  - Adult females: 5 mg/day
  - Recommended intake for athletes: 4–5 mg/day
- **Functions**
  - Energy metabolism as part of acetyl-CoA
  - Gluconeogenesis
  - Synthesis of acetylcholine

- **Good food sources**
  - Widely present in all foods, with the exception of highly processed and refined foods
- **Deficiency**
  - Unknown in humans
- **Toxicity**
  - Tolerable ULs not established; DV is 10 mg

and insomnia. Supplemental doses of the vitamin are typically 10 mg/day or higher (double the DRI) and, at this level, have not been shown to produce toxic effects (81).

There are human studies suggesting that pantothenic acid may aid in the wound healing of skin (82,83). Early studies on animals also suggest that pantothenic acid supplementation is effective in improving time to exhaustion (84,85). However, human studies do not agree on the potential benefits of pantothenic acid supplementation. In one study using a double-blind protocol, there was no difference in time to exhaustion in conditioned runners given either a pantothenic acid supplement or a placebo (86). However, in another study that used a double-blind protocol, there was a lowering of lactate (−16.7%) and an increase in oxygen consumption (+8.4%) in subjects given a pantothenate supplement versus those given a placebo prior to riding a cycle ergometer to exhaustion (87).

Although a possible relationship between increasing the intake of pantothenic acid and exercise performance may exist, more information is needed before a sound recommendation can be made on pantothenate intake for athletes. In studies that have experimented with pantothenic acid supplements to determine a requirement level, the typical dosage has been 10 mg/day. When this level is provided, 5–7 mg/day is excreted in the urine (44). Therefore, it appears that taking supplements at or above this level is excessive and is not associated with improved athletic performance.

Vitamin C (Ascorbic Acid, Ascorbate, Dehydroascorbate, L-Ascorbate)

Fresh fruits and vegetables are the best sources of vitamin C. Cereal grains contain no vitamin C (unless fortified with vitamin C), and meats and dairy products are low in vitamin C. Vitamin C is easily destroyed by cooking

(heat) and exposure to air (oxygen). It is also highly water soluble, which means it is easily removed from foods by water. The vitamin C deficiency disease, *scurvy*, is caused by a long-term dietary deficiency of the vitamin. For a variety of reasons (fresh food availability, supplement intake, use of vitamin C as an antioxidant in packaged foods), scurvy is almost nonexistent now. Toxicity from high, regular supplemental intakes of the vitamin is rare, but may include a predisposition to developing kidney stones and a reduced tissue sensitivity to the vitamin. Doses of 100–200 mg/day will saturate the body with vitamin C, yet many people take supplemental doses of 1,000–2,000 mg/day (44). This level of supplemental vitamin C intake represents doses that are many times higher than the DRI of 75–90 mg/day (Box 5.10). Consider that 70%–90% of vitamin C is absorbed with typical food intakes of 30–180 mg/day, but at doses above 1,000 mg/day the absorption rate falls to less than 50% with the unabsorbed vitamin C excreted in urine (88).

A number of studies have evaluated the relationship between vitamin C intake and athletic performance, and the results from these studies are inconsistent. Part of the problem with many of the studies performed on vitamin C is a lack of standardization between subjects and a general lack of comparative controls. Nevertheless, according to reviews of studies that used controls and provided vitamin C supplements at or below 500 mg/day (a level that is 5× the DRI), there was no measurable benefit in athletic performance (89,90). One study noted that when a 500-mg dose of vitamin C was provided shortly (4 hours) before testing, athletes experienced a significant improvement in strength and a significant reduction in maximal oxygen consumption (VO$_{2max}$)—which is a good thing—but there was no impact on muscular endurance (91). (VO$_{2max}$ is the maximum volume of oxygen that the lungs can bring into the system. Working at a lower level of VO$_{2max}$ means the person is not working as hard as

---

Box 5.10 — Vitamin C (Ascorbic Acid, Ascorbate, Dehydroascorbate, L-Ascorbate) Basic Information

- **DRI**
  - Adult males: 90 mg/day
  - Adult females: 75 mg/day
  - Recommended intake for athletes: 100–200 mg/day
- **Functions**
  - Antioxidant
  - Synthesis of carnitine (a transport molecule that carries fatty acids into mitochondria for energy metabolism)
  - Production of epinephrine and norepinephrine (neurotransmitters that rapidly degrade glycogen to make glucose available to working muscles)
  - Facilitates absorption of nonheme iron from fruits and vegetables
  - Synthesis of cortisol, a powerful catabolic hormone
  - Resynthesis of vitamin E to its active antioxidant state
  - Collagen formation (a connective tissue protein)
- **Good food sources**
  - Fresh fruits (particularly citrus and cherries)
  - Fresh vegetables
- **Deficiency**
  - Rare
  - Disease: Scurvy
  - *Deficiency symptoms:* bleeding gums, deterioration of muscles and tendons, sudden death
- **Toxicity**
  - Tolerable ULs:
    - 400–650 mg/day for young children (age 1–8 y)
    - 1.2–2.0 g/day for children and adults (age 9–70+ y)
    - Increased risk of kidney stone formation with chronic intake of 1 g/day (1,000 mg) or more

Source: Institute of Medicine, Food and Nutrition Board. Dietary reference intakes (DRIs): recommended intakes for individuals, vitamin. Washington (DC): National Academies Press; 2004.

---

maximal aerobic capacity.) However, when participants were provided with the same amount for 7 days, there was an improvement in strength with a *decrease* in endurance. When these same subjects were provided with 2,000 mg each day for 7 days, there was only a lowering of VO_{2max}, but no change in endurance performance. There may be a benefit in consuming a slightly higher level of vitamin C for athletes involved in concussive sports where muscle soreness occurs or there is an injury. Studies on animals generally indicate that having more vitamin C improves the healing process and that inadequate vitamin C inhibits healing (92). Although there is some evidence that muscle soreness may be more rapidly relieved with consumption of moderate supplemental doses of vitamin C and other antioxidants, it should be noted that the current scientific evidence to support the use of supplemental doses of antioxidant vitamins, including vitamin C, to enhance tendon and muscle healing in athletes is limited (93,94).

Given these inconsistent results, it is difficult to make a rational recommendation on vitamin C and athletic performance. However, slightly increasing vitamin C intake may reduce muscle soreness faster and may also improve healing because of its involvement in producing the connective tissue protein collagen. The enhanced collagen formation associated with adequate vitamin C intake may also enhance muscular force development resulting from training (95). The question is: How much

is just right? Unfortunately, it is impossible to know the correct answer for every person. Because studies demonstrate that high doses may cause endurance problems, it is important to keep the level of intake below one that may result in performance deficits. An early study reported on three deaths that were due to iron overload. Vitamin C is known to enhance iron absorption because it reduces iron to a more absorbable form, and the people who died were taking large daily doses of vitamin C (96). Also consider that athletes already typically consume more than 250 mg of vitamin C each day from food alone because of the high intake of fresh fruits and vegetables. A reasonable recommendation is to consume an abundant amount of fresh fruits and vegetables (wonderful sources of carbohydrates and many other nutrients besides vitamin C). It has been found that vitamin C supplementation is popular with athletes, with up to 77% of assessed athletes reportedly taking multivitamins containing vitamin C or vitamin C. Recommendations for consuming these supplements, however, did not come from health professionals, and over 80% reported being unaware that supplemental intake could negatively affect performance (97).

Choline

Although not officially a vitamin, choline has water-soluble vitamin-like characteristics that is considered

Box 5.11	Choline Basic Information

- **There is no DRI, only an AI level.**
  - AI adult males: 550 mg/day
  - AI adult females: 425 mg/day
  - Recommended intake for athletes: Unknown
- **Functions**
  - Structure of cell membranes
  - Signaling for cell membranes
  - Acetylcholine synthesis and neurotransmission
  - Methyl-group donor for protein synthesis
- **Good food sources**
  - Beef liver
  - Egg
  - Fish
  - Cauliflower, broccoli, and other cruciferous vegetables

- **Deficiency**
  - Fatty liver disease
  - Kidney disease
  - Easy fatigue
- **Toxicity**
  - Toxicity symptoms (seen with daily high doses of 10,000–16,000 mg/day):
    - Fishy body odor from excess production of trimethylamine (a choline metabolite)
    - May result in low blood pressure and fainting
- **Tolerable ULs**
  - 1,000 mg/day for children 1–8 y
  - 2,000 mg/day for children 9–13 y
  - 3,000 mg/day for adolescents 14–18 y
  - 3,500 mg/day for males and females 19 y and older

Sources: Busby MG, Fischer L, da Costa KA, Thompson D, Mar MH, Zeisel SH. Choline- and betaine-defined diets for use in clinical research and for the management of trimethylaminuria. J Am Dietet Assoc. 2004;104(12):1836–45; Institute of Medicine, Food and Nutrition Board. Dietary reference intakes for thiamin, riboflavin, niacin, vitamin B6, folate, vitamin B12, pantothenic acid, biotin, and choline. Washington (DC): National Academies Press; 1998. p. 390–422.

an essential nutrient and is related to the formation of the neurotransmitter *acetylcholine*, which is involved in muscle control, mood, nervous system functions, cell membrane signaling, and lipid transport and metabolism (98) (Box 5.11). It is often grouped together with B-complex vitamins. Some animal species require choline to sustain health, but humans can manufacture choline through a metabolic pathway that involves the amino acid *methionine* and the vitamin *folate*. Therefore, periodic consumption of high-protein foods that are excellent contributors of the amino acid *methionine* is a way to ensure adequate choline availability. In 1998, choline was determined to be an essential nutrient by the Institute of Medicine (99,100). It is present in many foods and is particularly high in beef liver, eggs, human breast milk, and cruciferous vegetables (cauliflower, broccoli, etc.). Choline is also naturally present in breast milk and, because of its importance in brain tissue formation and function, is fortified in most infant formulas (101). Lecithin, an emulsifying agent (causes fats to mix in water, as in creamy Italian dressing versus regular oil and vinegar dressing with the oil rising to the top), may contain anywhere from 20% to 90% choline, depending on its source (soybean, sunflower, rapeseed, etc.). Although the lecithin content of processed foods is small, consumption of lecithin-containing foods may

increase the choline intake in an average adult by only 1.5 mg/kg (78).

Although rare, possibly because of a small level of body synthesized choline, choline deficiency can result in muscle and liver damage, and nonalcoholic fatty liver disease (102). Common clinical signs of severe choline deficiency include liver, heart, and kidney disease (100,103). It is still being assessed, but there are early studies suggesting that endurance athletes and people who heavily consume alcohol may benefit from higher choline intakes (104,105). However, a more recent study on army rangers found no benefit of choline supplementation on endurance, injury rates, or shooting accuracy (106).

Even moderately high levels of **homocysteine** in the blood may increase cardiovascular disease risk, and there is evidence that choline deficiency may be a factor in higher homocysteine levels (107,108). One of the clinical problems seen with inadequate choline intake is *nonalcoholic fatty liver disease*. Choline is needed for the manufacture of the liver protein that carries liver-derived fat to the blood, called very–low-density lipoproteins (VLDL). Without sufficient choline, the protein carrier cannot be manufactured and the fat in the liver cannot be removed. A study of postmenopausal women with low estrogen found that they developed liver and/or muscular damage if provided a choline-deficient diet (109).

> ### 📖 Homocysteine
>
> An intermediary amino acid used to manufacture needed proteins through the interaction with vitamin B_{12}, vitamin B_6, and folic acid. Because of this conversion to needed proteins, there is typically a low level of circulating homocysteine in the blood. Elevated levels of homocysteine are typically the result of low thyroid hormone, or deficiency of folic acid, vitamin B_6, or vitamin B_{12}.

FAT-SOLUBLE VITAMINS

Fat-soluble vitamins are delivered in a fat solute and represent one of the important reasons why athletes should not attempt placing themselves on a diet that is excessively low in fat. (Going below 10% of total calories from fat is dangerous, whereas athletes do very well when fat intake is between 20% and 35% of total calories.) There are four fat-soluble vitamins, including vitamins A, D, E, and K, which can be efficiently stored for later use, so the intake of fat-soluble vitamins can be more periodic than water-soluble vitamins to satisfy needs. However, the storage capacity for these vitamins does have limitations, and providing a level of these vitamins that exceeds the storage capacity may quickly lead to symptoms of toxicity and, in extreme cases, death. The most potentially toxic substance in human nutrition is vitamin A. Achieving toxic-level doses of this vitamin is difficult if consuming typically consumed foods, but toxic doses may be easily achieved if supplemental intakes exceed recommended doses. In general, the storage capabilities we have for these vitamins eliminate the need for supplemental intake in most circumstances.

Vitamin A (Retinol and Its Precursor, β-Carotene)

The active form of vitamin A is *retinol* (Box 5.12). We obtain the active form from foods of animal origin, including liver, egg yolks, dairy products that have been fortified with vitamin A (*e.g.*, vitamin A and D milk), margarine, and fish oil. The DRI ranges between 700 retinol activity equivalents (RAE) for women and 900 RAE for men. One RAE equals:

- 1 mcg of retinol
- 12 mcg of β-carotene
- 24 mcg of α-carotene
- 24 mcg of β-cryptoxanthin

Vitamin A has a well-established relationship to normal vision; helps keep bones, skin, and RBCs healthy; and is needed for the immune system to function normally.

Box 5.12 — Vitamin A (Active Form: Retinol; Precursor Form: β-carotene) Basic Information

- **DRI**
  - Adult males: 900 mcg/day
  - Adult females: 700 mcg/day
  - Recommended intake for athletes: 700–900 mcg/day
- **Functions**
  - Maintaining healthy epithelial (surface) cells
  - Eye health
  - Immune system health
- **Good food sources**
  - Retinol:
    - Liver
    - Butter
    - Cheese
    - Egg yolks
    - Fish liver oils
  - β-Carotene:
    - Dark green and brightly pigmented fruits and vegetables
- **Deficiency**
  - Dry skin
  - Headache
  - Irritability
  - Vomiting
  - Bone pain
  - Night blindness
  - Increased risk of infection
  - Blindness
- **Toxicity** (high toxicity potential)
  - Tolerable ULs:
    - 600–900 mcg/day for young children (age 1–8 y)
    - 1.7–3.0 mg/day for children and adults (age 9–70+ y)
    - *Toxicity symptoms:* liver damage, bone malformations, death

There is no evidence that taking extra vitamin A aids athletic performance. In an early study performed in the 1940s, supplementation of vitamin A produced no improvement in endurance (110). In the same study, subjects provided with a diet deficient in vitamin A noted no decrease in performance, probably because a deficit state of the vitamin was not reached because of ample vitamin storage. Inadequate levels of vitamin A intakes have been reported in a small proportion of adolescent athletes, and given that the adolescent period is important for bone development/growth, some attention should be given to adolescent athletes to ensure the intake of vitamin A is adequate (111,112).

Because vitamin A (retinol) has clearly toxic side effects when chronically taken in excess of the DRI, athletes should be cautioned against taking supplemental doses of this vitamin. Toxicity of vitamin A manifests itself in several ways, including dry skin, headache, irritability, vomiting, bone pain, and vision problems. Excess vitamin A intake during pregnancy is also associated with an increase in birth defects (44).

A precursor to vitamin A is β-carotene. A precursor is a substance that, under the proper conditions, is converted to the active form of the vitamin. Therefore, consuming foods with β-carotene is an indirect way of obtaining vitamin A. β-Carotene is found in all red-, orange-, yellow-, and dark green–colored fruits and vegetables (carrots, sweet potatoes, spinach, apricots, cantaloupes, tomatoes, etc.). It is a powerful antioxidant, protecting cells from oxidative damage and, of course, can be converted to vitamin A as it is needed. Unlike preformed vitamin A (retinol), β-carotene has not been found to exhibit the same clear toxic effects if excess doses are consumed. However, a consistently high intake of carrots, sweet potatoes, and other foods high in β-carotene may cause a person to develop a yellowish skin tone. It should be noted that two research trials in smokers and former asbestos workers found that β-carotene supplementation for 4–6 years *increased* lung cancer risk by 16%–28% when compared with a placebo (113). These trials suggest that, although there is no current evidence of higher disease risk in nonsmokers, reasonable intakes that do not breach the all-important nutrient balance rule should be warranted.

Athlete surveys suggest that different sports have different vitamin A/β-carotene intake risks. Young wrestlers, gymnasts, combat sport athletes, and ballet dancers, all of whom may restrict food intakes in an attempt to achieve a desired weight, had average intakes that were below 60%–70% of the recommended intake, whereas other male and female athletes appear to have typical intakes that meet the recommended level (114–118). The difference may be the food restriction common in the sports with lower intakes.

It is conceivable that β-carotene may, as an antioxidant, prove to be effective in reducing postexercise muscle soreness and may aid in postexercise recovery. However, this is a theoretical connection only; no study makes a direct link between β-carotene intake and reduced soreness and improved recovery. One study has found that β-carotene reduced exercise-induced asthma, and another found that it was a useful antioxidant for reducing DNA damage in humans (119–121). A recent study found that consuming foods with elevated levels of β-carotene and other antioxidants enabled better tissue adaptation to elevated resistance training (122).

Vitamin D (Cholecalciferol)

There has been a great deal of work and rethinking about the role of vitamin D in human health. It is the most potentially toxic vitamin in human nutrition, with an upper limit (UL) of 50 mcg/day (Box 5.13) (123). We can obtain the vitamin in an inactive form from food and sunlight exposure. Ultraviolet radiation (sunlight) exposure of the skin alters a cholesterol derivative (7-dehydrocholesterol) to an inactive form of vitamin D called *cholecalciferol.* To be functional, this inactive form of vitamin D must be activated by the kidneys. Therefore, kidney disease may be the cause of vitamin D–related disorders. Dietary sources of vitamin D include eggs, vitamin D–fortified milk, liver, butter, and margarine. Cod liver oil, which was once given commonly as a supplement, is a concentrated source of the vitamin. The adult DRI for vitamin D is 15 mcg/day of cholecalciferol or 600 IU of vitamin D. The UL for vitamin D was set at a level that was intended to avoid calcium infusion and excess mineralization of soft (*i.e.*, muscle and organ) tissues. Because the current knowledge of vitamin D has increased, many scientists and qualified practitioners now recommend an intake that is at least 1,000–2,000 IU/day, or three to five times higher than the currently recommended intake level (124).

There is a great deal of current science suggesting that the vitamin D promotes growth and mineralizes bones and teeth by increasing the absorption of calcium and phosphorus. But vitamin D also has other important characteristics that may influence both health and athletic performance. Vitamin D activity includes (125–129):

- *Bone health* (through regulation of calcium and phosphorus absorption)
- *Muscle contraction* (through activation of enzymes for muscle stimulation)

Box 5.13   Vitamin D (Cholecalciferol) Basic Information

- **DRI**
  - Adult males: 15 mcg/day
  - Adult females: 15 mcg/day
  - Recommended intake for athletes: 15–20 mcg/day
- **Functions**
  - Absorption of calcium
  - Absorption of phosphorus
  - Healthy skin
- **Good sources**
  - Ultraviolet light exposure
  - Fish liver oil
  - Lesser amounts in:
    - Eggs
    - Canned fish
    - Fortified milk
    - Fortified margarine

- **Deficiency**
  - Disease: Rickets (children)
  - Disease: Osteomalacia (adults)
  - Increased risk of stress fractures
  - Increased risk of osteoporosis
- **Toxicity** (high toxicity potential)
  - Tolerable ULs:
    - 50 mcg/day for all age groups
  - *Symptoms:*
    - Nausea
    - Diarrhea
    - Loss of muscle function
    - Organ damage
    - Skeletal damage

- *Intestinal absorption* (through facilitation of calcium absorption in the intestines)
- *Muscle protein anabolism* (through both an increase in muscle mass and a decrease in muscle breakdown; muscle increase is for type II—power muscle fibers)
- *Improved immune function* (through accumulation of fluid and immune cells in injured and inflamed tissues and through release of antimicrobial peptides. Outcome is reduced risk of cancer, intestinal disease, cardiovascular disease, muscle soreness)
- *Improved anti-inflammatory action* (through increase production of anti-inflammatory cytokines and interleukin-4 and decreased production of inflammatory agents interleukin-6, interferon-γ, and interleukin-2)

Vitamin D functions to promote growth and mineralize bone and teeth by increasing the absorption of calcium and phosphorus. A diet with an AI of calcium and phosphorus, but without adequate vitamin D, will thus lead to calcium and phosphorus deficiency. The childhood deficiency disease rickets and the adult deficiency disease osteomalacia are diseases of calcium deficiency that are due to either inadequate levels of vitamin D or the inability to convert vitamin D to the active (functional) form.

There is a long history of ultraviolet light (*i.e.,* vitamin D) therapy for athletes (125). In the mid-1920s, sunlamps were used by swimmers in Germany, and the effect was sufficiently positive that it was considered a form of illegal doping by some. Ultraviolet light therapy was also used by Russian

and German athletes in the 1930s and 1940s, where it was found that it improved performance. In the mid-1940s in the United States, the combined effect of a fitness program plus ultraviolet irradiation produced significantly better fitness results than in those undergoing athletic training without the ultraviolet irradiation. The general consensus during these years was that ultraviolet irradiation had a positive impact on speed, strength, endurance, reaction time, and reduced pain. The muscle enhancing impact of adequate vitamin D was found in a study that supplemented vitamin D (4,000 IU) with whey protein (25 g) either before or after bedtime in a group of males undergoing resistance training. This supplementation resulted in beneficial increases in muscle mass when compared to a placebo (130).

Vitamin D may play an indirect role in resistance to injury. Athletes in some sports may have dramatically lower sunlight exposure because all training takes place inside. This lower sunlight (*i.e.,* ultraviolet) exposure may reduce vitamin D availability to a point where both growth and bone density are affected. Lower bone densities are known to place athletes at higher risk for developing stress fractures, an injury that can end an athletic career (131–133). In a survey of US national team gymnasts, it was found that the factor most closely related to bone density was sunlight exposure. Those with higher densities had the greatest exposure (134). Also, sunlight exposure was more important as a predictor of bone density in this group than vitamin D or calcium intake from food. A study did find that professional basketball players were at higher risk of vitamin D deficiency following the winter months, likely from reduced sunlight exposure (135). And another study also found a high prevalence of vitamin D inadequacy in athletes and dancers who have little sunlight exposure (136). It has been recommended, to lower the risk of developing a stress fracture in athletes, it has been recommended that the vitamin D blood level of ≥30 ng/mL should be sustained through a combination of adequate food intake and/or adequate sunlight exposure to equal approximately 800 IU/day (137). This is a level slightly higher than the 600 IU DRI for vitamin D.

Vitamin E (Tocopherol)

Vitamin E is a generic term for several substances (tocopherols) that have similar activity, and the unit of measure is based on the level of tocopherol with an activity equivalent to that of α-tocopherol (Box 5.14). For instance, β-tocopherol has a lower level of activity than α-tocopherol, so more of it would be necessary to get the same effect (44). Vitamin E is found in green leafy vegetables, vegetable oils, seeds, nuts, liver, and corn. It is difficult to induce a vitamin E deficiency in humans, and it also appears to be a relatively nontoxic vitamin. Vitamin E is a potent antioxidant that serves to protect membranes from destruction by peroxides. Peroxides are formed when fats (especially polyunsaturated fats) become oxidized (rancid). These peroxides are called free radicals because they bounce around unpredictably inside cells, altering or destroying them. Because vitamin E is an antioxidant, it helps to capture oxygen, thereby limiting the oxidation of fats to protect cells.

Several studies on vitamin E and physical performance have been conducted, but none has found an improvement in either strength or endurance with vitamin E supplementation (138–141). Several studies evaluating whether vitamin E supplementation reduced exercise-induced peroxide damage had mixed findings. Some suggest that a clear reduction in peroxidative damage occurs, but others suggest that vitamin E has no benefit (142–144). It was found that vitamin E (800 IU for 1–2 months) compared with placebo ingestion before a competitive triathlon race event actually promoted lipid peroxidation and inflammation during exercise, which was precisely the opposite of the expectation (12). However, another study found that low doses of vitamin E supplementation (less than 500 IU/day) protected against exercise-induced muscle damage and oxidative stress, while higher doses did not (145). This is yet another example of how too great an intake of a vitamin may produce results contrary to the potential benefits that an AI provides.

Vitamin K (Phylloquinone, Menaquinone)

Vitamin K is found in green leafy vegetables and also, in small amounts, in cereals, fruits, and meats. Intestinal bacteria also produce vitamin K, so the absolute dietary requirement is not known (Box 5.15). The phylloquinone form of the vitamin (vitamin K1) is found primarily in green leafy vegetables, and the menaquinone form of the vitamin (vitamin K2) is of bacterial origin from fermented foods and the form produced by intestinal bacteria. This vitamin is needed for the formation of prothrombin, which is required for blood to clot, and is also needed to sustain normal nervous system function and to sustain bone mineral density (146,147). It is possible for people who regularly take antibiotics that destroy the bacteria in the intestines to be at increased risk for vitamin K deficiency. A deficiency would cause an increase in bleeding and

---

Box 5.14 Vitamin E (Tocopherol) Basic Information

- **DRI**
  - Adult males: 15 mg/day
  - Adult females: 15 mg/day
  - Recommended intake for athletes: 15 mg/day
- **Functions**
  - Antioxidant protection of cell membranes
- **Good food sources**
  - Polyunsaturated and monounsaturated vegetable and cereal oils and margarines (corn, soy, safflower, olive)

- Lesser amounts in fortified cereals
- Lesser amounts in eggs
- **Deficiency**
  - Rare; if it occurs, possible increased risk of cancer and heart disease
- **Toxicity**
  - Tolerable ULs:
    - 200–300 mg/day for young children (age 1–8 y)
    - 600–1,000 mg/day for children and adults (age 9–70+ y)

Box 5.15   Vitamin K (Phylloquinone) Basic Information

- **DRI**
  - Adult males: 120 mcg/day
  - Adult females: 90 mcg/day
  - Recommended intake for athletes: 700–900 mcg/day
- **Functions**
  - Formation of blood clots
  - Enhancement of osteocalcin function to aid in bone strengthening
- **Good food sources**
  - Phylloquinone:
    - Variety of vegetable oils
    - Dark green leafy vegetables (cabbage, spinach)
  - Menaquinone:
    - Formed by the bacteria that line the GI tract
- **Deficiency**
  - Rare; if it occurs, results in hemorrhage
- **Toxicity**
  - Tolerable ULs not established

---

hemorrhages. Vitamin K appears to be relatively nontoxic, but high intakes of synthetic forms may cause jaundice.

Several studies have now found that vitamin K deficiency caused from inadequate dietary intake, albeit rare in human populations, results in low bone mineral density and/or an increase in skeletal fractures (148). It has been found that vitamin K–associated lower bone density can be improved with vitamin K supplementation (147,148). In addition, women obtaining a minimum of 110 mcg of vitamin K were found to be at significantly lower hip fracture risk than women with lower intakes (149). The Framingham Heart Study also found a relationship between higher vitamin K intake and reduced hip fracture risk (150,151).

There are no studies on the relationship between vitamin K and athletic performance, but for athletes involved in contact sports, normal vitamin K status is necessary to avoid excessive bruising and bleeding. In addition, there is evidence of a relationship between low vitamin K status and bone loss in female endurance athletes. In one study, amenorrheic females had lower bone densities that were not improved with 2 years of vitamin K supplementation (152). In another study, amenorrheic female athletes experienced an increase in bone formation when taking vitamin K supplements (153). The contrast in these studies highlights the difficulty for any single study to control for all the important nutritional factors that could influence the results, including energy intake adequacy, vitamin D status, estrogen status (in females), and calcium intake.

A word of caution for athletes involved in any form of *blood doping*, which refers to strategies that increase RBC numbers in the circulating blood. The purpose of blood doping is to increase oxidative capacity to enable an enhanced metabolism of fat for energy. Most blood doping strategies, which include taking erythropoietin or reinserting previously drawn blood, are considered illegal

by virtually all athletic organizations. Some forms of blood doping, however, are commonly practiced and are not considered illegal (*i.e.*, living at high altitude to enable a greater red cell formation or using a hypoxic tent to sleep in). Because of the elevated blood clotting potential that vitamin K produces, having a higher RBC density may predispose these athletes to unwanted clots. This would be particularly true for athletes who do blood doping and who become dehydrated, which would cause RBC density to increase still further. Whether legal or illegal, blood doping coupled with excess vitamin K may pose clotting risks, especially when coupled with dehydration.

SUMMARY

Vitamins enable normal cellular metabolic reactions inside the cell. As an example, vitamin D stimulates intestinal cells to absorb calcium and phosphorus, and the B-vitamins enable chemical reactions that help cells burn the fuel derived from carbohydrate, protein, and fat. A summary of the exercise-associated involvement of vitamins is given in Table 5.2.

- Vitamins are either fat soluble (vitamins A, D, E, and K) or water soluble (all others).
- The fat-soluble vitamins are delivered in the fats of consumed foods and can be stored in special storage depots. These stored vitamins can be called upon for long periods of time to satisfy cellular needs for these vitamins.
- The water-soluble vitamins are stored throughout the body in many tissues, but because their storage is limited, they must be consumed with more frequency.
- Both fat- and water-soluble vitamins are potentially toxic if consumed in excess.

Table 5.2	Summary of Exercise-Associated Involvement of Vitamins					
Vitamin	Energy Metabolism	Central Nervous System Function	Red Blood Cell Manufacture	Immune Function	Antioxidant Function	Bone Metabolism
Vitamin B$_1$	X	X				
Vitamin B$_2$	X	X	X			
Niacin	X	X				
Vitamin B$_6$	X	X	X	X	X	
Folic acid		X	X			
Vitamin B$_{12}$		X	X			
Pantothenic acid	X					
Biotin	X					
Vitamin C		X	X	X	X	
Vitamin A				X	X	X
Vitamin D				X	X	X
Vitamin E			X	X	X	
Vitamin K						X

- Because the amounts needed are relatively small, few people require vitamin supplements to satisfy dietary weaknesses, particularly if they consume a reasonably good and balanced diet that includes fresh and whole foods. Some issues to consider:
  - The chronic consumption of too much of any vitamin may result in just as poor an outcome as the consumption of too little.
  - Athletes who satisfy total energy requirements from the consumption of a variety of foods are also likely to satisfy vitamin requirements.
  - Athletes should not shy away from eating fat, as about 20%–25% of total calories from fat is needed to satisfy the need for the fat-soluble vitamins and the essential fatty acids.
  - The B-vitamins are associated with energy metabolism. The more energy you burn, the more B-vitamins you need. However, the B-vitamins are fortified in grains, so even high-energy burners are unlikely to achieve a deficiency.
  - Athletes who feel they eat a poor diet and may need vitamins should consult a registered dietitian to help determine what they need and in what amounts.

To maximize vitamin intake from your diet, try the following:

- Eat a wide variety of colorful fruits and vegetables.
- When possible eat fresh fruits and vegetables, especially those in season.
- Do not overcook vegetables, as long cooking times reduce nutrient content.
- Steam or microwave your vegetables rather than boiling them—nutrients seep out in boiling water only to be poured down the drain.

Practical Application Activity

The DRI values represent the recommended intake of each vitamin. You can assess the vitamin content of consumed foods using the same strategy followed in earlier chapters, accessing the online USDA Food Composition Database (https://fdc.nal.usda.gov), but this time create a spreadsheet with at least two water-soluble vitamins (e.g., vitamins C and B$_6$) and at least two fat-soluble vitamins (e.g., vitamins A and E).

1. Enter the foods/beverages with amounts consumed for an entire day, and create totals for each vitamin.
2. When completed, assess how your total intake compares with the recommended intake (recommended dietary allowance) for each selected vitamin.
3. Review which foods contribute most to your intake for each vitamin.
4. If any of the values are below the recommended levels, modify your food intake to see what changes you would make in your diet to reach the recommended intake level.

CHAPTER QUESTIONS

1. Of the following, which is a function of ascorbic acid?
   a. Antifungal agent
   b. Collagen producer
   c. Antioxidant
   d. Antibacterial
   e. b and c
   f. All of the above

2. Which of the following vitamins is associated with deamination and transamination reactions in protein metabolism?
   a. Thiamin
   b. Riboflavin
   c. Niacin
   d. Pyridoxine
   e. Cobalamin

3. This vitamin is involved in oxidation–reduction reactions for ATP production and is associated with photophobia.
   a. Vitamin B_1
   b. Vitamin B_2
   c. Vitamin B_6
   d. Vitamin B_{12}

4. This vitamin has hormone-like actions.
   a. Vitamin A
   b. Vitamin C
   c. Vitamin D
   d. Vitamin E

5. This vitamin is part of the intermediary product of energy metabolism, CoA:
   a. Thiamin
   b. Folate
   c. Niacin
   d. Pantothenate

6. A deficiency of this vitamin results in megaloblastic anemia.
   a. Vitamin B_1
   b. Vitamin B_6
   c. Vitamin B_{12}
   d. Niacin

7. Vitamin E is an effective
   a. Antioxidant
   b. Agent for increasing bone mineral density
   c. Substance for maintaining eye health
   d. Agent for reducing muscle soreness

8. Chronic, high doses of this vitamin may result in peripheral neuropathy.
   a. Vitamin C
   b. Vitamin B_6
   c. Vitamin Q_{10}
   d. Vitamin B_{12}

9. Consumption of sufficient B-vitamins generally occurs when athletes eat enough
   a. Vegetables
   b. Fruits
   c. Organ meats
   d. Energy

10. These two vitamins work together as antioxidants:
    a. Folic acid and thiamin
    b. Thiamin and riboflavin
    c. Vitamin C and vitamin E
    d. Niacin and thiamin

ANSWERS TO CHAPTER QUESTIONS

1. e
2. d
3. b
4. c
5. d
6. c
7. a
8. b
9. d
10. c

Case Study Considerations

1. **Case Study Answer 1:** Advertisements often focus on a little basic science, making them sound convincing, but typically fail to provide information on potential toxicity if an excess amount is consumed in a single high dose, and fail to describe consumption strategies that help to assure optimal cellular function. For instance, supplements that suggest the b-complex vitamins contained in the bottle may correctly indicate that these vitamins are involved in energy metabolism, but they fail to indicate that consuming 100 times the recommended dietary allowance in a single pill (an all-to-common level dosage level provided) is likely to compromise cellular function and may result in cellular rejection of these high doses. The result would be a cellular deficiency in the presence of extremely high doses. They may also advertise that the vitamin C and vitamin E in the bottle are antioxidants involved in protecting cells. However, they fail to mention that the chronic consumption of very high doses of these vitamins may result in the opposite of the desired effect by compromising cellular adaptation to training. It is important to consider that cells have a finite storage capacity for vitamins and minerals, making it far more

effective to provide, for instance, 400 mg in four 100 mg doses spread out throughout the day rather than 400 mg in a single dose. Eating a variety of good foods throughout the day nicely resolves this issue by providing cells with vitamin concentrations that the cells can deal with. So, it's not just how much is consumed, but how the nutrients can be consumed throughout the day to sustain optimal cellular function. More than enough is not better than enough.

2. **Case Study Answer 2:** When you access the NIH website, access the link that takes you to "Dietary Supplements for Exercise and Athletic Performance" under the "Health Professional" link. Once there, you can access "Ingredients in Supplements for Exercise and Athletic Performance." This section contains a long list of ingredients used in supplements that are advertised as enhancing athletic performance. For instance, selecting "Antioxidants" (Vitamin C, Vitamin E, and Coenzyme Q_{10}) will provide the following information: "Does it Work?"; "Is it Safe?"; "Bottom Line." Explore this section and you will quickly see that a good eating strategy is likely to be far superior to excess reliance on supplements to obtain nutrients.

REFERENCES

1. United States Department of Health and Human Services, National Institutes of Health, Office of Dietary Supplements. Dietary supplement fact sheets. Bethesda (MD): USDHHS. Accessed 2018 April 23. https://ods.od.nih.gov
2. Schaumberg H, Kaplan J, Windebank A, Vick N, Ragmus S, Pleasure D, Brown MJ. Sensory neuropathy from pyridoxine abuse. A new megavitamin syndrome. N Engl J Med. 1983;309(8):445–8.
3. Mursu J, Robien K, Harnack LJ, Park K, Jacobs DR Jr. Dietary supplements and mortality rate in older women: the Iowa Women's Health Study. Arch Intern Med. 2011;171(18):1625–33.
4. Knudson AG, Rothman PE. Hypervitaminosis A; a review with a discussion of vitamin A. AMA Am J Dis Child. 1953;85(3):316–34.
5. Penniston KL, Tanumihardjo SA. The acute and chronic toxic effects of vitamin A. Am J Clin Nutr. 2006;83(2):191–201.
6. Heikkinen A, Alaranta A, Helenius I, Vasankari T. Dietary supplementation habits and perceptions of supplement use among elite Finnish athletes. Int J Sports Nutr Exerc Metab. 2011;21:271–9.
7. Garthe I, Ramsbottom R. Elite athletes, a rationale for the use of dietary supplements: a practical approach. PharmaNutrition. 2020;14:100234.
8. Heikkinen A, Alaranta A, Helenius I, Vasankari T. Use of dietary supplements in Olympic athletes is decreasing: a follow-up study between 2002 and 2009. J Int Soc Sports Nutr. 2011;8:1.
9. Maughan RJ, Depiesse F, Geyer H; International Association of Athletics Federations. The use of dietary supplements by athletes. J Sports Sci. 2007;25(Suppl 1):S103–13.
10. Dascombe BJ, Karunaratna M, Cartoon J, Fergie B, Goodman C. Nutritional supplementation habits and perceptions of elite athletes within a state-based sporting institute. J Sci Med Sport. 2010;13(2):274–80.
11. Maughan RJ, Shirreffs SM, Vernac A. Making decisions about supplement use. Int J Sport Nutr Exercise Metab. 2018;28:212–9.
12. Nieman DC, Henson DA, McAnulty SR, McAnulty LS, Morrow JD, Ahmed A, Heward CB. Vitamin E and immunity after the Kona Triathlon World Championship. Med Sci Sports Exerc. 2004;36(8):1328–35.
13. Gleeson M, Nieman DC, Pedersen BK. Exercise, nutrition, and immune function. J Sports Sci. 2004;22:115–25.

14. Weight LM, Noakes TD, Labadarios D, Graves J, Jacobs P, Berman PA. Vitamin and mineral status of trained athletes including the effects of supplementation. Am J Clin Nutr. 1988;47(2):186–91.

15. Ramsey D. Vitamins deficiencies and mental health: how are they linked? Current Psychiatry. 2013;12(1):37–44.

16. Christensen N, van Woerden I, Aubuchon-Endsley NL, Fleckenstein P, Olsen J, Blanton C. Diet quality and mental health status among Division 1 female collegiate athletes during the COVID-19 pandemic. Int J Environ Res Public Health. 2021;18:13377.

17. United States Department of Agriculture, Food and Drug Administration. Are foods that contain added nutrients considered "enriched"? Accessed 2018 June 4. https://www.fda.gov/Food/GuidanceRegulation/GuidanceDocuments RegulatoryInformation/ucm470756.htm

18. Jessica P. Danh JP, Nucci A, Doyle JA, Feresin RG. Assessment of sports nutrition knowledge, dietary intake, and nutrition information source in female collegiate athletes: a descriptive feasibility study. J Am Coll Health. 2021;71(9):2717–25.

19. Winston AP, Jamieson CP, Madira W, Gatward NM, Palmer RL. Prevalence of thiamin deficiency in anorexia nervosa. Int J Eat Disord. 2000;28(4):451–4.

20. Gonçalves AC, Portari GV. The b-complex vitamins related to energy metabolism and their role in exercise performance: a narrative review. Sci Sports. 2021;36:433–40.

21. Hanninen SA, Darling PB, Sole MJ, Barr A, Keith ME. The prevalence of thiamin deficiency in hospitalized patients with congestive heart failure. J Am Coll Cardiol. 2006;47(2):354–61.

22. Shill AA, Ramadurai D, Gergen D, Reynolds PM. Dry beri-beri due to thiamine deficiency associated with peripheral neuropathy and Wernicke's encephalopathy mimicking Guillaine-Barré syndrome: a case report and review of the literature. Am J Case Rep. 2019;20:330–4.

23. Therrien A, Kelly CP, Silvester JA. Celiac disease: extraintestinal manifestations and associated conditions. J Clin Gastroenterol. 2021;54(1):8–21.

24. Lakhani S, Surti NK, Doshi MV, Panchasera SR, Vasvani VN, Bapna MR, Raval RC, Billimoria FE, Lakhani JD. Nutritional dermatoses and its association with anemia and systemic illness. Int J Res Dermatol. 2018;4(3):1–7.

25. Rodriguez NR, DiMarco NM, Langley S; American Dietetic Association, and Dietitians of Canada; Dietitians of Canada; American College of Sports Medicine. American College of Sports Medicine position stand. Nutrition and athletic performance. Med Sci Sports Exerc. 2009;41;709–31.

26. Thomas DT, Erdman KA, Burke LM. American College of Sports Medicine Joint Position Statement. Nutrition and athletic performance. Med Sci Sports Exerc. 2016;48(3):543–68.

27. Sato A, Shimoyama Y, Ishikawa T, Murayama N. Dietary thiamin and riboflavin intake and blood thiamin and riboflavin concentrations in college swimmers undergoing intensive training. Int J Sports Nutr Exerc Metab. 2011;21:195–204.

28. National Institutes of Health Office of Dietary Supplements. Riboflavin. Accessed 2022 June. https://ods.od.nih.gov/factsheets/Riboflavin-HealthProfessional/

29. Woolf K, Manore MM. B-vitamins and exercise: does exercise alter requirements? Int J Sports Nutr Exerc Metab. 2006;16(5):453–84.

30. Belko AZ, Meredith MP, Kalkwarf HJ, Obarzanek E, Weinberg S, Roach R, McKeon G, Roe DA. Effects of exercise on riboflavin requirements: biological validation in weight-reducing young women. Am J Clin Nutr. 1985;41(2):270–7.

31. Belko AZ, Obarzanek E, Kalkwarf JH, Rotter MA, Bogusz S, Miller D, Haas JD, Roe DA. Effects of exercise on riboflavin requirements of young women. Am J Clin Nutr. 1983;37(4):509–17.

32. Belko AZ, Obarzanek MP, Roach R, Urgan G, Weinberg S, Roe DA. Effects of aerobic exercise and weight loss on riboflavin requirements of moderately obese, marginally deficient young women. Am J Clin Nutr. 1984;40(3):553–61.

33. Tremblay A, Boiland F, Breton M, Bessette H, Roberge AG. The effects of a riboflavin supplementation on the nutritional status and performance of elite swimmers. Nutr Res. 1984;4(2):201–8.

34. Casazza GA, Tovar AP, Richardson CE, Cortez AN, Davis BA. Energy availability, macronutrient intake, and nutritional supplementation for improving exercise performance in endurance athletes. Curr Sports Med Rep. 2018;17(6):215–23.

35. Janssen JJE, Lagerwaard B, Nieuwenhuizen AG, Timmers S, de Boer VCJ, Keijer J. The effect of a single bout of exercise on vitamin B2 status is not different between high- and low-fit females. Nutrients. 2021;13:4097.

36. Borrione P, Grasso L, Quaranta F, Parisi A. Vegetarian diet and athletes. Sport Präventivmed. 2009;39(1):20–4.

37. Shaw KA, Zello GA, Rodgers CD, Warkentin TD, Baerwald AR, Chilibeck PD. Benefits of a plant-based diet and considerations for the athlete. Eur J Appl Physiol. 2022;122(5):1163–78.

38. Tambalis KD. Special nutritional needs for athletes and exercisers. Eur J Physiother. 2022;3(1).

39. Lukaski HC. Vitamin and mineral status: effects on physical performance. Nutrition. 2004;20:632–44.

40. Close GL, Hamilton DL, Philp A, Burke LM, Morton JP. New strategies in sport nutrition to increase exercise performance. Free Radic Biol Med. 2016;98:144–58.

41. Bergström J, Hultman E, Jorfeldt L, Pernow B, Wahren J. Effect of nicotinic acid on physical working capacity and on metabolism of muscle glycogen in man. J Appl Physiol. 1969;26(2):170–6.

42. Carlson LA, Havel RJ, Ekelund LG, Holmgren A. Effect of nicotinic acid on the turnover rate and oxidation of the free fatty acids of plasma in man during exercise. Metabolism. 1963;12:837–45.

43. Hilsendager D, Karpovich PV. Ergogenic effect of glycine and niacin separately and in combination. Res Q. 1964;35:389–92.

44. Institute of Medicine (US) Food and Nutrition Board. Dietary reference intakes (DRIs): recommended intakes for individuals, vitamins. Washington (DC): National Academies Press (US); 2004.

45. Stover PJ, Field MS. Vitamin B-6. Adv Nutr. 2015;6(1):132–3.

46. Brown MJ, Ameer MA, Daley SF, Beier K. Vitamin, B6 (Pyridoxine), deficiency. [Updated 2017 December 8]. In: StatPearls [Internet]. Treasure Island (FL): StatPearls Publishing; 2018. Accessed 2018 April 20. https://www.ncbi.nlm.nih.gov/books/NBK470579/

47. Halsted CH, Medici V. Vitamin B regulation of alcoholic liver disease. In: Patel VB, editor. Molecular aspects of alcohol and nutrition. London: Academic Press; 2016. p. 95–106.

48. Dalton K, Dalton MJ. Characteristics of pyridoxine overdose neuropathy syndrome. Acta Neurol Scand. 1987;76:8–11.

49. Manore MM. Vitamin B-6 and exercise. Int J Sports Nutr. 1994;4:89–103.

50. Fogelholm M, Ruokonen I, Laakso JT, Vuorimaa T, Himberg JJ. Lack of association between indices of vitamin B-1, B-2, and B-6 status and exercise-induced blood lactate in young adults. Int J Sports Nutr. 1993;3:165–76.

51. Guilland JC, Penarand T, Gallet C, Boggio V, Fuchs F, Klepping J. Vitamin status of young athletes including the effects of supplementation. Med Sci Sports Exerc. 1989;21:441–9.

52. Telford RD, Catchpole EA, Deakin V, McLeay AC, Plank AW. The effect of 7 to 8 months of vitamin/mineral supplementation on the vitamin and mineral status of athletes. Int J Sports Nutr. 1992;2:123–34.

53. Suboticanec K, Stavljenic A, Schalch W, Buzina R. Effects of pyridoxine and riboflavin supplementation of physical fitness in young adolescents. Int J Vitam Nutr Res. 1990;60:81–8.

54. Choi EY, Cho YO. Effect of vitamin B(6) deficiency on antioxidative status in rats with exercise-induced oxidative stress. Nutr Res Pract. 2009;3(3):208–11.

55. Delitala G, Masala A, Alagna S, Devilla L. Effect of pyridoxine on human hypophyseal trophic hormone release: a possible stimulation of hypothalamic dopaminergic pathway. J Clin Endorinol Metab. 1976;42:603–6.

56. Virk R, Dunton N, Young J, Leklem J. Effect of vitamin B-6 supplementation on fuels, catecholamines, and amino acids during exercise in men. Med Sci Sports Exerc. 1999;31(3):400–8.

57. Moretti C, Fabbri A, Gnessi L, Bonifacio V, Fraioli F, Isidori A. Pyridoxine (B6) suppresses the rise in prolactin and increases the rise in growth hormone induced by exercise. N Engl J Med. 1982;307(7):444–5.

58. Brancaccio M, Mennitti C, Cesaro A, Fimiani F, Vano M, Gargiulo B, Caiazza M, Amodio F, Coto I, D'Alicandro G, Mazzaccara C, Lombardo B, Pero R, Terracciano D, Limongelli G, Calabrò P, D'Argenio V, Frisso G, Scudiero O. The biological role of vitamins in athletes' muscle, heart and microbiota. Int J Environ Res Public Health. 2022;19:1249.

59. Dreon DM, Butterfield GE. Vitamin B-6 utilization in active and inactive young men. Am J Clin Nutr. 1986;43:816–24.

60. Rokitzki L, Sagredos AN, Reuss F, Büchner M, Keul J. Acute changes in vitamin B-6 status in endurance athletes before and after a marathon. Int J Sports Nutr. 1994;4:154–65.

61. Albert MJ, Mathan VI, Baker SJ. Vitamin B12 synthesis by human small intestinal bacteria. Nature. 1980;283:781–2.

62. Froiland K, Koszewski W, Hingst J, Kopecky L. Nutritional supplement use among college athletes and their sources of information. Int J Sports Nutr Exerc Metab. 2004;14(1):104–10.

63. United States Senate. Proper and improper use of drugs by athletes: hearings before the subcommittee to investigate juvenile delinquency of the committee. Washington (DC): U.S. Government Printing Office; 1973 June 18 and July 12–13.

64. Read M, McGuffin S. The effect of B-complex supplementation on endurance performance. J Sports Med Phys Fitness. 1983;23(2):178–84.

65. Tin-May T, Ma-Win M, Khin-Sann A, Mya-Tu M. The effect of vitamin B-12 on physical performance capacity. Br J Nutr. 1978;40(2):269–73.

66. Volpe SL. Micronutrient requirements for athletes. Clin Sports Med. 2007;26:119–30.

67. Morales-Gutierrez J, Díaz-Cortés S, Montoya-Giraldo MA, Zuluaga AF. Toxicity induced by multiple high doses of vitamin B_{12} during pernicious anemia treatment: a case report. Clin Toxicol. 2020;58(2):129–31.

68. Pawlak R, James PS, Raj S, Cullum-Dugan D, Lucas D. Understanding vitamin B12. Am J Lifestyle Med. 2013;7(1):60–5. doi:10.1177/1559827612450688.

69. NIH, National Institutes of Health Office of Dietary Supplements. Folate. Accessed 2022 June. https://ods.od.nih.gov/factsheets/Folate-HealthProfessional/

70. Williams J, Mai CT, Mulinare J, Isenburg J, Flood TJ, Ethen M, Frohnert B, Kirby RS; Centers for Disease Control and Prevention. Updated estimates of neural tube defects prevented by mandatory folic acid fortification—United States, 1995–2011. Morb Mortal Wkly Rep. 2015;64(1):1–5.

71. Figueiredo JC, Grau MV, Haile RW, Sandler RS, Summers RW, Bresalier RS, Burke CA, McKeown-Eyssen GE, Baron JA. Folic acid and risk of prostate cancer: results from a randomized clinical trial. J Natl Cancer Inst. 2009;101(6):432–5.

72. Mason JB, Dickstein A, Jacques PF, Haggarty P, Selhub J, Dallal G, Rosenberg IH. A temporal association between folic acid fortification and an increase in colorectal cancer rates may be illuminating important biological principles: a hypothesis. Cancer Epidemiol Biomarkers Prev. 2007;16(7):1325–9.

73. Wycoff KF, Ganji V. Proportion of individuals with low serum vitamin B-12 concentrations without macrocytosis is higher in the post folic acid fortification period than in the pre folic acid fortification period. Am J Clin Nutr. 2007;86(4):1187–92.

74. Danh JP, Nucci A, Doyle JA, Feresin RG. Assessment of sports nutrition knowledge, dietary intake, and nutrition information source in female collegiate athletes: a descriptive feasibility study. J Am Coll Health. 2023;71(9):2717–25.

75. Ruiz-Iglesias P, Gorgori-González A, Massot-Cladera M, Castell M, Pérez-Cano FJ. Does flavonoid consumption improve exercise performance? Is it related to changes in the immune system and inflammatory biomarkers? A systematic review of clinical studies since 2005. Nutrients. 2021;13:1132.

76. Matter M, Stittfall T, Graves J, Myburgh K, Adams B, Jacobs P, Noakes TD. The effect of iron and folate therapy on maximal exercise performance in female marathon runners with iron and folate deficiency. Clin Sci (Lond). 1987;72:415–22.

77. León-Del-Río A. Biotin in metabolism, gene expression, and human disease. J Inherit Metab Dis. 2019;42:647–54.

78. Institute of Medicine, Food and Nutrition Board. Dietary reference intakes for thiamin, riboflavin, niacin, vitamin B6, folate, vitamin B12, pantothenic acid, biotin, and choline. Washington (DC): National Academies Press; 1998. p. 390–422.

79. Combs GF Jr. Biotin. In: Combs GF Jr, editor. The vitamins: fundamental aspects in nutrition and health. 3rd ed. Burlington (MA): Elsevier Academic Press; 2008:331–44.

80. Miller JW, Rucker RB. Pantothenic acid. In: Erdman JW, Macdonald IA, Zeisel SH, editors. Present knowledge in nutrition. 10th ed. Washington (DC): Wiley-Blackwell; 2012:375–90.

81. Evans M, Rumberger JA, Azumano I, Napolitano JJ, Citrolo D, Kamiya T. Pantethine, a derivative of vitamin B5, favorably alters total, LDL and non-HDL cholesterol in low to moderate cardiovascular risk subjects eligible for statin therapy:

a triple-blinded placebo and diet-controlled investigation. Vasc Health Risk Manag. 2014;10:89–100.

82. Weimann BI, Hermann D. Studies on wound healing: effects of calcium D-pantothenate on the migration, proliferation and protein synthesis of human dermal fibroblasts in culture. Int J Vitam Nutr Res. 1999;69(2):113–9.

83. Wiederholt T, Heise R, Skazik C, Marquardt Y, Joussen S, Erdmann K, Schröder H, Merk HF, Baron JM. Calcium pantothenate modulates gene expression in proliferating human dermal fibroblasts. Exp Dermatol. 2009;18(11):969–78.

84. Bialecki M, Nijakowski F. Pantothenic acid in the tissues and blood of white rats after brief and prolonged physical exercise. Acta Physiol Polonica. 1967:18;33–8.

85. Shock NW, Sebrell WH. The effects of changes in concentration of pantothenate on the work output of perfused frog muscles. Am J Physiol. 1944;142(2):274–8.

86. Nice C, Reeves AG, Brinck-Hohnsen T, Noll W. The effects of pantothenic acid on human exercise capacity. J Sports Med. 1984;24(1):26–9.

87. Litoff D, Scherzer H, Harrison J. Effects of pantothenic acid on human exercise. Med Sci Sports Exerc. 1985;17(2):287.

88. NIH, National Institutes of Health Office of Dietary Supplements. Vitamin C. Accessed 2022 June. https://ods.od.nih.gov/factsheets/VitaminC-HealthProfessional/

89. Clarkson PM. Antioxidants and physical performance. Crit Rev Food Sci Nutr. 1995;35(1–2):131–41.

90. Hickson JF, Wolinsky I, editors. Nutrition in exercise and sport. Boca Raton (FL): CRC Press; 1989. 121 p.

91. Bramich K, McNaughton L. The effects of two levels of ascorbic acid on muscular endurance, muscular strength, and on V_{O2max}. Int J Clin Nutr Rev. 1987;7:5–10.

92. Schwartz PL. Ascorbic acid in wound healing—a review. J Am Diet Assoc. 1970;56(6):497–503.

93. Kanter MM. Free radicals, exercise, and antioxidant supplementation. Int J Sports Nutr. 1994;4:205–20.

94. Tack C, Shorthouse F, Kass L. The physiological mechanisms of effect of vitamins and amino acids on tendon and muscle healing: a systematic review. Int J Sports Nutr Exerc Metab. 2018;28(3):294–311.

95. Lis DM, Jordan M, Lipoma T, Smith T, Schaal K, Baar K. Collagen and vitamin C supplementation increases lower limb rate of force development. Int J Sport Nutr Exerc Metab. 2022; 32:65–73.

96. Herbert V. Does mega-C do more good than harm, or more harm than good? Nutr Today. 1993;28:28–32.

97. Tian HH, Ong WS, Tan CL. Nutritional supplement use among university athletes in Singapore. Singapore Med J. 2009;50:165–72.

98. Zeisel SH, Corbin KD. Choline. In: Erdman JW, Macdonald IA, Zeisel SH, editors. Present knowledge in nutrition. 10th ed. Washington (DC): Wiley-Blackwell; 2012. p. 405–18.

99. Zeisel SH. A brief history of choline. Ann Nutr Metab. 2012; 61(3):254–8.

100. Zeisel SH, da Costa KA. Choline: an essential nutrient for public health. Nutr Rev. 2009;67(11):615–23.

101. Zeisel SH. Choline. In: Ross AC, Caballero B, Cousins RJ, Tucker KL, Ziegler TR, editors. Modern nutrition in health and disease. 11th ed. Baltimore (MD): Lippincott Williams & Wilkins; 2014. p. 416–26.

102. Hollenbeck CB. An introduction to the nutrition and metabolism of choline. Cent Nerv Syst Agents Med Chem. 2012; 12(2):100–13.

103. Machlin LJ, editor. Handbook of vitamins: nutritional, biochemical, and clinical aspects. New York (NY): Marcel Dekker; 1984.

104. Klatskin G, Krehl WA, Conn HO. The effect of alcohol on the choline requirement. I. Changes in the rat's liver following prolonged ingestion of alcohol. J Exp Med. 1954;100(6): 605–14.

105. von Allwörden HN, Horn S, Kahl J, Feldheim W. The influence of lecithin on plasma choline concentrations in triathletes and adolescent runners during exercise. Eur J Appl Physiol Occup Physiol. 1993;67(1):87–91.

106. Azad A, Parsa R, Ghasemnian A. Lack of effect of choline supplement on inflammation, muscle endurance and injury indices, and shooting accuracy following simulated army ranger operation. J Arch Mil Med. 2017;5(3):e14902.

107. Leach NV, Dronca E, Vesa SC, Sampelean DP, Craciun EC, Lupsor M, Crisan D, Tarau R, Rusu R, Para I, Grigorescu M. Serum homocysteine levels, oxidative stress and cardiovascular risk in non-alcoholic steatohepatitis. Eur J Intern Med. 2014;25(8):762–76.

108. Zhou J, Austin RC. Contributions of hyperhomocysteinemia to atherosclerosis: causal relationship and potential mechanisms. Biofactors. 2009;35(2):120–9.

109. Fischer LM, da Costa KA, Kwock L, Galanko J, Zeisel SH. Dietary choline requirements of women: effects of estrogen and genetic variation. Am J Clin Nutr. 2010;92(5):1113–9.

110. Wald G, Brouha L, Johnson R. Experimental human vitamin A deficiency and ability to perform muscular exercise. Am J Physiol. 1942;137(3):551–6.

111. Garrido G, Webster AL, Chamorro M. Nutritional adequacy of different menu settings in elite Spanish adolescent soccer players. Int J Sports Nutr Exerc Metab. 2007;17:421–32.

112. Martinez S, Pasquarelli BN, Romaguera D, Cati A, Pedro T, Aguiló A. Anthropometric characteristics and nutritional profile of young amateur swimmers. J Strength Cond Res. 2011;25(4):1126–33.

113. Moyer VA; U.S. Preventive Services Task Force. Vitamin, mineral, and multivitamin supplements for the primary prevention of cardiovascular disease and cancer: U.S. Preventive services Task Force recommendation statement. Ann Intern Med. 2014;160(8):558–64.

114. Benson J, Gillien DM, Bourdet K, Loosli AR. Inadequate nutrition and chronic calorie restriction in adolescent ballerinas. Phys Sportsmed. 1985;13(10):79–90.

115. Cohen JL, Potosnak L, Frank O, Baker H. A nutritional and hematological assessment of elite ballet dancers. Phys Sportsmed. 1985;13(5):43–54.

116. Kim JY, Lee JS, Cho SS, Park H, Kim KW. Nutrient intakes of male college combat sport athletes by weight control status. Korean J Commun Nutr. 2017;22(6):495–506.

117. Steen NS, Mayer K, Brownell KD, Wadden TA. Dietary intake of female collegiate heavy weight rowers. Int J Sports Nutr. 1995;5(3):225–31.

118. Welsh PK, Zager KA, Endres J, Poon SW. Nutrition education, body composition and dietary intake of female college athletes. Phys Sportsmed. 1987;15(1):63–74.

119. Khanna S, Atalay M, Laaksonen DE, Gul M, Roy S, Sen CK. Alpha-lipoic acid supplementation: tissue glutathione homeostasis at rest and after exercise. J Appl Physiol. 1999; 86:1191–6.

120. Murray R, Horsun CA II. Nutrient requirements for competitive sports. In: Wolinsky E, editor. Nutrition in exercise and sport. 3rd ed. Boca Raton (FL): CRC Press; 1998.550 p.

121. Neuman I, Nahum H, Ben-Amotz A. Prevention of exercise-induced asthma by a natural isomer mixture of beta-carotene. Ann Allergy Asthma Immunol. 1999;82:549–53.

122. Kawamura A, Ali W, Abe R, Kobayashi Y, Kuwahata M, Higashi A. Astaxanthin-, β-carotene-, and resveratrol-rich foods support resistance training-induced adaptation. Antioxidants. 2021;10:113.

123. Institute of Medicine, Food and Nutrition Board. Dietary reference intakes for calcium and vitamin D. Washington (DC): National Academies Press; 2011.

124. Maughan RJ, Burke LM, Dvorak J, Larson-Meyer DE, Peeling P, Phillips SM, Rawson ES, Walsh NP, Garthe I, Geyer H, Meeusen R, van Loon LJC, Shirreffs SM, Spriet LL, Stuart M, Vernec A, Currell K, Ali VM, Budgett RG, Ljungqvist A, Mountjoy M, Pitsiladis YP, Soligard T, Erdener U, Engebretsen L. IOC consensus statement: dietary supplements and the high-performance athlete. Br J Sports Med. 2018;52(7):439–55.

125. Cannell JJ, Hollis BW, Sorenson MB, Taft TN, Anderson JJ. Athletic performance and vitamin D. Med Sci Sports Exerc. 2009;41(5):1102–10.

126. Hamilton B. Vitamin D and human skeletal muscle. Scand J Med Sci Sports. 2010;20(2):182–90.

127. Schubert L, DeLuca HF. Hypophosphatemia is responsible for skeletal muscle weakness of vitamin D deficiency. Arch Biochem Biophys. 2010;500(2):157–61.

128. Williams MH. Dietary supplements and sports performance: introduction and vitamins. J Int Soc Sports Nutr. 2004;1:1–6.

129. Williams MH. Dietary supplements and sports performance: minerals. J Int Soc Sports Nutr. 2005;2:43–9.

130. Chen Y, Liang Y, Guo H, Meng K, Qiu J, Benardot D. Muscle-related effect of whey protein and vitamin D3 supplementation provided before or after bedtime in males undergoing resistance training. Nutrients. 2022;14:2289.

131. Barr SI, Prior JC, Vigna YM. Restrained eating and ovulatory disturbances: possible implications for bone health. Am J Clin Nutr. 1994;59:92–7.

132. Chesnut CH III. Theoretical overview: bone development, peak bone mass, bone loss, and fracture risk. Am J M. 1991; 91(5B):2S–4S.

133. Heaney RP. Effect of calcium on skeletal development, bone loss, and risk of fractures. Am J Med. 1991;(Suppl 5B):23–8.

134. Benardot D. Unpublished data from USOC research project on national team gymnasts. Laboratory for Elite Athlete Performance. Georgia State University. 1997.

135. Bescós García R, Rodríguez Guisado FA. Low levels of vitamin D in professional basketball players after wintertime: relationship with dietary intake of vitamin D and calcium. Nutr Hosp. 2011;26(5):945–51.

136. Constantini NW, Rakefet A, Chodick G, Dubnov-Raz G. High prevalence of vitamin D insufficiency in athletes and dancers. Clin J Sport Med. 2010;20(5):368–71.

137. Knechte B, Jastrzębski Z, Hill L, Nikolaidis PT. Vitamin D and stress fractures in sport: preventive and therapeutic measures—a narrative review. Medicina (Kaunas). 2021;57:223.

138. Bunnell RH, DeRitter E, Rubin SH. Effect of feeding polyunsaturated fatty acids with a low vitamin E diet on blood levels of tocopherol in men performing hard physical labor. Am J Clin Nutr. 1975;28(7):706–11.

139. Sharman IM, Down MB, Norgan NG. The effects of vitamin E on physiological function and athletic performance of trained swimmers. J Sports Med Phys Fitness. 1976;16(3):215–25.

140. Sharman IM, Down MG, Sen RN. The effect of vitamin E and training on physiological function and athletic performance in adolescent swimmers. Br J Nutr. 1971;26(2):265–76.

141. Talbot D, Jamieson J. An examination of the effect of vitamin E on the performance of highly trained swimmers. Can J Appl Sport Sci. 1977;2:67–9.

142. Brady PS, Brady LJ, Ullrey DE. Selenium, vitamin E, and the response to swimming stress in the rat. J Nutr. 1979; 109(6):1103–9.

143. Dillard CJ, Liton RE, Savin WM, Dumelin EE, Tappel AL. Effects of exercise, vitamin E, and ozone on pulmonary function and lipid peroxidation. J Appl Physiol Respir Environ Exerc Physiol. 1978;45(6):927–32.

144. Shephard RJ, Campbell R, Pimm P, Stuart D, Wright GR. Vitamin E, exercise, and the recovery from physical activity. Eur J Appl Physiol Occup Physiol. 1974;33(2):119–26.

145. Kim M, Eo H, Lim JG, Lim H, Lim Y. Can low-dose of dietary vitamin E supplementation reduce exercise-induced muscle damage and oxidative stress? A meta-analysis of randomized controlled trials. Nutrients. 2022;14:1599.

146. Suttie JW. Vitamin K. In: Coates PM, Betz JM, Blackman MR, Cragg GM, Levine M, White JD, Moss J, editors. Encyclopedia of dietary supplements. 2nd ed. London and New York: Informa Healthcare; 2010:851–60.

147. Crintea A, Dutu AG, Masalar AL, Linga E, Constatin A-M, Crăciun A. Vitamin K in sport activities: a less considered benefit for athletic training. Health, Sports & Rehabil Med. 2021;22(2):127–32.

148. Bügel S. Vitamin K and bone health. Proc Nutr Soc. 2003; 62(4):839–43.

149. Feskanich D, Weber P, Willett WC, Rockett H, Booth SL, Colditz GA. Vitamin K intake and hip fractures in women: a prospective study. Am J Clin Nutr. 1999;69(1):74–9.

150. Booth SL, Pennington JA, Sadowski JA. Food sources and dietary intakes of vitamin K-1 (phylloquinone) in the American diet: data from the FDA Total Diet Study. J Am Diet Associ. 1996;96(2):149–54.

151. Booth SL, Tucker KL, Chen H, Hannan MT, Gagnon DR, Cupples LA, Wilson PW, Ordovas J, Schaefer EJ, Dawson-Hughes B, Kiel DP. Dietary vitamin K intakes are associated with hip fracture but not with bone mineral density in elderly men and women. Am J Clin Nutr. 2000;71(5):1201–8.

152. Braam LA, Knapen MHJ, Geusens P, Brouns F, Vermeer C. Factors affecting bone loss in female endurance athletes. Am J Sports Med. 2003;31(6):889–95.

153. Craciun AM, Wolf J, Knapen MHJ, Brouns F, Vermeet C. Improved bone metabolism in female elite athletes after vitamin K supplementation. Int J Sports Med. 1998;19(7):479–84.

CHAPTER

6

Minerals: Important for Health and Performance

CHAPTER OBJECTIVES

- Understand the primary functions of each mineral, including the macrominerals and microminerals.
- Know the minerals that have the highest prevalence of deficiency.
- Identify good food sources for each macro- and micromineral.
- Comprehend the digestion and absorption factors associated with each mineral where there is a high prevalence of deficiency.
- Describe the issue of competitive absorption, and how the consumption of a high level of one mineral may have a negative impact on the absorption of another mineral.

- Apply your understanding of minerals to increase the likelihood of good athletic performance and decrease the likelihood of poor health.
- Explain the interactive effects of energy, calcium, vitamin D, and estrogen (in females) in the development of bone mineral density (BMD).
- Analyze the factors and justifications for why certain macro- and microminerals may be appropriately taken as supplements.
- Identify the micro- and macrominerals that are most associated with athletic performance, and how to lower the risk that an athlete may develop a deficiency of each of these minerals.

Case Study

Alice, a 26-year-old elite female ultraendurance Ironman competitor, was undergoing a nutrition and health assessment when she said, "I am just not doing as well as I believe I should be doing, and I am so stressed about my poor performance in my most recent competitions that my stomach is bothering me." Psychological stress and gastrointestinal (GI) issues are clearly related, but there are also other possibilities. To investigate one of the possibilities, Alice was asked to provide a listing of all the vitamin/mineral supplements and "ergogenic aids" she was currently taking. Luckily, Alice had arrived for her assessment carrying a bag full of the supplements and ergogenic aids she was regularly consuming, making an assessment of potential problems far easier and accurate. Alice was taking everything from amino acids to creatine monohydrate to vitamins and minerals. The vitamin

and mineral supplements were all being taken in large megadoses, all well above 300% of the recommended dietary allowances (RDAs). When asked why she was taking these, Alice indicated she felt this was the best way to prepare for her competitions. She also mentioned that a number of other highly competitive athletes she knew were also taking these same products and she felt if she did not take them she would be at a disadvantage compared with those who were. Alice was then asked to describe a typical day of eating and workouts, with special emphasis and clarity on her food/beverage/supplement consumption. It caught the attention of the assessment staff that she was taking 120 mg of iron (the RDA is 18 mg, best consumed spread out over the day from consumed meals). Then she clarified that she had been so miserable lately that she thought she should take more iron, so increased the intake to 120 mg in the morning, 60 mg at noon, 60 mg in the evening, and 60 mg before bedtime (a whopping 300 mg/day!). This was particularly interesting because a history of blood tests on Alice, since she was 14 years old (a 12-year span) confirmed that she never had iron deficiency or iron deficiency anemia. When asked about her GI problems, she just could not understand it—she *never* had a gut problem, with good appetite and normal bowel function her entire life. Nevertheless, because of her GI problem, she thought she should take *more* supplements because she was afraid the GI problem would cause her to limit her food intake.

Alice then got a quick lesson on heavy metal toxicity and the potential medical problems she could be creating with the high-dose supplemented iron she was consuming. It was explained that most iron is not absorbed because the body is trying to protect itself. Excess absorbed iron could have a serious effect on the liver, and since 1979 supplement containers having more than 250 mg of elemental iron have warnings that severe toxicity can result from excess consumption. Symptoms of iron overdosing (toxicity) include vomiting, diarrhea, abdominal pain, irritability, and sleepiness. The GI symptoms result from the irritating effect of all the unabsorbed iron in the intestines, which has also been found to increase the risk of colon cancer. It was suggested to Alice that she eat "clean" for 2 weeks (no supplements, plenty of fluids, and reintroduction of regular small frequent meals that were not excessively spicy to let her gut heal), and then come back for a chat on an eating and activity strategy that would dynamically match her workout schedule.

Two weeks later, Alice returned feeling far better, with many of the GI symptoms gone. The lesson was learned, that "more than enough is not better than enough." Alice was provided an eating plan to satisfy her nutritional needs and returned at regular intervals to ensure that there were no sequelae from her prior excess supplementation.

CASE STUDY DISCUSSION QUESTIONS

1. Describe why it is important to consider the implications of iron deficiency in athletes.
2. It is commonly believed that there is no limit to how much of a nutrient can be consumed because "if a little bit is good then more must be better." What strategy would you use if working with a team of athletes to help them understand that consumption of more than the body can effectively utilize causes problems that can turn into serious disease states?
3. If supplements rather than foods are being used to satisfy the need for nutrients, what other health/nutrition/performance risks might the athlete encounter?
4. Many minerals are competitively absorbed. That is, if too much of one mineral is accessing the site of absorption, less of other minerals that are absorbed in the same site will get absorbed. Iron is competitively absorbed with calcium, magnesium, and zinc. With so much iron intake, what other problems (deficiencies) might this athlete experience?

Iron Deficiency

Characterized by low serum ferritin but normal hemoglobin and hematocrit (Hct). This is an initial sign that iron status is poor and, if it continues, will result in iron deficiency anemia. The body places a high priority on maintaining red blood cells (RBCs), so it is possible that other iron-containing molecules (*i.e.*, myoglobin in muscle tissue) are depleted of iron as a strategy to sustain RBCs. An athlete with iron deficiency is likely to feel weak and easily fatigued but will have normal hemoglobin and Hct.

Anemia

A below-normal hemoglobin and/or Hct in the blood. It may be caused by blood loss, inadequate production of RBCs, or a fast rate of red cell breakdown. Common causes of anemia are iron deficiency, folate deficiency, and vitamin B_{12} deficiency. Athletes are at higher risk of anemia because of faster red cell breakdown and loss of iron through sweat.

Iron Deficiency Anemia

A microcytic (small red cells), hypochromic (pale red rather than deep red) anemia (insufficient red cells) that is characteristic of chronic iron deficiency. The most common sign is easy fatigue, but may also be associated with cold hands and feet, chest pain, weakness, headache, and shortness of breath. The immune system is also affected, with increased illness frequency and infections.

INTRODUCTION

Consumed minerals play a variety of critically important roles, ranging from helping to strengthen bones (calcium), assuring optimal oxygen delivery to working tissues (iron), sustaining good blood volume (sodium), and even helping the immune system function properly (zinc). Minerals are unique in that, unlike other nutrients, they are inorganic compounds (*i.e.*, they contain no carbon or living matter). However, minerals are functionally similar to the organic nutrients in that they *work together* to produce the desired outcome. As an example, vitamin D works to enhance the absorption of consumed calcium. Another example is that iron is part of the protein **hemoglobin**, found inside red cells and involved in cellular respiration.

> ### 📕 Hemoglobin
>
> Abbreviated as Hb or Hgb, this is the iron-containing protein in RBCs that picks up (inhaled) oxygen from the lungs, delivers oxygen to tissues, and takes carbon dioxide from tissues to be exhaled through the lungs. In adult males, normal hemoglobin is 14–18 g/dL; in adult females, normal hemoglobin is 12–16 g/dL.

Minerals have numerous major functions, including:

- Adding to the strength and structure of the skeleton and keeping it strong and resistant to fracture.
- Helping to maintain the relative acidity or alkalinity of the blood and tissue. For athletes, hard physical activity has the tendency to lower the pH level because of lactic acid production (*i.e.*, the effect is to increase the relative acidity), so having a healthy system to control acid–base balance is critical for athletic performance.
- Serving as a pathway for electrical impulses that stimulate muscle contraction. *All* athletic endeavors rely on efficient and effective muscular movement and coordination, making this function critically important.
- Minerals are involved in energy metabolic processes. Because physical activity increases the rate at which fuel is burned, it is important to have the right minerals in the right amounts at the cellular level to enable this elevated rate of energy metabolism.

All of these functions are important for athletes. Athletes with weak, lower-density bones are at increased risk of stress fractures; poor fluid buffering (acid–base imbalance) leads to poor endurance; poor nerve and muscle function leads to poor coordination; and altered cell metabolism limits a cell's ability to obtain and store energy (1).

The established roles of minerals in the development of optimal physical performance include involvement in glycolysis (obtaining energy from stored glucose), lipolysis (obtaining energy from fats), proteolysis (obtaining energy from proteins), and help in obtaining energy from phosphocreatine (1). Inorganic mineral nutrients are required in the structural composition of hard (bones

and teeth) and soft (muscles and organs) body tissues. They also participate in such processes as the action of enzyme systems, the contraction of muscles, nerve reactions, and the clotting of blood. These mineral nutrients, all of which must be supplied in the diet, have two classes: the *macrominerals* have a higher requirement and a greater presence in the body and the *microminerals* have a lower dietary requirement and a lower presence in the body (2,3). Do not mistake the difference in amount as a difference in importance, because all minerals discussed in this chapter are highly important for sustaining health.

MACROMINERALS

Important Factors to Consider

- Minerals have many functions related to keeping the skeleton, muscles, heart, and brain working as they should. Although there can be daily fluctuations in mineral intakes, the human system does poorly with a chronic deficiency of any of the minerals. To obtain all of the minerals needed for good health, a wide variety of foods must be consumed to ensure tissues are exposed to all of the minerals. Monotonous eating patterns (*i.e.*, patterns where people continuously eat the same few foods) increase the risk of developing a mineral deficiency because no single food has all of the minerals needed to sustain health and performance.
- Supplements of minerals are commonly taken. However, even the seemingly most benign minerals, such as calcium, may create problems if taken in excess. For instance, calcium is a powerful buffer that may lower gastric pH and make it more difficult to digest certain foods, and calcium competes with other bivalent minerals (*i.e.*, magnesium, iron, and zinc) for absorption. All of the bivalent minerals are absorbed in the proximal duodenum (a portion of the small intestine that immediately follows the stomach and remains acidic because pancreatic juice, which buffers the acidity, enters later), so having too much calcium may interfere with the absorption of these other minerals and increases deficiency risk. The competitive absorption of the bivalent minerals results in the same outcome if any of the other bivalent minerals is taken in excess, with reduced absorption of the others. The key to mineral nutrition is balance.

Macrominerals are those minerals that are present in the body in relatively large quantities (compared with **microminerals**) and perform important physiologic functions. By accepted definition, macrominerals are required at a level of 100 mg/day or more, or the body content of the mineral is greater than 5 g (5,000 mg). The macrominerals include calcium, phosphorus, magnesium, potassium, sodium, chloride, and sulfur. Calcium comprises ~1.75% of total body weight, phosphorus makes up ~1.10% of total body weight, and magnesium makes up ~0.04% of total body weight, with even smaller weight contributions for potassium, sodium, chloride, and sulfur.

Macrominerals

Minerals required in amounts greater than 100 mg/day. These include potassium, calcium, magnesium, sodium, chloride, sulfur, and phosphorus. (Note: Although the macrominerals are required in greater daily amounts than microminerals, it makes them no longer important in human health.)

Microminerals

Minerals required by the body in amounts less than 100 mg/day. These include iron, zinc, iodine, selenium, copper, manganese, fluoride, chromium, and molybdenum. (Note: Although the microminerals are required in smaller daily amounts than macrominerals, it makes them no less important in human health.)

Calcium

Calcium is an important mineral for bone and tooth structure, blood clotting, nerve transmission, vasoconstriction and vasodilation of blood vessels, muscle contraction, and insulin secretion (Box 6.1) (4). The adult **dietary reference intake (DRI)** for calcium ranges from 1,000 to 1,200 mg/day, depending on age and gender. Calcium absorption and the uptake of calcium by bones and other tissues are regulated by vitamin D and parathyroid hormone. Even a small drop in circulating serum calcium increases the secretion of parathyroid hormone, which reduces the urinary excretion of calcium and releases calcium from bone to stabilize serum calcium. Parathyroid hormone also converts the inactive form of vitamin D to the active form, which enhances the absorption of both calcium and phosphorus from the diet. It is important to consider that both female and male athletes commonly suffer from calcium and vitamin D deficiencies, particularly if they fail to satisfy energy needs and/or are involved in indoor sports that limit sunlight (vitamin D) exposure (5–7). A return of serum calcium to the normal level causes a cessation of parathyroid hormone secretion. The high consumption of several substances may increase urinary calcium losses stimulating parathyroid hormone release. These include (8–11):

- High sodium intake
- High protein intake (above 2.0 g/kg/day)

Box 6.1   Calcium Basic Information (Chemical Symbol Ca)

- RDA
  - Adult males (ages 19–70 years): 1,000 mg/day (1,200 mg/day for older males, ages 70+ years)
  - Adult females (ages 19–50 years): 1,000 mg/day (1,200 mg/day for older females, ages 51–70+ years)
  - Recommended intake for athletes: 1,300–1,500 mg/day
- Functions
  - Bone structure and strength
  - Acid–base balance
  - Nerve function
  - Muscle contraction
  - Enzyme activation
- Good food sources
  - Dairy products
  - Dark green leafy vegetables
  - Calcium-fortified orange juice and other calcium-fortified foods
  - Soy milk
  - Legumes
- Deficiency
  - Osteoporosis
  - Rickets/osteomalacia
  - Muscle dysfunction
  - *Symptoms of deficiency*
    - Fractures and stress fractures
    - Muscle weakness
- Toxicity
  - Tolerable UL: 2,000–3,000 mg/day depending on age/gender of group
  - *Symptoms of toxicity*
    - Constipation
    - Malabsorption of other bivalent minerals (iron, magnesium, and zinc)
    - Kidney stones
    - Cardiac dysrhythmia

- High phosphorus intake (associated with high protein intake and processed foods)
- High caffeine intake

Dietary Reference Intakes

Nutrient reference values are established as scientific guides for planning and assessing nutrient intakes of healthy people. The DRI values, established by the Food and Nutrition Board of the Institute of Medicine, National Academy of Sciences, are composed of the following:

- **RDA:** The average daily level of intake sufficient to meet the nutrient requirements of nearly all (97%–98%) healthy people.
- **Adequate Intake** (AI): Established when evidence is insufficient to develop an RDA and is set at a level assumed to ensure nutritional adequacy.
- **Tolerable Upper Intake Level** (UL): The maximum daily intake unlikely to cause adverse health effects, above which toxicity reactions are possible/likely.

Table 6.1	Calcium Content of Commonly Consumed Foods	
Food	Serving Size	Calcium (mg)
Broccoli (cooked)	½ cup	31
Bok choy	½ cup	79
Cheddar cheese	1.5 oz	303
Figs (dried)	¼ cup	61
Kale (boiled)	½ cup	90
Milk	1 cup	300
Orange	1 medium	60
Pinto beans	½ cup	39
Red beans	½ cup	25
Sardines (canned)	8 oz	325
Spinach (boiled)	½ cup	122
Tofu (made with calcium sulfate)	½ cup	434

Food Sources of Calcium

Many foods provide ample amounts of calcium (Table 6.1), including legumes, dairy products, and green leafy vegetables. This list should make it clear that dairy products are *not* the only way to supply calcium in the diet. In fact, many cultures have adequate calcium intakes with no or limited consumption of dairy products. Here are some common examples:

- In Asia, sweet and sour sauces are made by putting a stock bone in water that has vinegar added. The vinegar leaches out the calcium from the bone and is consumed as part of the sauce.
- In Mexico, Central America, and South America, *masa* is used to make corn tortillas. Masa is lime-soaked corn flour, and lime is calcium salt. Consumption of the tortilla provides calcium through the lime in the corn flour.

Green leafy vegetables (particularly spinach and rhubarb) are high in oxalic acid, which has a high binding affinity for calcium and other bivalent minerals (*i.e.*, zinc, magnesium, iron). The bioavailability of calcium and these minerals may be poor unless the oxalic acid is removed. However, it is possible to improve the bioavailability of these oxalate-bound minerals through an easy food preparation technique called blanching. Oxalate is highly water-soluble, so by dipping the vegetables for a few seconds into boiling water a good deal of the oxalate is removed but the minerals remain (12). You can then prepare the vegetables as you like. This technique dramatically improves the delivery of calcium from vegetables

and has been used by cultures (especially in Asia) that traditionally have not consumed dairy products for thousands of years (13). As a side benefit, vegetables that are blanched may also be more acceptable for children to eat. Children are more sensitive to bitter tastes than adults (we lose some of our taste sensitivities as we age), and oxalic acid has a bitter taste. Therefore, by removing the oxalate you also remove some of the bitter taste that children find unacceptable.

Phytic acid, which is present in wheat bran and dried beans, also inhibits the bioavailability of calcium and other bivalent minerals (14). The phytic acid of wheat bran can be reduced when yeast is used in food preparation (as in bread, rolls, etc.). Yeast contains phytase, which enzymatically breaks down the phytic acid in grains, making minerals more bioavailable. Regular consumption of whole-grain flat breads, crackers, and so forth may provide enough phytic acid to lower the bioavailability of all of the bivalent minerals, including calcium.

Bone Density

Important Factors to Consider

Ensuring an optimal bone density takes many factors to occur simultaneously and is more than simply consuming enough calcium (Figure 6.1). Sustaining good bone density requires avoiding consumption of too much protein at one time (the excreted nitrogen

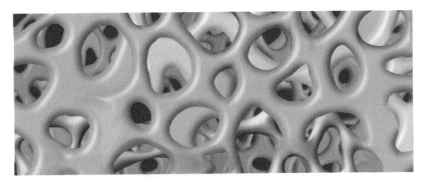

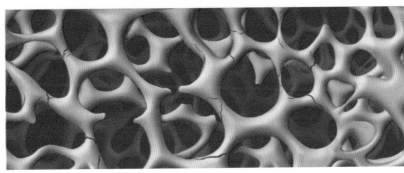

FIGURE 6.1: Normal and low bone mineral density. (Sources: Anatomical Chart Company. Understanding osteoporosis anatomical chart. LWW (PE); 2003; Weksler B, Schecter GP, Ely S. Wintrobe's atlas of clinical hematology. 2nd ed. LWW (PE); 2018; Higdon J, Drake VJ. An evidence-based approach to vitamins and minerals: health benefits and intake recommendations. 2nd ed. Thieme; 2011.)

causes calcium to be lost, lowering bone density); sustaining a good calcium intake; sustaining good energy balance and blood sugar to limit cortisol production (cortisol breaks down bone); providing stress (exercise) on the skeleton to provide a reason to sustain good density; having enough vitamin D to ensure that the consumed calcium will be absorbed; and if a female, sustaining normal menstrual status as estrogen helps to limit the activity of cells (osteoclasts) that break down bone.

It is important to consider that any factors, either individual or combined, that result in below-optimal peak **BMD** in growing children may contribute to increased risk of **osteoporosis** (extremely low BMD) later in life. **Osteopenia** is low BMD above the threshold for normal BMD but below the threshold for osteoporosis. A major risk factor for low BMD in athletic children and adolescents is insufficient energy (calorie) consumption. The inadequate consumption of energy stimulates excess production of cortisol, which lowers both metabolic mass (*i.e.*, muscle and organ mass) and BMD. Because food is more than the carrier of just "energy" (*i.e.*, calories), inadequate energy consumption is also associated with lower nutrient intake, including lower calcium intake. Female athletes are at an even higher risk of low bone density if they fail to consume sufficient energy, as this results in higher risk for amenorrhea, which is associated with lower estrogen levels. Estrogen inhibits the activity of osteoclasts, the cells that break

down bone. Therefore, low estrogen is related to amenorrhea, which is related to poor bone development (15).

Bone Mineral Density (BMD) Measurement

A common unit of measurement (g/cm²) for determining bone mineral density (BMD) is typically obtained with a Dual-Energy X-Ray Absorptiometer (DEXA), which is considered the gold standard for determining BMD. DEXA uses two X-ray beams of different intensities that pass through the skeletal tissue and determines BMD by assessing the relative absorbance of the X-ray beams. Higher-density bones have greater X-ray absorbance (*i.e.*, less X-ray passes through the bone). DEXA is the best way to determine if an individual has osteoporosis or osteopenia.

Dual-Energy X-Ray Absorptiometry (DEXA)

The current gold standard methodology for determining BMD. DEXA uses two X-ray beams of different intensities that pass through the skeletal tissue and determines BMD by assessing the relative absorbance of the X-ray beams. Higher-density bones have greater X-ray absorbance (*i.e.*, less X-ray passes through the bone). DEXA is the best way to determine if an individual has osteoporosis or osteopenia.

Osteoporosis

Extremely low BMD, 2.5 standard deviations below the young adult standard (the point of peak BMD). Osteoporosis, by definition, is the point at which bones cannot adequately support body weight and may spontaneously fracture. Osteoporotic fractures typically occur in late adulthood but are often the result of a failure to reach an optimal peak BMD following the adolescent growth spurt/young adulthood.

📕 Osteopenia

Low BMD between −1.0 and −2.5 standard deviations below the young adult standard (the point of peak BMD). This level of low bone density may place an athlete at risk for developing stress fractures and is a sign that energy, calcium, and/or vitamin D may not be adequate. In females, low estrogen associated with dysmenorrhea (abnormal menstrual status) is also a factor in osteopenia.

Because of greater torsional forces placed on bones owing to higher relative muscle mass and sports activities, athletes require higher bone densities and, therefore, higher calcium intakes than nonathletes. Physical activity in children and adolescents has been found to aid the attainment of higher BMD, making the bone more resistant to later fracture (16). In individuals who consume inadequate calcium, the skeletal bone density may be reduced to sustain normal blood calcium, which is an important blood buffer that must be maintained within a narrow range of 1.16–1.32 mmol/L (17). High protein consumption, typical of the diets of many athletes, results in higher nitrogen excretion which is also associated with higher serum calcium excretion. This condition is also associated with lower BMD, as calcium is taken from the skeleton to sustain normal serum calcium (referred to as **serum ionized calcium**). These higher urinary calcium losses that athletes may experience, higher sweat losses than nonathletes, and higher BMD requirements all contribute to a higher calcium recommended intake for athletes (18). The current recommendation is for athletes to consume 1,500 mg/day, or ~33% more calcium than the nonathlete requirement (15,19). The threshold for absorption is ~1,500 mg/day, making it unnecessary to consume amounts greater than this amount (20).

📕 Serum Ionized Calcium

The calcium in the blood serum (also called *free calcium*), acts as an important blood buffer (controls pH) and remains relatively constant (1.16–1.32 mmol/L).

Since 1993, there has been an increased availability of an accurate bone density measuring device, DEXA, which has dramatically improved the ability to measure bone density and determine risk of fracture. Studies that have used DEXA appear to indicate that children and adolescents who have a calcium intake at or slightly above the DRI (up to 1,500 mg) may improve bone density. However, the relationship between calcium supplementation and bone density in adults is less clear (*i.e.*, taking calcium supplements by themselves does not necessarily

lead to a greater bone density). Despite this, it seems prudent to make certain that calcium intake is maintained at the RDA level, that adequate physical activity is maintained (not a problem for most athletes), and that there is an AI of vitamin D. A recent survey of the U.S. Gymnastics team indicated that sunlight exposure was more highly correlated (and significantly so) to BMD than calcium intake. Even in gymnasts with an inadequate calcium intake (*i.e.*, below the DRI), having more sunlight exposure was associated with higher bone densities (21).

Another concern with many female athletes is amenorrhea (cessation of menses) because this is strongly associated with either poor bone development (in young athletes) or bone demineralization (in older athletes). The causes of amenorrhea are complex and include inadequate energy intake, eating disorders, low body fat levels, poor iron status, psychological stress, high cortisol levels, and overtraining. It is known that estrogen is lower in a state of amenorrhea and estrogen lowers the activity of osteoclasts. Osteoclasts are the bone cells that break down bone and osteoblasts are the cells that build up bone. Without estrogen to lower the activity of osteoclasts the osteoblast activity may not be sufficient to sustain BMD (22). In other words, hard-working elite female athletes are at risk. Anything that might lower risk, such as maintaining a good iron status and consuming enough energy, is useful for lowering the risk of developing amenorrhea. Even if an amenorrheic athlete has sufficient calcium intake, that alone would not suffice to maintain or develop healthy bones because the lower level of circulating estrogen associated with amenorrhea would inhibit normal bone development or maintenance.

Other Calcium-Related Issues

Obesity

Calcium consumption, primarily through the consumption of dairy products, has also been inversely associated with overweight and obesity in a number of studies (23,24). Although dairy products are an excellent source of calcium, they contain much more than just calcium. Therefore, there remains a question about whether calcium alone or a combination of calcium, protein, and, perhaps, other dairy product content, such as protein or vitamin D, works together to help lower body fat levels. A recent study found, for instance, that better vitamin D status (vitamin D is commonly a fortified vitamin in dairy products) is inversely associated with obesity (25). There is also some evidence that the increase in parathyroid hormone, which is associated with inadequate calcium intake, could increase fat storage (26).

Blood Pressure

There is evidence that adequate calcium intake, through the **D**ietary **A**pproaches to **S**top **H**ypertension (DASH) diet, may help to control blood pressure (BP) (27). The DASH diet is high in fruits, vegetables, and low-fat dairy products. According to the National Heart, Lung, and Blood Institute of the National Institutes of Health, the DASH diet has the following components:

- Eating vegetables, fruits, and whole grains
- Including fat-free or low-fat dairy products, fish, poultry, beans, nuts, and vegetable oils
- Limiting foods that are high in saturated fat, such as fatty meats, full-fat dairy products, and tropical oils such as coconut, palm kernel, and palm oils
- Limiting sugar-sweetened beverages and sweets

Nerve Transmission

Calcium plays a major role in nerve impulse transmission and muscle contraction. Nerve and muscle cells contain calcium channels that enable calcium ions to pass through membranes rapidly, thereby transferring the nerve impulse and stimulating muscle fiber contraction. The same type of calcium-mediated system is involved in breaking down glycogen to glucose and stimulating the secretion of insulin (4,28).

Calcium Deficiency

Calcium deficiencies are associated with skeletal malformations in children (as in the disease **rickets**, which is how it appears in children or **osteomalacia**, which is how it appears in adults), increased skeletal fragility (as in osteoporotic fracture and stress fractures), and BP abnormalities. There are few reports of toxicity from taking high doses of calcium, but it is conceivable that a high and frequent intake of calcium supplements may alter the acidity of the stomach (making it more alkaline), thereby interfering with protein digestion. Because of a competitive absorption between many minerals (particularly the bivalent minerals calcium, zinc, iron, and magnesium) in the small intestine, it is also possible that having a high amount of calcium may interfere with the absorption of these other minerals if they are present in the gut at the same time. Taking high-dose calcium supplements at the same time an iron-containing food is consumed, for example, may result in the malabsorption of iron and eventually could contribute to the development of iron deficiency anemia.

 Rickets

Refers to an inadequate mineralization of the growth plate of bones resulting in low BMD. It is a disease of children representing inadequate calcium deposition in bones that is most likely the result of vitamin D deficiency but may also be related to insufficient calcium intake. In many cases, rickets is the result of a young child's inability to convert vitamin D to the active form in the kidneys, commonly due to the delayed maturation of the kidneys (29). It is associated with low BMD and misshaped bones (bowed legs, knock-knees, etc.). See Table 6.2.

Table 6.2	Common Factors Associated With Rickets
Factor	**Explanation**
Dark skin pigmentation	Darker skin requires regular almost daily exposure to sunlight exposure to create adequate inactive vitamin D.
Living at high altitude or cold environments	These environments are likely to inhibit vitamin D creation as the necessary warm clothing worn inhibits skin exposure to sunlight.
Cultural environments that require skin covering	Cultures may require that most skin is covered when in outside public settings.
Poor vitamin D intake from foods	When insufficient sunlight exposure occurs, it becomes more necessary to obtain vitamin D from foods (*e.g.*, vitamin D–fortified foods, salmon, cod liver oil, tuna, beef liver).
Excessively long breastfeeding	Breastfeeding as an exclusive source of nutrients beyond 6 months may not fully satisfy the vitamin D and calcium requirements of a growing infant.
Vitamin D deficiency in a breastfeeding mother	Poor vitamin D status in a breastfeeding mother translates into poor delivery of adequate vitamin D to the breastfed infant.

Information from: Gentile C, Chiarelli F. Rickets in children: an update. Biomedicines. 2021;9:738. https://doi.org/10.3390/biomedicines9070738

📖 **Osteomalacia**

A disease of adults that is similar to rickets (see above) that is most likely the result of vitamin D deficiency but that may also be related to insufficient calcium consumption. (Note: Rickets and osteomalacia are really the same condition. "Rickets" is the name used when it occurs in children, and "osteomalacia" is the term used when it occurs in adults.)

Calcium Toxicity

There have been numerous studies looking at the relationships among calcium intake, physical activity, and bone density. However, the relationship between calcium supplementation and physical performance has not been well studied. In fact, when athletes take calcium supplements it is typically for the purpose of reducing the risk of fracture (*i.e.*, improving bone density) and not for the purpose of improving physical performance. The higher skeletal stress associated with physical activity (often referred to as higher gravitational forces) is known to enhance bone density, just as physical inactivity is known to lower bone density. However, the mineralization of bone is complex and involves several factors including:

- Growth phase (childhood and adolescence are associated with faster bone development)
- Hormonal status (especially estrogen for women)
- Energy adequacy
- Vitamin d availability
- Calcium intake

Hypercalcemia (too much calcium in the blood) has been reported in people regularly consuming calcium supplements and/or calcium-containing antacids (30). Because calcium and several other minerals are all absorbed in the same place in the GI tract (upper duodenum), having too much calcium may take up all the absorption space, leaving little space for the absorption of other minerals and resulting in compromised absorption and increased deficiency risk. Symptoms of calcium toxicity include appetite loss, constipation, fatigue, and confusion (4).

Phosphorus

Phosphorus is present in most foods and is especially high in protein-rich foods (meat, poultry, fish, and dairy products) and cereal grains (Box 6.2). It combines with calcium (about two parts calcium for every part phosphorus) to produce healthy bones and teeth. It also plays an important role in energy metabolism, affecting carbohydrates, lipids, and proteins. The energy derived for muscular work comes largely from phosphorus-containing compounds called adenosine triphosphate (ATP) and creatine phosphate. Phosphorus is also important for maintaining acid–base balance and is a component of phosphorylation relations that transfer a phosphate group (PO_4) from ATP to another molecule. As with calcium, the absorption of phosphorus is largely dependent on vitamin D, and the adult DRI is 700 mg/day. The goal of dietary intake is to sustain serum calcium in the range of 2.5–4.5 mg/dL. Pregnancy and breastfeeding nearly

---

Box 6.2	Basic Phosphorus Information (Chemical Symbol P)

- RDA
  - Adult males (ages 19–70+ years): 700 mg/day
  - Adult females (ages 19–70+ years): 700 mg/day
  - Recommended intake for athletes: 1,250–1,500 mg/day
- Functions
  - Bone structure and strength
  - Component of nucleic acids
  - Phosphorylation reactions
  - Acid–base balance
  - B-vitamin function
  - Component of ATP (energy)
- Good food sources: All high-protein foods, whole-grain products, carbonated beverages

- Deficiency
  - Deficiency unlikely, but if it occurs, results in:
    - Low BMD
    - Muscle weakness
- Toxicity
  - Tolerable UL
    - 3,000 mg for young children (1–8 years), and adults over 70 years
    - 4,000 mg for children and adults (9–70 years)
  - Toxicity is unlikely, but if it occurs, results in:
    - Low BMD
    - GI distress

double the phosphorus requirement (1,250 mg/day) in pre–18-year-old girls (31).

Metabolism of Phosphorus

Blood phosphorus concentration is maintained via para-thyroid hormone and vitamin D and is tied to calcium metabolism. Low serum calcium results in parathyroid secretion, which decreases urinary calcium excretion but *increases* phosphorus excretion to achieve a calcium–phosphorus balance. Parathyroid hormone also causes the kidneys to activate vitamin D, which increases the absorption of both calcium and phosphorus.

Food Sources of Phosphorus

Phosphorus is widespread in the food supply and is mostly well absorbed. If excess phosphorus is consumed, it is also easily excreted. The phosphorus in beans, cereals, and nuts is part of phytic acid, which is only about 50% available to humans. Yeast contains an enzyme, phytase, that can break down phytic acid and make the phosphorus more bioavailable for absorption. Therefore, consuming yeast breads/rolls delivers more bioavailable phosphorus than the equivalent volume of flatbreads, crackers, or cereals that are not leavened (31). Phytic acid has a high binding affinity for iron, zinc, calcium, and magnesium, so lowering the phytic acid content of foods also improves the absorption of these minerals.

Athletes and Phosphorus

There is a long history of supplementing with phosphorus-containing substances to improve physical performance. In World War I, Germany provided its soldiers with foods and supplements high in phosphorus with the aim of improving strength and endurance (32). This experience with phosphorus suggests that relatively large amounts are well tolerated over time, but there is no evidence that strength and endurance are actually improved. The results of more recent studies on the effect of phosphorus supplementation are mixed. A study on runners, rowers, and swimmers who took 2 g of sodium dihydrogen phosphate 1 hour prior to exercise all showed performance improvements, whereas only half of the unsupplemented athletes also showed improvements (33). In another study, VO_{2max} was improved on a treadmill test following short-term phosphorus supplementation (34). However, in yet another study evaluating the effect of phosphate supplementation on muscular power, there was no apparent benefit from taking the phosphate (35). Taken together, the mixed results of these studies make it difficult to say whether a small pre-exercise supplement of phosphorus will improve performance. Clearly, more studies are needed before an answer to this question can be attempted.

Phosphorus Deficiency

Because phosphorus is nearly everywhere in the food supply, a deficiency is rare and typically occurs only in starvation. However, it has been seen in people taking antacids that contain aluminum hydroxide for long periods of time (36). This type of antacid binds with phosphorus, making it unavailable for absorption (31,37). Symptoms of deficiency include poor appetite, weakness, fragile bones, and numb fingers and toes. If it occurs in children, a phosphorus deficiency may result in rickets (38). It is also important to note that athletes in different sports may be more or less likely to restrict food intake in an attempt to achieve a sport-specific "ideal" body profile, and athletes with restrictive intakes are more likely to have inadequate phosphorus intakes. A study assessing the nutrient intakes of gymnasts and swimmers found a statistically significant difference between them, with gymnasts consuming below the recommended phosphorus intake and swimmers consuming the recommended level (39).

Phosphorus Toxicity

Kidney disease may be associated with excess blood serum phosphorus (hyperphosphatemia), which is made more likely with supplemental consumption of phosphate salt. Low-functioning kidneys may lose their capacity to excrete excess phosphorus. Regardless of the cause, hyperphosphatemia may result in higher cardiovascular disease risk and a higher risk of bone disease (40). There is evidence that phosphoric acid in some sodas and phosphate-containing additives in some processed foods if chronically consumed, may result in high serum phosphorus, which could have a negative impact on bone health (41).

Magnesium

The average human body has 25 g of magnesium, with the majority in bones and the remaining amount in soft tissue (42). Magnesium is the second most prevalent intercellular mineral, after potassium, and has numerous functions (Box 6.3). Carbohydrate and fat metabolism for the production of ATP energy involves chemical reactions that require magnesium, and ATP itself exists mainly as a magnesium-containing compound. Magnesium is

---

Box 6.3   Magnesium Basic Information (Chemical Symbol Mg)

- RDA
  - Adult males (ages 19–30 years): 400 mg/day
  - Adult males (ages 31–70+ years): 420 mg/day
  - Adult females (ages 19–30 years): 310 mg/day
  - Adult females (ages 31–70+ years): 320 mg/day
  - Recommended intake for athletes:
    - 400–450 mg/day if from food sources
    - 350 mg/day if from supplements
- Functions
  - Protein synthesis
  - Glucose metabolism
  - Bone structure
  - Muscle contraction
- Good food sources
  - Milk and milk products
  - Meats

- Nuts
- Whole grains
- Dark green leafy vegetables
- Fruits
- Deficiency
  - Unlikely, but if it occurs, results in:
    - Muscle weakness
    - Muscle cramps
    - Cardiac dysrhythmia
- Toxicity
  - Tolerable UL: 350 mg if taken as supplements
  - *Symptoms of toxicity*
    - Nausea
    - Vomiting
    - Diarrhea

---

required for the synthesis of the genetic material deoxyribonucleic acid (DNA), and also for the synthesis of the cellular antioxidant glutathione (43). Magnesium is also a part of many enzymes, is a structural component of bones and cell membranes, and is also needed for protein synthesis, muscle function, calcium absorption, normal heart rhythm, and nerve impulse conduction (cell signaling) (31,44). Taken together, magnesium is an important substance in over 300 metabolic systems (42).

Food Sources of Magnesium

Dark green leafy vegetables are high in magnesium because chlorophyll contains magnesium. Whole grains and nuts also are good sources of magnesium, whereas meats and dairy products contain lower amounts. Processed and refined foods have the lowest concentration of magnesium, as the processing may remove the germ and bran of the grain, where the magnesium resides. People who live in areas with hard water obtain an important amount of magnesium from the water they drink, and some bottled waters also contain magnesium. However, there is a large range in the magnesium content of bottled water, ranging from 1 to 120 mg/L (45). Table 6.3 contains magnesium content of commonly consumed foods.

Several factors may affect magnesium absorption, including:

- High zinc consumption, primarily from supplements, interferes with the absorption of magnesium (46).

High intakes of grain-based dietary fiber, likely from associated phytic acid, interfere with the absorption of magnesium (31,43).

- Low protein intakes (<30 g/day) may lower magnesium absorption in young boys, whereas higher

Table 6.3	Magnesium Content of Commonly Consumed Foods	
Foods	**Serving Size**	**Magnesium (mg)**
Almonds	1 oz	77
Apple, raw	1 medium	9
Banana	1 medium	32
Beef, ground (90% lean)	3 oz	20
Bread, whole wheat	2 slices	46
Cereal, all bran	½ cup	112
Cereal, shredded wheat	1 serving	61
Hazelnuts	1 oz	46
Lima beans	½ cup	37
Okra, cooked	½ cup	37
Peanuts	1 oz	48
Rice, brown, cooked	1 cup	86
Spinach, cooked	½ cup	78

protein intakes (~93 g/day) may increase magnesium absorption in young boys (47). The form of magnesium impacts its ability to dissolve in water, which affects absorption. Supplements come in several forms (magnesium oxide, sulfate, citrate, aspartate, lactate, and chloride), with better absorption from the forms that dissolve well in liquid (the citrate, aspartate, lactate, and chloride forms) (48–50).

Magnesium Requirements

Magnesium is present in most foods, is essential for human metabolism, and is important for maintaining the electrical potential in nerve and muscle cells. A deficiency in magnesium among malnourished people, especially alcoholics, leads to tremors and convulsions. It is involved in more than 300 reactions in which food is synthesized into new products, and it is a critical component in the processes that create muscular energy from carbohydrates, protein, and fat (51). The adult DRI for magnesium is 280–350 mg/day. Dietary surveys indicate that large proportions of the U.S. population have magnesium intake below the recommended level (52). Chronically low magnesium intakes may increase the risk of several chronic disorders, including hypertension and cardiovascular disease, type 2 diabetes, and osteoporosis (53–56). There is also evidence that sustaining acceptable magnesium status may help to avoid migraine headaches (57).

Athletes and Magnesium

It is possible that athletes training in hot and humid environments could lose a large amount of magnesium in sweat. Were this to occur, a magnesium deficiency could, given the importance of magnesium in muscle function processes, cause athletes to underachieve athletically. In one study where magnesium supplements were given to athletes, there was an improvement in physical performance (58). There is some limited evidence that consuming low-dose magnesium supplements at the level of the DRI (about 350 mg/day) may have a beneficial effect on endurance and strength performance in athletes who have blood magnesium levels at the low end of the normal range (59,60). A study of athletes competing in a half-marathon found that those consuming a sodium-magnesium electrolyte beverage experienced less than half the muscle cramping than those who consumed water (61). However, with the exception of these studies, there is little other research evidence that magnesium deficiency is common among athletes or

that supplementation improves performance. In fact, with the exception of athletes who are known to reduce total energy intake in an attempt to maintain or lower weight (wrestlers, gymnasts, skaters, etc.), it appears as if most male and female athletes have adequate magnesium intakes (2,3,62). There has also been an expressed concern that vegetarian/vegan athletes may be at risk of certain nutrients that are more easily obtained from animal–food-based sources, including magnesium. However, a review of studies has found that, with proper dietary planning, these athletes are not at higher risk of magnesium deficiency (63).

Magnesium Deficiency

In otherwise healthy people, the risk of magnesium deficiency is relatively low because the urinary excretion of magnesium is reduced when dietary intake is low. However, heavy and chronic alcohol consumption causes a high urinary loss of magnesium, overriding the normal system for sustaining body magnesium levels, resulting in high risk of magnesium deficiency in alcoholics (42). Other groups that are also at risk of deficiency include type II diabetics and people with GI disorders (celiac disease, Crohn disease, irritable bowel syndrome). Symptoms of mild magnesium deficiency include the following:

- Loss of appetite
- Nausea
- Vomiting
- Fatigue
- Weakness

Symptoms of severe magnesium deficiency include the following:

- Numbness and tingling in the fingers and toes
- Muscle cramps and seizures
- Abnormal heart rhythm
- Personality changes
- Osteoporosis
- Migraine headaches

Magnesium Toxicity

The body's capacity to systematically excrete excess magnesium via the urine helps to avoid toxicity reactions that theoretically could result from supplements and/or drugs that are high in magnesium (64). (This assumes, of course, that the kidneys are healthy and functioning normally and that a state of dehydration does not compromise urine production.) There are reports that high

---

Box 6.4   Sodium Basic Information (Chemical Symbol Na)

- AI
  - Adult males (ages 19–50 years): 1.5 g/day
  - Adult males (ages 51–70 years): 1.3 g/day
  - Adult males (ages 70+ years): 1.2 g/day
  - Adult females (ages 19–50 years): 1.5 g/day
  - Adult females (ages 51–70 years): 1.3 g/day
  - Adult females (ages 70+ years): 1.2 g/day
  - Recommended intake for athletes:
    - ◆ >1.5 g/day; high sweat losses of sodium may increase requirement to >10 g/day (Whatever it takes to replace losses. Athletes may have a requirement that far exceeds the general AI.)
- Functions
  - Water balance
  - Nerve function
  - Acid–base balance
  - Muscle contraction
- Foods high in sodium
  - Processed and canned foods
  - Pickles
  - Potato chips
  - Pretzels
  - Soy sauce
  - Cheese
- Deficiency
  - Hyponatremia (low blood sodium)
    - ◆ Muscle cramping
    - ◆ Nausea
    - ◆ Vomiting
    - ◆ Anorexia
    - ◆ Seizures
    - ◆ Coma (extremely dangerous)
- Toxicity
  - Tolerable UL:
    - ◆ 2.3 g/day (about 5.8 g of table salt)
    - ◆ Major symptom: hypertension

---

supplemental intakes of magnesium may result in diarrhea and GI distress (48). It is due to this very laxative effect of magnesium salts that it is included in laxatives meant to resolve constipation. Although rare, there are reports in both the young and old that excess and chronic consumption of laxatives that contain magnesium may result in fatal magnesium toxicity (65,66).

Sodium

Sodium is an essential mineral commonly referred to as *salt*, which is actually sodium chloride (Box 6.4). Although these two minerals are discussed separately, humans consume the vast majority of sodium with chloride in the form of table salt. There is no question that salt is required in multiple processes that support life, but it is also clear that excess salt consumption creates health risks in large numbers of people (67). Once again, *more than enough is not better than enough.*

Salt is involved in body water balance and acid–base balance, and the sodium (Na^+, which is a **cation**) and chloride (Cl^-, which is an **anion**) that constitute salt are the main extracellular (outside the cell, including blood and fluid) mineral **electrolytes**. The other major functions of sodium and chloride include:

Cation

A positively charged ion that has more protons than electrons. Typically, cations are illustrated with a "+" sign. *Examples*: sodium (Na^+), calcium (Ca^+), magnesium (Mg^+), and potassium (K^+).

Anion

A negatively charged ion that has more electrons than protons. Typically, anions are illustrated with a "−" sign. *Examples*: chloride (Cl^-), sulfur (S^{2-}), and hydroxide (OH^-).

Electrolytes

Electrolytes are minerals that are dissociated into ions (charged particles) in solutions, making them capable of conducting electricity. They also help to regulate fluid balance, transport nutrients into cells, help normal muscle and mental function, help convert food calories into cellular energy and regulate pH. The main extracellular (outside the cell; mainly blood) electrolyte is positively charged (cation) sodium, and the main intracellular (inside the cell) electrolyte is positively charged (cation) potassium.

- *Maintaining cell membrane function:* The balance between sodium and chloride outside the cell and potassium inside the cell creates an electrical charge that helps cells bring in the nutrients they require and excrete metabolic by-products (68).

- *Absorption of protein (amino acids), glucose, and water:* Sodium chloride is needed to maintain sufficient fluid in the GI tract and the blood so that consumed nutrients can be absorbed into the blood (69).

- *Maintaining blood volume:* Maintenance of adequate blood volume is important for delivery of nutrients to cells and for removal of metabolic by-products away from cells. For athletes, the blood volume does double duty because the blood volume must also "feed" the sweat glands so that body temperature can be maintained. Insufficient sodium chloride consumption is associated with low blood volume, poor sweat rates, and higher risk of muscle cramping (69). Importantly, taking salt tablets as a strategy for sustaining hydration state is not likely to be a satisfactory solution for athletes who are involved in high-sweat activities. It is important to replace the volume of water lost while simultaneously considering the ideal sodium concentration in the water consumed to sustain blood volume (70).

The following terms are used when discussing sodium and conditions relevant to low or high levels of sodium:

- *Hypo* = Low
- *Hyper* = High
- *Emia* = Blood
- *Na* = Symbol for sodium
- *Hyponatremia* = Low (hypo) sodium (Na) in the blood (emia)
- *Hypernatremia* = High (hyper) sodium (Na) in the blood (emia)

Food Sources of Sodium

Sodium is present in small quantities in most natural foods and is found in high amounts in processed, canned, cooked, and fast foods. Although most people are capable of excreting excess sodium, some are sensitive to sodium, because they do not have this capability. In these individuals, the retention of sodium causes an overaccumulation of extracellular fluid and contributes to high BP. The intake of sodium can be limited by consuming natural, whole foods and avoiding commercially prepared foods that are likely to be high in sodium. Food labels provide information about sodium content (Table 6.4). The Food and Drug Administration's (FDA) daily reference values for the sodium content of 2,500-calorie diets are less than 2,400 mg. The estimated daily sodium requirement is 500 mg.

Table 6.4	Sodium on Food Labels: Understanding What the Labels Mean
Term	**Definition**
Sodium free	Less than 5 mg sodium per serving (serving size listed on label)
Low sodium	140 mg sodium or less per serving size listed on label. If the serving weighs 30 g or less, 140 mg sodium or less per 50 g of food. If the serving is two tablespoons or less, 140 mg sodium or less per 50 g of the food
Very low sodium	35 mg sodium or less per serving size listed on the label. If the serving weighs less than 30 g, 35 mg sodium or less per 50 g of food. If the serving is two tablespoons or less, 35 mg sodium or less per 50 g of the food
Reduced or less sodium	A minimum of 25% lower sodium content than the food with which it is compared

1 teaspoon of salt = 6 g = 2,325 mg sodium.

A sample of the salt content of commonly consumed foods can be found in Table 6.5. In general, the lowest salt consumption is found in fresh, whole, unprocessed foods including fruits, vegetables, and legumes. Processed foods are considerably higher in salt content.

Sodium Requirements

The DRIs established by the Food and Nutrition Board of the Institute of Medicine established an AI level for sodium that is an estimate of the amount required by moderately active people to replace sodium loss in sweat and to ensure that the diet is adequate for other nutrients. This recommended intake level, which ranges from 1 g/day in young children to 1.5 g/day in adults, is far below the level commonly consumed by most people living in Western societies. In 2015, the Dietary Guidelines Advisory Committee found that only two nutrients, sodium and saturated fat, are commonly overconsumed by large segments of the United States and pose a health risk (71). The recommendations established by this advisory group are for the general population to consume less than 2,300 mg of dietary sodium per day, which although more than the AI, is still significantly less than the current U.S. sodium consumption.

Table 6.5	Salt and Sodium Content of Commonly Consumed Foods (Listed from Low to High Sodium)		
Food	Amount	Salt (mg)	Sodium (mg)
Olive oil	1 tbsp	0	0
Orange juice	1 cup	0	0
Pear (fresh)	1 med	5	2
Tomato (fresh)	1 med	15	6
Carrot (fresh)	1 med	105	42
Bread, whole wheat	2 slices	660	264
Corn flakes cereal	1 cup	665	266
Bread, white	2 slices	850	340
Hot dog (beef)	1 hot dog	1,300	510
Ham	3 oz	2,500	1,000
Pretzels (salted)	2 oz (10 pretzels)	3,000	1,200
Potato chips (salted)	8 oz (1 bag)	3,300	1,300
Macaroni and cheese (canned)	1 cup	3,400	1,400

5 g salt = 2 g sodium.

Athletes and Sodium

One of the key ingredients of sports beverages is sodium because it helps to drive the desire to drink and to maintain blood volume. Maintenance of blood volume is an important factor in athletic performance because it is related to the ability to deliver nutrients to cells, remove metabolic by-products from cells, and maintain the sweat rate to avoid overheating. Because sweat contains sodium and athletes can lose a large volume of sweat, the general sodium recommendation for athletes is to consume whatever amount of sodium is needed to stay in sodium balance. The recommended level of sodium intake by athletes, therefore, is likely to be significantly higher than that of nonathletes.

During prolonged exercise in hot and humid environments, *hyponatremia* (low sodium in the blood) may occur. The common causes of hyponatremia are high fluid consumption that contains insufficient sodium to satisfy sweat loss, or possibly the consumption of nonsteroidal anti-inflammatory drugs, such as aspirin and Motrin, which may cause a sweat loss that is highly concentrated in sodium (72). Additional information on sodium, chloride, and hydration strategies is included in Chapter 7.

Sodium Deficiency

With the exception of hyponatremia (see below), which may occur in athletes who consume sodium-free beverages, sodium chloride deficiency is not commonly observed, even in individuals who are purposefully on low-salt dietary intakes (69).

Hyponatremia

Low (hypo) sodium (Na) in the blood (emia) is most likely to occur in people who spend long periods of time in a hot environment with heavy sweating but consume beverages that fail to adequately supply sufficient sodium to recover the amount lost in sweat. It is also seen when fluid consumption exceeds fluid losses (73). The normal serum sodium concentration is 135–145 mmol/L, whereas hyponatremia is typically diagnosed with serum sodium concentrations of lower than 135 mmol/L. A serum sodium concentration lower than 120 mmol/L is considered dangerous. It is a relatively common water–electrolyte imbalance that occurs in ~10% of people who participate in endurance events. A recent study found an extremely high incidence of hyponatremia during 28 days of high-volume rowing training (74). Of the 30 junior elite rowers studied, 70% achieved hyponatremia at least one time during the 28 days of training. Because the symptoms of hyponatremia may be similar to those of dehydration (*i.e.*, hyponatremia may occur when hydration state is poor), care should be taken so that they are not confused (75). Athletes should consider that hyponatremia may induce both muscular and kidney damage, and should encourage them to establish sodium-containing fluid protocols that avoid hyponatremia (76).

Important Factors to Consider

It is possible for physicians caring for those they believe to be dehydrated, but are actually suffering from hyponatremia, to be incorrectly treated with rapid infusion of large volumes of hypotonic solutions. This treatment in someone with hyponatremia may result in coma and death (77).

Sodium Toxicity

A number of population-based studies suggest that a chronically high intake of salty foods may increase the risk of developing stomach cancer (78). Because high salt intakes stimulate an increase in urinary excretion of calcium, high salt consumption has been found to be associated with greater risk of developing osteoporosis (low BMD resulting in higher fracture risk) (79). The increased loss of calcium may also play a role in the development of **kidney stones.** Although all of these potential problems are important, the greatest toxicity associated with excess sodium intake is hypertension (high BP). Although humans not suffering from primary hypertension have an effective mechanism for excreting excess sodium, high sodium intakes do increase BP, and lowering sodium intake decreases BP, even in those without primary hypertension (80). Taken together, the problems associated with excess salt intake can have a profoundly negative impact on health and should encourage people to carefully manage salt consumption.

Kidney Stones

Kidney stones are composed of calcium oxalate or calcium phosphate and occur in up to 15% of adults who have high urine calcium. Extremely high levels of animal protein (>2.0 g/kg/day), common among certain groups of athletes, may increase urinary calcium excretion and, therefore, the risk of kidney stones. Other risk factors for kidney stones include dehydration (forcing the kidneys to produce a concentrated urine with lower urinary volume) and chronically high intakes of calcium, oxalate (often from excess consumption of some raw dark greens that are high in oxalate), sodium, and vitamin C. Chronically low intakes of citrate (high in citrus fruits but also in other fruits and vegetables) and low calcium intake may also elevate kidney stone risk. Certain medical conditions also result in high risk for kidney stones, including gout (high uric acid), Crohn disease and colitis (both of which often result in dehydration), and some inherited disorders that affect kidney function.

Chloride

Chloride, another extracellular mineral, is essential for the maintenance of fluid balance and is also an important component of gastric juices (Box 6.5). Combining with hydrogen, chloride is an important component of hydrochloric acid in the stomach. Hydrochloric acid lowers gastric pH (*i.e.*, makes the stomach more acidic) to aid in the digestion of protein, the activation of intrinsic factor (needed for absorbing vitamin B_{12}), and the absorption of iron, zinc, magnesium, and calcium. Chloride also works

---

Box 6.5 Chloride Basic Information (Chemical Symbol Cl)

- AI
  - Adult males (ages 19–50 years): 2.3 g/day
  - Adult males (ages 51–70 years): 2.0 g/day
  - Adult males (ages 70+ years): 1.8 g/day
  - Adult females (ages 19–50 years): 2.3 g/day
  - Adult females (ages 51–70 years): 2.0 g/day
  - Adult females (ages 70+ years): 1.8 g/day
  - Recommended intake for athletes:
    - 2.3 g/day or more to match the increase in sodium intake with high sweat losses
- Functions
  - Water balance
  - Nerve function
  - Parietal cell (stomach) HCl production
- Good food sources
  - Table salt (~60% chloride and 40% sodium)
  - Any food high in "salt/table salt"
- Deficiency (rare)
  - Associated with frequent vomiting
  - May lead to convulsions
- Toxicity
  - Tolerable UL
    - 3,500 mg/day, or the equivalent of 5,800 mg of table salt
    - Cl intake is associated with Na intake, so an excess intake is typically associated with hypertension (from the excess sodium)

Box 6.6   Potassium Basic Information (Chemical Symbol K)

- RDA
  - Adult males (ages 19–70+ years): 4.7 g/day
  - Adult females (ages 19–70+ years): 4.7 g/day
  - Recommended intake for athletes:
    - 4.7 g/day or more with high levels of sweat loss
- Functions
  - Water balance
  - Glucose delivery to cells
- Good food sources
  - Citrus fruits
  - Potatoes
  - Vegetables
- Milk
- Meat
- Fish
- Bananas
- Deficiency
  - Hypokalemia, which is associated with anorexia, dysrhythmias, and muscle cramping
- Toxicity
  - Hyperkalemia, a condition that may lead to arrhythmias and altered heart function (may lead to death). Potassium supplements are generally NOT recommended for this reason

---

with sodium and potassium in transporting nervous system electrical charges throughout body tissues.

Virtually all the chloride we consume is associated with table salt (sodium chloride), so there is a parallel between sodium and chloride intakes. In addition, chloride losses are closely linked to sodium losses, so a deficiency of one is likely to be related to a deficiency of the other. Because most people consume excessive amounts of sodium as a result of a heavy table salt intake, chloride intake is also high (estimated at 6,000 mg/day) and well above normal requirements, which is 750 mg/day (81).

Chloride Deficiency

Although rare, chloride deficiencies typically occur with heavy sweating, frequent diarrhea, or frequent vomiting (81). Sweat losses are likely to deplete both chloride and sodium to a greater degree than other minerals that are lost in sweat (82–84). Therefore, heavy fluid loss through sweating that is not adequately replaced with a salt-containing beverage may result in chloride deficiency. The symptoms of deficiency are similar to those of sodium deficiency (as they would occur simultaneously) and include muscle weakness, irritability, lethargy, and appetite loss (85). Please see the section on sodium for additional information on chloride, sodium chloride, and table salt.

Potassium

Potassium is the main mineral found inside cells (an intracellular electrolyte) at a concentration that is 30 times greater than the concentration of potassium found outside cells (Box 6.6). It is involved in water balance,

nerve impulse transmission, and muscular contractions. It is also a cofactor in a number of enzymes necessary for carbohydrate metabolism (86).

The differences in concentrations between sodium (outside the cell) and potassium (inside the cell) create an electrical energy gradient that pumps sodium outside the cell in exchange for potassium. The energy requirement for these electrical energy pumps is estimated to account for between 20% and 40% of the total energy required while in a state of rest (68,86).

Food Sources of Potassium

The best food sources for potassium include fruits and vegetables (Table 6.6). Supplements in the United States

Table 6.6	Some Commonly Consumed Foods High in Potassium	
Food	**Serving**	**Potassium (mg)**
Baked potato (with skin)	1 medium potato	926
Raisins	½ cup	598
Prune juice	6 oz	528
Banana	1 medium	422
Spinach (cooked)	½ cup	420
Tomato juice	6 oz	417
Orange	1 medium	237
Almonds	1 oz	200

Source: United States Department of Agriculture, Agricultural Research Service, Food Composition Database [Internet]. Accessed 2018 April 24. Available from: https://fdc.nal.usda.gov

do not contain more than 99 mg of potassium because a high single dose of excess potassium may result in hyperkalemia, which is associated with cardiac arrhythmia and heart failure (87).

The typical intake of potassium ranges from 1,000 to 11,000 mg/day (1–11 g/day), with people consuming large amounts of fresh fruits and vegetables having the highest intakes. It has been found that regular consumption of more potassium (*i.e.*, through greater consumption of fruits and vegetables) is associated with lower stroke risk, lower risk of osteoporosis, and lower risk of kidney stones (88–90).

Potassium Requirements

There is good evidence that relatively high levels of potassium (~3,500 mg/day) are beneficial in controlling high BP (81). However, excess intake may lead to toxicity, which occurs with intakes of ~18,000 mg (18 g) potassium, hyperkalemia, and sudden cardiac arrest (81). The DRI estimated that daily potassium requirement is 4,700 mg.

Athletes and Potassium

Although it is well established that potassium is critical to heart and skeletal muscle function, the amount of potassium lost in sweat during exercise is relatively small and does not seriously affect the body's potassium stores. Therefore, sweat-related losses of potassium should not seriously affect athletic performance in the well-nourished athlete (82). Some terms used in the discussion of potassium are as follows:

- *Hypo* = Low
- *Hyper* = High
- *Emia* = Blood
- *K* = Symbol for potassium
- *Hypokalemia* = Low (hypo) potassium (K) in the blood (emia)
- *Hyperkalemia* = High (hyper) potassium (K) in the blood (emia)

Potassium Deficiency

Low plasma potassium is referred to as *hypokalemia*. Dietary deficiency is rare and typically only occurs with chronic diarrhea and vomiting or laxative abuse. Individuals taking medications for high BP force the loss of sodium, and in this process potassium is also lost. These individuals are encouraged to replace this lost potassium through the intake of potassium supplements or foods high in potassium (fruits, vegetables, and meats). Symptoms of deficiency include early fatigue, muscle weakness, muscle cramps, bloating, constipation, and pain. If severe, hypokalemia may result in abnormal heart function (cardiac arrhythmia) (68). Higher risk of potassium deficiency occurs with chronic alcohol consumption, severe diarrhea, excess use of laxatives, eating disorders (anorexia nervosa and bulimia), and congestive heart failure (91).

Potassium Toxicity

Although rare, high serum potassium (hyperkalemia) occurs in people taking diuretics or in those with chronic renal failure. Symptoms include tingling fingers and toes, muscle weakness, and heart arrhythmia that may result in death. There is no established tolerable UL for potassium by the Institute of Medicine (69). However, supplemental intake of potassium has been reported to cause GI problems, including diarrhea, nausea, and vomiting (91).

MICROMINERALS

The microminerals (trace elements) are present in extremely small amounts but have important roles to play in human nutrition. These microminerals are needed in amounts less than 100 mg/day and have body contents of less than 5 g. They include iron, iodine, zinc, copper, fluorine, manganese, molybdenum, selenium, and chromium.

Iron

A primary requirement for iron is to form the oxygen-transporting compounds *hemoglobin* (in blood) and *myoglobin* (in muscle) and is also found in a number of other compounds involved in normal tissue function (Box 6.7). These functions include (92):

- *Energy metabolism.* Iron-containing compounds are involved in electron transport which is critical to the production of ATP energy.
- *Detoxification reactions.* Enzymes that are iron-containing are involved in removal of toxic pollutants.
- *Antioxidant protection.* Peroxidases are iron-containing substances that protect cells from being damaged by reactive oxygen species (free radicals), such as hydrogen peroxide.

Box 6.7	Iron Basic Information (Chemical Symbol Fe)

- RDA
  - Adult males (ages 19–70+ years): 8 mg/day
  - Adult females (ages 19–50 years): 18 mg/day
  - Adult females (ages 51–70+ years): 8 mg/day
  - Recommended intake for athletes:
    - 15–18 mg/day
- Functions
  - Oxygen delivery (as hemoglobin and myoglobin)
  - Part of numerous oxidative enzymes
  - Essential for aerobic metabolism
- Good food sources
  - Meat, fish, poultry, and shellfish
  - Lesser amounts in:
    - Legumes

- Dark green leafy vegetables
- Dried fruit
- Note: Cast-iron cookware increases iron content of cooked foods
- Deficiency
  - Fatigue
  - Lower infection resistance
  - Poor ability to concentrate
  - Low energy metabolism (with possible hypothermia).
- Toxicity
  - Toxic levels of tissue iron (hemochromatosis)
  - Liver damage

- *DNA synthesis.* Iron-dependent enzymes are needed for the synthesis of DNA, a critical genetic substance for all cell functions.
- *Enzymes.* Iron is literally in hundreds of protein substances, including enzymes.

Iron is reused and conserved when iron-containing substances, such as heme, break down. However, iron is lost through bleeding, sweating, and urination. The total body content of iron is ~2–5 g, and only a small amount of iron must be absorbed (~1–2 mg/day) to compensate for small losses (93). The daily iron exposure from food and fluids is regulated through controlled absorption, which typically can vary from 3% to 23% of dietary intake, depending on physiologic need (higher when body stores are low or erythropoiesis is high), bioavailability of the iron in the consumed foods, and relative absorption competition from other minerals (82,94). To satisfy requirements that may arise from fluctuations in dietary intake, humans store iron in the form of **ferritin**, which is found in the liver, bone marrow, and spleen. Serum ferritin is a marker of stored iron because a proportion of stored iron "leaks" into the serum and can be measured (95). The amount in serum is proportionate to the amount in storage, so serum ferritin provides a satisfactory marker of stored iron. When iron is required by tissues, an iron-transporting protein, transferrin, takes iron from storage (ferritin) and transports it to the tissue requiring it. In the case of hemoglobin, transferrin picks up iron from ferritin, and transports it to a copper-containing protein, ceruloplasmin, that picks up iron

from transferrin and hands off the iron to heme to produce hemoglobin.

 Ferritin

An iron storage protein that releases it for tissue use on an as-needed basis. Serum ferritin is an indirect marker of the total stored iron in the body. In adult males, normal ferritin concentration is 12–300 ng/mL; in adult females normal ferritin concentration is 12–150 ng/mL (96).

Food Sources of Iron

Iron is available in a wide variety of foods, including meats, eggs, vegetables, and iron-fortified cereals. A typical balanced diet for an omnivore supplies ~6 mg/1,000 kcal of iron. Milk and other dairy products are poor sources of iron. The most easily absorbed form of iron is *heme* iron, which comes from meats and other foods of animal origin. Interestingly, heme iron also enhances the absorption of nonheme iron from nonmeat sources (97). Nonheme iron, which is not as easily absorbed as heme iron, is found in fruits, vegetables, and cereals. However, nonheme iron absorption may be enhanced by consuming foods high in vitamin C, which can reduce ferric iron to a more elemental form, ferrous iron, that has better bioavailability. The absorption of nonheme iron found in nonmeat foods may be inhibited by phytic acid (a substance associated with bran in cereal grains), antacids, and calcium phosphate. In general, red meats are considered to provide the most abundant and easily absorbable source of iron. It is for this reason that vegetarians are considered to be at increased risk for iron deficiency anemia. Nevertheless, with proper planning, the consumption of vegetables and fruits high in iron, and sound cooking techniques that enhance iron absorption, vegetarians can obtain sufficient iron.

Maximizing Iron Intake in a Vegetarian Diet

For vegetarians who want to improve iron absorption from foods, consider the following:

- Dark green vegetables have iron, but they also have oxalic acid, which reduces iron availability. To remove the oxalic acid from the vegetables, blanch them by putting them in a pot of boiling water for 5–10 seconds. Much of the oxalate is removed but the iron remains.
- High-fiber cereals (those with a high bran content) have large amounts of phytic acid, which binds with iron and reduces iron availability. Switch to whole-grain cereals rather than consuming bran-added cereals.

Iron in vegetables is in a form that has a lower rate of absorption than iron in meats. To improve the rate of absorption, add vitamin C to the vegetables by squeezing lemon or orange juice on them before eating.

Iron Requirements

The recommended intake for iron ranges from 8 mg/day for adult men to 18 mg/day for adult women. The requirement for pregnancy, because of the significant expansion of the blood volume, is 27 mg/day. Given the usual concentration of iron in an omnivorous diet (~6 mg/1,000 kcal), an adult woman would require ~3,000 kcal/day to be exposed to the recommended 18 mg. Surveys indicate that the average female daily intake of iron is 12 mg/day, or 33% below the recommended level (97). These same surveys indicate that the average daily intake for men is 16–18 mg/day, or well above the recommended level.

Athletes and Iron

Regular and intense athletic training may increase blood loss from the GI tract and may also increase red cell breakdown (hemolysis) of RBCs to a significant degree. The Food and Nutrition Board has estimated that these factors may raise the iron requirement for athletes by 30% above regular requirements (97). Athletes have good reason to be concerned about iron status because oxygen-carrying capacity (via hemoglobin in blood and myoglobin

in muscles) is a critical factor in physical endurance. It is also important to consider that nutrients work together. A recent study assessing the impact of low-carbohydrate high-fat diet found unfavorable iron, immune, and stress responses to exercise (98). In addition, it was also found that very high carbohydrate diets commonly consumed by endurance athletes have no negative impact on iron status (99). Iron deficiency is one of the most common nutrient deficiencies, and it appears as if athletes have about the same rate of iron deficiency anemia as the general public (82,100). Two types of anemia are **macrocytic hypochromic anemia** and **microcytic hypochromic anemia**.

Macrocytic Hypochromic Anemia

Literally, insufficient RBCs that are large (macro) and low in color (hypochromic) because of low hemoglobin content. This form of anemia, commonly referred to as *pernicious anemia*, is specific to insufficient vitamin B_{12}, insufficient folic acid, or inadequate amounts of both.

Microcytic Hypochromic Anemia

Literally, insufficient RBCs that are small (micro) and low in color (hypochromic) because of low hemoglobin content. This form of anemia is associated with insufficient iron.

There may be several reasons why some athletes suffer from low iron levels. These include:

- *Low dietary intake of iron.* It is possible that some athletes may consume foods with an inadequate total intake of iron. This may be especially true with athletes who are limiting total energy intake as a means (albeit ineffective) of maintaining or reducing weight.
- *Consumption of foods with low iron absorption rates.* Many athletes consume large amounts of carbohydrates and are limiting the intake of red meat. Although iron exists in nonmeat sources, the absorption rate of iron in these foods is typically less, as well as the total iron content.
- *Increased iron losses (hematuria).* Some forms of exercise, particularly long-distance running and concussive sports, cause small amounts of hemoglobin and/or myoglobin to be lost in the urine because of a rupturing of RBCs (101).
- *Loss of iron in sweat.* Although iron losses in sweat are low (about 0.3–0.4 mg/L of sweat), a typical absorption rate of iron from food of about 10% would require that 3–4 mg of additional dietary iron be consumed for each liter of sweat produced. Runners commonly

Table 6.7	How Iron Deficiency or Iron Deficiency *Anemia* Affect Sports Performance	
Anemia	**Iron Deficiency**
Lower oxygen delivery to cells	Higher rate of glucose oxidation
Decreased oxygen uptake (lower VO_{2max})	Higher lactic acid production
Lower endurance performance	Higher respiratory quotient (higher proportion of carbohydrate consumed to meet energy needs)
Lower oxidative metabolism	
Higher glucose oxidation	
Higher lactic acid production	
Higher respiratory quotient (higher proportion of carbohydrate consumed to meet energy needs)	

One of the major impacts of both iron deficiency and iron deficiency anemia is compromised fat metabolism (an oxygen-dependent metabolic pathway), which increases the reliance on carbohydrates as an energy substrate. Because carbohydrate storage in humans is limited, the result is lower endurance at all exercise intensities.

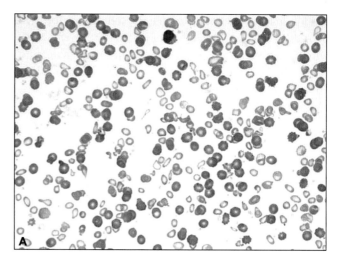
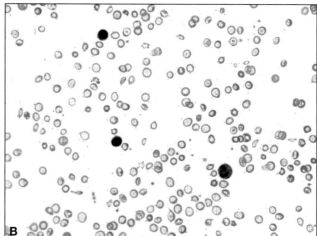

FIGURE 6.2: Difference between normal (**A**) and abnormal (**B**) red blood cells seen in iron deficiency anemia. (From Weksler B, Schecter GP, Ely S. Wintrobe's atlas of clinical hematology. 2nd ed. LWW (PE); 2018.)

lose, particularly in hot and humid environments, up to 2 L of sweat per hour (100,102).

■ *Increased RBC breakdown.* A number of studies have documented higher rates of intravascular hemolysis in athletes than in nonathletes (103). Hemolysis occurs when exertional forces cause a ballistic and premature breakdown of RBCs. Athletes have RBCs with a life expectancy of ~80 days, whereas in nonathletes RBCs last ~120 days (Table 6.7).

■ *Sports anemia.* It is common for many athletes to appear as if they are anemic at the beginning of training season because there is a large increase in blood volume at the initiation of training. This increase in blood volume has the effect of diluting the constituents of the blood, including RBCs, making it appear as though there is an anemia. However, after a short time, the body increases the production of RBCs to remove the appearance of anemia (104).

There are differences in how an athlete might respond in the presence of frank anemia (reduction in the number and size of RBCs) versus iron deficiency (low serum iron and low stored iron, but normal RBCs) anemia (Figure 6.2) (105).

Although iron-deficient athletes are known to experience a performance deficit, there appears to be no benefit in providing iron supplements to athletes who have a normal iron status (32). Further, iron supplementation is often associated with nausea, constipation, and stomach irritation. However, in athletes who have had blood tests that demonstrate either an anemia or a marginal level of stored iron, iron supplementation is warranted. The best means of providing iron supplements to reduce the chance of potential negative side effects is to provide 25–50 mg every third or fourth day rather than daily doses (106).

Iron Deficiency

There are multiple health risks from poor iron status. In children with iron deficiency, poor mental development, underachievement in school, and behavior problems have been documented (107). Because lead binds to the same molecules as iron, an iron deficiency increases the risk that more lead can be taken up by tissues, resulting in lead toxicity (108). During pregnancy, there is a large enlargement of the blood volume, with a requirement that the components of the blood, including iron-containing RBCs, also increase. A failure to consume sufficient iron during pregnancy has been found to increase the risk of premature birth, low–birth-weight infants, and maternal death (109). It should be noted that having excessively high hemoglobin is also associated with pregnancy outcomes, including hypertension and preeclampsia (109). Poor iron status is also associated with ineffective immune function, leading to higher risk of infectious disease (110). Worldwide, the most common nutrient deficiency is iron deficiency. There are three levels of iron deficiency (Table 6.8):

■ Depleted ferritin (stored iron), but functional iron (*i.e.*, hemoglobin, myoglobin muscle iron, iron-containing enzymes) remains normal.
■ Depleted ferritin, myoglobin, and iron-containing enzymes, but normal hemoglobin.
■ Depleted ferritin, myoglobin, iron-containing enzymes, and low hemoglobin result in microcytic, hypochromic anemia (low number of RBCs, and remaining cells are small and low in red color).

As can be seen, it is possible to be in an iron-compromised state that could have an impact on both a sense of well-being and athletic performance without actually being diagnosed with anemia. The diagnosis of anemia is typically made through an evaluation

---

Table 6.8   Stages of Iron Deficiency (Too Little Iron) and Measured Values

The three stages leading from iron deficiency to iron deficiency anemia are as follows:
1. An insufficient supply of dietary iron causes iron stores in bone marrow to be depleted. (This stage is typically without symptoms except for muscle weakness and is associated with depleted myoglobin and low serum ferritin.)
2. Iron deficiencies develop, with reduced hemoglobin production. (This stage shows very low serum ferritin, low hematocrit, and normal hemoglobin.)
3. Iron deficiency anemia from inadequate hemoglobin production and a failure to produce sufficient RBCs with adequate hemoglobin content. (This stage shows absent myoglobin, very low serum ferritin, very low hematocrit, and low hemoglobin.)

Measured Value	Normal	Stage 1 Depleted Stores	Stage 2 Iron-Deficient Erythropoiesis	Stage 3 Iron-Deficiency Anemia
Tissue iron (myoglobin)	Normal ■ 10–95 ng/mL for men ■ 10–65 ng/mL for women	Depleted	Absent	Absent
Stored iron (serum ferritin)	Normal ■ 20–500 ng/mL for men ■ 20–200 ng/mL for women	Low	Very low	Very low
Serum iron (hematocrit)	Normal ■ 39–54% for men ■ 34–47% for women	Normal	Low	Very low
Red cell iron (hemoglobin)	Normal ■ 14–18 g/dL for men ■ 11–16 g/dL for women	Normal	Normal	Low

Camaschella C. New insights into iron deficiency and iron deficiency anemia. Blood Rev. 2017;31:225–33.

Clénin GE, Cordes M, Huber A, Schumacher YO, Noak P, Scales J, Kreimler S. Iron deficiency in sports-definition, influence on performance and therapy: Consensus statement of the Swiss Society of Sports Medicine. Swiss Med Wkly. 2015;145:w14196.

Cowell BS, Rosenbloom CA, Skinner R, Summers SH. Policies on screening female athletes for iron deficiency in NCAA Division I-A institutions. Int J Sport Nutr Exerc Metab. 2003;13:277–85.

of hemoglobin and **hematocrit** (Figure 6.3). However, iron is stripped from myoglobin and iron-containing enzymes to keep hemoglobin normal if storage iron (ferritin) is low (95). Because of this, it may *appear* that iron status is normal when it is actually low. For this reason, the assessment of iron status in athletes should include the evaluation of ferritin in addition to hemoglobin and Hct.

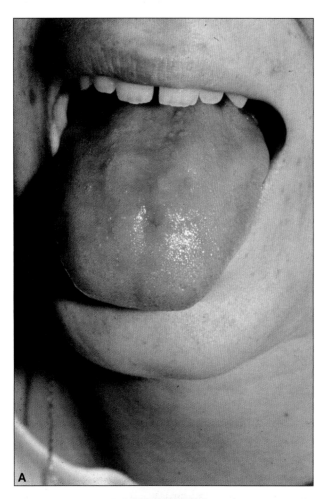

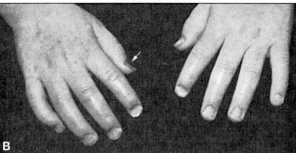

FIGURE 6.3: Commonly observed signs of iron deficiency. In addition to illustrated glossitis (red tongue; **A**) and koilonychias (transverse ridging and spoon nails; **B**), the most common signs are early fatigue and poor concentration as well as whitish lower eyelids. (From Weksler B, Schecter GP, Ely S. Wintrobe's atlas of clinical hematology. 2nd ed. LWW (PE); 2018.)

> **Hematocrit**
>
> Abbreviated as Hct, it is also referred to as *packed cell volume* and is the volume percentage of RBCs in the blood. In adult males, normal Hct is 45%; in adult females normal Hct is 40%.

The lower the storage level, the higher the absorption; however, the absorption rate rarely goes above 10%–15% of the iron content of consumed food. This variable absorption mechanism is aimed at maintaining a relatively constant level of iron and avoiding an excess uptake, which is a health risk. Despite this variable absorption rate, people with marginal intakes of iron are at risk for developing iron deficiency and eventual anemia.

Iron deficiency anemia is characterized by poor oxygen-carrying capacity, a condition that is known to cause performance deficits in athletes. Iron deficiency is also associated with poor immune function, short attention span, irritability, and poor learning ability. Children experiencing fast growth, women of menstrual age, vegetarians, and pregnant women are at increased risk for developing iron deficiency anemia. Periods of growth and pregnancy are associated with a higher requirement of iron because of a fast expansion of the blood volume, and iron is an essential component of RBCs. Women of menstrual age have higher requirements because of the regular blood (and iron) losses associated with the menstrual period. For this reason, women of childbearing age have a higher requirement for iron (18 mg) than men of the same age (10 mg). Symptoms of iron deficiency anemia are listed in Box 6.8.

Box 6.8	**Symptoms of Iron Deficiency Anemia**

Eyes: Yellowing
Skin: Paleness, coldness, yellowing
Respiratory: Shortness of breath
Muscular: Weakness
Intestinal: Changed color of stool
Central nervous system: Fatigue, dizziness, fainting (severe anemia)
Blood vessels: Low blood pressure
Heart: Palpitations, rapid heart rate, chest pain (severe anemia), angina (severe anemia), heart attack (severe anemia)
Spleen: Enlargement

Iron Toxicity

Some people are at risk of developing iron toxicity because they are missing the mechanisms for limiting absorption. Young children, in particular, may be at risk for iron toxicity if they ingest supplements intended for adults. According to the Food and Nutrition Board, the accidental consumption of high doses of iron-containing products is the largest cause of poison-related fatalities in children under 6 years of age (97). Many iron supplements intended for adults have levels of iron that are more than 300% of the recommended daily level, and iron overload may be fatal (111).

Zinc

Zinc has many functions, including forming enzymes, involvement in the structure of tissues, and multiple regulatory activities (Box 6.9). Enzymes help chemical reactions—such as the healing of wounds—occur at a proper rate, and zinc is present in over 300 enzymes (112,113). Zinc-containing enzymes are also involved in the metabolism of carbohydrates, fats, and proteins. The structures of many proteins and cell membranes are also zinc-dependent, and insufficient zinc increases the risk that cell membranes will be oxidatively damaged, as it is part of an important antioxidant enzyme called copper–zinc superoxide dismutase (97). It appears that the absorption of dietary folate is reduced with poor zinc status

(114). In addition, zinc is related to vitamin A metabolism, with insufficient dietary intake of zinc causing a variety of health problems that may be related to vitamin A, including stunted growth, slow wound healing, and failure of the immune system (115). Zinc is competitively absorbed with other bivalent minerals (iron, magnesium, calcium, copper), so high levels of zinc consumption may result in malabsorption of these minerals (114,116).

Food Sources of Zinc

The content and bioavailability of zinc in meats, eggs, and seafood are high, but zinc is also available in pumpkin seeds, nuts, and legumes (Table 6.9). The sulfur-containing amino acids (cysteine and methionine) found in foods of animal origin enhance zinc absorption, whereas phytic acid in whole grains/bran products that are unleavened inhibits zinc absorption (114).

Zinc Requirements

The adult RDA for zinc is 12–15 mg/day, whereas surveys indicate that the average zinc intake for adult women is 9 mg/day and for adult men 13 mg/day (97).

Athletes and Zinc

Zinc levels at the lower end of the normal range, or lower, have been observed in male and female endurance

---

Box 6.9 Zinc Basic Information (Chemical Symbol Zn)

- RDA
  - Adult males (ages 19–70+ years): 11 mg/day
  - Adult females (ages 19–70+ years): 8 mg/day
  - Recommended intake for athletes:
    - 11–15 mg/day
- Functions
  - Part of numerous enzymes involved in energy metabolism
  - Protein synthesis
  - Immune function
  - Sensory function
  - Sexual maturation
- Good food sources
  - Meat, fish, poultry, shellfish, eggs
  - Whole-grain foods
  - Vegetables
  - Nuts
  - Note: Pumpkin seeds are a good vegetarian source of zinc

- Deficiency
  - Impaired wound healing
  - Impaired immune function
  - Loss of appetite (anorexia)
  - Failure to thrive (in children)
  - Dry skin
- Toxicity
  - Tolerable UL: 40 mg/day.
  - *Symptoms:*
    - Impaired immune system
    - Slow wound healing
    - Hypogeusia (loss of taste sensation)
    - Hyposmia (loss of smell sensation)
    - High low-density lipoprotein:high-density lipoprotein cholesterol ratio
    - Nausea

Table 6.9	Zinc Content of Commonly Consumed Foods	
Food	Serving	Zinc (mg)
Beef, broiled	3 oz	6.64
Pumpkin seeds, dried	½ cup	5.04
Milk, 2% fat	1 cup	1.17
Chicken, baked	3 oz	1.05
Beans, cooked	½ cup	0.94
Salmon, cooked	3 oz	0.70
Spinach, cooked	½ cup	0.68
Potato, baked (skin and flesh)	1 medium	0.53
Peanut butter	1 tbsp	0.40

runners. Athletes with lower serum zinc values had lower training mileage (*i.e.*, could probably not train as hard) than those who had higher values (117–119). Therefore, there appears to be a performance deficit in the small number of athletes who have poor zinc status. It is important to note that athletes undergoing regular physical training have elevated plasma concentrations compared to individuals who do not train. This may be due to the muscle damage commonly experienced as a result of training, which would result in zinc release from muscle cells (120).

The effect of zinc supplementation on performance has not been extensively studied, and the level of supplementation in these studies has been extremely high (around 135 mg/day). Also, the athletes tested were never assessed for zinc status prior to the initiation of the research protocol. Nevertheless, this level of intake did lead to an improvement in both muscular strength and endurance (121). Athletes should be cautioned that this level of zinc intake has never been tested over time for safety, so it may well have negative side effects. Toxicity and malabsorption of other nutrients are both likely and possible with this level of intake (122–124).

Because oxygen-carrying capacity, and therefore iron status, is essential for helping athletes perform up to their conditioned capacity, many athletes consume high levels of iron. However, iron supplementation may interfere with zinc absorption. For athletes supplementing with zinc, a malabsorption of copper may occur that could develop into anemia. Therefore, any athlete considering supplementation with either iron or zinc should be careful that the amount consumed is not excessive (125).

A safer and less expensive approach is to consume an adequate amount of a wide variety of foods to optimize tissue exposure to all nutrients in a balanced way.

Zinc Deficiency

Zinc deficiency, while rare, is associated with multiple diseases and conditions, including:

■ *Growth impairment:* Failure to thrive (*i.e.*, poor linear growth and weight gain) in young children is associated with zinc deficiency, perhaps because zinc regulates a hormone, insulin-like growth factor-1 (IGF-1), that is involved in muscle and bone development (126).
■ *Poor neurologic development:* Zinc deficiency is associated with poor attention and poor motor development in newborns and young children (127).
■ *Inadequate functioning of the immune system:* Adequate zinc status is necessary for the normal functioning of cells that help protect tissues from invasion of foreign substance, including bacteria and viruses (128).
■ *Macular degeneration of the eye in older adults*: A high level of zinc is found in the macula (a portion of the retina in the back portion of the eye), and the zinc content of the macula declines with age. Antioxidants, zinc, and copper are part of the standard formula provided for helping older adults lower the risk of macular degeneration (129).

The people most at risk of zinc deficiency include the following (114,130):

■ Young children
■ Pregnant and lactating women (particularly adolescents)
■ People with malabsorption syndromes, including celiac disease, Crohn disease, and ulcerative colitis
■ Alcoholics (increased urinary zinc excretion)
■ Diabetics (frequent urination increases urine zinc losses)
■ People with chronic renal disease
■ People 65 years of age and older
■ Strict vegans (high phytic and oxalic acid associated with cereals and vegetables reduces zinc absorption)

Zinc Toxicity

The tolerable UL for zinc has been established and is set at 40 mg/day for adult males and females. Excessive intake can cause anemia, vomiting, and immune system failure. Some toxicity has occurred as a result of zinc contamination from food containers, while there are also cases of toxicity from nasal sprays containing high levels of zinc (97).

The zinc-containing nasal sprays may produce an irreversible loss of the sense of smell (anosmia) and an irreversible loss of the sense of taste (hypogeusia) and should, therefore, be avoided (131).

Iodine

Iodine is an essential component of thyroid hormones *triiodothyronine* (T3) and *thyroxine* (T4), which control energy metabolism, growth, and nervous system development (Box 6.10). Thyroid hormone production involves both the pituitary gland and the hypothalamus. When thyrotropin-releasing hormone (TRH) is created by the hypothalamus, the pituitary gland secretes thyroid-stimulating hormone (TSH). TSH stimulates the thyroid gland to trap iodine and release thyroid hormones thyroxine (T4) and triiodothyronine (T3) into the circulating blood. When there is sufficient consumption of iodine, there is adequate T4 and T3, and this results in lower levels of TRH and TSH. When the circulating T4 level is low, the pituitary gland increases secretion of TSH to stimulate greater iodine trapping and greater release of both T3 and T4. When there is a chronic iodine deficiency, the resulting persistently elevated TSH may result in an enlargement of the thyroid gland, which is referred to as goiter. (See Figure 6.4.) Goiter was once common in the United States because certain geographic areas have foods grown in soils with a low iodine content. It remains a prevalent nutritional deficiency disease in certain parts of Asia, Africa, and South America. Pregnant women with low iodine intakes may give birth to cretinous or mentally retarded infants. In the United States, an early public health measure to ensure that everyone had an AI of iodine was to add iodine to salt, a strategy that eliminated goiter (132). An excessive intake of iodine has the effect of depressing thyroid activity, so taking additional supplemental doses of iodine is not recommended.

Food Sources of Iodine

A major source of iodine in Western countries is iodized salt. In some countries, such as Canada, iodized salt is mandated. In the United States, however, iodized salt is voluntary. As a result, only about half of the salt sold in the United States is iodized, and a smaller proportion of consumed salt is iodized (133). Sea water also has high levels of iodine, making salt-water seafood a good source as well. It is possible that other foods, including vegetables and fruits, are also good dietary sources of iodine, but this depends on the iodine content of the soil in which the food was grown. Other sources of iodine include eggs and poultry. See Table 6.10 for the iodine content of commonly consumed foods, but consider that, except for iodized salt which has a predictable amount of iodine, other foods vary depending on the preparation and the soil in which they were grown.

Iodine Requirements

The recommended intake of iodine for adult males and females is 150 mcg/day (97). Surveys suggest that the dietary intake of iodine in the United States is adequate, ranging from 138 to 268 mcg/day. In the extremely rare case of people living near a nuclear accident or a nuclear blast, consumption of potassium iodide (a supplemental form of iodine) in very high doses (130 mg/day) may help to saturate the thyroid with nonradioactive iodine, thereby reducing the uptake by the thyroid of radioactive

---

Box 6.10   Iodine Basic Information (Chemical Symbol I)

- RDA
  - Adult males (ages 19–70+ years): 150 mcg/day
  - Adult females (ages 19–70+ years): 150 mcg/day
  - Recommended intake for athletes: 150 mcg/day
- Functions
  - Forms thyroid hormone T4, which is involved in metabolism control
- Good food sources
  - Iodized salt and seafood
  - Depending on soil, some vegetables may also be good sources
- Deficiency
  - Goiter (enlarged thyroid gland with inadequate T4 production), with low metabolic rate and associated obesity
  - Note: Inadequate iodine intake with associated lower T4 production was once relatively common in the United States, but the use of iodized salt effectively eliminated this condition.
- Toxicity
  - An excessive intake of iodine depresses thyroid activity, so taking supplemental doses of iodine is not recommended.

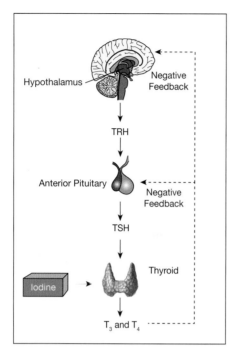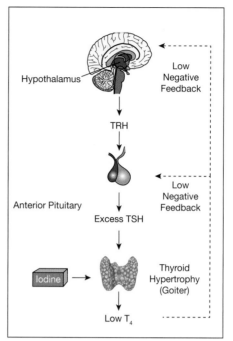

FIGURE 6.4: Thyroid function demonstrating the different production of T3 and T4 associated with adequate and inadequate iodine intakes. (Higdon J, Drake VJ. An evidence-based approach to vitamins and minerals: health benefits and intake recommendations. 2nd ed. Thieme; 2011.)

iodine-131. Studies suggest that this strategy successfully reduces the risk of radiation-causing thyroid cancer (134).

Athletes and Iodine

There are no data suggesting that the iodine intake of athletes is inadequate, and no data suggesting that elevating iodine intake would have a positive impact on performance. On the contrary, the normal absorption of minerals is competitive, so elevating the intake of iodine may have the effect of reducing the absorption of other minerals (iron, copper, etc.), which would have a negative impact on performance. Although there are no studies to confirm that this is so, athletes who chronically restrict food intake can be expected to have a chronically low intake of all nutrients, including iodine. There are data to suggest that inadequate energy intake does suppress T3 and IGF-1, both of which are associated with energy metabolism and tissue development and repair (135).

Iodine Deficiency

Approximately 80 mcg/day of iodine is used to synthesize the thyroid hormones and, while a relatively small requirement, iodine deficiency exists. Countries with large proportions of the population suffering from iodine deficiency have made efforts to reduce iodine deficiency disease through improved availability of iodized salt. On a worldwide basis, however, iodine deficiency is still sufficiently prevalent that it is widely believed to be the most common cause of brain damage (132). The primary condition associated with deficiency is the disease goiter, although hypothyroidism without goiter is still responsible for developmental problems, particularly in children (136). It should be noted that the United States is not a country currently suffering from a high prevalence of

Table 6.10	Iodine Content of Commonly Consumed Foods (in mcg)	
Food	Serving Size	Iodine (mcg)
Iodized salt	1 g (1,000 mg)	77
Cod fish (cooked)	3 oz	99
Milk (2%)	8 oz (1 cup)	99
Potato with skin (baked)	1 medium	60
Shrimp (boiled)	3 oz	35
Turkey breast (baked)	3 oz	34
Navy beans (cooked)	½ cup	32
Egg (chicken, boiled)	1 large egg	12

iodine deficiency. However, recent surveys suggest that the average per capita intake of iodine has decreased in recent years, perhaps because of an increased availability of nonionized "designer" salts on the market, and a public health effort to lower salt consumption because of its well-known association with hypertension (137).

Iodine Toxicity

Although toxicity from iodine is rare, there is an established tolerable UL, which is 1,100 mcg/day for adult males and females. There are some conditions that are associated with iodine sensitivity, including Graves disease and Hashimoto thyroiditis. Individuals who have had a portion of the thyroid surgically removed may also be sensitive to iodine (97). There is no evidence that excess iodine is beneficial for health, so the consumption of foods that provide sufficient iodine should help to avoid excess exposure and toxicity to those who are sensitive and should satisfy the iodine requirement for those who are not.

Selenium

Selenium is an important antioxidant mineral in human nutrition. It is part of glutathione peroxidase and other antioxidants that protect cells from oxidative damage (Box 6.11). It is difficult to determine dietary adequacy, however, because the selenium content of food is determined by soil and water where the food is grown. Nutritional supplements, including sodium selenite and high-selenium yeast, are effective sources of selenium, but excessive intake may be toxic, so proper care in taking appropriate levels of selenium is important.

Food Sources of Selenium

The foods with the highest concentrations of selenium are organ meats (*e.g.*, liver), seafood, and red meats (muscle).

Table 6.11	Sources of Selenium from Commonly Consumed Foods	
Food	Serving	Selenium (mcg)
Brazil nuts (from high-selenium soil)	6 nuts	544
Tuna fish (cooked)	3 oz	92
Shrimp (cooked)	3 oz	42
Pork (roasted)	3 oz	33
Beef (grilled)	3 oz	31
Chicken (roasted)	3 oz	26
Sunflower seeds	¼ cup	19
Bread, whole wheat	2 slices	16

Soils where foods are grown vary widely in selenium content, making it difficult to specify which vegetables are good sources. The food with the highest selenium concentration, assuming they are grown in selenium-rich soil, is Brazil nuts. This is followed by seafood, beef, and seeds (Table 6.11).

Selenium Requirements

The recommended intake of selenium ranges from 20 mcg/day in children to 70 mcg/day in breastfeeding women. Surveys suggest that selenium requirements are adequate in nearly all the U.S. population, with intakes in U.S. adults ranging from 100 to 159 mcg/day from the consumption of foods, or two to three times above the recommended intake of 55 mcg/day (138).

Athletes and Selenium

Because exercise (particularly endurance exercise) is associated with an increased production of potentially

---

Box 6.11 Selenium Basic Information (Chemical Symbol Se)

- RDA
  - Adult males (ages 19–70+ years): 55 mcg/day
  - Adult females (ages 19–70+ years): 55 mcg/day
  - Recommended intake for athletes: 50–55 mcg/day
- Functions
  - Antioxidant (part of glutathione peroxidase)
- Good food sources
  - Meat, fish, seafood
  - Whole-grain foods
- Nuts
- Depending on soil, some vegetables may also be good sources
- Deficiency
  - Unlikely; if it occurs, results in heart damage
- Toxicity
  - Tolerable UL: 400 mcg/day for adults (lower for children)
  - Toxicity is rare; if it occurs, results in nausea, GI distress, and hair loss

---

Box 6.12 **Copper Basic Information (Chemical Symbol Cu)**

- RDA
  - Adult males (ages 19–70+ years): 900 mcg/day
  - Adult females (ages 19–70+ years): 900 mcg/day
  - Recommended intake for athletes: 900 mcg/day
- Functions
  - Part of iron-transport protein ceruloplasmin
  - Oxidation reactions
- Good food sources
  - Meat, fish, poultry, shellfish, eggs
  - Nuts

- Whole-grain foods
- Bananas
- Deficiency
  - Rare; if it occurs, results in anemia (inability to transport iron to RBCs)
- Toxicity
  - Tolerable UL: 10 mg/day. Toxicity is rare; if it occurs, leads to nausea and vomiting

---

damaging oxidative by-products (peroxides and free radicals) in muscle fibers, it has been theorized that selenium plays a role in reducing muscular oxidative stress (139). There is evidence that regular exercise may be protective by helping to maintain the serum selenium level (140). It has also been theorized that selenium deficiency may result in muscle weakness and increased recovery time from exhaustive exercise (32). There is no evidence, however, that consumption of additional selenium, either through foods or supplements, has a beneficial impact on exercise performance (141,142).

Selenium Deficiency

Although rare, poor selenium status will negatively affect selenium-related antioxidant status, increasing susceptibility to oxidative stress, tissue damage, and, potentially, cancer. Those most at risk of selenium deficiency include people who, because of GI surgery, receive their nutrition through a vein (total parenteral nutrition), bypassing normal food consumption and nutrient absorption through the gut. People with compromised GI tracts (*e.g.*, celiac disease and Crohn disease) appear also to be at risk. In these individuals, selenium deficiency is associated with heart damage and muscular weakness (143). There are no data to suggest that athletes are at high risk of selenium deficiency.

Selenium Toxicity

Excessive intake of selenium is toxic and may be fatal (138). The tolerable UL for selenium in adult males and females is set at 400 mcg/day. Early signs of chronic selenium toxicity include brittle nails and hair and hair loss. In addition, excess selenium exposure may negatively impact the central nervous system by disrupting several neurotransmitters (144).

Copper

Copper-containing enzymes are involved in iron metabolism, production of ATP energy, bone formation, collagen production, and neurotransmission (145) (Box 6.12). The important role copper plays in iron metabolism has been long recognized. The copper-containing protein, *ceruloplasmin*, can convert ferrous iron to ferric iron, making it possible to transfer iron for RBC formation (146). It is interesting that individuals with inadequate ceruloplasmin are more at risk for developing iron overload disease, which can be fatal, at similar levels of iron consumption. This is likely because the iron cannot be efficiently transferred to manufacture hemoglobin in RBCs, resulting in an increased storage in the liver and other tissues (147).

Food Sources of Copper

Copper is widely distributed in the food supply and is particularly high in beef liver, shellfish, nuts, seeds, and whole grains (Table 6.12). Copper intake for the adult U.S. population is slightly above the recommended intake (900 mcg/day), with adult men having an average daily intake of between 1,000 and 1,100 mcg, and adult women having 1,200–1,600 mcg.

Copper Requirements

The recommended intake of copper ranges from 340 mcg/day in young children to 1,300 mcg/day in breastfeeding women. The recommended intake amount is based on multiple studies to ensure avoidance of any copper-related deficiencies (97). As another good example of why nutritional balance is important, excessive consumption of calcium, phosphate, iron, zinc, and vitamin C reduces copper absorption and, therefore, alters the requirement. It has been suggested that physically active individuals

Table 6.12	Copper Content of Commonly Consumed Foods	
Foods	Serving Size	Copper (mcg)
Beef liver, cooked	1 oz	4,128
Oysters, cooked	6 medium	2,397
Clams	3 oz	585
Hazelnuts, dry roasted	1 oz	496
Mushrooms, raw white, sliced	1 cup	223
Shredded wheat	2 biscuits	167

require additional copper, primarily to efficiently manufacture the higher requirement for hemoglobin in RBCs (148). However, a well-balanced diet providing the extra energy required by athletes should satisfy this higher need.

Athletes and Copper

Very few studies have been performed on the relationship between copper and athletic performance. Studies of blood copper concentrations in athletes and nonathletes have not revealed any significant differences, but the athletes have a slightly higher (3%–4%) concentration of serum copper than nonathletes (2,3). In a study evaluating the copper status of swimmers during a competitive season, there was no difference in preseason and postseason copper status. In this study, the majority of swimmers were consuming adequate levels of copper (more than 1 mg/day) from food (149). An evaluation of elite athletes involved in different types of activities found normal copper status in these athletes (150).

Copper Deficiency

Copper deficiency resulting in a disease state is extremely rare, and mainly seen in individuals who have inborn errors of copper metabolism. The most common indication of copper deficiency is iron deficiency anemia which does not improve following strategies to improve iron status (97). In a relatively low number of cases, newborn infants fed cow's milk formula, which is low in copper, may not have a normal growth velocity (151).

Copper Toxicity

Toxicity of copper is rare, but when it occurs it may result in liver and kidney failure, coma, and death. The U.S. tolerable UL for copper in adults is ~10 times the recommended intake level and is set at 10,000 mcg/day. In people with genetic intolerance to copper (Wilson disease), the UL is likely to be excessive and result in copper accumulations in tissues that would be damaging. Recent findings suggest that copper toxicity results in liver accumulation that causes oxidative damage and negatively impacts zinc metabolism. In addition to the negative impact on the immune system, copper toxicity may also be associated with neurodegenerative diseases such as Alzheimer and Parkinson disease (152).

Manganese

Although there is still much to learn about manganese, current information has established that it is a trace mineral involved in energy metabolism, bone formation, immune function, antioxidant activity, and carbohydrate metabolism (105) (Box 6.13). In the mitochondria (the oxygen-using energy factories of cells), manganese

---

Box 6.13   Manganese Basic Information (Chemical Symbol Mn)

- AI
  - Adult males (ages 19–70+ years): 2.3 mg/day
  - Adult females (ages 19–70+ years): 1.8 mg/day
  - Recommended intake for athletes: 2.0–2.5 mg/day
- Functions
  - Energy metabolism
  - Fat synthesis
  - Bone structure
- Good food sources
  - Whole-grain foods
  - Legumes
- Green leafy vegetables
- Bananas
- Deficiency
  - Poor growth and development in children
- Toxicity
  - Tolerable UL: 11 mg/day
  - Symptoms:
    - Neurologic problems
    - Confusion
    - Easy fatigue

superoxide dismutase is the primary protective antioxidant (153). In addition, muscles have elevated manganese superoxide dismutase after vigorous exercise, which is likely an adaptation to the elevated tissue oxygen exposure associated with exercise (154). Animals that suffer from manganese deficiency develop fragile skeletons, and production of the same protein that helps to stabilize bone joints, collagen, is manganese (and vitamin C) dependent (155,156).

Food Sources of Manganese

Food sources of manganese include coffee, tea, chocolate, whole wheat, nuts, seeds, soybeans, dried beans (*e.g.*, navy beans, lentils, split peas), liver, and fruits. As with several other minerals, the intake of foods high in oxalic acid (present in dark green leafy vegetables) may inhibit manganese absorption (See section on calcium for ways of reducing the oxalic acid content of foods.) Much like iron, manganese absorption is enhanced with vitamin C and meat intake.

Manganese Requirements

The AI for manganese in the United States for adult men is 2.3 mg/day and for adult women 1.8 mg/day. The AI level of intake level is higher for pregnancy (2.0 mg/day) and breastfeeding (2.6 mg/day), an amount that should be easily obtained with the increase food consumption associated with both pregnancy and lactation.

Athletes and Manganese

There are no current studies suggesting that athletes are at higher risk of manganese deficiency, and no studies suggesting that athletic performance would be enhanced with higher intake of manganese.

Manganese Deficiency

Although manganese deficiency is rare, deficiencies are associated with skeletal problems (undermineralized bone and increased risk of fracture) and poor wound healing. There is also some indication from animal studies that manganese deficiency could be associated with impaired glucose tolerance and poor carbohydrate and lipid metabolism (155). However, there are currently no human studies with similar findings. It appears that those at greatest risk for deficiency are those on diets (inadequate intake) or where malabsorption occurs. Manganese is in competition with calcium, iron, and zinc for absorption, so an excess intake of these other minerals may decrease manganese absorption and lead to deficiency symptoms.

Manganese Toxicity

Welders are at risk of inhaling manganese dust, which has been recognized as a health risk that can result in central nervous system problems (157). Chronic toxicity from excess manganese can worsen the neurologic disorders and make them permanent, with physical symptoms that mimic Parkinson disease, and psychological symptoms that include hallucinations (158). Besides welders, people most at risk for manganese toxicity include those with iron deficiency (manganese replaces iron and accumulates in the brain) and children (they have less absorption protection for heavy metals than adults) (159). The tolerable UL for manganese is relatively low because of the relatively high risk of developing neurologic problems with excess manganese exposure. For this reason, individuals should be cautious about consuming manganese supplements. For adult males and females, the UL is 11 mg/day, or ~5 times greater than the average daily intake of adults living in the United States.

Chromium

The trace mineral chromium is widespread in the food supply and environment (Box 6.14). Chromium is also known as *glucose tolerance factor* because of its involvement in helping cells use glucose through normal insulin function. It appears to improve insulin function by enhancing insulin sensitivity in cells, thereby aiding the transportation of glucose out of the blood and into cells (160). A deficiency of chromium is known to be associated with poor blood glucose maintenance (either hypoglycemia or hyperglycemia), an excessive production of insulin (hyperinsulinemia), excessive fatigue, and a craving for sweet foods. It is also associated with irritability, which is commonly associated with poor blood glucose control, weight gain, type 2 diabetes, and higher cardiovascular disease risk (105). There is limited evidence that frequent and intense exercise may increase chromium deficiency risk.

Food Sources of Chromium

The best food sources of chromium include whole grains and meats. Nutritional supplements, commonly in the form of chromium picolinate, are taken as a means of reducing weight or body fat, but the results of studies on this supplement have produced mixed results. Initial studies of chromium picolinate supplementation suggested that this supplement was effective at increasing muscle mass and decreasing body fat in bodybuilders

---

Box 6.14   Chromium Basic Information (Chemical Symbol Cr)

- AI
  - Adult males (ages 19–50 years): 35 mcg/day
  - Adult males (ages 51–70+ years): 30 mcg/day
  - Adult females (ages 19–50 years): 25 mcg/day
  - Adult females (ages 51–70+ years): 20 mcg/day
  - Recommended intake for athletes: 30–35 mcg/day
- Functions
  - Glucose tolerance (glucose–insulin control)
- Good food sources
  - Brewer yeast
  - Mushrooms
  - Whole-grain foods
  - Nuts
  - Legumes
  - Cheese
- Deficiency
  - Glucose intolerance
- Toxicity
  - Unlikely

---

and football players (161). However, subsequent controlled studies have failed to reach the same conclusions (162,163). Other supplements for chromium include chromium polynicotinate, chromium chloride, and high-chromium yeast. Dietary sources include whole-grain bread and cereals, meats, and high-chromium yeast.

Chromium Requirements

There is insufficient information on chromium status to set a recommended intake level or an estimated average requirement, so the current standard of intake is based on the AI estimation, which is based on the average chromium content of healthy diets (97). The AI for chromium ranges from 25 mcg/day in adult females to 35 mcg/day in adult males, with higher recommendations for pregnant and breastfeeding women.

Athletes and Chromium

Because chromium is not well absorbed, there is little evidence to suggest that an excessive intake of chromium will result in toxicity. However, the toxicity of chromium has not been directly tested, so athletes should be cautious about taking supplements. One study suggests that chromium picolinate has the potential of altering DNA, and thus producing mutated, cancerous cells (164). Taken together, these studies suggest that, to maintain an optimal chromium status, athletes should consume foods low in sugar and a diet that contains whole grains and, if the athlete is not a vegetarian, some meat. It is important to consider that insulin, besides being closely associated with carbohydrate metabolism, is also involved in protein and fat metabolism (165). Normal metabolism of these energy substrates is critically important for all athletes. A number of studies have investigated whether chromium

supplementation enhances fat-free mass in people who do and do not exercise. The results of these studies suggest that chromium supplementation does not contribute to an improved body composition (more muscle mass, less fat mass) (166,167).

Chromium Deficiency

Deficiency of chromium is rare, but it has been described in people who have been fed intravenously for long periods of time (168). High consumption of simple sugars (sweets) may also place people at risk for deficiency. It appears, from a number of surveys, that a large proportion of the U.S. population consumes inadequate levels of chromium, a factor that may be associated with the excess weight commonly found in greater numbers of the population.

Chromium Toxicity

The usual form of chromium that is consumed (trivalent chromium; Cr^{3+}) is not considered to be highly toxic because of its relatively low rate of absorption and rapid urinary excretion (169). Although there is no current tolerable UL for chromium currently set by the Food and Nutrition Board, the Board has stated that high supplemental intakes of chromium may be toxic (97). A usual form of chromium that is taken as a supplement is chromium picolinate. Although there has been some concern from laboratory studies that chromium picolinate may cause cancer, there are no studies on humans indicating that cancer is a risk factor when taking 400 mcg/day (a level well above the AI) (97,170). At higher levels (600 mcg/day), however, chromium picolinate taken over a 5-month period was associated with the development of chronic renal failure (171).

SUMMARY

- Minerals are inorganic substances that have multiple functions. They are attached to proteins to provide strength and structure to the skeleton (such as calcium and phosphorus); they help to sustain the pH of the blood and tissues; they are involved in creating nerve impulses that stimulate muscle movement, and they are integral parts of hormones that control the rate of energy metabolism.

- A large number of athletes, particularly female athletes, are at risk for calcium and iron deficiency, both of which are essential for health and athletic performance. Low bone density that results from poor calcium intake may increase stress fracture risk, and poor iron status lowers the capacity to deliver oxygen to working cells and remove carbon dioxide from these cells, resulting in reduced aerobic endurance and early fatigue. Other minerals are equally important for athletic performance, mental acuity, muscle function, and nerve function.

- Minerals must be consumed regularly to ensure good health. Mineral deficiencies take a long time to correct (for instance, iron deficiency may take more than 6 months to resolve), so athletes could suffer poor performance for long periods of time if mineral deficiencies are allowed to occur.

- Of all the minerals, iron and calcium have been found by multiple studies to be the most likely to be deficient in athletes.

- Because of limited absorption capacity, it is typically better to spread out the intake of minerals during the day, rather than by consuming minerals in single, large doses. Eating good foods throughout the day is a preferred strategy.

- One cup of milk provides about 240 mg of calcium. With a calcium requirement of 1,200–1,500 mg/day, an athlete would have to consume ~5 cups of milk or an equivalent amount from other foods to satisfy this daily requirement.

- Meat is the *easiest* way to obtain iron and zinc, so vegetarians may be at increased risk without careful planning to consume well-prepared dark green vegetables and enriched grains to obtain these minerals. However, good dietary planning can dramatically reduce the risk that vegetarians have from iron and/or zinc deficiency.

- Sodium is critically important for maintaining blood volume and the sweat rate. The current general population sodium recommendation does not apply to athletes. The more an athlete sweats the more sodium they require in a sports beverage, with the normal range of between 50 and 200 mg/cup. The athlete's goal is to replace *all* the sodium lost through sweat.

Practical Application Activity

Iron deficiency is one of the most common nutrient deficiencies, with high prevalence among the general population and athletes. Using the procedure described in earlier chapters, create a spreadsheet with iron, calcium, zinc, and potassium, and the RDA for each of these minerals. Look up the mineral content of the foods consumed by accessing the online USDA Food Composition Database (172) (https://fdc.nal.usda.gov). Analyze your food intake for the mineral content of the foods you consume and determine their adequacy using the procedure described below.

- Create three new analysis days and plug in your foods and activities for each hour of the day for each day.
- When completed, "analyze" the average daily iron consumed over the 3 days, and see how it compares with the DRI/RDA for your age and gender.
- If not adequate, try modifying your diet by eating more of the foods that are good sources of iron.
- Once done, now assess the adequacy of other minerals, including calcium, zinc, and potassium, to see if the intake of these minerals meets the DRI/RDA standard.

CHAPTER QUESTIONS

1. The primary cation in extracellular fluid is:
   a. Sodium
   b. Potassium
   c. Calcium
   d. Chloride

2. The primary cation in intracellular fluid is:
   a. Sodium
   b. Potassium
   c. Calcium
   d. Chloride

3. Of the following foods, which are good sources of potassium?
   a. Orange
   b. Banana
   c. Blueberries
   d. Bread
   e. a, b, and c
   f. All of the above

4. Which of the following nutrients are associated with BMD?
   a. Calcium and vitamin C
   b. Sodium and vitamin D
   c. Vitamin D and calcium
   d. Potassium and sodium

5. Which mineral listed below is most associated with immune function?
   a. Selenium
   b. Magnesium
   c. Zinc
   d. Calcium

6. Without _____, consumed calcium is likely to be excreted in the _____.
   a. Vitamin E, urine
   b. Vitamin D, fecal matter
   c. Thiamin, urine
   d. Niacin, fecal matter

7. In industrialized nations, the most common nutrient deficiencies are:
   a. Potassium and iron
   b. Selenium and iodine
   c. Calcium and iron
   d. Zinc and manganese

8. Severe and chronic iron deficiency will result in:
   a. Macrocytic, hyperchromic anemia
   b. Microcytic, hypochromic anemia
   c. Pernicious anemia
   d. Macrocytic, normochromic anemia

9. Production of cortisol is likely to aid vitamin D activity and increase BMD.
   a. True
   b. False

10. Iron absorption is limited for the following reason:
    a. Excess iron absorption is toxic and associated with liver disease.
    b. People commonly consume excess iron, so the controlled absorption helps to limit tissue exposure.
    c. Most people have subtle zinc deficiency, which negatively impacts iron absorption.
    d. a and c

ANSWERS TO CHAPTER QUESTIONS

1. a
2. b
3. f
4. c
5. c

6. b
7. c
8. b
9. b
10. a

Case Study Considerations

1. **Case Study Answer 1: Iron deficiency, anemia, and iron deficiency anemia** represent the most common nutrient deficiencies found in both male and female athletes. Female athletes are at particularly high risk because of the blood (and iron) loss associated with monthly menstrual periods. Iron deficiency anemia is a problem for athletic performance as it is impossible for an athlete to perform up to his or her conditioned capacity when in a state

of iron deficiency, and it also represents a significant health problem because of associated higher disease risks. Iron deficiency/anemia also affects a general sense of well-being because of easy fatigue and poor concentration ability.

2. **Case Study Answer 2:** The cellular capacity to take up and productively use nutrients is finite. Imagine that a cell is the size of a cup, and the typical daily requirement is the size of a quart. It is impossible

to put the entire quart in the cell at once. Rather, it must be spread out over the day to provide what the cell requires and not exceed the cell's capacity to use it productively. It is important to emphasize to athletes that the "gas tank" for nutrients is finite. You shouldn't overfill the tank by providing too much at once, and you shouldn't let the tank run to empty. To achieve optimal nutrient delivery requires well-distributed and highly nourishing meals that are spaced well throughout the day.

3. **Case Study Answer 3:** Supplements typically provide a level of nutrient that is at or well above the recommended daily requirement, and at this level taken in a single dose may result in toxicity. In addition, there is evidence that chronically high doses of nutrients may also cause cells to lower absorption as a means of survival. Importantly, supplements do not provide either the fluid or the energy that should be high on the list of needed nutrients required by athletes. Far too often athletes believe

that taking a supplement satisfies their nutritional needs. It does not.

4. **Case Study Answer 4:** Taking a high chronic dose of iron has the effect of saturating a large portion of the primary absorption site in the intestines, the proximal duodenum, which makes it difficult for other nutrients to be absorbed in the same site. The bivalent minerals include iron, magnesium, zinc, and copper, all of which are absorbed in the same area. If you have too much of one, you can logically predict that this will negatively impact the absorption of the other minerals. Doing this chronically (*i.e.*, daily) has the predictable impact of increasing deficiency risks. In the case of iron, the supplemental doses taken are often so high that a large proportion of the iron cannot be absorbed, and there is evidence that the unabsorbed portion of this potentially inflammatory mineral may increase colon cancer risk as it passes through the intestines.

REFERENCES

1. Rodriguez NR, DiMarco NM, Langley S; American Dietetic Association, and Dietitians of Canada. American College of Sports Medicine position stand. Nutrition and athletic performance. Med Sci Sports Exerc. 2009;41;709–31.
2. Lukaski HC. Micronutrients (magnesium, zinc, and copper): are mineral supplements needed for athletes? Int J Sport Nutr. 1995;5:S74–83.
3. Lukaski HC. Prevention and treatment of magnesium deficiency in athletes. In: Vecchiet L, editor. Magnesium and physical activity. Parthenon; 1995:211–26.
4. Weaver CM. Calcium. In: Erdman JJ, Macdonald I, Zeisel S, editors. Present knowledge in nutrition. 10th ed. John Wiley & Sons, Inc.; 2012.
5. Holtzman B, Ackerman KE. Recommendations and nutritional considerations for female athletes: health and performance. Sports Med. 2021;51(Suppl 1):43–57.
6. Schroeder N, Evidence-based nutritional strategies to enhance athletic performance. Strength Cond J. 2022;44(2):33–44.
7. Beck KL, von Hurst PR, O'Brien WJ, Badenhorst CE. Micronutrients and athletic performance: a review. Food Chem Toxicol. 2021;158:112618.
8. Ferraro PM, Taylor EN, Gambaro G, Curhan GC. Caffeine intake and the risk of kidney stones. Am J Clin Nutr. 2014;6(1):1596–1603.
9. Gutiérrez OM, Luzuriaga-McPherson AL, Lin Y, Gilbert LC, Ha S-W, Beck GR Jr. Impact of phosphorus-based food additives on bone and mineral metabolism. J Clin Endocrinol Metab. 2015;100(11):4264–71.
10. Kerstetter JE, O'Brien KO, Insogna KL. Dietary protein, calcium metabolism, and skeletal homeostatis revisited. Am J Clin Nutr. 2003;78(3):584S–92S.
11. Park SM, Jee J, Joung JY, Cho YY, Sohn SY, Jin S-M, Hur KY, Kim JH, Kim SW, Chung JH, Lee MK, Min Y-K. High dietary sodium intake assessed by 24-hour urine specimen increase urinary calcium excretion and bone resorption marker. J Bone Metab. 2014;21(3):189–94.
12. Akhtar MS, Israr B, Bhatty N, Ali A. Effect of cooking on soluble and insoluble oxalate contents in selected Pakistani vegetables and beans. Int J Food Properties. 2011;14(1):241–49.
13. Amalraj A, Pius A. Bioavailability of calcium and its absorption inhibitors in raw and cooked green leafy vegetables commonly consumed in India—an in vitro study. Food Chem. 2015;170(1):430–6.
14. Kumar V, Sinha AK, Makkar HPS, Becker K. Dietary roles of phytate and phytase in human nutrition: a review. Food Chem. 2010;120(4):945–59.
15. Mountjoy M, Sundgot-Borgen J, Burke L, Carter S, Constantini N, Lebrun C, Meyer N, Sherman R, Steffen K, Budgett R, Ljungqvist A. The IOC consensus statement: beyond the Female Athlete Triad-Relative Energy Deficiency in Sport (RED-S). Br J Sports Med. 2014;48:491–97.
16. Rizzoli R, Bianchi ML, Garabedian M, McKay HA, Moreno LA. Maximizing bone mineral mass gain during growth for the prevention of fractures in the adolescents and the elderly. Bone. 2010;46(2):294–305.
17. Fischbach F, Dunning MB. A manual of laboratory and diagnostic tests. Wolters Kluwer/Lippincott Williams & Wilkins; 2009.

18. Larson-Meyer E. Calcium and vitamin D. In: Maughan RJ, ed. Sports nutrition. Wiley Blackwell; 2014:242–62.

19. Thomas DT, Erdman KA, Burke LM. Position of the Academy of Nutrition and Dietetics, Dietitians of Canada, and the American College of Sports Medicine: nutrition and athletic performance. J Acad Nutr Diet. 2016;116(3):501–28.

20. Chesnut CH 3rd. Theoretical overview: bone development, peak bone mass, bone loss, and fracture risk. Am J Med. 1991;91(5B):S2–4.

21. Benardot D. Nutrition for gymnasts. In: Marshall NT, editor. The athlete wellness book. USA Gymnastics; 1999:12–13.

22. McNamara LM. Osteocytes and estrogen deficiency. Curr Osteoporos Rep. 2021;19:592–603.

23. Dougkas A, Reynolds CK, Givens ID, Elwood PC, Minihane AM. Associations between dairy consumption and body weight: a review of the evidence and underlying mechanisms. Nutr Res Rev. 2011;24(1):72–95.

24. Zemel MB, Thompson W, Milstead A, Morris K, Campbell P. Calcium and dairy acceleration of weight and fat loss during energy restriction in obese adults. Obes Res. 2004; 12(4):582–90.

25. Mallard SR, Howe AS, Houghton LA. Vitamin D status and weight loss: a systematic review and meta-analysis of randomized and nonrandomized controlled weight-loss trials. Am J Clin Nutr. 2016;104(4):1151–59.

26. Zemel MB, Shi H, Greer B, Dirienzo D, Zemel PC. Regulation of adiposity by dietary calcium. FASEB J. 2000;14(9):1132–8.

27. Appel LJ, Moore TJ, Obarzanek E, Vollmer WM, Svetkey LP, Sacks FM, Bray GA, Vogt TM, Cutler JA, Windhauser MM, Lin PH, Karanja N. A clinical trial of the effects of dietary patterns on blood pressure. DASH Collaborative Research Group. N Engl J Med. 1997;336(16):1117–24.

28. Clapham DE. Calcium signaling. Cell. 2007;131(6):1047–58.

29. Gentile C, Chiarelli F. Rickets in children: an update. Biomedicines. 2021;9:738. https://doi.org/10.3390/biomedicines9070738

30. Moe SM. Disorders involving calcium, phosphorus, and magnesium. Prim Care. 2008;35(2):215–37.

31. Institute of Medicine, Food and Nutrition Board. Dietary reference intakes (DRIs): calcium, phosphorus, magnesium, vitamin d, and fluoride. National Academy Press; 1997:146–89.

32. Bucci L. Nutrients as ergogenic aids for sports and exercise. CRC Press; 1993.

33. Keller WD, Kraut HA. Work and nutrition. World Rev Nutr Diet. 1961;3:65–81.

34. Cade R, Conte M, Zauner C, Mars D, Peterson J, Lunne D, Hommen N, Packer D. Effects of phosphate loading on 2,3-diphosphoglycerate and maximal oxygen uptake. Med Sci Sports Exerc. 1984;16(3):263–8.

35. Duffy DJ, Conlee RK. Effects of phosphate loading on leg power and high intensity treadmill exercise. Med Sci Sports Exerc. 1986;18:674–77.

36. Lotz M, Zisman E, Bartter FC. Evidence for a phosphorus-depletion syndrome in man. N Engl J Med. 1968;278(8):409–15.

37. Cervelli MJ, Shaman A, Meade A, Carroll R, McDonald SP. Effect of gastric acid suppression with pantoprazole on the efficacy of calcium carbonate as a phosphate binder in haemodialysis patients. Nephrology (Carlton). 2012;17(5):458–65.

38. Amanzadeh J, Reilly RF Jr. Hypophosphatemia: an evidence-based approach to its clinical consequences and management. Nat Clin Pract Nephrol. 2006;2(3):136–48.

39. Jakše B, Jakše B, Mis NF, Jug B, Šajber D, Godnov U, Čuk I. Nutritional status and cardiovascular health in female adolescent elite-level artistic gymnasts and swimmers: a cross-sectional study of 31 athletes. J Nutr Metab. 2021;8810548. https://doi.org/10.1155/2021/8810548

40. Calvo MS, Uribarri J. Public health impact of dietary phosphorus excess on bone and cardiovascular health in the general population. Am J Clin Nutr. 2013;98(1):6–15.

41. Calvo MS, Park YK. Changing phosphorus content of the US diet: potential for adverse effects on bone. J Nutr. 1996;126 (4 Suppl):1168S–80S.

42. Rude RK. Magnesium. In: Ross AC, Caballero B, Cousins RJ, Tucker KL, Ziegler TR, editors. Modern nutrition in health and disease. 11th ed. Lippincott Williams & Wilkins; 2012:159–75.

43. Rude RK, Shils ME. Magnesium. In: Shils ME, Shike M, Ross AC, Caballero B, Cousins RJ, editors. Modern nutrition in health and disease. 10th ed. Lippincott Williams & Wilkins; 2006:223–47.

44. Hunt G, Sukumar D, Volpe SL. Magnesium and vitamin D supplementation on exercise performance. Transl J ACSM. 2021;6(4):e000179.

45. Fine KD, Ana CAS, Porter JL, Fordtran JS. Intestinal absorption of magnesium from food and supplements. J Clin Invest. 1991;88:396–402.

46. Spencer H, Norris C, Williams D. Inhibitory effects of zinc on magnesium balance and magnesium absorption in man. J Am Coll Nutr. 1994;13(5):479–84.

47. Schwartz R, Walker G, Linz MD, Mackellar I. Metabolic responses of adolescent boys to two levels of dietary magnesium and protein. I. Magnesium and nitrogen retention. Am J Clin Nutr. 1973;26(5):510–18.

48. Firoz M, Graber M. Bioavailability of US commercial magnesium preparations. Magnes Res. 2001;14:257–62.

49. Mühlbauer B, Schwenk M, Coram WM, Antonin KH, Etienne P, Bieck PR, Douglas FL. Magnesium-L-aspartate-HCl and magnesium-oxide: bioavailability in healthy volunteers. Eur J Clin Pharmacol. 1991;40:437–8.

50. Ranade VV, Somberg JC. Bioavailability and pharmacokinetics of magnesium after administration of magnesium salts to humans. Am J Ther. 2001;8:345–57.

51. Shils ME. Magnesium. In: Shils ME, Olson JA, Shike M, editors. Modern nutrition in health and disease. 8th ed. Lea & Febiger; 1993:164–84.

52. Rosanoff A, Weaver CM, Rude RK. Suboptimal magnesium status in the United States: are the health consequences underestimated? Nutr Rev. 2012;70(3):153–64.

53. Del Gobbo LC, Imamura F, Wu JHY, de Oliveira Otto MC, Chiuve SE, Mozaffarian D. Circulating and dietary magnesium and risk of cardiovascular disease: a systematic review and meta-analysis of prospective studies. Am J Clin Nutr. 2013;98:160–73.

54. Larsson SC, Wolk A. Magnesium intake and risk of type 2 diabetes: a meta-analysis. J Intern Med. 2007;262:208–14.

55. Peacock JM, Ohira T, Post W, Sotoodehnia N, Rosamond W, Folsom AR. Serum magnesium and risk of sudden cardiac

death in the Atherosclerosis Risk in Communities (ARIC) study. Am Heart J. 2010;160(3):464–70.

56. Tucker KL. Osteoporosis prevention and nutrition. Curr Osteoporos Rep. 2009;7(4):111–7.

57. Holland S, Silberstein SD, Freitag F, Dodick DW, Argoff C, Ashman E. Evidence-based guideline update: NSAIDs and other complementary treatments for episodic migraine prevention in adults. Neurology. 2012;78:1346–53.

58. Steinacker JM, Grunert-Fuchs M, Steininger K, Wodick RE. Effects of long-time administration of magnesium on physical capacity. Int J Sports Med. 1987;8:151.

59. Brilla LR, Haley TF. Effect of magnesium supplementation on strength training in humans. J Am Coll Nutr. 1992;11:326–9.

60. Golf SW, Bohmer D, Nowacki PE. Is magnesium a limiting factor in competitive exercise? A summary of relevant scientific data. In: Golf S, Dralle D, Vecchiet L, editors. Magnesium. John Libbey; 1993:209–20.

61. Kharait S. A magnesium-rich electrolyte hydration mix reduces exercise associated muscle cramps in half-marathon runners: direct original research. J Exerc Nutr. 2022;5(3). https://doi.org/10.53520/jen2022.103126

62. Hickson JF Jr, Schrader J, Trischler LC. Dietary intake of female basket- all and gymnastics athletes. J Am Diet Assoc. 1986;86:251–4.

63. Vitale K, Hueglin S. Update on vegetarian and vegan athletes: a review. J Sports Med Phys Fitness. 2021;10(1):1–11.

64. Musso CG. Magnesium metabolism in health and disease. Int Urol Nephrol. 2009;41(2):357–62.

65. McGuire JK, Kulkarni MS, Baden HP. Fatal hypermagnesemia in a child treated with megavitamin/megamineral therapy. Pediatrics. 2000;105:E18.

66. Onishi S, Yoshino S. Cathartic-induced fatal hypermagnesemia in the elderly. Int Med. 2006;45(4):207–10.

67. Harper ME, Willis JS, Patrick J. Sodium and chloride in nutrition. In: O'Dell BL, Sunde RA, editors. Handbook of nutritionally essential minerals. Marcel Dekker; 1997:93–116.

68. Sheng H-W. Sodium, chloride and potassium. In: Stipanuk M, editor. Biochemical and physiological aspects of human nutrition. W. B. Saunders Company; 2000:686–710.

69. Institute of Medicine, Food and Nutrition Board. Dietary reference intakes for water, potassium, sodium, chloride, and sulfate. National Academies Press; 2005:269–423.

70. Veniamakis E, Kaplan's G, Voulgaris P, Nikolaidis PT. Effects of sodium intake on health and performance in endurance and ultra-endurance sports. Int J Environl Res Public Health. 2022;19:3651.

71. United States Department of Agriculture. Scientific Report of the 2015 Dietary Guidelines Advisory Committee. Part A: Executive summary. USDA, February 2015.

72. Ayus JC, Varon J, Arieff AI. Hyponatremia, cerebral edema, and noncardiogenic pulmonary edema in marathon runners. Ann Intern Med. 2000;132(9):711–4.

73. Whatmough S, Mears S, Kipps C. Exercise associated hyponatremia (EAH) and fluid intake during the 2016 London marathon. Br J Sports Med. 2017;51(4):409.

74. Mayer CU, Treff G, Fenske WK, Blouin K, Steinacker JM, Allolio B. High incidence of hyponatremia in rowers during a four-week training camp. Am J Med. 2015;128:1144–51.

75. Filippatos TD, Liamis G, Christopoulou F, Elisaf MS. Ten common pitfalls in the evaluation of patients with hyponatremia. Eur J Intern Med. 2016;29:22–5.

76. Lecina M, López I, Castellar C, Pradas F. Extreme ultra-trail race induced muscular damage, risk for acute kidney injury and hyponatremia: a case report. Int J Environ Res Public Health. 2021;18:11323.

77. Noakes TD. Hyponatremia of exercise. In. Maughan RJ, editor. Sports nutrition: volume XIX of the encyclopaedia of sports medicine. Wiley Blackwell; 2014:539–50.

78. Tsugane S. Salt, salted food intake, and risk of gastric cancer: epidemiologic evidence. Cancer Sci. 2005;96(1):1–6.

79. Cohen AJ, Roe FJ. Review of risk factors for osteoporosis with particular reference to a possible aetiological role of dietary salt. Food Chem Toxicol. 2000;38(2–3):237–53.

80. Intersalt Cooperative Research Group. Intersalt: an international study of electrolyte excretion and blood pressure. Results for 24 hour urinary sodium and potassium excretion. BMJ. 1988;297(6644):319–28.

81. Institute of Medicine, Food and Nutrition Board. Dietary reference intakes (DRIs): recommended intakes for individuals. National Academy Press; 2004.

82. Clarkson P. Vitamins, iron, and trace minerals. In: Lamb D, Williams M, editors. Ergogenics: enhancement of performance in exercise and sport. Benchmark Press; 1991.

83. Pivarnik JM. Water and electrolytes during exercise. In: Hickson JF, Wolinsky I, editors. Nutrition in exercise and sport. CRC Press; 1989:185–200.

84. Turner MJ, Avolio AP. Does replacing sodium excreted in sweat attenuate the health benefits of physical activity? Int J Sport Nutr Exerc Metab. 2016;26(4):377–89.

85. Mielgo-Ayuso J, Maroto-Sánchez B, Luzardo-Socorro R, Palacios G, Gil-Antuñano NP, González-Gross. Evaluation of nutritional status and energy expenditure in athletes. Nutr Hosp. 2015;31(Suppl 3):227–36.

86. Brody T. Nutritional biochemistry. 2nd ed. Academic Press; 1999.

87. Mandal AK. Hypokalemia and hyperkalemia. Med Clin North Am. 1997;81(3):611–39.

88. Green DM, Ropper AH, Kronmal RA, Psaty BM, Burke GL. Serum potassium level and dietary potassium intake as risk factors for stroke. Neurology. 2002;59(3):314–20.

89. Trinchieri A, Zanetti G, Curro A, Lizzano R. Effect of potential renal acid load of foods on calcium metabolism of renal calcium stone formers. Eur Urol. 2001;39(Suppl 2):33–6.

90. Tucker KL, Hannan MT, Chen H, Cupples LA, Wilson PW, Kiel DP. Potassium, magnesium, and fruit and vegetable intakes are associated with greater bone mineral density in elderly men and women. Am J Clin Nutr. 1999;69(4):727–36.

91. Gennari FJ. Hypokalemia. N Engl J Med. 1998;339(7):451–8.

92. Wood RJ, Ronnenberg AG. Iron. In: Shils ME, Shike M, Ross AC, Caballero B, Cousins RJ, editors. Modern nutrition in health and disease. 10th ed. Lippincott Williams & Wilkins; 2006:248–70.

93. Ganz T. Does pathological iron overload impair the function of human lungs? EBioMedicine. 2017;20:13–14.

94. Gulec S, Anderson GJ, Collins JF. Mechanistic and regulatory aspects of intestinal iron absorption. Am J Physiol Gastrointest Liver Physiol. 2014;307(4):G397–409.

95. Wang W, Knovich MA, Coffman LG, Torti FM, Torti SV. Serum ferritin: past, present and future. Biochim Biophys Acta. 2010;1800(8):760–9.

96. Brittenham GM. Disorders of iron homeostasis: iron deficiency and overload. In: Hoffman R, Benz EJ Jr, Silberstein LE, Heslop H, Weitz J, Anastasi J, editors. Hematology: basic principles and practice. 6th ed. Elsevier; 2013.

97. Institute of Medicine, Food and Nutrition Board. Dietary reference intakes (DRIs): vitamin A, vitamin K, boron, chromium, copper, iodine, iron, manganese, molybdenum, nickel, silicon, vanadium, and zinc. National Academy Press; 2001:290–393.

98. McKay AKA, Peeling P, Pyne DB, Tee N, Whitfield J, Sharma AP, Heikura IA, Burke LM. Six days of low carbohydrate, not energy availability, alters the iron and immune response to exercise in elite athletes. Med Sci Sports Exerc. 2022;54(3):377–87.

99. McKay AKA, Peeling P, Pyne DB, Tee N, Welveart M, Heikura IA, Sharma AP, Whitfield J, Ross ML, van Swelm RPL, Laarakkers CM, Burke LM. Sustained exposure to high carbohydrate availability does not influence iron-regulatory responses in elite endurance athletes. Int J Sport Nutr Exerc Metab. 2021;31(2):101–8.

100. Aruoma OI, Reilly T, MacLauren D, Halliwell B. Iron, copper, and zinc concentrations in human sweat and plasma: the effect of exercise. Clin Chim Acta. 1988;177:81–7.

101. Baska RS, Moses FM, Graeber G, Kearney G. Gastrointestinal bleeding during an ultramarathon. Dig Dis Sci. 1990;35(2):276–9.

102. Waller M, Haymes E. The effects of heat and exercise on sweat iron loss. Med Sci Sports Exerc. 1996;28(2):197–203.

103. Shaskey DJ, Green GA. Sports haematology. Sports Med. 2000;29(1):27–38.

104. Balaban EP. Sports anemia. Clin Sports Med. 1992;11(2):313–25.

105. Wolinsky I, Driskell JA. Sports nutrition: vitamins and trace elements. CRC Press; 1997:148.

106. Stephenson LS. Possible new developments in community control of iron-deficiency anemia. Nutr Rev. 1995;53(2):23–30.

107. McCann JC, Ames BN. An overview of evidence for a causal relation between iron deficiency during development and deficits in cognitive or behavioral function. Am J Clin Nutr. 2007;85(4):931–45.

108. Wright RO. The role of iron therapy in childhood plumbism. Curr Opin Pediatr. 1999;11(3):255–8.

109. Yip R. Significance of an abnormally low or high hemoglobin concentration during pregnancy: special consideration of iron nutrition. Am J Clin Nutr. 2000;72(1 Suppl):272S–9S.

110. Oppenheimer SJ. Iron and its relation to immunity and infectious disease. J Nutr. 2001;131(2S-2):616S–33S.

111. Zhao L, Yang N, Song Y, Si H, Qin Q, Guo Z. Effect of iron overload on endothelial cell calcification and its mechanism. Ann Transl Med. 2021;9(22):1658.

112. McCall KA, Huang C, Fierke CA. Function and mechanism of zinc metalloenzymes. J Nutr. 2000;130(5S Suppl):1437S–46S.

113. O'Dell BL. Role of zinc in plasma membrane function. J Nutr. 2000;130 (5S Suppl):1432S–6S.

114. King JC, Cousins RJ. Zinc. In: Shils ME, Shike M, Ross AC, Caballero B, Cousins RJ, editors. Modern nutrition in health and disease. 10th ed. Lippincott Williams & Wilkins; 2006:271–85.

115. Boron B, Hupert J, Barch DH, Fox CC, Friedman H, Layden TJ, Mobarhan S. Effect of zinc deficiency on hepatic enzymes regulating vitamin A status. J Nutr. 1988;118(8):995–1001.

116. McKenna AA, Ilich JZ, Andon MB, Wang C, Matkovic V. Zinc balance in adolescent females consuming a low- or high-calcium diet. Am J Clin Nutr. 1997;65(5):1460–4.

117. Dressendorfer RH, Sockolov R. Hypozincemia in runners. Phys Sportsmed. 1980;8:97–100.

118. Haralambie G. Serum zinc in athletes during training. Int J Sports Med. 1981;2(3):135–8.

119. Singh A, Deuster PA, Moser PB. Zinc and copper status of women by physical activity and menstrual status. J Sports Med Phys Fitness. 1990;30:29–36.

120. Toro-Román V, Siquier-Coll J, Bartolomé I, Grijota FJ, Muñoz D, Maynar-Mariño M. Influence of physical training on intracellular and extracellular zinc concentrations. J Int Soc Sports Nutr. 2022;19(1):110–25.

121. Krotkiewski M, Gudmundsson M, Backstrom P, Mandroukas K. Zinc and muscle strength and endurance. Acta Physiol Scand. 1982;116:309–11.

122. Fischer PWF, Giroux A, L'Abbe MR. Effect of zinc supplementation on copper status in adult man. Am J Clin Nutr. 1984;40:743–46.

123. Hooper PL, Visconti L, Garry PJ, Johnson GE. Zinc lowers high-density lipoprotein cholesterol levels. JAMA. 1980; 244(17):1960–1.

124. Spencer H. Minerals and mineral interactions in human beings. J Am Diet Assoc. 1986;86(7):864–7.

125. McDonald R, Keen CL. Iron, zinc and magnesium nutrition and athletic performance. Sports Med. 1988;5(3):171–84.

126. MacDonald RS. The role of zinc in growth and cell proliferation. J Nutr. 2000;130(5S Suppl):1500S–08S.

127. Black MM. Zinc deficiency and child development. Am J Clin Nutr. 1998;68(2 Suppl):464S–9S.

128. Shankar AH, Prasad AS. Zinc and immune function: the biological basis of altered resistance to infection. Am J Clin Nutr. 1998;68(2 Suppl):447S–63S.

129. Evans JR, Henshaw K. Antioxidant vitamin and mineral supplements for preventing age-related macular degeneration. Cochrane Database Syst Rev. 2006;19(2):CD000254.

130. Krebs NF. Update on zinc deficiency and excess in clinical pediatric practice. Ann Nutr Metab. 2013;62(Suppl 1):19–29.

131. DeCook CA, Hirsch AR. Anosmia due to inhalational zinc: a case report. Chem Senses. 2000;25(5):659.

132. Zimmermann MB. Iodine and iodine deficiency disorders. In: Erdman JWJ, Macdonald IA, Zeisel SH, editors. Present knowledge in nutrition. 10th ed. John Wiley & Sons; 2012:554–67.

133. Leung AM, Braverman LE, Pearce EN. History of U.S. iodine fortification and supplementation. Nutrients. 2012;4(11): 1740–6.

134. Zanzonico PB, Becker DV. Effects of time of administration and dietary iodine levels on potassium iodide (KI) blockade of thyroid irradiation by 131I from radioactive fallout. Health Phys. 2000;78(6):660–7.

135. Koehler K, Achtzehn S, Braun H, Joachim M, Schaenzer W. Comparison of self-reported energy availability and metabolic hormones to assess adequacy of dietary energy intake in young elite athletes. Appl Physiol Nutr Metab. 2013;38(7): 725–33.

136. de Benoist B, McLean E, Andersson M, Rogers L. Iodine deficiency in 2007: global progress since 2003. Food Nutr Bull. 2008;29(3):195–202.

137. Caldwell KL, Makhmudov A, Ely E, Jones RL, Wang RY. Iodine status of the U.S. population, National Health and Nutrition Examination Survey, 2005–2006 and 2007–2008. Thyroid. 2011;21(4):419–27.

138. Institute of Medicine, Food and Nutrition Board. Dietary reference intakes (DRIs): selenium. Dietary reference intakes for vitamin C, vitamin E, selenium, and carotenoids. National Academy Press; 2000:284–324.

139. Zamora AJ, Tessier F, Marconnet P, Margaritis I, Marini JF. Mitochondria changes in human muscle after prolonged exercise, endurance training, and selenium supplementation. Eur J Appl Physiol Occup Physiol. 1995;71(6):505–11.

140. Ozan M, Buzdagli Y, Baygutalp NK, Yüce N, Baygutalp F, Bakan E. Serum BDNF and selenium levels in elite athletes exposed to blows. Medicina. 2022;58(5):608.

141. Packer L. Oxidants, antioxidant nutrients and the athlete. J Sports Sci. 1997;15(3):353–63.

142. Tessier F, Margaritis I, Richard MJ, Moynot C, Marconnet P. Selenium and training effects on the glutathione system and aerobic performance. Med Sci Sports Exerc. 1995;27(3):390–6.

143. Cooper A, Mones RL, Heird WC. Nutritional management of infants and children with specific diseases and other conditions. In: Ross AC, Caballero B, Cousins RJ, Tucker KL, Ziegler TR, editors. Modern nutrition in health and disease. 11th ed. Lippincott Williams & Wilkins; 2012:988–1005.

144. Naderi M, Puar P, Zonouzi-Marand M, Chivers DP, Niyogi S, Kwong RWM. A comprehensive review on the neuropathophysiology of selenium. Sci Total Environ. 2021;767:144329. https://doi.org/10.1016/j.scitotenv.2020.144329

145. Uauy R, Olivares M, Gonzalez M. Essentiality of copper in humans. Am J Clin Nutr. 1998;67(5 Suppl):952S–9S.

146. Vashchenko G, MacGillivray RT. Multi-copper oxidases and human iron metabolism. Nutrients. 2013;5(7):2289–313.

147. Kono S. Aceruloplasminemia. Curr Drug Targets. 2012;13(9):1190–9.

148. Toro-Román V, Siquiera-Coll J, Bartolemé I, Grijota FJ, Muñoz D, Maynar-Mariño M. Copper concentration in erythrocytes, platelets, plasma, serum and urine: influence of physical training. J Int Soc Sports Nutr. 2021;18(1):28.

149. Lukaski HC, Hoverson BS, Gallagher SK, Bolonchuk WW. Physical training and copper, iron, and zinc status of swimmers. Am J Clin Nutr. 1990;51(6):1093–9.

150. Koury JC, de Oliveira AV Jr, Portella ES, de Oliveira CF, Lopes GC, Donangelo CM. Zinc and copper biochemical indices of antioxidant status in elite athletes of different modalities. Int J Sport Nutr Exerc Metab. 2004;14(3):358–72.

151. Shaw JC. Copper deficiency and non-accidental injury. Arch Dis Child. 1988;63(4):448–55.

152. Barber RG, Grenier ZA, Burkhead JL. Copper toxicity is not just oxidative damage: zinc systems and insight from Wilson disease. Biomedicines. 2021;9(3):316.

153. Leach RM, Harris ED. Manganese. In: O'Dell BL, Sunde RA, eds. Handbook of nutritionally essential minerals. Marcel Dekker, Inc; 1997:335–55.

154. Yones MS, Shikara M, Almusawi YK, Munshid HQ. Effect of aerobic-anaerobic exercises on serum cobalt, chromium, manganese, molybdenum and phosphorous elements. Biochemical Cellular Archives. 2022;1:127–32.

155. Keen CL, Zidenberg-Cherr S. Manganese. In: Ziegler EE, Filer LJ, editors. Present knowledge in nutrition. 7th ed. ILSI Press; 1996:334–43.

156. Muszynska A, Palka J, Gorodkiewicz E. The mechanism of daunorubicin-induced inhibition of prolidase activity in human skin fibroblasts and its implication to impaired collagen biosynthesis. Exp Toxicol Pathol. 2000;52(2):149–55.

157. Keen CL, Ensunsa JL, Watson MH, Baly DL, Donovan SM, Monaco MH, Clegg MS. Nutritional aspects of manganese from experimental studies. Neurotoxicology. 1999;20(2–3):213–23.

158. Pal PK, Samii A, Calne DB. Manganese neurotoxicity: a review of clinical features, imaging and pathology. Neurotoxicology. 1999;20(2–3):227–38.

159. Wright RO, Amarasiriwardena C, Woolf AD, Jim R, Bellinger DC. Neuropsychological correlates of hair arsenic, manganese, and cadmium levels in school-age children residing near a hazardous waste site. Neurotoxicology. 2006;27(2):210–6.

160. Hua Y, Clark S, Ren J, Srccjayan N. Molecular mechanisms of chromium in alleviating insulin resistance. J Nutr Biochem. 2012;23(4):313–9.

161. Evans GW. The effect of chromium picolinate on insulin controlled parameters in humans. Int J Biosoc Res. 1989;11:163.

162. Clancy SP, Clarkson PM, DeCheke ME, Nosaka K, Freedson PS, Cunningham JJ, Valentine B. Effects of chromium picolinate supplementation on body composition, strength, and urinary chromium loss in football players. Int J Sport Nutr. 1994;4:142–53.

163. Hasten DL, Rome EP, Franks BD, Hegsted M. Effects of chromium picolinate on beginning weight training students. Int J Sport Nutr. 1992;2:343–50.

164. Stearns D, Wise JP, Patierno SR, Wetterhahn KE. Chromium (III) picolinate produces chromosome damage in Chinese hamster ovary cells. FASEB J. 1995;9(15):1643–8.

165. Saltiel AR, Kahn CR. Insulin signaling and the regulation of glucose and lipid metabolism. Nature. 2001;414(6865):799–806.

166. Kobla HV, Volpe SL. Chromium, exercise, and body composition. Crit Rev Food Sci Nutr. 2999;40(4):291–308.

167. Lukaski HC. Chromium as a supplement. Ann Rev Nutr. 1999;19:279–302.

168. Rech M, To L, Tovbin A, Smoot T, Mlynarek M. Heavy metal in the intensive care unit: a review of current literature on trace element supplementation in critically ill patients. Nutr Clin Pract. 2014;29(1):78–89.

169. Nielsen FH. Manganese, molybdenum, boron, chromium, and other trace elements. In: Erdman JJ, Macdonald I, Zelssel S, editors. Present knowledge of nutrition. John Wiley & Sons, Inc.; 2012.

170. Kato I, Vogelman JH, Dilman V, Karkoszka J, Frenkel K, Durr NP, Orentreich N, Toniolo P. Effect of supplementation with chromium picolinate on antibody titers to 5-hydroxymethyl uracil. Eur J Epidemiol. 1998;14(6):621–6.

171. Wasser WG, Feldman NS, D'Agati VD. Chronic renal failure after ingestion of over-the-counter chromium picolinate. Ann Intern Med. 1997;126(5):410.

172. United States Department of Agriculture, Agricultural Research Service, FoodDataCentral [Internet]. Accessed 2024 May 19. https://fdc.nal.usda.gov

CHAPTER 7

Hydration Issues in Athletic Performance

CHAPTER OBJECTIVES

- Explain the different compartments that hold body water and the factors that cause water shifts between these compartments.
- Know the mechanisms (organs, hormones, etc.) available to the human system for sustaining a state of water balance.
- Explain the major factors associated with causing a state of dehydration and hypohydration.
- Demonstrate how acclimated athletes are at lower risk of developing dehydration and hypohydration.
- Recognize how and why some people develop hypertension, and identify dietary strategies that can be followed to lower blood pressure (BP) in some individuals.

- Describe the reasons why some people are at higher risk of developing hypohydration.
- Describe the reasons why some people are at higher risk of developing hyponatremia.
- Explain how to induce shifts in extracellular osmolarity, and how these shifts can have an impact on blood volume and sweat rates.
- Analyze the current strategies available to endurance athletes for achieving a state of hyperhydration.
- Distinguish between **heat index** (HI), relative humidity, and temperature and how these may affect dehydration risk.

Case Study

Sally was an amazing, hard-working runner. She successfully ran 5Ks for her university, but was trying to run longer distances to try to compete for a spot on her country's 10K or marathon Olympic roster. She started training longer distances and found that her 10K time was getting gradually better. Sally entered her first 10K race and, to everyone's amazement, finished in the top three. With that success, she decided to work toward going the 26.2 miles for the marathon.

Her country was not known for producing top-notch marathoners, and Sally saw this as an excellent opportunity to make a name for herself. To prepare, Sally followed her proven formula for the 5K (3.1 miles) and 10K (6.2 miles) by gradually increasing her practice mileage in her morning run and her late afternoon run. To her surprise, she started "hitting the wall" after 10K, but figured if she persisted she

could eventually pass that barrier and go the distance. To her dismay, it did not happen. She just could not get her body to go past 10K without stopping, and she knew that stopping was a terrible way to win a race. She decided to call a retired elite marathoner to see if she could get some ideas for how to do better, and the marathoner asked her to write down her training protocol: "Sleep, Wake up, Glass of Orange Juice, Morning Practice Run, Shower, Dress, Breakfast . . . ." The marathoner realized right away what was happening, and asked the key question: "What do you drink during your morning run?" The answer was "Nothing . . . I never drink anything during my practice runs." The response was immediate: "You are trying to emulate your 5K training, but you are increasing the distance dramatically. You are running out of fuel and fluid, making it difficult to sustain normal blood sugar, normal

(continued)

blood volume, and the normal sweat rate, and making it impossible to adequately cool yourself. Try drinking a suitable fluid in the same pattern that you are able to drink during the Olympic marathon . . . every 5 kilometers."

So, Sally figured out how to put some beverages on the trunk of her car, run 2.5 km out and 2.5 km back, grab a drink, and repeat this pattern. Almost immediately the carbohydrates, electrolytes, and water in the beverage started helping and Sally was soon able to go the distance. She learned something critically important. It takes more than a desire to compete—you also must do the right things.

CASE STUDY DISCUSSION QUESTIONS

Background: Consider the nutrients Sally uses/loses quickly during a training run of approximately 10 km. Sally weighs 105 lb, is 25 years of age, and trains in typical environment of 70 °F with moderate humidity. Her practice time for the 10K is approximately 45 minutes, and she loses 4 lb of body weight from beginning to end of her training.

1. How much liquid should she consume to prevent the negative performance effects of dehydration? Use the sweat rate calculator below to predict how much she should drink, and the optimal volume to consume at timed intervals.

2. What are Sally's liquid needs during the practice run? Create a consumption/drinking pattern with a sports beverage of your making (you create the contents) that will satisfy Sally's needs during her 10K practice run, with a drinking frequency and volume that would be necessary. Consider the following:
   - Volume and drinking frequency of fluid
   - Electrolytes and their concentration
   - Carbohydrates and their concentration
   - Problems the runner may encounter
     - Gastric emptying
     - Delayed drinking
     - Diarrhea

Sweat Rate Calculator		
A. Body weight pre-exercise		[lb]
B. Body weight postexercise		[lb]
C. Change in body weight (an estimate of sweat loss)		["A" – "B", lb]
D. Conversion of sweat loss in lb to oz		[1 lb = 16 oz] "C" × 16
E. Volume of fluid consumed during exercise		[oz]
F. Unreplaced sweat loss in oz		"D" – "E"
G. Exercise time		[min]
H. Sweat rate per minute		[oz/min] "D"/"G"
I. Amount of *additional* fluid to be consumed per minute to match sweat rate (oz)		"F"/"H"
J. Calculate the volume of *additional* fluid to be consumed every 15 minutes to match sweat rate		"I" × 15
K. Calculate the total volume of fluid that should be consumed every 15 minutes to match sweat rate		"H" × 15

INTRODUCTION

It is difficult to imagine any nutrient more important for sustaining health and athletic performance than body water. A good hydration state ensures not only adequate total body water but also a good balance of **extracellular fluid (ECF)** and **interstitial fluid (ISF)**. Although all nutrients are required for sustaining health, the performance deficit that occurs in a poorly hydrated person, resulting in either **hypohydration** or **hyponatremia**, may occur more quickly and is more noticeable than with any other nutritional substance. Water is the single biggest component of human weight, ranging from ~50%–70% of body weight, depending on body composition. Athletes typically have more body water than nonathletes because of a greater proportion of lean tissue, which is composed of more water than

Table 7.1	Body Fat Percent and Body Water as Percent of Total Weight	
Body Fat Percent	**Body Water Percent**	
Females		
4–20	58–70	
21–29	52–58	
30–32	49–52	
33+	37–49	
Males		
4–14	63–70	
15–21	57–63	
22–24	55–57	
25+	37–55	

Source: Wang Z, Deurenberg P, Wang W, Pietrobelli A, Baumgartner RN, Heymsfield SB. Hydration of fat-free body mass: review and critique of a classic body-composition constant. Am J Clin Nutr. 1999;69(5):833–841.

fat tissue (fat tissue is essentially anhydrous) (Table 7.1) (1). People who live in moderate climates typically lose ~2.5 L (2.6 quarts) of water per day performing normal activities (2). Men working in hot climates can lose as much as 12 L (12.7 quarts) of water per day (3). Ultraendurance cyclists performing in a hot environment were found to lose up to 12.7 L (13.4 quarts) of water per day (4).

Extracellular Fluid (ECF)

This represents the fluid outside the cell and includes blood (*intravascular fluid [IVF]*) and interstitial water. The primary electrolyte controlling the volume of extracellular water is sodium. Blood-associated extracellular water is necessary as a transport agent for nutrients and oxygen to muscle, organs, fat, and skeletal cells and is necessary for transporting fluid to sweat glands. Low extracellular water is associated with low sweat rates and poor cooling capacity.

Interstitial Fluid (ISF)

The fluid that surrounds cells and is part of the ECF and that is not a component of blood (another component of the ECF). Excess interstitial water results in edema.

Intracellular Fluid (ICF)

ICF represents the fluid inside cells, which contains water, sugars, neurotransmitters, amino acids, and other small proteins involved in cellular function. The primary electrolyte controlling the volume of intercellular water is potassium.

Hypohydration

This represents the result of losing more body water than is replaced (*i.e.*, dehydration), resulting in a state of hypohydration. Severe hypohydration is associated with body water deficits of 6%–10% of body weight and is associated with reduced exercise performance, decreased cardiac output, lower sweat production, and reduced muscle blood flow. The urine osmolality when in a state of hypohydration is >900 mOsm/kg, whereas **euhydration** (definition follows) is <700 mOsm/kg. Although muscle cramps have multiple causes, including muscular fatigue, they may be associated with hypohydration and electrolyte imbalances.

Hyponatremia

The condition refers to low (hypo) sodium (na) in the blood (emia), which results in lower blood volume, poor blood flow to working muscles, lower sweat rates, headaches, nausea, and loss of balance. Blood sodium in a state of hyponatremia is <135 mmol/L. Blood volume is normalized on the main extracellular electrolyte, sodium, and when sodium is low, water leaves the blood to normalize the sodium concentration. The water goes to the surrounding tissue and creates edema, and if the edema occurs in the brain, it can cause serious confusion and a coma. In athletes, the likely cause of hyponatremia is overconsumption of fluids in excess of sweat and urinary losses or high consumption of sodium-free or hypotonic sports beverage (typically water), and as sodium is lost in the sweat but not replaced, hyponatremia occurs. Women typically are smaller than men and have lower sweat rates than men and may be at greater risk of overdrinking that could result in hyponatremia.

Euhydration

Also referred to as *normohydration*, this refers to being in a state of adequate or normal hydration that is associated with normal sweating capacity, good control of body temperature, adequate delivery potential of nutrients to body tissues, and adequate removal potential of metabolic by-products from body tissues. A euhydrated state is associated with a urinary osmolality of <700 mOsm/kg.

The elevated water loss in physical activity is the result of a basic reality: More energy is used by working tissues per unit of time during physical activity than when not active, and humans are relatively inefficient (typically ranging from 20% to 40%) at converting "burned" fuel to muscle movement. Therefore, about 60%–80% of this burned energy creates heat (5). Because humans must maintain a relatively stable body temperature of ~98.6 °F (37 °C), sweat is produced to dissipate this excess heat. The greater the intensity of activity, the greater the heat production and the greater the sweat loss to maintain body temperature. The requirement for water and associated

Table 7.2	Concentrations of Electrolytes in Sweat, Plasma, and Intracellular Water		
	Sweat (mmol/L)	Plasma (mmol/L)	Intracellular Water (mmol/L)
Sodium	**20–80**	130–155	10
Potassium	4–8	3.2–5.5	150
Calcium	0–1	2.1–2.9	0
Magnesium	<0.2	0.7–1.5	15
Chloride	**20–60**	96–110	8
Bicarbonate	0–35	23–28	10
Phosphate	0.1–0.2	0.7–1.6	65
Sulfate	0.1–2.0	0.3–0.9	10

Source: Maughan RJ. Fluid and electrolyte loss and replacement in exercise. In: Harries M, Williams G, Stanish WD, Micheli LL, editors. Oxford textbook of sports medicine. New York (NY): Oxford University Press; 1994, p. 82–93.

Table 7.3	Typical Daily Water Loss in an Inactive Man Weighing 70 kg (154 lb)	
Source of Water Loss	Amount (L)	Amount (oz)
Kidneys (urine)	1.40	47.3
Breathing (expired air)	0.32	10.8
Gastrointestinal tract (fecal matter)	0.10	3.4
Skin (perspiration/sweat)	0.65	22.0
Skin (insensible loss)	0.53	17.9
Total	**3.0**	**101.4**

The loss of body water increases dramatically through physical activity, with even greater water losses if the activity is of high intensity and performed in high heat and humidity. Water losses may also be increased through diarrhea and conditions that increase urinary volume output.

Source: Maughan RJ, Burke LM. Handbook of sports medicine and science, sports nutrition. Oxford: Wiley Blackwell; 2002, p. 52.

elements found in sweat is, therefore, determined by the amount of sweat that has been lost. (Table 7.2 shows the element concentrations typically found in sweat.)

Besides sweat, water is also lost through urine, fecal matter, breathing (expired air), and tears. However, unless someone is losing a great deal of water from diarrhea or following the consumption of a diuretic that induces increased urinary volume, nothing compares with the amount of water that can be lost through sweat (Table 7.3).

The *electrolytes* (the major intracellular electrolyte is potassium and the major extracellular electrolyte is sodium) influence the hydration state by determining the distribution of body water. By definition, electrolytes are substances that conduct electrical currents, such as a nerve impulse, and have either a negative charge (*anion*) or a positive charge (*cation*). The major electrolytes are sodium, chloride, potassium, magnesium, calcium, bicarbonate, and sulfate. As with all nutrients, *balance* is important. Providing too much of any of these electrolytes is just as problematic as providing too little. Because sodium, chloride, and potassium are of particularly high importance to water balance and in helping to determine where body water goes, these electrolytes are the focus of this chapter.

WATER HAS MANY FUNCTIONS

It is hard to imagine any normal body function that can take place without sufficient water in the system.

Body tissues require water for many essential functions, including:

- *Regulation of body temperature:* Because humans are not efficient at converting metabolized energy into muscular movement, with ~60%–80% of metabolized energy creating heat rather than participating in muscle movement. We cannot acquire the additional heat associated with higher energy metabolism (*i.e.,* we must sustain a nearly stable body temperature), so the excess heat is dissipated through the evaporation of sweat. As exercise is associated with more energy utilization per unit of time than when in a nonexercise state, having a strategy to efficiently dissipate the added heat creation is critical to training and avoiding early fatigue.

- *Nutrient transport:* Nutrients are transported to tissues via blood, which is primarily water. A drop in blood volume through inadequate replacement of water inhibits the normal transportation of nutrients to tissues and compromises tissue function. Lower blood volume requires that the heart work harder to deliver the needed nutrients and oxygen to tissues.

- *Joint lubrication:* Water is the major lubricant in joints, including the spine, helping to reduce stiffness and soreness. As an added benefit, sustaining a good hydration state helps to diminish the concentration in joints of potential inflammatory agents, such as uric acid. It has been reported that many novice runners fail to adequately hydrate themselves stop exercising after 1–2 months because of muscle and joint problems (6). It was also determined that hydration status is an independent predictor of joint function and athletic performance (7).

- *Metabolic waste removal:* Tissues are constantly producing metabolic waste products that must be removed, as they are potentially toxic. Nitrogenous waste, for instance, is highly toxic and requires chronic removal through urine. This removal takes place primarily through the kidneys, but waste products are also removed through the skin. Both urine (kidneys) and sweat (skin) production are water dependent. This is a multifactorial issue, as the lower blood volume associated with dehydration results in a hyperosmolar state (*i.e.,* more molecules/unit of blood), that makes it difficult for tissues to remove metabolic byproducts. In addition, the lower blood volume requires the production of highly concentrated urine as the body attempts to preserve as much body water as possible. This concentrated urine production may limit efficient metabolic by-product removal (8,9).
- *Digestion:* The digestion of foods into component nutrients and nonnutrient waste is highly water dependent from the very beginning (saliva) to the end (producing a lubricated stool that avoids constipation). Poor hydration inhibits digestion, absorption, and normal bowel function.
- *Absorption:* Absorption of nutrients through the intestinal wall and into the blood is water dependent. A poor hydration state inhibits the transfer of nutrients through the intestinal mucosa, negatively impacting nutrient absorption, and limiting the potential multiple benefits that are received from consumed foods. There is also evidence that the absorption of specific nutrients may be negatively impacted when in a state of dehydration. As an example, there is evidence that calcium absorption is reduced when dehydrated, increasing the risk of low bone mineral density if chronic (10,11).
- *Immunity:* Through blood and lymph, water distributes white blood cells, minerals, vitamins, and glucose to cell for normal cell function. The white blood cells and other immune system cells that are distributed to tissues improve disease resistance.

Other Functions of Water

Central Nervous System Function

The central nervous system (CNS) does not have a nutrient storage capacity, so must be fed continuously by nutrients and oxygen transported by blood, which is water based. Minor interruptions in blood flow to the CNS (brain ischemia) have the potential of causing neurologic damage and if the blood flow interruption continues, potentially, death. *Brain ischemia* is also referred to as cerebral ischemia or cerebrovascular ischemia and describes a condition in which insufficient blood flows to the brain to satisfy the brain's metabolic demands. The insufficient blood flow results in inadequate oxygen delivery (hypoxia) that may result in death of brain tissue and, potentially, cerebral infarction (ischemic stroke).

Cardiovascular Health

Sustaining a good hydration state enables the heart to more effectively pump blood to working muscles and other tissues. Maintenance of a good hydration state is an important principle for sustaining athletic performance and, importantly, reducing heart stress.

Sustaining Water Balance

Humans have multiple systems for sustaining water balance, but these systems can easily be strained with a gross failure to consume sufficient water and associated electrolytes. It has been estimated that, for sedentary people living in a temperate client, daily water turnover is ~2–2.5 L, but men and women working in hot environments may experience far higher sweat losses of up to 8–12 L (12,13).

Ideally, athletes should avoid a state of **dehydration** by consuming an appropriate mix of water and electrolytes in a timely manner. The goal should be to sustain a state of normal hydration rather than wait to drink to recover from dehydration. Water comes from multiple sources, including the fluids that are directly consumed, the water in fresh fruits and vegetables, and the water produced from energy metabolism (*e.g.,* Carbohydrate + Oxygen = Energy + Carbon Dioxide + Water), which provides ~1 mL water for each kilocalorie of energy expended (Table 7.4).

Dehydration

This represents a state of low body water, often the result of losing more water via sweat, vomiting, or diarrhea than was replaced, or simply a failure to consume sufficient fluids doing regular daily activities. Dehydration refers to the process of losing body water and, if it continues, results in a state of hypohydration. Dehydration is likely to be associated with a drop in blood volume, which results in lower cooling capacity as a result of lower sweat rate.

Table 7.4	The Water Content (Percent of Total Weight) of Foods Commonly Consumed
Very high water content (over 80%)	Plain oatmeal, soy milk, tofu, cooked brussels sprouts, cucumber, carrots, watermelon
High water content (65%–80%)	Cooked barley, hard-boiled egg, low-calorie salad dressings, bananas, most fish
Medium water content (50%–65%)	Cooked pinto beans, broiled ground beef, roasted chicken
Low water content (30%–50%)	Plain bagel, cheddar cheese, regular salad dressings
Very low water content (15%–30%)	Toasted whole wheat bread
Extremely low water content (below 15%)	Most ready-to-eat cereal, baked taco shell, regular peanut butter, fruit leather, sun dried tomatoes, raisins
No water content	White granulated sugar, oils

Source: USDA. Nutrition value of foods. Available from: https://www.ars.usda.gov/is/np/NutritiveValueofFoods/NutritiveValueofFoods.pdf

As physical activity is heat producing, requiring greater amounts of heat to be dissipated via sweat, athletes who become dehydrated must diminish the energy expended (*i.e.*, they must slow down) to produce less heat. Put simply, dehydrated athletes with fluid deficits >2% body weight can experience compromised cognitive function and reduced aerobic exercise performance, particularly if the exercise occurs in hot weather. Anaerobic performance deficits are more commonly seen with dehydration associated with 3%–5% loss of body weight. A failure to adequately consume fluids during exercise can easily ready these levels of performance impacting dehydration. Both power and endurance athletes who exercise for >2 hours can easily achieve a dehydration level of 5% loss of body weight with an associated decline in performance (14,15). There is concern that purposefully dehydrating to "make weight" prior to a competition may also negatively affect both health and performance (16). Common signs of dehydration include:

- Thirst
- Dry mouth and lips
- Flushed skin
- Headache
- Dizziness
- Dark-colored and strong-smelling urine
- Increased heart rate

Approximately 33% of total body water is in blood plasma and the spaces between cells (ECF), whereas ~66% of total body water is inside cells (ICF). The amount of water held in the body is affected by several factors, including body composition. The fat-free mass in a well-hydrated state is composed of about 72%–75% water, whereas the fat mass contains much less water of about 10%–20%, which is mainly from the plasma running through fat tissue (12). Fat itself is essentially anhydrous (*i.e.*, without water). Because females typically have higher body fat levels than

men, female bodies hold proportionately less water. A 70 kg (154 lb) male with average body composition has ~42 L (44.4 quarts) of water. (Note: 1 L of water = 1 kg, so 42 L = 42 kg or 92.4 lb water.) In this example, 60% of weight in the 70-kg male is water (Figure 7.1).

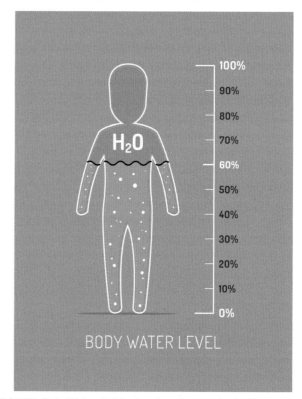

FIGURE 7.1: Water distribution in a human body. The average adult male body is approximately 60% water. Average adult females have slightly less body water, and average children have slightly more body water. Higher body fat levels are associated with lower total body water as a percent of weight. (From Szlyk PC, Sils IV, Francesconi RP, Hubbard RW, Armstrong LE. Effects of water temperature and flavoring onvoluntary dehydration in men. Physiol Behav. 1989;45(3):639–47. Zoran Milic/Shutterstock.com)

- 66% of a person's total body weight is from water
- 65% of total body water is intracellular
- 35% of total body water is extracellular
- Well-hydrated muscles are about 75% water
- Bones are about 22% water
- Fat is essentially anhydrous, having only about 10% water content
- Blood is about 83% water
- Average males are about 60% water weight
- Average females are about 50% water weight
- Obese individuals are about 40% water weight
- Athletes are about 70% water weight

The loss of body water is also affected by a number of factors, including:

- *Ambient temperature:* Higher temperature results in greater water loss through higher sweat rates. The body has to remove heat associated with higher energy metabolism and also must remove heat associated with higher temperature.
- *Ambient humidity:* Higher humidity results in greater loss through higher sweat rates. It is difficult to evaporate water (sweat) into a high-water (high-humidity) environment. As a result, cooling capacity is less efficient so more sweat is produced in an attempt to improve cooling (Figure 7.2).
- *Age:* Several studies have suggested that the temperature regulation of preadolescent children is as effective as an adult (17,18). However, most studies have found that temperature thermoregulation in young (preadolescent) children and older adults is less effective as that in young adults (19–23). A recent study found that young boys and adult men had similar thermoregulatory responses to 80 minutes of exercise in the heat performed at a fixed metabolic heat production. However, sweat volume was found to be lower in boys, despite similarities in the absolute metabolic heat production and the evaporative heat balance requirement (24).
- *Urinary loss:* Urine is always being produced to excrete metabolic by-products and as a means of adjusting the concentration of intercellular (inside the cell) and extracellular (outside the cell, including blood plasma) electrolytes and total body water volume. Certain substances may induce a diuretic effect, including high-potassium foods (*e.g.*, fresh fruits and vegetables) and drugs consumed for the purpose of lowering blood volume (*e.g.*, Lasix, Aldactone, Dyazide).
- *Gastrointestinal (GI) (fecal) loss:* The typical loss of water from the GI tract is relatively low (~0.10 L/day). However, a state of diarrhea can dramatically increase GI tract water loss to 100× more. Any number of conditions may result in diarrhea, including bacterial infection (*e.g.*, rotavirus, *Escherichia coli*), consumption of foods/food substances that the individual has an intolerance to (*e.g.*, lactose intolerance), or heavy consumption of high osmolar substances that have a slow absorption rate (*e.g.*, the food additive sorbitol or the sweetener high-fructose corn syrup [HFCS]).

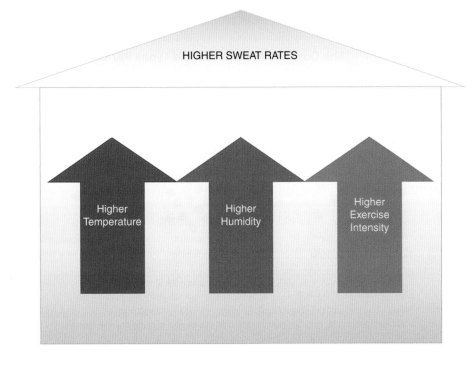

FIGURE 7.2: Sweat rates during different climatic conditions. Combinations of any of these three result in even higher sweat rates.

HFCS is a commonly used sweetener in sodas and other sweetened beverages. Because fructose requires absorption in the small intestine through a specialized receptor (GLUT-5 transporter), the absorptive capacity is limited and may result in delayed absorption. This delayed absorption may protect the liver from excessive fructose exposure but contributes to a high level of free molecules in the small intestine (25).

■ *Protein consumption:* Excess protein consumption, either in a single meal or over the course of a day, is associated with dehydration, even in athletes who consume the same amount of fluid as athletes consuming less protein. The dehydration is caused by the requirement to remove nitrogen from the excess protein. The resulting elevated blood urea nitrogen (BUN) must be removed via urine, resulting in an increased urine formation and fluid loss (26,27).

■ *Salt consumption:* Blood volume is, to a great degree, determined by the availability of sodium. Low salt (sodium chloride) consumption has the effect of lowering blood volume and increasing water loss. High salt consumption requires the formation of more urine to excrete the excess, as the body attempts to maintain urine osmolarity (28) (Figure 7.3).

■ *Clothing:* The type of clothing worn may influence the ability to dissipate heat via sweat. Clothing made of material (*e.g.*, cotton) that traps water results in ineffective cooling because of lower evaporation, resulting in more sweat formation and greater water loss. Some athletic clothing is made of materials specifically designed to release water and enhance evaporative cooling. These moisture-wicking materials help to transport liquid to the surface, thereby enhancing evaporation and cooling.

■ *Conditioned state:* People who are physically fit and well acclimated to the environmental conditions are capable of producing more sweat to enhance cooling, and the sodium content of the sweat produced is lower than that in less well-conditioned people, enabling better maintenance of plasma volume.

Athletes exercising *intensely* for 45 minutes or longer, particularly in high heat and humidity, will experience some degree of dehydration. For athletes exercising most days, as is common for elite athletes, postexercise fluid consumption becomes a critically important part of the exercise regimen because it allows the athlete to begin each subsequent day of activity in a well-hydrated state. The less time there is to rehydrate, the lower the likelihood that the athlete will be capable of becoming optimally hydrated by the beginning of the next exercise session. Because maximal absorption rates are lower than maximal sweat rates, athletes consuming fluids during intense exercise are, at best, only likely to provide 70% of fluid lost via sweat. Studies have shown that most athletes replace sweat losses at a rate significantly lower than this (29,30). Therefore, athletes require a planned rehydration strategy *before* the next exercise session begins. Despite this need, athletes are known to remain in an underhydrated state even when fluids are made available to them (31). This resulting voluntary dehydration suggests that athletes should be placed on a fixed fluid replacement schedule that will decrease the degree to which this dehydration is maintained. A way of encouraging this is to make certain that good-tasting fluids are easily available to the athlete as soon as the exercise session is over (32).

FIGURE 7.3: Osmolality: Illustration of different concentrations of particles in solution. Dehydration, which often occurs in athletes from a failure to consume a sufficient volume of an electrolyte/fluid beverage (*i.e.*, a sports beverage) commonly results in a high particle concentration in the blood (a hyper-osmolar solution). A hyper-osmolar solution may also occur in athletes who consume a high level of electrolytes without consuming sufficient water. A hypo-osmolar solution may occur in athletes who consume large volumes of water without consuming sufficient electrolytes.

The Concentration of Particle Types Per Unit Volume of Fluid Determines Osmolarity and Osmolality

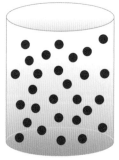

Normal Osmolar Solution

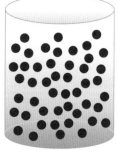

Hyper-Osmolar Solution

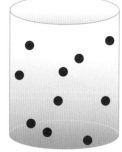

Hypo-Osmolar Solution

Osmolarity: The total concentration of all active solute particles in solution, typically expressed as osmoles/liter of solution.

Osmolality: The total dissolved particles in solution, typically reflecting the concentration of sodium, potassium, chloride, glucose, and urea in a sample of blood or urine, typically expressed as osmoles/liters of solution.

Systems for Regulating Water Balance

Important Factors to Consider

- Total body water volume = ~60% of total body weight
- Extracellular Fluid (ECF) volume = ~20% of body weight
  - *IVF:* On average, ~3.5 L (~20% of ECF) of fluid that is inside the blood vessels (*i.e.,* the blood plasma) and the fluid that makes up lymph.
  - *ISF:* On average, ~10.5 L (~80% of ECF) of fluid in the space that surrounds cells, but does not include blood plasma or lymph.
- Intracellular Fluid (ICF) volume = ~40% of body weight
  - *ICF:* On average, ~28 L of fluid contained inside cells.
  - The approximate volume of the different fluid compartments is provided only for relative comparison purposes. Fluid shifts occur between compartments because of hydrostatic and osmotic pressure and because of changes in body temperature. As an example, water shifts to the skin to enhance the sweat rate when body temperature rises.

Fluid Balance

Sustaining water balance involves assuring the volume of water lost equals the amount of water that is replaced. Water is always being lost through breathing, insensible (not noticed) skin loss, sweat (noticeable water on the skin), urine, and the GI tract (fecal loss). We replace water through the drinks we consume, from the water in foods we consume, and through the water created from energy

Table 7.5	Water Balance	
Water out = Water in		
Air (breathing)	Drinks	
Skin loss (insensible)	Foods	
Skin loss (sweat)	Water of metabolism	
Urine		
Feces		

Source: United States Department of Agriculture, Agricultural Research Service, 2012. Accessed 2016 November 4. Available from: http://www.ars.usda.gov/ba/bhnrc/ndl

metabolism (Table 7.5). It is important to consider how different beverages compare to water in their capacity to sustain or improve the hydration state. Referred to as the Beverage Hydration Index (BHI), it has been established that the combination of electrolytes and carbohydrate in water helps to enhance the hydration state (33).

ELECTROLYTES

Sodium and Chloride (Salt)

Sodium and chloride are consumed as salt, and both of these electrolytes are involved in multiple body functions (see Table 7.6). Importantly, sodium (Na^+) and chloride (Cl^-)

Table 7.6	Electrolyte Functions and Homeostasis
General functions	■ Distribution of body fluids through osmosis and the sodium–potassium pump ■ Acid–base balance (pH and buffers) ■ Regulation of nerve impulse transmission ■ Muscle contractility
Sodium (Na^+)	■ The main extracellular fluid (ECF) electrolyte ■ 40% found in bones, 10% in intracellular fluid (ICF), and 50% in ECF ■ Kidneys regulate excretion (the aldosterone system) ■ Lost through both sweat and urine
Potassium (K^+)	■ The main ICF electrolyte ■ Maintains fluid balance in the ICF environment ■ In enzymatic reactions involving protein and glycogen synthesis ■ Nerve and muscle activity ■ Kidneys excrete K even when dietary intake is low ■ Excessive loss of K may lead to cardiac dysrhythmias that can be fatal ■ High potassium may be protective against hypertension ■ Very high potassium intake may result in cardiac dysrhythmias that can be fatal
Chloride (Cl^-)	■ The main anion (–) in ECF ■ Required for acid–base balance ■ Required for nerve impulse transmission ■ Part of HCl produced in the stomach and required for normal digestion

are the main electrolytes of the ECF, which includes blood plasma (34). The main cation (positively charged ion) inside the cells is potassium, whereas sodium is the primary cation outside the cell in the ECF. Although both potassium and sodium exist inside and outside cells, the concentration of sodium is ten times higher outside the cell than inside, and the concentration of potassium is thirty times higher inside the cell than outside. Pumps in the cell membrane use energy to remove sodium from inside the cell in exchange for potassium. The energy usage in this process is significant, accounting for ~20%–40% of the resting energy used by average adults (35). These concentration differences between the primary intercellular and extracellular electrolytes impact cell membranes and account for multiple functions that include fluid shifts between the intercellular and extracellular environments, muscle contraction (including cardiac function), and nerve impulse transmission (Table 7.6) (36).

Sodium absorption influences the absorption of other nutrients, including amino acids, monosaccharides (primarily glucose), chloride, and water. Chloride is a major component of the hydrochloric acid in the stomach and lowers the gastric pH to enable the digestion of proteins and other nutrients (37).

Because sodium is the primary cation in the ECF (including blood volume), blood volume is, to a large extent, controlled through processes that regulate sodium. Greater sodium consumption results in either higher blood volume or higher urinary sodium losses. Receptors that monitor BP and blood osmolarity communicate changes to the hypothalamus, which forms vasopressin (arginine vasopressin and antidiuretic hormone [ADH]). The two main actions of vasopressin are (36):

■ Regulation of ECF volume by influencing renal processing of water. Vasopressin results in decreased urine formation (hence the name "ADH") that ultimately results in greater blood volume and BP (Figure 7.4).
■ Vasoconstriction that serves to compensate for low blood volume by increasing vascular resistance.

The release of vasopressin results primarily from the following conditions:

■ *Hypovolemia (low blood volume).* The decrease in blood volume is detected by receptors in the arterial wall, which signals the hypothalamus to release vasopressin by the pituitary gland.
■ *Hypotension (low BP).* The lower BP stimulates vasopressin release through sympathetic nerve activity.

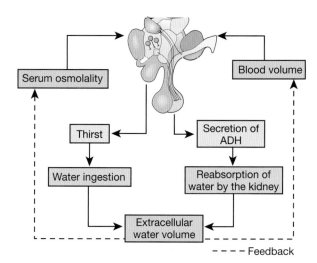

FIGURE 7.4: Production of antidiuretic hormone (ADH). (From Lippincott Professional Development. Philadelphia [PA]: LWW; 2014 August.)

■ *Rise in osmolarity (high blood sodium).* The increase in osmolarity, typical of what occurs in dehydration, stimulates vasopressin release.

When osmolarity is low (low blood sodium), aldosterone is produced through a cascade of reactions that are stimulated through the release of renin. Renin converts angiotensinogen to angiotensin I, which is then converted to angiotensin II. Angiotensin II not only constricts blood vessels to increase BP but also stimulates the production of aldosterone (Figure 7.5). Aldosterone causes the kidneys to retain sodium, which eventually results in higher blood osmolarity and an increase in plasma volume and BP (36). See Figure 7.5.

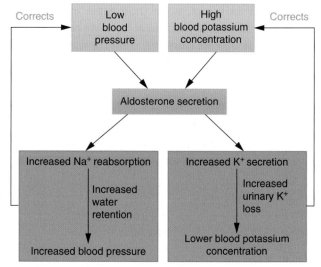

FIGURE 7.5: Production of aldosterone. (From Cohen BJ, Hull K. Memmler's the human body in health and disease. 13th ed. Philadelphia [PA]: LWW (PE); 2015.)

Table 7.7		Adequate Intake for Sodium and the Equivalent Salt (Sodium Chloride) Required to Achieve This Level of Intake	
Group	Age (Y)	Male and Female Sodium Intake (g/day)	Male and Female Salt Intake (g/day)
Adolescents	14–18	1.5	3.8
Adults	19–50	1.5	3.8
Adults	51–70	1.3	3.3
Adults	71+	1.2	3.0
Pregnancy	14–50	1.5	3.8
Breastfeeding	14–50	1.5	3.8

The full table that included the recommended intake levels for infants and children is included in the online Appendix.

Source: Institute of Medicine, Food and Nutrition Board. Sodium and chloride. dietary reference intakes for water, potassium, sodium, chloride, and sulfate. Washington (DC): National Academies Press; 2005. p. 269–423.

It is not common for people to experience a salt (sodium chloride) deficiency as a result of inadequate dietary intake. However, it has been found that hyponatremia (hypo = low; NA = sodium; emia = blood plasma; low plasma sodium) may occur in athletes who exercise for long periods in a hot environment and fail to consume sufficient sodium during the exercise (38). Severe vomiting and/or diarrhea and the use of some diuretics (chlorthalidone) that induce sodium loss may also result in hyponatremia (39). More information on hyponatremia is included later in this chapter.

The recommended intake for sodium is based on the adequate intake (AI) level to replace the loss of sodium through sweat in moderate activity (Table 7.7). Please note that the average consumption of sodium is well above the level recommended by the Food and Nutrition Board (37).

Disease Risks With Excess Intake of Salt

There are several disease risks associated with chronic consumption of excess sodium, which is far more prevalent than underconsumption of sodium. The 2015–2020 Dietary Guidelines for Americans recommend that Americans consume less than 2,300 mg of sodium per day as part of a healthy eating pattern. According to the Centers for Disease Control and Prevention (40), 90% of children and 89% of adults aged 19 and older consume more than 3,400 mg/day, or over 1,000 mg more per day than the recommended maximum. Recent findings indicate that the global sodium intake is 3,960 mg/day (41). Reading the label to help understand the level of sodium in packaged foods is useful (Table 7.8). Please note that the label refers to the *per serving* amount, which may be a lower amount than people are accustomed to eating.

Important Factors to Consider

- Most people have effective mechanisms for excreting excess sodium in the urine. However, about 10% of the population is missing these mechanisms, putting them at high risk of retaining too much sodium with a resultant high BP (hypertension). Sustained high BP is a risk factor for cardiovascular and kidney disease, making it important for *everyone* to have BP checked periodically to determine if he or she is hypertensive.
- People with hypertension must be cautious about how much salt they consume and are also encouraged to eat foods high in potassium to help pull fluid out of the blood and into cells to help control blood volume/BP.

Table 7.8	Interpreting the Sodium Content on Nutrition Facts Label in Packaged Foods	
Label	Meaning	
Sodium free	Less than 5 mg sodium per serving	
Salt free	Less than 5 mg sodium per serving	
Very low sodium	35 mg sodium or less per serving	
Low sodium	140 mg sodium or less per serving	
Reduced sodium or less sodium	At least 25% lower sodium than the regular product	
No salt added	The amount of sodium per serving must be listed on the label	

Hypertension

There is clear evidence that chronic consumption of a high level of salt increases the risk of high BP, whereas lowering salt consumption lowers BP (42,43). Chronic high BP is associated with heart disease and early death (44,45). Some individuals are more sensitive to sodium intake than others, including those with diagnosed hypertension. Higher sodium sensitivity risk is also seen in people who are overweight, African-Americans, and older adults (46). It is likely that many of these high-risk individuals have a genetic predisposition to sustaining an elevated aldosterone production, which inhibits sodium excretion (47). The type of foods consumed may have a desirable change in BP. Consumption of the Dietary Approaches to Stop Hypertension (DASH) diet, which is high in fruits, vegetables, whole grains, poultry, fish, low-fat dairy, and nuts, has been effective in lowering BP in people who have hypertension (48).

Kidney Stones

Elevated dietary intake of salt is associated with greater excretion of urine calcium, and kidney stones are strongly associated with high calcium in the urine. It has been found that high sodium intakes (~5,000 mg/day) result in a 30% increase in developing kidney stones when compared with people consuming less sodium (~1,500 mg/day) (49). Other studies have found that lowering sodium intake lowers the risk of developing kidney stones (50).

Gastric Cancer

The chronic consumption of high-salt foods (Table 7.9) has been found to increase gastric cancer risk. High-salt foods may inflame the stomach lining, which increases the possibility of bacterial infection (*Helicobacter pylori*) that is associated with gastric ulcers and cancer (51). The original associations between salt intake and gastric cancer were found in Asian populations, where the consumption of high-salt foods is common (52,53).

Osteoporosis

The development of strong bones involves many factors, including adequate availability of calcium and vitamin D, adequate bone stress, estrogen availability (in women), and adequate energy intake. Any single factor may compromise bone mineral density, and there is concern that high sodium consumption may be a negative factor in bone health. Because high levels of sodium intake are known to elevate calcium excretion, there is concern that this calcium loss may increase the risk of developing low bone density. Although more studies are needed to confirm this risk, a study has found that postmenopausal women with high-salt consumption had lower bone mineral density in the hip (54).

Potassium

Although sodium is the primary cation (positively charged electrolyte) outside cells, potassium (K^+) is the primary cation inside cells. The different concentrations of potassium and sodium inside and outside cells create an electrochemical "charge" in the cell membrane. The cell's membrane uses this electrical charge to pump sodium out of the cell and potassium into the cell and,

Table 7.9	A Sampling of Sodium and Salt Content in Foods Commonly Consumed		
Foods	Amount	Sodium (mg)	Sodium Chloride (Salt) (mg)
Orange juice	1 cup	0	0
Almonds (unsalted)	1 cup	1	3
Tomato	1 medium (fresh)	6	15
Carrot	1 medium (fresh)	42	105
Bread, whole wheat	2 slices	264	660
Cereal, cornflakes	1 cup	266	665
Dill pickle	1 spear	300	800
Hot dog (beef)	1 hot dog	510	1,300
Ham	3 oz	1,000	2,500
Pretzels (salted)	2 oz or 10 pretzels	1,000	2,500
Macaroni and cheese	1 cup (from canned)	1,300	3,300

Source: United States Department of Agriculture. National Nutrient Database for Standard Reference, Release 28.

Table 7.10	A Sampling of Potassium Sources in Foods Commonly Consumed	
Foods	Serving Size	Potassium (mg)
Almonds	1 oz	200
Orange	1 medium (fresh)	237
Sunflower seeds	1 oz	241
Tomato	1 medium (fresh)	292
Raisin bran cereal	1 cup	362
Banana	1 medium (fresh)	422
Acorn squash	½ cup (cooked)	448
Lima beans	½ cup (cooked)	485
Raisins	½ cup	598
Plums, dried (prunes)	½ cup	637
Potato (with skin)	1 medium (baked)	926

Source: United States Department of Agriculture. National Nutrient Database for Standard Reference, Release 28.

in doing so, is involved in muscle contraction and nerve impulse transmission.

Besides this critically important cell membrane function, potassium is also involved in carbohydrate metabolism through the enzyme *pyruvate kinase* (55). The AI level, established by the Food and Nutrition Board of the Institute of Medicine, is 4,700 mg/day for all adolescents and adults, both male and female, and is found to satisfy potassium needs while having the effect of lowering BP and lowering the risk for kidney stones. The recommended potassium intake for breastfeeding women is slightly higher (5,100 mg/day). (See the online Appendix for the full recommended intakes, including infants and children.) Dietary surveys of the US population indicate that potassium intake is approximately half of the recommended level (Table 7.10) (56). As a general rule, fruits and vegetables are an excellent source of dietary potassium.

Potassium Deficiency

Potassium deficiency is referred to as *hypokalemia* (hypo = low; k = potassium; emia = blood) and typically results from excess potassium loss rather than inadequate intake (57). Conditions associated with high potassium losses include diarrhea and vomiting, excess use of laxatives, high alcohol consumption, some prescribed diuretics (thiazide and/or furosemide), and depletion of magnesium. Congestive heart failure is associated with

hypokalemia, as is high consumption of black licorice or drinks and products containing licorice. Licorice contains an acid (glycyrrhizic acid) that increases urinary excretion of potassium while retaining sodium (58).

Several studies suggest that the combination of excess salt consumption, coupled with inadequate potassium intake, increases the risk for several diseases, including hypertension, kidney stones, osteoporosis, and stroke. The current recommendations for greater consumption of fresh fruits and vegetables are, to a large degree, to lower sodium intake and elevate potassium intake to reduce these disease risks.

Hypertension

Studies examining the dietary intakes of Americans have found that those with higher intakes of potassium have lower BP than those with lower intakes of potassium (56). The DASH diet has provided additional evidence that higher potassium intakes help to lower BP (59).

Kidney Stones

High levels of calcium loss via urine increase kidney stone risk, and it has been found that low potassium intakes increase urinary calcium (60). This is a powerful relationship, as several studies found that diets high in potassium or with a high potassium intake relative to animal protein consumption significantly reduced the incidence of kidney stone development (60,61).

Osteoporosis

There is strong evidence that higher potassium intakes are protective of bones, likely because potassium helps to develop bicarbonate, which buffers acidity. A failure to provide sufficient potassium lowers bicarbonate formation, forcing the removal of calcium from bone to use calcium as a buffer. Greater consumption of fruits and vegetables has the effect of buffering system acidity, helping to keep calcium in bones (62,63).

Potassium Toxicity

Although it is more common for people to consume insufficient potassium, potassium toxicity may occur when the intake of potassium is greater than the capacity of the kidneys to clear the excess (1). This condition, referred to as *hyperkalemia*, is most likely to occur with intakes of prescribed supplements that exceed 18,000 mg in a single dose. Hyperkalemia may also occur with severe trauma, such as a burn that covers a large proportion of the body, damages cells, and causes a sudden elevated plasma potassium. Some nonprescription medications, including nonsteroidal anti-inflammatory drugs (NSAIDs), are associated with hyperkalemia, as are some prescription antihypertensive agents (β-blockers, etc.) (64).

EXERCISE AND THE BALANCE OF FLUIDS AND ELECTROLYTES

Important Factors to Consider

- Exercise increases the *rate* at which energy is burned. Greater energy expenditure results in more heat production, and because humans are only ~30% efficient at converting metabolized fuel to energy, ~70% of all metabolized energy burned creates heat that must be dissipated to avoid a potentially dangerous rise in body temperature.
- The primary system humans have for removal of heat is the evaporation of sweat. Because exercise increases the necessity to remove heat, the *rate* at which fluids are lost is increased to maintain body temperature. The greater the energy expenditure per unit of time (*i.e.*, the greater the exercise intensity), the greater the heat production, and the greater the sweat rate to dissipate the produced heat.

FIGURE 7.6: Systems for adding and removing heat in an exercising athlete. (From Sawka MN, Latzka WA, Montain SJ. Effects of dehydration and rehydration on performance. In: Maughan RJ, editor. Nutrition in sport. London: Blackwell Science; 2000. p. 205–17.)

Systems for Adding and Removing Heat

There are multiple ways that an athlete can acquire heat and multiple ways that an athlete can dissipate the acquired heat (Figure 7.6).

Factors That Affect Body Temperature

The following factors affect body temperature in humans:

- Solar radiation
- Air temperature
- Air humidity
- Ground thermal radiation
- Ground-reflected solar radiation
- Energy metabolism (contracting muscle, etc.)
- Sweat
- Respiration
- Convection
- Clothing or protective equipment
- Wind
- Conditioned state

Regardless of the source of heat or cooling, the body must maintain a relatively constant temperature to avoid thermal stress (too cold or too hot) (Figure 7.7).

Physical activity creates heat, which must be dissipated for the athlete to continue the activity. Failure to dissipate

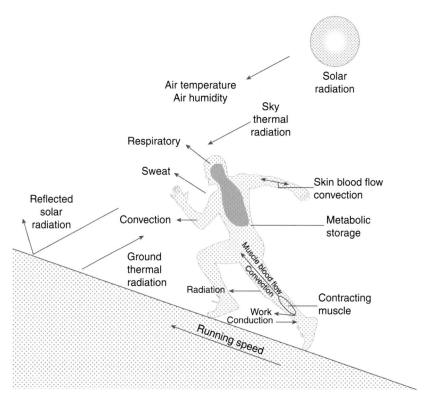

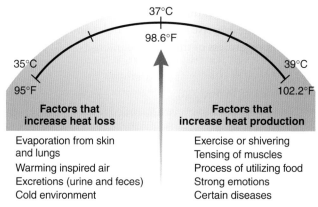

FIGURE 7.7: Heat balance equation. (From Kronenberger J, Ledbetter J. Lippincott Williams & Wilkins' comprehensive medical assisting. 5th ed. Philadelphia [PA]: WK Health and Pharmacy; 2016.)

sufficient heat may elevate core body temperature to a point that results in heat illness and, if severe, death. The primary system for dissipating heat is the production of sweat, the evaporation of which has a cooling effect. It should be obvious that inadequate sweat production results in poor heat removal and heat stress. Temperature regulation represents the balance between heat produced or gained (heat in) and heat removed (heat out), and when working correctly, these are in balance and body temperature is maintained. Both internal and external factors can contribute to body heat. Radiant heat from the sun contributes to body temperature, and the heat created from burning fuel also contributes to body temperature. Somehow, the body must dissipate the same amount of heat that has been acquired to sustain constant body temperature.

Exercise increases heat production significantly, requiring the loss of this excess heat. The body moves heat from the muscles to the skin where the heat can be removed to the surrounding environment. This makes blood flow to the skin important during physical activity (65). Once at the skin, heat can be removed via evaporation, conduction, radiation, and convection (see Figure 7.7):

- *Conduction: Heat transfer driven by temperature difference.* Because air has a high thermal resistance, heat transfer from the body to the air is a minor mechanism for heat loss in humans. This is also a minor contributor to body temperature maintenance, except where athletes are exposed to cold surfaces, such as figure skaters and hockey players.
- *Convection: Heat transfer via movement of fluids.* When a fluid passes by tissue, it absorbs the higher heat of the tissue and transfers the heat via convection to cooler tissue. This is a minor contributor to body temperature maintenance, except in athletes who

are exposed to cold air, such as mountain climbers, or cold water, such as swimmers. When the ambient temperature is very high (above body temperature), convection can *add* heat to the body.

- *Moving more blood to the skin to allow heat dissipation through radiation.* Heat is removed from all hot objects (hotter than the environment) via radiation, much like a heat radiator in the home. Sun radiation can add heat to the body, whereas radiative cooling occurs when the athlete is in an environment cooler than the body temperature. This is typically a minor contributor to body temperature maintenance, except when the athlete is in direct sunlight or in a cold environment.
- *Increasing the rate of sweat production and evaporation.* This involves changing the state of the heat transfer vehicle (fluid) to a vapor (evaporation) and is the major contributor to body temperature maintenance during exercise. Approximately 80% of the heat removal during vigorous exercise is the result of sweat evaporating off the skin (65).

These systems account for the majority of thermoregulation, but during exercise, the majority of all heat loss occurs via the evaporation of sweat. Sustaining the sweat rate relies on maintenance of the plasma (blood) volume. Lowering the blood volume results in lower blood flow to the skin with a reduction in sweat production. Exercise increases the requirement for blood that goes beyond the production of sweat. Exercise also increases the blood flow requirement to working muscles to satisfy the demand for energy and nutrients and to remove the metabolic by-products of burned fuel. Lower blood volume compromises that capacity to satisfy all of these requirements, resulting in decreased athletic performance. The maintenance of blood volume is sufficiently important for athletic performance that many consider it to be the primary factor determining if physical work can continue at a high intensity.

The metabolism of energy is only about 20%–40% efficient, resulting in a high level of heat production. As the rate of energy metabolism increases (*i.e.*, more intense work per unit of time), heat creation is also increased. This heat cannot be acquired and must be dissipated, so the heat-removal systems must be turned up. High-intensity activity may increase heat production to a level 20 times greater than the heat produced while at rest (66). Failure to dissipate this higher level of exercise-associated heat production may put the athlete at risk for heat illness, with an even higher risk of heat illness if environmental heat and humidity are additional contributors to heat stress. There is a large variability in sweat rates during physical activity, depending on exercise duration and intensity, fitness of the athlete, and how well the athlete has acclimatized to the environment (*e.g.*, heat, altitude, humidity). Consider that a well-trained athlete who is training in a hot and humid environment commonly loses 1–1.5 L of fluid per hour and may lose 2.4 L of fluid per hour or more (67–69).

Heat Index

The HI (also called the apparent temperature) combines the temperature and relative humidity in the immediate surroundings to provide a value of how humans *perceive* the temperature. A high HI results in greater sweat rates because high humidity results in less effective cooling from sweat evaporation (it is difficult to evaporate the water of sweat into high water content of the environment). As a result, the sweat volume is increased in an attempt to achieve better cooling. High HI values may make it extremely difficult or impossible to achieve adequate sweat-related cooling, making activities dangerous because of the higher risk of heat illness (Figure 7.8; also see Figure 7.2). As demonstrated in Figure 7.2, exercising

in higher heat and humidity results in higher sweat rates than when the exercise occurs in a cooler and dryer environment, regardless of the exercise intensity.

> **Heat Index**
>
> A measure of the combined temperature and humidity is calculated for shady areas.

Wet Bulb Globe Temperature

The **wet bulb globe temperature** (WBGT) represents the relative heat stress experienced from a combination of direct sunlight, temperature, humidity, wind speed, sun angle, and cloud cover, which affects solar radiation. Although the multiple factors used to predict the WBGT may be difficult to simultaneously measure, the factors used to predict WBGT make it an important index for predicting the heat stress that may be faced by an athlete (70). It is for this reason that the WBGT method of predicting heat stress is recommended by the American College of Sports Medicine (71,72).

> **Wet Bulb Globe Temperature**
>
> A measure of the heat stress in direct sunlight, which simultaneously considers temperature, humidity, wind speed, sun angle, and cloud cover (affecting solar radiation).

Factors Affecting Loss of Fluids and Electrolytes

The following factors that affect fluid and electrolyte loss are considered when discussing athletes and exercise:

- *Ambient temperature:* Higher temperature results in greater sweat rates.
- *Ambient humidity:* Higher humidity results in greater sweat rates.
- *Clothing/equipment:* Clothing that traps moisture against the skin results in ineffective evaporation and greater sweat rates and may also lower convective heat loss through the increase in skin blood flow.
- *Body surface area:* Enhanced sweat production capacity is seen in adults with larger body surface areas.
- *Conditioning:* Well-conditioned athletes have enhanced sweating capability (*i.e.*, can sweat a greater volume per unit of time to enhance evaporative cooling).
- *Fluid balance:* Better fluid balance states are associated with higher sweat rates. Dehydration reduces the

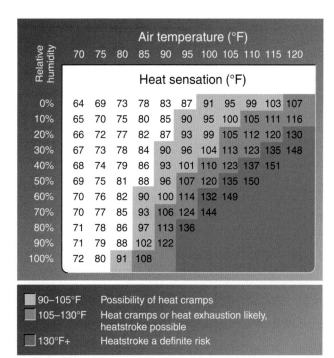

Relative humidity	Air temperature (°F)										
	70	75	80	85	90	95	100	105	110	115	120
	Heat sensation (°F)										
0%	64	69	73	78	83	87	91	95	99	103	107
10%	65	70	75	80	85	90	95	100	105	111	116
20%	66	72	77	82	87	93	99	105	112	120	130
30%	67	73	78	84	90	96	104	113	123	135	148
40%	68	74	79	86	93	101	110	123	137	151	
50%	69	75	81	88	96	107	120	135	150		
60%	70	76	82	90	100	114	132	149			
70%	70	77	85	93	106	124	144				
80%	71	78	86	97	113	136					
90%	71	79	88	102	122						
100%	72	80	91	108							

■ 90–105°F	Possibility of heat cramps
■ 105–130°F	Heat cramps or heat exhaustion likely, heatstroke possible
□ 130°F+	Heatstroke a definite risk

FIGURE 7.8: The heat index with heat stress risks at different heat index values. Individual reactions to heat will vary. Heat illnesses can occur at lower temperatures than indicated on this chart. Exposure to full sunshine can increase values up to 15 °F. (From Anderson MK, Parr GP. Fundamentals of sports injury management. 3rd ed. Philadelphia [PA]: WK Health and Pharma; 2011.)

sweat rate by ~15% and can be elevated to a normal sweat rate via restoration of water balance (73,74).

- *Activity intensity:* Higher-intensity activities are associated with more energy utilization per unit of time with more metabolic heat production, which requires greater sweat rates to dissipate this heat.
- *Gender:* Women not only have lower sweat rates than men but also have lower rates of energy expenditure than men because of (typically) lower muscle mass, and possibly other gender-specific variability in sweat glands and the adaptation to exercise (75,76).
- *Age:* Children have fewer sweat glands and produce less sweat per gland than adults. Therefore, children are at high risk of heat stress.

Ideally, athletes will learn to consume fluids during exercise to mediate the inevitable loss of fluids and electrolytes through sweat and to replace the inevitable use of carbohydrates (both blood sugar and muscle glycogen) during exercise. The benefits associated with consuming fluids, electrolytes, and energy during exercise are clear and include:

- *Attenuation of elevated heart rate through improved stroke volume:* Maintaining blood volume during physical activity helps the heart function more efficiently by improving stroke volume. For each beat of the heart, the heart can deliver more blood and associated oxygen/nutrients to cells. Avoiding a higher heart rate through sustained stroke volume lowers exercise stress and improves time to fatigue. Sweat results in a lowering of the blood volume, making consumption of fluids and electrolytes during exercise an effective means of maintaining efficient heart stroke volume, especially during prolonged exercise bouts of >30 minutes.
- *Attenuation of increased core temperature:* Maintaining adequate hydration sustains skin blood flow, which helps to sustain sweat rates and heat dissipation. This makes it easier for athletes to cool themselves from energy-metabolism–associated heat production and environmental heat through sustained sweat rates.
- *Attenuation of higher plasma sodium, osmolality, and adrenaline:* Sweat is composed of more water and a lower concentration of electrolytes than the concentration of electrolytes in plasma. The greater the fitness level of the athlete, the lower the concentration of sodium in sweat. This ability to maintain plasma osmolality is one of the reasons more fit individuals can exercise longer. Once plasma volume becomes lower, sweat rates are reduced. Blood sugar, the primary fuel for the brain, is also an important factor

in fatigue. Low blood sugar results in an increase in adrenaline (epinephrine), which causes a fast breakdown of liver glycogen, which quickly increases blood sugar. However, the resultant depleted liver glycogen makes it difficult to sustain blood sugar, resulting in fatigue. Maintaining the hydration states with adequate sodium and sugar helps to avoid this outcome.

- *Reduction in net muscle glycogen usage:* The failure to provide sufficient fluid, electrolytes, and carbohydrates during physical activity increases muscle glycogen usage, which results in early fatigue. As a simple rule: if three elements are being reduced during exercise (water, electrolytes, blood sugar), then all three should be replaced during exercise in an attempt to maintain normal tissue function. Replacing just one of these three (for instance, just water or just salt) fails to adequately sustain the hydration state.

Systems for Regulating Body Temperature

The control of body temperature is a function of the body's thermostat: the *preoptic anterior hypothalamus.* Receptors that monitor changes in temperature, called thermoreceptors, are located in the brain, muscles, spine, and skin and provide body temperature information to the preoptic anterior hypothalamus and also to the cerebral cortex, which lets us be aware of whether body temperature is too high (hot) or too low (cold). A primary response to high body temperature is the production of sweat for evaporation off the skin's surface as a means of dissipating body heat. Being well hydrated is an important component of sweat production. Should body temperature become too low, a primary response is involuntary muscle shivering, which has the effect of increasing heat production (65).

Hydration

There are multiple important functions related to health and athletic performance associated with maintaining an adequate hydration state. Despite the importance of hydration, however, studies have found that athletes tend to replace less fluid than the amount lost in sweat, leading to a gradual reduction in performance and reducing the potential benefits that should be derived from exercise (68). Some of this difference is due to the fact that the rate of water lost through sweat can exceed the maximal rate of water absorption from consumed fluids. It has been noted that 50 mL of fluid/min may be lost through sweat, but only 20–30 mL of fluid may be absorbed by intestines (77). But some of this inadequate fluid replacement is due to poor hydration strategies followed by people who exercise.

We have systems for controlling body water levels that involve forcing an increased retention of body water or an increased loss of body water, all mediated through a series of hormones that monitor blood osmolality (the molecular concentration in the blood of electrolytes, including sodium, chloride, and potassium, and other substances), and baroreceptors in blood vessels that sense shifts in BP and signal the brain with the information to sustain appropriate BP.

Excretion of fluids and metabolic by-products is a primary function of the kidneys, which are stimulated by hormones and enzymes to adjust the volume of water and electrolytes excreted or retained. The concentration of sodium is a primary influence on the osmolality of ECF, which is maintained within a narrow range. Because sweat is hypotonic (the concentration of sodium in sweat is lower than the concentration of sodium in plasma), prolonged exercise results in a higher plasma osmolality because more water is lost than sodium. As a means of preserving body water volume, urine production during and shortly after exercise is slightly decreased (66,78). As shown in Table 7.2, sodium chloride (salt) in sweat far surpasses all other electrolytes in sweat and is a primary reason why sports beverages contain salt.

Poor hydration habits in athletes are due to several reasons, including:

- The drinking tradition in the sport
- Failure to take advantage of opportunities to consume fluids
- The lack of a timely thirst mechanism (the athletes driven to drink *after* the fluid is needed)
- Poor fluid availability
- Fluids that do not taste good to the exercising athlete

All of these factors can be overcome with training and planning and will go a long way toward sustaining the athlete's performance over the entire practice or competition.

Issues Related to Hydration

There are several situations and conditions that are related to hydration and fluid consumption, as follows:

- Exercise in hot and humid environments causes more sweat production to maintain body temperature, so requires more fluid consumption.
- Some conditions, such as diabetes, cause an increase in urinary water loss, increasing the requirement for

water. Cystic fibrosis increases the loss of salt through sweat, increasing the requirement for salt in the water that is consumed.

- Some people take drugs for the treatment of high BP, glaucoma, osteoporosis, kidney disease, and heart failure, for example, which increase urinary frequency. Careful monitoring of the hydration state with the intake of appropriate amounts of water to avoid dehydration is important when these water-losing drugs are taken.
- Athletes who exercise while wearing heavy protective clothing (*e.g.*, football players) sweat more heavily because the clothing inhibits evaporative cooling. Sweating more increases the need for more water.
- High-intensity exercise increases the amount of energy used to satisfy muscle energy requirements. Approximately 70% of the burned energy is heat creating. This extra energy cannot be acquired, as that would increase body temperature to an unsafe level, so the sweat rate increases to dissipate the extra heat. The higher the exercise intensity, the greater the need for water per unit of time.

Fluid Balance and Exercise

Exercise results in faster loss of water and electrolytes as well as a fast utilization of blood glucose and muscle glycogen. Therefore, optimal hydration requires replacement of all three: water, electrolytes, and carbohydrate (WEC). When not exercising, the rate of WEC reduction is relatively slow and, therefore, it is relatively easy to maintain a state of hydration. Because the WEC level drops so slowly, consuming an occasional glass of water, other fluid, and/or high–water-content foods (that also contain carbohydrate and electrolytes) may be sufficient to adequately maintain the state of hydration. Physical activity, however, makes the rate of WEC reduction proceed extremely quickly. Depending on exercise intensity and environmental temperature and humidity, it is possible to have sufficient sweat losses within a relatively short period of time, resulting in difficulty in adequately replacing WEC. This could affect exercise performance and, if allowed to continue, could result in serious heat illness. Particularly when sweat rates are high, *waiting* to drink an appropriately composed fluid makes it virtually impossible to return to a well-hydrated state while the exercise continues and sweat loss remains high. Therefore, athletic endeavors resulting in high sweat rates require that the athlete begin the activity in a well-hydrated state, and initiate a frequent fluid (WEC) consumption pattern that minimizes the difference between fluid lost and fluid consumed (72).

The usual nonathlete recommendation for sustaining hydration in people experiencing relatively low sweat rates is to consume ~3.7 L (3.9 quarts) of water per day, including beverages and the water contained in foods (37). The athlete's requirement for fluid is higher (sufficient to replace fluids lost in sweat), and surveys have found that both male and female athletes fail to accurately estimate the total volume of sweat loss and fail to create a strategy that minimizes the difference between sweat loss and fluids consumed. The result is often the consumption of fluids far less than needed to sustain an optimal state of hydration and performance (79).

Even relatively small changes in hydration state can manifest significant reductions in performance. The goal for athletes, therefore, is to initiate exercise well hydrated and to stay within at least 2% of pre-exercise body weight, while avoiding weight gain (68,72). Regardless of the activity, it appears that losing significantly more water than this marginal level results in performance deficits. Therefore, a strategy for maintaining hydration during exercise should be developed and practiced to allow the body systems to adapt to the strategy. It is also important to consume fluids that are appropriately composed to ensure that fluids are distributed appropriately. It has been found that poor hydration (68,80,81):

- results in inadequate ICF and ECF;
- affects muscle and skin (sweat glands) and lowers the sweat rate potential;
- decreases cardiac stroke volume (the heart has to work harder);
- decreases athlete cognitive performance;
- lowers plasma volume, diminishes fluid delivery to working muscles, decreases delivery of energy to working muscles, and lowers the removal of metabolic by-products from working muscles;
- negatively affects athletic performance; and
- elevates core temperature to a degree that is particularly serious in hot and humid environments.

If the frequency of drinking when not exercising is once every 2 hours, then the frequency of drinking during exercise could easily be imagined to be every 10–15 minutes. Waiting too long between drinking opportunities is a bad strategy because it allows WEC to decrease in such a way that it cannot be adequately replaced. If you wait to drink, you may be able to stabilize the body's hydration state, but that state will be too low.

How the Body Acclimatizes to Exercise

Conditioned athletes who have acclimatized to exercise in more hot and humid environments do better than athletes who have not acclimatized. The typical body adaptations to exercise in the heat include the following (55):

- Plasma volume expands to increase total blood volume, making it easier for the heart to pump more blood per stroke (stroke volume improves).
- More blood flows to the muscles and skin.
- Less muscle glycogen is used as an energy source during exercise, improving endurance (82,83).
- The sweat glands hypertrophy (enlarge) and produce 30% more sweat.
- Salt in sweat decreases by about 60% to conserve electrolytes, which helps to maintain blood volume.
- Sweat is initiated at a lower core temperature, which helps to keep body temperature normal.

The psychological feeling of stress is reduced, lowering the production of adrenalin and cortisol and resulting in improved endurance.

Monitoring Fluid Balance During Training

Without sufficient WEC intake, blood volume can quickly lower to have a negative impact on the sweat rate, causing body temperature to rise quickly. However, it is difficult to consume sufficient fluids during hard physical work, mandating that athletes and/or their coaches have a well-developed hydration plan. For instance, an athlete who loses 1 L of water per hour should have a plan for consuming about four cups of WEC per hour. Although it is difficult to know precisely how much fluid is being lost during exercise, this simple strategy can help provide athletes with an estimate of how much is lost and, therefore, how much should be consumed. One liter of water weighs ~2 lb, and 1 pint (16 oz) of water weighs ~1 lb. Knowing these weights can provide an estimate of how much fluid is lost and how much the athlete should try to consume during activity. To estimate the water requirement during activity, do the following:

- Write down the ambient temperature and humidity (HI).
- Write down the time just before the exercise session.
- Write down body weight (preferably nude weight) in pounds. Using kg is much easier as no calculations are necessary (1 kg lost = 1 L).

- Perform the exercise and monitor how much fluid (in ounces) *is consumed* during the exercise period.
- When the exercise is completed, calculate the time of exercise by subtracting ending time from beginning time.
- Take off the sweaty clothing and towel dry.
- Once completely dry, write down body weight (preferably nude weight) in pounds.
- Calculate the amount of fluid lost via sweat by subtracting your body weight at the end of exercise from your body weight at the beginning of exercise (1 lb = 16 oz).
- The amount of extra fluid that should be consumed is equivalent to 16 oz of fluid for each pound lost, provided in volumes that range from 2 to 8 oz and in time intervals that range from 10 to 20 minutes.

Differences in the amount to drink and the frequency of drinking are related to the total amount of fluid that must be replaced. It is easiest to have the lowest amount with the least frequency (*i.e.*, 2 oz every 20 minutes), but athletes should try to never go longer than 20 minutes without drinking something during exercise (Example 7.1).

Example 7.1: Consuming Fluid During Exercise

- Thomas weighs 160 lb at the beginning of his 2-hour football practice and drinks 1 pint (2 cups; 16 oz) of fluid during the practice.
- At the end of practice, Thomas weighs 158 lb, so he needs to calculate how to consume an *additional* 2 pints of water during the practice for a total of 3 pints (6 cups or 48 oz) over 2 hours.
- There are 12 10-minute increments in 2 hours, so Thomas has 12 opportunities to consume a total of 48 oz of fluids if he chooses to drink some fluids once every 10 minutes.
- Forty-eight ounces divided by 12 equals 4 oz of fluid (1/2 cup) every 10 minutes.
- It may be difficult to consume that much fluid if the athlete is unaccustomed to it, so Thomas should try training himself to drink that much by *gradually* increasing the fluid consumption over several weeks to try to achieve an equal pre- and postexercise weight. The main point is this: any fluid amount greater than the current amount consumed is beneficial if the athlete experiences weight loss during the activity.

All of this is made more complex by environmental conditions and the level of conditioning an athlete has.

Better-conditioned athletes are better able to cool themselves because they have developed more efficient sweat systems. This allows better-conditioned athletes to perform longer, but it also requires that they consume more fluids. When the environment is hot and humid, water does not evaporate off the body easily, so it does not have the desired cooling effect.

- The higher the temperature, the more the athlete sweats.
- The higher the humidity, the more the athlete sweats, but with reduced cooling efficiency.
- Clothing that traps sweat against the skin (*i.e.*, does not breathe) has a reduced cooling efficiency, so it forces the athlete to sweat more.
- Well-conditioned athletes sweat more volume per unit of time, resulting in improved cooling potential. However, this higher sweat rate requires a greater during-exercise fluid consumption.
- Several factors affect fluid intake and the rate consumed fluids leave the stomach (gastric emptying) and enter the small intestine. The two main factors for fluid intake are *thirst* experienced by the athlete and *taste* of the beverage consumed (84). It has been found that many athletes fail to consume sufficient fluids even if ample fluids are available (referred to as voluntary dehydration), but most athletes fail to consume sufficient fluids simply because they are not thirsty (85,86). The thirst sensation, therefore, should not be considered an appropriate indicator of the need for fluids in athletes (87). It appears that thirst in athletes occurs only after the loss of 1.5–2.0 L of water (88). Should an athlete begin drinking at the point of thirst, there is little chance of achieving an adequately hydrated state during exercise. This delay in the sensation of thirst is a strong argument for athletes to train themselves to consume fluids on a fixed schedule, regardless of whether they are thirsty.

The *appeal* (color, odor, temperature, mouth feel, etc.) of a beverage is another important factor in whether it will be consumed. In general, it appears that athletes prefer cool beverages with a slightly sweet flavor (89,90). Heavily sweetened beverages of around a 12% carbohydrate solution, including sodas and fruit juices, are not as widely tolerated during exercise as beverages with a 6% or 7% carbohydrate solution (91,92). It appears, however, that when in a relaxed and nonexercising state, more highly sweetened beverages are preferred. This points to an interesting phenomenon of exercise: The organoleptic properties (*i.e.*, the perception of taste) of foods and beverages differ when exercising than when not exercising (93). Given the extensive research on the benefits of consuming a sports drink with a 6%–7% carbohydrate solution and electrolytes, regardless of whether the activity lasts half an hour or longer than 4 hours, it appears clear that athletes should adapt to drinking a sports beverage in a way that optimizes tolerance and hydration. Consumption of sports beverages results in better performance than water whether you do sprints or endurance work (94,95).

Dehydration

When significantly more fluids are lost than are consumed, dehydration occurs. By definition, hypohydration means that total body water is below the optimal state, with as little as a 2% drop in body weight from sweat loss resulting in a measurable reduction in athletic performance (96). It has also been found that 76.3% of male athletes involved in different sports, including basketball, gymnastics, swimming, running, and canoeing, were hypohydrated, with an average training-related body weight loss of −1.1% (97). Importantly, interventions that encourage fluid intake clearly improve hydration status and exercise performance (98). Common risks for dehydration include the following (71,96,99):

- Vomiting
- Diarrhea
- Inadequate fluid replacement
- Poor fluid availability
- High sweat rates due to environmental heat/humidity
- Induced high sweat rates (as in saunas)
- Delayed drinking (waiting until thirsty)
- Laxatives
- Diuretics (and substances with a diuretic effect)
- Dieting
- Febrile illness (illness with high body temperature)
- Purposeful weight loss
- Fluid avoidance to "make weight"

The only logical strategy for avoiding dehydration during exercise is to correctly assume that there is a constant output of fluids that must be balanced through the constant consumption of an equal volume of fluids. Athletes should recognize the signs of dehydration, including thirst, urine volume, and urine color (Figure 7.9). Thirst may be an obvious sign, but both low urine output and dark urine color are signs of dehydration that may precede the sensation of thirst.

The tradition in some sports is for athletes to purposefully dehydrate themselves in an attempt to improve

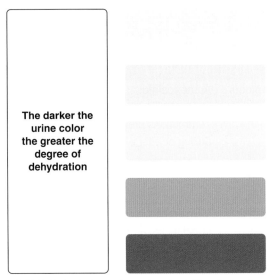

The darker the urine color the greater the degree of dehydration

FIGURE 7.9: Dehydration urine color chart. The darker the urine color the greater the degree of dehydration.

their appearance or to try to make a competitive weight classification. Other athletes simply fail to consume fluids even when they are readily available to them (*voluntary dehydration*) and become dehydrated, whereas other athletes become dehydrated as a result of heavy training, particularly in hot and humid environments, when adequate fluid consumption is difficult (referred to as *involuntary dehydration*) (100). Regardless of the dehydration cause, athletes can be certain that dehydration results in inferior performance outcomes and reduced mental function (101,102).

Exertional Heat Illnesses That May Be Related to Poor Hydration

Exertional heat illnesses that may be related to poor hydration include heat cramps, heat exhaustion, heat syncope, and heatstroke/sunstroke (Table 7.11).

Heat Cramps

Exercise-associated muscle cramps, often referred to as **heat cramps**, occur suddenly and may occur both during and following physical activity (103). The most likely reasons for these cramps include dehydration coupled with electrolyte imbalance, fatigue, altered muscle control, and any combination of these (104–106). Heat cramps are most likely to occur in people who sweat heavily and who lose a higher-than-normal amount of sodium and other electrolytes (including potassium, calcium, and magnesium) in the sweat (106). For these individuals, drinking adequate amounts of salt-containing beverages during

Table 7.11   **Differences in Exertional Heat Illnesses**

	Muscle (Heat) Cramps	Heat Syncope	Heat Exhaustion	Heatstroke
Symptoms	Acute, painful, involuntary muscle contractions presenting during or after exercise	Collapsing in the heat, resulting in loss of consciousness	Inability to continue exercise because of cardiovascular insufficiency	Severe hyperthermia leading to overwhelming of the thermoregulatory system with possible central nervous system dysfunction and core temperature >104.9 °F (40.5 °C)
Cause(s)	Dehydration, electrolyte imbalances, and/or neuromuscular fatigue	Standing erect in a hot environment, causing postural pooling of blood in the legs	High skin blood flow, heavy sweating, and/or dehydration, causing reduced venous return	High metabolic heat production and/or reduced heat dissipation
Treatment(s)	Stop exercising, provide sodium-containing beverages	Lay patient supine and elevate legs to restore central blood volume	Cease exercise, remove from hot environment, elevate legs, provide fluids	Immediate whole-body cold-water immersion to quickly reduce core body temperature
Recovery	Often occurs within minutes to hours	Often occurs within hours	Often occurs within 24 hr; same-day return to play not advised	Highly dependent on initial care and treatment; further medical testing and physician clearance required before return to activity

Source: Adapted from Casa DJ, DeMartini JK, Berjeron MF, Csillan D, Eichner ER, Lopez RM, Ferrara MS, Miller KC, O'Connor F, Sawka MN, Yeargin SW. National Athletic Trainers' Association position statement: exertional heat illnesses. J Athl Train. 2015;50(9):986–1000.

exercise is particularly useful. Heat cramps also appear to occur late in the day after consumption of large volumes of plain water (107). Severe muscle cramps affect athletic performance, with the recommendation that there should be no further exercise (103).

Heat Cramps

Skeletal muscle cramps are most often associated with muscular fatigue and may occur in athletes participating in all sports and in all environmental conditions. There is evidence that muscle cramps may be associated with a state of hypohydration and electrolyte imbalances. Profuse sweating, particularly when not well acclimatized to hot/humid environments and coupled with high sweat sodium losses, appears to place athletes at greatest risk for cramping (68,72).

It has been recommended that athletes experiencing exertional heat cramps consume 16–20 oz (~0.5 L) of a sports beverage with 0.5 teaspoon (3 g) of salt added over a 10-minute period, followed by additional fluid and electrolytes to restore fluid balance (108). As muscle cramping may be associated with muscle fatigue separate from hydration issues, however, these recommendations may not universally apply to athletes experiencing muscle cramps. Care must also be taken to ensure that excess fluid consumption does not occur, as this may increase the risk of hyponatremia (68,72). To help meet the needs of athletes who experience frequent cramping, companies have developed products that provide a measured amount of sodium, potassium, calcium, and magnesium for adding to a given volume of sports beverages. The common sports beverage contains between 50 and 110 mg sodium/240 mL (1 cup) of fluid. Endurance sports beverages typically contain more sodium, at the level of between 150 and 200 mg sodium/240 mL.

Heat Exhaustion

Heat exhaustion refers to the athlete's inability to continue exercising in the current heat and humidity environment. Symptoms include weakness, red skin rash, cold/clammy skin, a feeling of faintness, muscle cramping, fatigue,

Table 7.12	Exertional Heatstroke Extrinsic and Intrinsic Risk Factors
Extrinsic Factors	**Intrinsic Factors**
■ High ambient temperature, solar radiation, and high humidity ■ Athletic gear or uniforms ■ Peer or organizational pressure ■ Inappropriate work-to-rest ratios based on intensity, wet bulb globe temperature, clothing, equipment, fitness, and athlete's medical condition ■ Predisposing medical conditions ■ Lack of education and awareness of heat illnesses among coaches, athletes, and medical staff ■ No emergency plan to identify and treat exertional heat illnesses ■ Minimal access to fluids before and during practice and rest breaks ■ Delay in recognition of early warning signs	■ High intensity of exercise and/or poor physical conditioning ■ Sleep loss ■ Dehydration or inadequate fluid intake ■ Use of diuretics or certain medications (i.e., antihistamines, diuretics, antihypertensives, attention-deficit hyperactive disorder drugs) ■ Overzealousness or reluctance to report problems, issues, or illnesses ■ Inadequate heat acclimatization ■ High muscle mass-to-body fat ratio ■ Presence of a fever ■ Skin disorder

Source: Adapted from Casa DJ, DeMartini JK, Berjeron MF, Csillan D, Eichner ER, Lopez RM, Ferrara MS, Miller KC, O'Connor F, Sawka MN, Yeargin SW. National Athletic Trainers' Association position statement: exertional heat illnesses. J Athl Train. 2015;50(9):986–1000.

nausea, dizziness, confusion, poor coordination, and a weak pulse (109). If there is severe body water depletion, the athlete may also stop sweating and the skin feels dry. The likely cause of these symptoms is poor blood flow to the brain, with the sufferer typically on the ground but semiconscious. Symptoms usually respond well to rapid cooling, so heat exhaustion victims should be cooled through whatever means are available. Applying wet, ice-cold cloths to the body or placing the victim in a cold water bath is effective (110). After a return to full consciousness, the athlete can be given sips of cool fluid, but this should not be forced as it may cause nausea. There is no reason for a heat-exhausted athlete to return to physical activity on the same day. Instead, the person should spend the remainder of the day staying cool and hydrating with sodium-containing fluids, including sports beverages (103).

CAUTION: Under no circumstances should an athlete who has stopped sweating continue exercising because this may cause a rapid and dangerous hyperthermia (a dangerous rise in core temperature).

Heat Syncope

Syncope refers to dizziness, which is likely to occur in individuals who are not well adapted to the current environmental heat and humidity (103). Thus, **heat syncope** is most likely to occur when people begin exercising in a hotter and more humid environment than they are accustomed to and is associated with inadequate sweat rates

(*i.e.*, poor cooling) from dehydration and an inadequate fitness level. Individuals taking diuretics, because of the lower blood volume, are also at higher risk of developing heat-related syncope (111).

Heatstroke (Sunstroke)

Exertion-related **heatstroke** is a dangerous condition associated with high body temperature (usually above 105 °F or 40.5 °C), hot/dry skin, and a rapid pulse (Table 7.12) (71). Although most likely to occur in environmental conditions of high heat and humidity, the athlete may also develop heatstroke with continued hard physical activity but compromised capacity to dissipate heat through sweat (103). It is also possible for the athlete to be in and out of consciousness. The first responder should call for emergency medical care and then do whatever possible to immediately cool the athlete (cold water, loosening clothing, cold water bath, etc.). Mortality risk increases the longer the body temperature remains elevated (112). Fluids should not be put into the mouth until the athlete returns to consciousness (113).

Heat Exhaustion

A heat illness characterized by a failure to sustain cardiac output and sweat rate, resulting in high skin temperature. Symptoms include a rapid pulse, dizziness, fainting, paleness, and anxiety. It is one of the heat-related conditions experienced by athletes.

Heat Syncope

Decreased relative blood volume coupled with excessive vasodilation results in lower cardiac output and decreased BP that, because of the increased sweat rate, lowers blood flow to the brain. The result is dizziness, mental confusion, and fainting.

Heatstroke

Also called *sunstroke*, heatstroke is a life-threatening exertional heat illness associated with overheating. When core temperature rises quickly, brain and muscle function are adversely affected. Typically, athletes respond to these signals by slowing down or ceasing exercise to allow core temperature to decrease. Failure to respond to these signals may result in heatstroke with an elevated body temperature (above 104 °F), which can damage neurologic tissue, heart, kidneys, and muscle. Heatstroke requires immediate emergency treatment and is considered the most serious of the heat injury conditions that can result in death.

Hyponatremia

Exercising for long periods may cause low blood sodium (hyponatremia), which is a potentially fatal condition (114). Low blood sodium can occur when drinking excessive amounts of water (*i.e.*, fluids with no or low sodium), causing a dilution of the blood sodium content. To normalize the concentration of sodium per unit volume of blood, water leaves the blood, causing edema, which may result in rapid and dangerous swelling of the brain (115). Low blood sodium is most likely to occur during prolonged exercise in dehydrated athletes who have experienced large sodium losses through sweat, but may also occur in athletes who habitually restrict sodium consumption in the foods and beverages they consume. Unless contraindicated because of a medical condition and the athlete is under the careful supervision of a physician, adding salt to meals and consuming salt-containing beverages is a desirable strategy for avoiding low blood electrolytes and reducing hyponatremia risk. Signs and symptoms of hyponatremia include (114):

- Headache
- Swollen fingers and ankles
- Bloated stomach
- Confusion
- Pulmonary edema
- Nausea
- Seizures
- Cramping
- Coma

Prior to the 2003 Boston Marathon, USA Track & Field announced fluid replacement guidelines for long-distance runners that are designed to lower hyponatremia risk. Earlier guidelines encouraged runners to drink as much as possible to "stay ahead" of their thirst, but the new guidelines advise runners to drink only as much fluid as they lose through sweat during a race. This recommendation suggests that athletes consume 100% of fluids lost through sweat and no more. Higher levels of consumption, particularly of plain water, could cause a drop in blood sodium concentration, leading to hyponatremia. Athletes who have an increased risk of developing hyponatremia (116):

- Take NSAIDs (*i.e.*, aspirin, ibuprofen);
- Are on a low-sodium diet;
- Drink water or other no-sodium beverages during exercise;
- Are not acclimatized to warm weather or are poorly trained;
- Are of small stature (more evidence documents this than documents poor training);
- Run slowly, taking longer than 4 hours to complete endurance events.

Hyponatremia risk appears highest in athletes with high sweat rates and with a relatively high concentration of sodium, but who fail to consume sodium-containing beverages during exercise (117). Commonly available sports beverages contain ~20 milliequivalents (mEq) of sodium chloride (table salt), but even higher levels of sodium are recommended by a number of researchers who have assessed plasma changes during prolonged exercise in the heat (118,119). These researchers have recommended 20–50 mEq/L. However, most athletes with normal sweat rates and normal sweat sodium concentrations who consume commercial sports beverages *and avoid consumption of plain water during endurance events* appear to be protected against developing hyponatremia (114,120).

Hyponatremia is a serious condition requiring the immediate attention of appropriately qualified health professionals. However, if no one is available, salt tablets can be used to recover from hyponatremia, but should not otherwise be used. A single salt tablet typically delivers 1 g (1,000 mg) of sodium. For recovery, 1–2 tablets should be consumed per cup of water taken every 15–20 minutes, depending on the degree to which hyponatremia symptoms appear. Salty foods (potato chips, pretzels, etc.) may also be consumed if salt tablets are unavailable. The total fluid consumed should return the athlete to pre-exercise weight, but not cause the athlete to increase body weight above that point (108). Common causes of hyponatremia include (121): Water intake exceeds water losses; Sodium loss exceeds sodium intake.

Factors That Influence Effectiveness of a Sports Beverage

Factors That Affect Gastric Emptying

A number of factors influence the rate at which fluids leave the stomach, but before these are reviewed, it is important to understand what slow or fast gastric emptying really means. When a food or drink is described as having a slower gastric emptying, it does not mean that all of the food stays in the stomach longer. It means that the food or drink trickles out of the stomach and into the intestines more slowly, so some of the food or drink remains in the stomach longer. Gastric emptying, therefore, describes the volume of food or drink that leaves the stomach per unit of time. Because athletes are more comfortable exercising without an extensive amount of food or fluid in the stomach, a beverage that leaves the stomach more quickly (*i.e.*, has a fast gastric emptying property) is considered desirable. In addition, fast gastric emptying offers the possibility for a faster delivery of energy and water to working muscles by more quickly presenting substances to the intestines for absorption. The speed of gastric emptying is important for three reasons: (i) athletes exercising with full stomach contents report GI distress; (ii) athletes are less likely to consume more fluid to replace fluid loss in sweat if fluid remains in the stomach; and (iii) faster gastric emptying translates into fluids, electrolytes, and carbohydrate that are more readily available for absorption and, therefore, can satisfy blood and tissue requirements more efficiently.

Carbohydrate Concentration of the Solution

Although there are individual tolerance differences, carbohydrate concentrations exceeding 7% have generally resulted in a slower gastric emptying rate, whereas in carbohydrate concentrations of ≤7%, gastric emptying time is not significantly affected (122). This is one of the reasons why the recommended carbohydrate concentration in sports beverages is below 8%. Studies assessing how carbohydrate concentration affects performance in team players have found that a 6% carbohydrate solution was significantly more effective than a 10% carbohydrate solution (123). Other studies have found similar performance benefits when the carbohydrate concentration does not rise above 7% in a sports beverage (124,125).

Type of Carbohydrate in the Solution

Carbohydrates come in different molecular sizes and in different molecular combinations. For instance, glucose is a monosaccharide (a single-molecule carbohydrate), sucrose is a disaccharide (two monosaccharides held together with a bond), and starch is a polysaccharide (many molecules of monosaccharides held together with bonds). The smaller the length of a carbohydrate chain, the slower the gastric emptying time. For instance, 100 kcal from sucrose has half the molecules as 100 kcal from glucose. Because of the higher molecular count, the osmolarity of the glucose solution is higher, resulting in slower gastric emptying. An equal caloric level of pure glucose (a monosaccharide) takes longer to leave the stomach than table sugar (a disaccharide), and table sugar takes longer to leave the stomach than a simple starch (a polysaccharide). The size of the sugar particle is so important that even if two beverages have the same carbohydrate concentration, the beverage with smaller carbohydrate molecules will take longer to leave the stomach than the beverage with larger carbohydrate molecules (126). The type of carbohydrate consumed may also affect performance. It has been found that a beverage containing glucose and fructose (sucrose) when compared with a beverage containing only glucose, resulted in higher carbohydrate oxidation and improved 100-km cycling performance (127). Pure glucose-containing beverages also result in delayed gastric emptying (128). Another study also found that cyclists exercising at moderate intensity completed a time trial 8% more quickly when a multiple-carbohydrate drink was consumed than when a glucose-only drink was consumed (129).

Amount of Solution Consumed

The amount of fluid consumed at one time has a major influence on gastric emptying time. When a large volume of fluid is consumed, gastric emptying time is initially faster. When the volume of fluid in the stomach is reduced, gastric emptying time slows. This suggests that to become more quickly hydrated prior to competition or practice, a relatively large volume of fluid should be consumed (approximately half a liter), followed by frequent sipping of fluid to maintain the fluid volume in the stomach and, therefore, a faster gastric emptying time (130).

Temperature of the Solution

Most studies indicate that the solution temperature only slightly affects gastric emptying time. When people are at rest, fluids at body temperature leave the stomach more quickly than either very hot or very cold fluids (131). There is evidence that, during exercise, cool fluids leave the stomach more quickly than fluids at room or body temperature (132).

Carbonation of the Solution

Although there are many athletes who believe that consuming a carbonated beverage will cause gastric distress and delayed gastric emptying (the first sports beverage was probably a "defizzed" cola), there is little scientific evidence that this occurs. However, the studies that have evaluated the impact of fluid carbonation on gastric emptying time have typically relied on few subjects. In general, the studies suggest that all other things being equal (carbohydrate concentration, volume, temperature, etc.), carbonation has little impact on gastric emptying (133,134). However, carbonation does lower voluntary fluid intake following exercise, which could impact hydration recovery and future exercise performance (135).

State of Hydration or Dehydration

With the increasing dehydration and higher body temperatures associated with high-intensity activity, the rate of gastric emptying slows (126). This is an excellent reason for athletes, as much as possible, to try to maintain their hydration state during activity. Allowing dehydration to occur makes it almost impossible for the athlete to return to an adequately hydrated state during exercise. If such hydration is attempted through consumption of a large volume of fluid, it will likely add to a sense of discomfort rather than faster rehydration.

Degree of Mental Stress

The mental stress and anxiety associated with athletic competition are major factors in gastric emptying. Higher levels of mental stress and anxiety are associated with a reduced gastric emptying that can have a serious impact on the athlete's ability to adequately rehydrate during competition (87,136). Obviously, the mental training techniques that may be learned from a sports psychologist to reduce stress are an important strategy for reducing the physiologic effects of sports-related stress and anxiety.

Type of Activity

Studies have suggested that high-intensity activity is associated with a slower gastric emptying rate than lower-intensity activity, but the differences appear to be minor. In addition, the type of activity (running, swimming, cycling, etc.) does not appear to have a large influence on gastric emptying rate (87).

Athlete's Conditioning and Adaptation

The human body has wonderful adaptive mechanisms, and the ability to adapt to higher or lower glucose concentrations and faster or slower rates of fluid ingestion is no exception. To a certain extent, athletes can find a system for optimal rehydration that suits them best by consistently practicing that system. Practicing a reasonable system allows the body to adapt to it and reduce the chance of any difficulties that could arise from trying something new just before an important competition. Therefore, it is important for athletes to start with general recommendations for fluid intake to maintain their hydration state, but to make modifications that are best suited to their own individual circumstances.

Intestinal Absorption

Once the solution (fluid) leaves the stomach and goes into the small intestine, the water and carbohydrate that make up the solution must be absorbed into the blood. The main factor that influences the speed with which water and carbohydrate are absorbed is the concentration of carbohydrate in the solution that enters the intestines (137). A solution that has a slightly lower concentration of carbohydrate and electrolytes, relative to the concentration of plasma, causes a faster absorption of water than a solution that has either a much higher or a much lower concentration (138). Consumption of highly concentrated carbohydrate solutions during exercise may cause a temporary shift of fluids away from the muscles and into the intestines to dilute the solution prior to absorption. This would have a negative impact on both muscle function and sweat rates because it would cause, at least temporarily, a shift of water away from muscle to cause tissue dehydration.

Palatability of the Beverage

The taste, flavor, and mouth feel of a beverage have an impact on voluntary hydration patterns and volume of fluid consumption. However, exercise affects the way fluids taste as compared with how the same fluid tastes when not exercising. In comparing commonly consumed beverages (homemade sports beverage, commercial sports beverage, diluted orange juice, and water), it was found that palatability varied widely, as did their voluntary consumption during exercise. It has been found that a commercially available 6% carbohydrate solution was significantly more palatable and desired over other beverages when consumed during exercise (139).

Optimal Sports Beverage Composition and Drinking Strategy

The evidence suggests that even a relatively minor level of hypohydration (as little as 2% of body weight) may result in a performance and endurance decrement, with greater levels of underhydration having a more significant performance impact (140,141). It is also important to consider that it takes time, often 24 hours or longer, to return a dehydrated athlete to a euhydrated state. Therefore, every effort should be made to help an athlete return to a normally hydrated state prior to the next exercise session. There is evidence that two per day practices may fail to provide sufficient time for dehydrated athletes to return to a hydrated state after the first practice and before the second (142) (Table 7.13).

The degree to which the cardiovascular and heat maintenance capacity is maintained is directly related to athlete's ability to avoid dehydration (143–145). A failure to consume sufficient fluids during exercise represents a major risk for developing heat exhaustion (146). It is clear that the best strategy for athletes to follow to avoid heat exhaustion and maintain athletic performance is to consume fluids during exercise.

Some sports require athletes to achieve a particular look (*i.e.*, figure skating, rhythmic gymnastics, diving) or to achieve a particular weight (*i.e.*, wrestling), which may cause them to restrict fluid intake. Many wrestlers have a regimen for fluid restriction to achieve a desired weight classification, followed by a rehydration protocol. Besides the inherent health dangers of doing this (there are well-documented deaths associated with this strategy), there is doubt that dehydrated wrestlers have sufficient time to achieve a state of adequate rehydration for competition (147).

Some athletes are on the other side of the continuum by trying to hyperhydrate before exercise. Long-distance runners, for instance, experience water loss during competition that is likely to be greater than their ability to replace it. The best-hydrated runner nearing the end of the 26.2-mile marathon has a major advantage over

Table 7.13	Composition of Commonly Consumed Hydration Beverages						
Beverage (8 oz; 240 mL; 1 cup)	Cal (Kcal)	Carb (g)	Carb (%)	Prot (g)	Na (mg)	K (mg)	Other
Water	0	0	0	0	0	0	0
Accelerade	80	21	6.2	4	220	90	**Contains:** whey protein, trehalose, lecithin, vitamin C, vitamin E, sucrose, fructose, maltodectrin, vitamins C (100%), E (100%), CA (2%), Mg (30%), 5% calories from fat
Powerade	55	15	6.0	0	100	23	**Contains:** Niacin (15%), Vit B6 (15%), Vit B12 (15%), high fructose corn syrup
Gatorade	50	14	6.0	0	110	30	**Contains:** sucrose, glucose, fructose
Gatorade Endurance	50	14	6.0	0	200	90	**Contains:** sucrose, glucose, fructose
All-Sport	67	16	6.5	0	55	60	**Contains:** vitamin C, high fructose corn syrup
Cytomax	57	14	6.0	0	55	30	**Contains:** chromium, vitamin C, sucralose, maltodextrin, fructose, dextrose
Glukose	70	17	7.0	0	40	0	**Contains:** glucose
Pedialyte Sport	20	6	3.0	0	327	313	**Contains:** dietary fiber, phosphorus, magnesium, chloride.

runners who are less well hydrated. They have greater blood (plasma) volume that helps to sustain the sweat rate and cooling capacity, and this results in lower core temperature and heart rate during activity (148,149). Although consumption of large fluid volumes may also associated with frequent urination, this may be mediated to a degree by consumption of sodium-containing fluids (140). The rate of voluntary fluid ingestion during physical activity is typically only 50% of the rate of fluid loss as sweat during exercise, but there is also evidence that developing a scheduled fluid intake to more closely match sweat loss results in better maintenance of core temperature and a significantly small decline in plasma volume (150).

Glycerol (a simple three-carbon lipid that is metabolized like a carbohydrate) has historically been used by some athletes to aid hyperhydration because it helps to retain water. There is some limited evidence that adding glycerol to pre-exercise fluids at the rate of 1 g/kg body weight improves endurance performance in hot and humid environments for two reasons: (i) the greater total body water helps to sustain sweat rates and cooling and (ii) the glycerol provides more carbohydrate-like metabolic fuel (140,151). Some athletes find that hyperhydrating with glycerol makes them feel stiff and uncomfortable, whereas others are more comfortable with this sensation (152).

NOTE: Please be aware that glycerol was on the banned substance list from 2010 to 2018 by the World Anti-Doping Agency (WADA). It is now no longer on the banned substance list and is used by some athletes as a hyperhydration aid. It is important for those working with athletes to be aware of its functionality and potential risks.

When banned, WADA established a level of 200 mcg/mL of urinary glycerol as the threshold for identifying athletes who have misused glycerol (153).

Most studies that have evaluated the interaction between hydration adequacy and athletic performance have used either plain water or sports beverages that contain, in differing degrees, carbohydrates, and electrolytes. The results of these studies are similar in confirming the importance of fluid consumption during exercise. However, the inclusion of carbohydrates and electrolytes in the fluids affords the athlete clear advantages over plain water. Studies suggest that including carbohydrates in the rehydration solution improves the athlete's ability to maintain or increase work output during exercise and increases the time to exhaustion (72,154–157). This occurs because consumed carbohydrates help to avoid

the depletion of muscle glycogen and actively provide a fuel to muscles when muscle glycogen is low. In simple terms, exercise results in a loss of body water and electrolytes and a lowering of blood sugar. All three should be replaced.

Different types of physical activity result in different rates of carbohydrate utilization, but consuming carbohydrate-containing fluid helps to maintain athletic performance regardless of the activity type. For instance, in strenuous cycling, the rate of muscle glycogen use is not affected when a carbohydrate solution is used (158). In long-distance running, there is a reduction in the rate of muscle glycogen usage when a carbohydrate-containing fluid is consumed (159). In stop-and-go intermittent exercise typical of team sports, there is a reduction in muscle glycogen usage when a carbohydrate-containing fluid is consumed (160–162). In each of these scenarios, carbohydrate depletion is considered to be the principal cause of reduced performance, and consuming a carbohydrate-containing beverage helps to avoid premature fatigue. There is even good evidence that consumption of a carbohydrate-containing beverage is also important for improving athletic performance in high-intensity activities, where there is no expectation for carbohydrate depletion because of the relatively short duration of the activity (124,160,163).

Carbohydrate energy, regardless of whether it is in liquid or solid form, aids athletic performance (164). However, because providing carbohydrates in liquid form allows the athlete to take care of multiple issues at once (energy and fluid, and preferably also electrolytes), carbohydrate-containing liquids are preferred. The type and concentration of carbohydrate in a sports beverage are important considerations. There appears to be no major differences among sucrose, maltodextrins, and starch (all different types of carbohydrates) on exercise performance (158,165,166). However, sports beverages relying extensively on either glucose or fructose for carbohydrates may cause a delay in gastric emptying, causing a delay in absorption (165,167). Maltodextrins are less sweet than sucrose and fructose, so they may be used to add carbohydrate energy to solutions without making them unpalatably sweet tasting (161).

HFCS is used as the source of carbohydrate in some sports beverages. HFCS is manufactured from cornstarch, which is processed into glucose, and then processed via enzymes to convert a proportion of glucose to fructose. The glucose and fructose are then blended to create HFCS 42 and HFCS 55 (commonly used in beverages). HFCS is commonly used by manufacturers because it has several characteristics that are useful in manufacturing processed foods, including:

- Retains moisture, helping keep the product from drying out
- Helps control bacterial growth, as the osmotic pressure created by HFCS is greater than that of sucrose
- It is a liquid, so more easily blends with other ingredients in the food
- It is highly sweet
- In many food manufacturing countries HFCS is lower in cost than sucrose

The composition of HFCS 55 is similar to sucrose but has more *free* fructose (168):

- Sucrose: 50% fructose, 50% glucose
- HFCS 42: 42% fructose, 52% glucose, 6% polysaccharide (used in beverages, processed foods, cereals, and baked goods)
- HFCS 55: 55% fructose, 42% glucose, 3% polysaccharide (used in soft drinks)
- HFCS 65: 65% fructose, 35% glucose (used in soft drinks)
- HFCS 90: 90% fructose, 10% glucose (typically mixed with HFCS 43 to make HFCS 55)

Once absorbed, fructose is transported to the liver with three possible pathways: (i) conversion to glucose and stored as liver glycogen; (ii) conversion to triglyceride with resultant elevated serum very low-density lipoprotein; and (iii) conversion to uric acid, which is associated with possible gout-like joint pain. Pathway 1 (conversion to glucose with storage as glycogen) is the preferred pathway, but excess liver exposure to fructose may overwhelm this pathway, resulting in more triglyceride and uric acid formation. Uric acid uses nitric oxide, which disturbs oxygen delivery to working tissues and creates another concern for athletes (169).

The volume of carbohydrate provided during exercise longer than 45 minutes is an important consideration, because providing too much carbohydrate too quickly may induce delayed gastric emptying and GI distress and, at least temporarily, take needed fluids away from blood (thereby lowering fluid availability to muscle and skin) to dilute this excessively concentrated solution. On the other hand, providing a fluid that delivers an excessively small amount of carbohydrate (<4% carbohydrate solution) may diminish the performance benefit. Athletes should strive to consume ~1 g carbohydrate/minute of exercise (*i.e.*, 4 kcal/minute). This level of intake can occur through consumption of sports beverages that contain between 4% and 8% carbohydrate, at a volume of ~0.6–1.2 L/hr (154,170). Some sports beverages have carbohydrates precisely within this range, whereas others have higher concentrations. Higher concentrations may cause a delay in gastric emptying, compromising speedy delivery of needed carbohydrate to working tissues during exercise (171). Another advantage of consuming a 4%–8% carbohydrate solution is that, if the carbohydrate source is mixed, it has a faster rate of intestinal *absorption* than water alone (127). This faster absorption can more efficiently deliver carbohydrate to the blood and, ultimately, working tissues.

The goals of drinking a sports beverage during exercise is to supply carbohydrate to avoid low blood sugar, supplement the glycogen stores in the liver and muscles, and to replace the electrolytes and water lost in sweat. There is evidence that commercial sports drinks containing both carbohydrate and sodium are more effective at restoring body water balance than plain water (172). It appears, however, that to maximize rehydration, a level of sodium greater than that provided in most sports drinks is desirable (173). This added sodium can be obtained through the normal consumption of foods, many of which have added salt (sodium) (174). Endurance sports beverages typically have higher levels of sodium.

FLUID INTAKE RECOMMENDATIONS

Fluid intake recommendations for athletes can be summarized as follows:

- Ideally, athletes should try to consume sufficient fluid to match fluid sweat losses.
- Humans have little comprehension of the rate of fluid loss during exercise, so fluids should be consumed on a fixed schedule, regardless of thirst. (The sensation of thirst occurs only following a large fluid deficit of 1%–2% of body mass and should be considered an "emergency" sensation rather than treated as the perfect time to drink.)
- With intense exercise and/or exercise during a hot and humid day, it is difficult to consume and absorb fluids at the same rate that fluids are lost via sweat. Therefore, athletes should begin exercise in a well-hydrated state, and drink fluids at opportunities that present themselves during exercise and/or competition.
- In some athletes, ingestion of relatively large fluid volumes may increase GI distress, which can result in

reduced performance. However, practicing drinking ever larger volumes of fluids improves fluid consumption tolerance. There is a maximum of gastric emptying rate (noted above).

■ Although a robust fluid replacement strategy is desirable, consumption of fluids in excess of sweat and urinary losses is a primary cause of hyponatremia (also referred to as water intoxication). Hyponatremia risk can be made worse when sweat sodium loss is heavy, with consumption of low-sodium beverages, and with excess fluid consumption prior to the exercise bout. The risk of hyponatremia appears to be particularly high in women, likely because of smaller body size and lower sweat rates than males (68,72).

Hydration Recommendations (31,72)

■ Fluid deficits of >2% body weight can compromise cognitive function and aerobic exercise performances, particularly in hot weather.

■ Fluid deficits of 3%–5% body weight can compromise performance in anaerobic, high-intensity, or skill-intensive activities, and aerobic activities performed in a cool environment.

■ Fluid deficits of 6%–10% body weight have pronounced negative impacts on exercise tolerance, decreases in cardiac output, sweat production, and skin and muscle blood flow. Common signs of hypohydration include thirst, flushed skin, apathy, dizziness, nausea, GI cramping, and loss of body weight.

■ Assuming the athlete is in a satisfactory state of energy balance, daily hydration state may be estimated by measuring body weight upon waking and after voiding. Significant daily changes that exceed 2% of body weight are likely representative of changes in total body water.

■ Prior to beginning exercise athletes should attempt to achieve euhydration through consumption of 5–10 mL/kg (2–4 mL/lb) fluids 2–4 hours prior to exercise. The goal is to achieve a urine color suggesting adequate hydration (see Figure 7.9).

■ Sweat rates vary during exercise from 0.3 to 2.4 L/hr (has been recorded up to 3.9 L/hr), depending on exercise intensity, duration, fitness, acclimatization to the heat, and environmental heat and humidity. Fluid consumption patterns should attempt to minimize net fluid loss to less than 2% of body weight. Routine measurements of body weight pre- and postexercise under different environmental conditions should help guide athletes on how well their hydration practices are achieving this goal.

■ Overhydration is seen in recreational athletes who achieve sweat rates lower than fluid consumption, increasing the risk of hyponatremia. Common signs of hyponatremia include altered mental status, mood changes, confusion, muscular twitching, muscular weakness, headache, swollen limbs.

■ Fluids containing both salt and carbohydrates should be consumed during exercise, particularly if longer than 45 minutes and/or if high sweat rates are achieved.

■ After exercise athletes should immediately initiate rehydration strategies that include water, salt, and carbohydrate. The volume consumed should be ~125%–150% of the measured fluid deficit (*i.e.*, the difference in weight between pre- and postexercise) because water loss through sweat and urination continues postexercise.

■ Alcohol is a diuretic and should be discouraged postexercise, at least until after the athlete has achieved a state of euhydration.

SUMMARY

■ There is perhaps no other factor that so clearly has an impact on performance than hydration state and no nutritional substance than water that can so quickly be inadequate to elevate the risk of serious illness.

■ Athletes in all sports can gain an immediate performance benefit by assuring that physical activity begins, continues, and ends with hydration state adequately maintained. To do this, athletes should practice consuming appropriately constituted fluids on a fixed schedule rather than by relying on thirst as the primary stimulus to drink. The thirst mechanism fails to occur until a substantial amount of body water (about 2% of body weight) has already been lost, assuring that athletes will perform in a poorly hydrated state that will negatively affect performance.

■ Well-formulated sports beverages that contain a sodium (about 100–200 mg/240 mL) and carbohydrate (about 4%–8% carbohydrate solution) and are appropriately consumed have been found to encourage fast absorption, sustain blood volume, sustain sweat rates, and provide fuel to the brain and muscles to minimize the impact of hydration deficits.

■ Athletes should find an appropriately formulated sports beverage that tastes good while they are physically active, and that they are willing to consume enough of to minimize body weight loss during exercise.

- Athletes should become accustomed to a sports beverage to ensure adequate gastric emptying, which is affected by fluid volume, osmolality, pH, type(s) and concentration of carbohydrates, exercise intensity, fluid temperature, environmental conditions, and the extent to which the athlete is hypohydrated.

- Entering physical activity in a well-hydrated state is important because improving hydration status while exercising is difficult during intense activity because the maximal sweat rate is higher than the maximal absorption rate for fluid.

- After exercise is completed, the athlete should continue to drink to replace any amount of fluid that was unreplaced during the exercise to return as quickly as possible to a well-hydrated state. Athletes should be cautious to not overconsume fluids because of the risk of hyponatremia.

- Athletes should practice to find themselves a refueling and hydration plan that suits their individual needs, based on their state of acclimatization, exercise intensity and duration, sweat fluid loss, and GI tolerance. They should find an appropriately constituted sports beverage before, during, and after exercise, with the confidence of knowing that an appropriate hydration strategy is critically important to performance and recovery (72).

- Before exercise athletes should strive to achieve euhydration by consuming a fluid volume equivalent to 5–10 mL/kg body weight (~2–4 mL/lb) in the 2–4 hours prior to exercise, with the goal of producing urine that is pale yellow and allowing sufficient time

for excess fluid consumed to be voided. Studies suggest an ergogenic benefit in athletes who consume a sports drink 1–4 hours prior to exercise to help ensure a good hydration state prior to the initiation of exercise (175–177).

- During exercise, athletes should drink sufficient fluids to replace fluid losses in a way that limits the total body fluid loss to no more than 2% of body weight. Different sports, different sweat rates, and different environmental conditions mandate that athletes find hydration strategies that are well suited to them.

After exercise, athletes typically finish with a fluid deficit, requiring that they establish an appropriate strategy to achieve euhydration during the recovery period. This generally involves consumption of water and sodium at a rate that minimizes diuresis.

Practical Application Activity

1. Measure your body weight just before you begin to exercise.
2. Measure how much fluid (in oz) you consume during the exercise.
3. Measure your body weight (dry off first) right after you finish your exercise.
4. The difference in weight is the fluid you should have consumed but did not consume (16 oz = 1 lb). (If there was more than a 2% difference in weight you have likely not benefited from the exercise as much as you might have.)

CHAPTER QUESTIONS

1. On average, the body of a physically active adult is composed of approximately _____ water weight.
   a. 20.0%
   b. 30.5%
   c. 60.0%
   d. 80.0%

2. The greatest proportion of total body fluid is found in the
   a. ISF
   b. Blood plasma
   c. ECF
   d. ICF

3. ISF refers to
   a. Fluids in and around the heart muscle
   b. Fluids that are mainly composed of anions rather than cations
   c. Fluids surrounding cells but not part of the cell or plasma
   d. Fluids in capillaries that nourish the periphery (toes, fingers, eyes, etc.)

4. The main cation in ECF is
   a. Calcium
   b. Chloride
   c. Potassium
   d. Sodium

5. The primary cation in ICF is
   a. Calcium
   b. Chloride
   c. Potassium
   d. Sodium

6. ICF osmolarity is higher than ECF osmolarity, so what is the tonicity of the blood?
   a. Isotonic to the ICF
   b. Hypotonic to the ICF
   c. Hypertonic to the ICF
   d. Hypertonic to the ECF

7. A heavily sweating athlete, particularly if he or she is well conditioned to the environment, is likely to experience the following osmolarity change in the blood:
   a. Osmolarity increases
   b. Osmolarity decreases
   c. Osmolarity does not change
   d. Osmolarity change is unpredictable

8. The greatest water loss that occurs when an athlete exercises intensely is from
   a. Kidneys (urine)
   b. Lungs (air)
   c. GI tract (feces)
   d. Skin (sweat)

9. In athletes, the sensation of "thirst" is a perfect indicator that it is a good time to consume fluids.
   a. True
   b. False

10. Of the following, which is present in the greatest concentration in sweat?
    a. Lactate
    b. Calcium
    c. Magnesium
    d. Sodium

ANSWERS TO CHAPTER QUESTIONS

1. c
2. d
3. c
4. d
5. c
6. b
7. a
8. d
9. b
10. d

Case Study Considerations

1. **Case Study Answer 1:** The goal of the sweat rate calculator is to determine how much additional fluid the athlete should consume to avoid a dehydration-associated weight loss that exceeds 2% of body weight. As she typically loses 4 lb during the 10K training run, which represents 3.8% of body weight, Sally needs to plan on adding approximately 2 lb more fluid during the training run. Since 16 oz of fluid = 1 lb, Sally would need to develop a strategy to consume approximately 32 oz of additional fluid during the training. So as to tolerate this level of fluid, Sally should practice sipping on a sports beverage during her run with a consumption pattern that provides approximately 16 oz every 5 km. This represents approximately 10 oz of consumed fluid every 15 minutes of the training run.

2. **Case Study Answer 2:** The primary nutrients of concern are carbohydrate, sodium, and water. Both sodium and water are lost through sweat, and carbohydrate found in the liver, blood, and muscles are used at a much faster rate during exercise.
   - **Volume and drinking frequency of fluid:** As discussed in answer 1 above, approximately 32 oz of fluid should be consumed to avoid reaching the >2% body weight loss associated with reduced performance. While this seems a relatively easy goal, it is important to give the body an opportunity to adapt to this level of fluid consumption during exercise. Therefore, while Sally should have this as a goal, it should not be instantly pursued. Instead, Sally should initially consume a smaller volume, perhaps 4–5 oz every 15 minutes, and add a couple of ounces each week until the volume goal is reached. This will

give the GI tract an opportunity to adapt to the fluid being consumed.

- **Electrolytes and their concentration:** Both water and electrolytes are important for maintaining athletic performance, but either too much or too little of either creates problems. The electrolyte lost in the greatest volume via sweat is sodium, making it the electrolyte that should be focused on the most. Low sodium can result in hyponatremia (low sodium in the blood), which has multiple negative effects. Importantly, as the main extracellular fluid electrolyte, low sodium results in low blood volume, even if a large volume of fluid is consumed. The typical sports beverage concentrations of sodium range from 50 to 200 mg/cup. Recommended concentration levels of sodium in a sports beverage range from 100 to 200 mg/cup, with the higher concentration levels recommended for endurance activities with relatively large sweat losses. Importantly, many sports beverage companies include magnesium and potassium in their beverage despite not being significantly lost in sweat. The result of adding these electrolytes is typically to lower the sodium concentration below desirable levels so as to help ensure that the high osmolarity resulting from the addition of these other electrolytes does not impede gastric emptying.

- **Carbohydrates and their concentration:** Carbohydrate consumption is critically important to sustain blood sugar so that the central nervous system continues to work normally, and also to help ensure hard-working muscles have a source of carbohydrate once muscle glycogen stores become depleted. The concentration of carbohydrate in the sports beverage is important, as is the composition of the carbohydrate. Studies indicate that a 6%–7% carbohydrate works well for most athletes. (To put this into perspective, orange juice is a 14% carbohydrate solution.) Having a concentration that exceeds 7% tends to delay gastric emptying, which has 2 negative impacts: (1) It can inhibit drinking more beverage because the stomach holds the beverage longer; (2) It slows the provision of needed electrolytes, carbohydrate, and fluid to the blood and tissues. The composition of the carbohydrate should be varied to optimize the utilization of receptors in the intestines. We have glucose and fructose receptors. So, if you have a beverage that is high in fructose, the glucose receptors are under used, delaying the provision of the carbohydrate to the blood. In addition, the delayed absorption may increase gut osmolarity, causing fluid to go from the blood into the gut to dilute the contents. This is the opposite of how you would like the consumed fluid to flow. The same problem occurs if you have a beverage with pure glucose, causing an underutilization of the fructose receptors. Having a mixture works best so that the carbohydrate receptors can all be well accessed.

- **Problems the runner may encounter:**
  - *Gastric emptying:* Anything that delays gastric emptying, including fiber, a high level of free glucose, a high level of electrolytes, etc., will delay gastric emptying, which results in a reduced fluid consumption.
  - *Delayed drinking:* Many athletes wait until they become thirsty before they drink, but the sensation of thirst typically doesn't occur until the athlete has already lost ~1.5 L of fluid. Athletes should take the approach that sustaining "normalcy" is better than recovering from "abnormalcy," and since sweating increase almost immediately when exercise is initiated, fluid intake should also occur at that time.
  - *Diarrhea:* There are many potential causes of diarrhea, but in athletes it is typically because too much fluid is consumed at once (a common occurrence with delayed drinking), consuming a beverage that has an excessively high osmolar concentration, and/or consuming a beverage that the athlete is unfamiliar with and they discover that, as a result of the diarrhea, it is a beverage they cannot tolerate.

REFERENCES

1. Jackson S. Anatomy & physiology for nurses: nurses' aids series. 9th ed. London: Bailliere Tindall; 1985.
2. European Food Safety Authority. European Food Safety Authority Panel on Dietetic Products, Nutrition, and Allergies (NDA). Scientific opinion on dietary reference values for water. ESFA J. 2010;8(3):1459.
3. Armstrong LE. Performing in extreme environments. Champaign (IL): Human Kinetics; 2000.

4. Armstrong LE, Johnson EC, McKenzie AL, Ellis LA, Williamson KH. Ultraendurance cycling in a hot environment: thirst, fluid consumption, and water balance. J Strength Cond Res. 2015;29(4):869–76.

5. Flouris AD, Schlader ZJ. Human behavioral thermoregulation during exercise in the heat. Scand J Med Sci Sports. 2015;25(Suppl 1):52–64.

6. Franko G, Acs P, Vari SG, Figler M. Dehydration of amateur long-distance runners and fluid consumption. Int J Sports Sci Med 2019;3(1):24–8.

7. Bhati P, Anand P, Das J, Comma K, Sen S, Hussain ME, Khanna GL. Predictors of physical performance in national level make Kho Kho players: a cross-sectional analysis. Sport Sci Health. 2022;19(2):589–96.

8. Zach K. Hydration and nutrition in athletes. In: Miranda-Comas G, Cooper G, Herrera J, Curtis S, editors. Essential sports medicine: A clinical guide for students and residents. 2nd ed. Cham: Springer; 2021.

9. Pryor JL, Johnson EC, Roberts WO, Pryor RR. Application of evidence-based recommendations for heat acclimatization: individual and team sport perspectives. Temperature (Austin). 2019;6(1):37–49.

10. Christo K, Prabhakaran R, Lamparello B, Cord J, Miller KK, Goldstein MA, Gupta N, Herzog DB, Klibanski A, Misra M. Bone metabolism in adolescent athletes with amenorrhea, athletes with eumenorrhea, and control subjects. Pediatrics. 2008;121:1127–36.

11. Kontele I, Vassilakou T. Nutritional risks among adolescent athletes with disordered eating. Children (Basel). 2021;8;715.

12. Maughan RJ. Water and electrolyte loss and replacement in training and competition. In: Maughan RJ, editor. Sports nutrition. Oxford: Wiley Blackwell; 2014. p. 174–84.

13. O'Neal E, Boy T, Davis B, Pritchett K, Pritchett R, Nepocatych S, Black K. Post-exercise sweat loss estimation accuracy of athletes and physically active adults: a review. Sports (Basel). 2020;8(8):113.

14. Ceylan B, Kons RL, Detanico D, Šimenko J. Acute dehydration impairs performance and physiological responses in highly trained judo athletes. Biology (Basel). 2022;11(6):872.

15. Urso C, Brucculeri S, Caimi G. Physiopathological, epidemiological, clinical and therapeutic aspects of exercise-associated hyponatremia. J Clin Med. 2014;3(4):1258–75.

16. Burke LM, Slater GJ, Matthews JJ, Langan-Evans C, Horswill CA. ACSM expert consensus statement on weight loss in weight-category sports. Curr Sports Med Rep. 2021;20(4):199–217.

17. Gullestad R. Temperature regulation in children during exercise. Acta Paediatr Scand. 1975;64(2):257–63.

18. Inbar O, Morris N, Epstein Y, Gass G. Comparison of thermoregulatory responses to exercise in dry heat among prepubertal boys, young adults and older males. Exp Physiol. 2004;89(6):691–700.

19. Davies CT. Thermal responses to exercise in children. Ergonomics. 1981;24(1):55–61.

20. Delamarche P, Bittel J, Lacour JR, Flandrois R. Thermoregulation at rest and during exercise in prepubertal boys. Eur J Appl Physiol Occup Physiol. 1990;60(6):436–40.

21. Drinkwater BL, Kupprat IC, Denton JE, Christ JL, Horvath SM. Response of prepubertal girls and college women to work in the heat. J Appl Physiol Respir Environ Exerc Physiol. 1977;43(6);1046–53.

22. Havenith G. Human surface to mass ratio and body core temperature in exercise heat stress—a concept revisited. J Therm Biol. 2001;26(4–5):387–93.

23. Wagner JA, Robinson S, Tzankoff SP, Marino RP. Heat tolerance and acclimatization to work in the heat in relation to age. J Appl Physiol. 1972;33(5):616–22.

24. Leites GT, Cunha GS, Obeid J, Wilk B, Meyer F, Timmons BW. Thermoregulation in boys and men exercising at the same heat production per unit body mass. Eur J Appl Physiol. 2016;116(7):1411–9.

25. Jang C, Hui S, Lu W, Cowan AJ, Morscher RJ, Lee G, Liu W, Tesz GJ, Birnbaum MJ, Rabinowitz JD. The small intestine converts dietary fructose into glucose and organic acids. Cell Metab. 2018;27(2):351–61.

26. Ko GJ, Rhee CM, Kalantar-Zadeh K, Joshi S. The effects of high-protein diets on kidney health and longevity. J Am Soc Nephrol. 2020;31(8):1667–79.

27. Wizard OC, Garthe I, Phillips SM. Dietary protein for training adaptation and body composition manipulation in track and field athletes. Int J Sport Nutr Exerc Metab. 2019; 29(2):165–74.

28. Heer M, Baisch F, Kropp J, Gerzer R, Drummer C. High dietary sodium chloride consumption may not induce body fluid retention in humans. Am J Physiol Renal Physiol. 2000; 278(4):F585–95.

29. Broad EM, Burke LM, Cox GR, Heeley P, Riley M. Body-weight changes and voluntary fluid intakes during training and competition sessions in team sports. Int J Sport Nutr. 1996;6(3):307–20.

30. Noakes TD, Adams BA, Myburgh KH, Greff C, Lotz T, Nathan M. The danger of inadequate water intake during prolonged exercise. A novel concept re-visited. Eur J Appl Physiol Occup Physiol. 1988;57(2):210–9.

31. McDermott BP, Anderson SA, Armstrong LE, Casa DJ, Cheuvront SN, Cooper L, Kenney WL, O'Connor FG, Roberts WO. National Athletic Trainers' Association position statement: fluid replacement for the physically active. J Athl Train. 2017;52(9):877–95.

32. Carter JE, Gisolfi CV. Fluid replacement during and after exercise in the heat. Med Sci Sports Exerc. 1989;21:532–9.

33. Millard-Stafford M, Snow TK, Jones ML, Suh HG. The beverage hydration index: influence of electrolytes, carbohydrate, and protein. Nutrients. 2021;13:2933.

34. Harper ME, Willis JS, Patrick J. Sodium and chloride in nutrition. In: O'Dell BL, Sunde RA, editors. Handbook of nutritionally essential mineral elements. New York (NY): Marcel Dekker; 1997. p. 93–116.

35. Brody T. Nutritional biochemistry. 2nd ed. San Diego (CA): Academic Press; 1999.

36. Sheng H-W. Sodium, chloride and potassium. In: Stipanuk MH, editor. Biochemical and physiological aspects of human nutrition. Philadelphia (PA): W.B. Saunders Company; 2000. p. 686–710.

37. Institute of Medicine, Food and Nutrition Board. Sodium and chloride. dietary reference intakes for water, potassium, sodium, chloride, and sulfate. Washington (DC): National Academies Press; 2005. p. 269–423.

38. Adrogue HJ, Madias NE. Hyponatremia. N Engl J Med. 2000; 342(21):1581–9.

39. van Blijderveen JC, Straus SM, Rodenburg EM, Zietse R, Stricker BH, Sturkenboom MC, Verhamme CM. Risk of hyponatremia with diuretics: chlorthalidone versus hydrochlorothiazide. Am J Med. 2014;127(8):763–71.

40. Centers for Disease Control and Prevention. New research: excess sodium intake remains common in the United States. 2016. Accessed 2016 May 12. Published 2016 January 7. Available from: http://www.cdc.gov/media/releases/2016/p0106-sodium-intake.html

41. Powles J, Fahimi S, Micha R, Khatibzadeh S, Shi P, Ezzati M, Engell RE, Lim SS, Danaei G, Mozaffarian D; Global Burden of Diseases Nutrition and Chronic Diseases Expert Group (NutriCoDE). Global, regional and national sodium intakes in 1990 and 2010: a systematic analysis of 24 h urinary sodium excretion and dietary surveys worldwide. BMJ Open. 2013;3:e003733.

42. Denton D, Weisinger R, Mundy NI, Wickings EJ, Dixson A, Moisson P, Pingard AM, Shade R, Carey D, Ardaillou R, Paillard F, Chapman J, Thillet J, Michel JB. The effect of increased salt intake on blood pressure of chimpanzees. Nat Med. 1995;1(10):1009–16.

43. Elliott P. Observational studies of salt and blood pressure. Hypertension. 1991;17(1 Suppl):I3–8.

44. Elliott P, Stamler J, Nichols R, Dyer AR, Stamler R, Kesteloot H, Marmot M. Intersalt revisited: further analyses of 24 hour sodium excretion and blood pressure within and across populations. Intersalt Cooperative Research Group. BMJ. 1996;312(7041):1249–53.

45. Franco V, Oparil S. Salt sensitivity, a determinant of blood pressure, cardiovascular disease and survival. J Am Coll Nutr. 2006;25(3 Suppl):247S–55S.

46. Vollmer WM, Sacks FM, Ard J, Appel LJ, Bray GA, Simons-Morton DG, Conlin PR, Svetkey LP, Erlinger TP, Moore TJ, Karanja N; DASH-Sodium Trial Collaborative Research Group. Effects of diet and sodium intake on blood pressure: subgroup analysis of the DASH-sodium trial. Ann Intern Med. 2001;135(12):1019–28.

47. Giner V, Poch E, Bragulat E, Oriola J, González D, Coca A, de la Sierra A. Renin-angiotensin system genetic polymorphisms and salt sensitivity in essential hypertension. Hypertension. 2000;35(1 Pt 2):512–7.

48. Akita S, Sacks FM, Svetkey LP, Conlin PR, Kimura G; DASH-Sodium Trial Collaborative Research Group. Effects of the Dietary Approaches to Stop Hypertension (DASH) diet on the pressure-natriuresis relationship. Hypertension. 2003;42(1):8–13.

49. Curhan GC, Willett WC, Speizer FE, Spiegelman D, Stampfer MJ. Comparison of dietary calcium with supplemental calcium and other nutrients as factors affecting the risk for kidney stones in women. Ann Intern Med. 1997;126(7):497–504.

50. Borghi L, Schianchi T, Meschi T, Guerra A, Allegri F, Maggiore U, Novarini A. Comparison of two diets for the prevention of recurrent stones in idiopathic hypercalciuria. N Engl J Med. 2002;346(2):77–84.

51. Tsugane S. Salt, salted food intake, and risk of gastric cancer: epidemiologic evidence. Cancer Sci. 2005;96(1):1–6.

52. Hirohata T, Kono S. Diet/nutrition and stomach cancer in Japan. Int J Cancer. 1997;(Suppl 10):34–6.

53. Liu C, Russell RM. Nutrition and gastric cancer risk: an update. Nutr Rev. 2008;66(5):237–49.

54. Devine A, Criddle RA, Dick IM, Kerr DA, Prince RL. A longitudinal study of the effect of sodium and calcium intakes on regional bone density in postmenopausal women. Am J Clin Nutr. 1995;62(4):740–5.

55. Sawka MN, Latzka WA, Montain SJ. Effects of dehydration and rehydration on performance. In: Maughan RJ, editor. Nutrition in sport. London: Blackwell Science; 2000. p. 205–17.

56. Hajjar IM, Grim CE, George V, Kotchen TA. Impact of diet on blood pressure and age-related changes in blood pressure in the US population: analysis of NHANES III. Arch Intern Med. 2001;161(4):589–93.

57. Gennari FJ. Hypokalemia. N Engl J Med. 1998;339(7):451–8.

58. Mumoli N, Cei M. Licorice-induced hypokalemia. Int J Cardiol. 2008;124(3):e42–4.

59. Appel LJ, Moore TJ, Obarzanek E, Vollmer WM, Svetkey LP, Sacks FM, Bray GA, Vogt TM, Cutler JA, Windhauser MM, Lin PH, Karanja N. A clinical trial of the effects of dietary patterns on blood pressure. DASH Collaborative Research Group. N Engl J Med. 1997;336(16):1117–24.

60. Ferraro PM, Mandel EI, Curhan GC, Gambaro G, Taylor EN. Dietary protein and potassium, diet-dependent net acid load, and risk of incident kidney stones. Clin J Am Soc Nephrol. 2016;11(10):1834–44.

61. Curhan GC, Willett WC, Rimm EB, Stampfer MJ. A prospective study of dietary calcium and other nutrients and the risk of symptomatic kidney stones. N Engl J Med. 1993;328(12):833–8.

62. Tucker KL, Hannan MT, Chen H, Cupples LA, Wilson PW, Kiel DP. Potassium, magnesium, and fruit and vegetable intakes are associated with greater bone mineral density in elderly men and women. Am J Clin Nutr. 1999;69(4):727–36.

63. Zhu K, Devine A, Prince RL. The effects of high potassium consumption on bone mineral density in a prospective cohort study of elderly postmenopausal women. Osteoporos Int. 2009;20(2):335–40.

64. Mandal AK. Hypokalemia and hyperkalemia. Med Clin North Am. 1997;81(3):611–39.

65. Kenney WL, Murray R. Chapter 2: Exercise physiology. In: Maughan RJ, editor. Sports nutrition: The encyclopaedia of sports medicine. 2014 International Olympic Committee. London: John Wiley & Sons, Ltd; 2014. p. 20–35.

66. Poortmans J. Exercise and renal function. Sports Med. 1984;1:125–53.

67. Coyle EF. Fluid and fuel intake during exercise. J Sports Sci. 2004;22(1):39–55.

68. American College of Sports Medicine; Sawka MN, Burke LM, Eichner ER, Maughan RJ, Montain SJ, Stachenfield NS. American College of Sports Medicine position stand. Exercise and fluid replacement. Med Sci Sports Exerc. 2007;39(2):377–90.

69. Williams MH. Nutrition for health, fitness and sport. 5th ed. New York (NY): WCB McGraw-Hill; 1999. p. 276–7; 285–7; 292–3; 317–8.

70. Bernard TE, Iheanacho I. Heat index and adjusted temperature as surrogates for wet bulb globe temperature to screen for occupational heat stress. J Occup Environ Hyg. 2015;12(5):323–33.

71. American College of Sports Medicine; Armstrong LE, Casa DJ, Millard-Stafford M, Moran DS, Pyne SW, Roberts WO.

American College of Sports Medicine position stand. Exertional heat illness during training and competition. Med Sci Sports Exerc. 2007;39(3):556–72.

72. Thomas DT, Erdman KA, Burke LM. American College of Sports Medicine joint position statement. Nutrition and athletic performance. Med Sci Sports Exerc. 2016;48:543–68.

73. de Souza Martins ND, Gonçalves LVS, Neto WK, Gama EF, da Silva Marinho PC. Effect of acute moderate-intense aerobic exercise on the state of hydration and sweat rate of trained individuals. Aust J Basic Appl Sci. 2015;9(11):124–7.

74. Pearcy M, Robinson S, Miller DI, Thomas JT Jr, Debrota J. Effects of dehydration, salt depletion and pitressin on sweat rate and urine flow. J Appl Physiol. 1956;8:621–6.

75. Inoue Y, Ichinose-Kuwahara T, Funaki C, Ueda H, Tochihara Y, Kondo N. Sex differences in acetylcholine-induced sweating responses due to physical training. J Physiol Anthropol. 2014;33:13.

76. Mee JA, Gibson OR, Doust J, Maxwell NS. A comparison of males and females' temporal patterning to short-and long-term heat acclimation. Scand J Med Sci Sports. 2015;25(S1): 250–8.

77. Candas V, Libert JP, Brandenberger G, Sagot JC, Amoros C, Kahn JM. Hydration during exercise. Effects on thermal and cardiovascular adjustments. Eur J Appl Physiol Occup Physiol. 1986;55(2):113–22.

78. Zambraski EJ. Renal regulation of fluid homeostasis during exercise. In: Gisolfi CV, Lamb DR, editors. Perspectives in exercise science and sports medicine. Vol. 3. Fluid homeostasis during exercise. Carmel (IN): Benchmark Press; 1990. p. 247–80.

79. Thigpen LK.Green JM, O'Neal EK. Hydration profile and sweat loss perception of male and female division II basketball players during practice. J Strength Cond Res. 2014; 28(12):3425–31.

80. Dube A, Gouws C, Breukelman G. Effects of hypo hydration and fluid balance in athletes' cognitive performance: a systematic review. Afr Health Sci. 2022;22(1):367–76.

81. Sawka MN. Physiological consequences of hypohydration: exercise performance and thermoregulation. Med Sci Sports Exerc. 1992;24(6):657–70.

82. King DS, Costill DL, Fink WJ, Hargreaves M, Fielding RA. Muscle metabolism during exercise in the heat in unacclimatized and acclimatized humans. J Appl Physiol (1985). 1985; 59(5):1350–4.

83. Périard JD, Racinais S, Sawka MN. Adaptations and mechanisms of human heat acclimation: applications for competitive athletes and sports. Scand J Med Sci Sports. 2015;25(Suppl 1): 20–38.

84. Szlyk PC, Sils IV, Francesconi RP, Hubbard RW, Armstrong LE. Effects of water temperature and flavoring on voluntary dehydration in men. Physiol Behav. 1989;45(3):639–47.

85. Greenleaf JE, Sargent F II. Voluntary dehydration in man. J Appl Physiol. 1965;20(4):719–24.

86. Passe D, Horn M, Stofan J, Horswill C, Murray R. Voluntary dehydration in runners despite favorable conditions for fluid intake. Int J Sport Nutr Exerc Metab. 2007;17(3):284–95.

87. Rehrer JN. Factors influencing fluid bioavailability. Austr J Nutr Diet. 1996;53(4):S8–12.

88. Maresh CM, Gabaree-Boulant CL, Armstrong LE, Judelson DA, Hoffman JR, Castellani JW, Kenefick RW, Bergeron MF,

Casa DJ. Effect of hydration status on thirst, drinking and related hormonal responses during low-intensity exercise in the heat. J Appl Physiol. 2004;97(1):39–44.

89. Wilk B, Rivera-Brown AM, Ramírez-Marrero AM, Bar-Or O. Voluntary drinking and hydration in trained, heat-acclimatized girls exercising in a hot and humid climate. Eur J Appl Physiol. 2008;103:109–16.

90. Wilk B, Bar-Or O. Effect of drink flavor and NaCL on voluntary drinking and hydration in boys exercising in the heat. J Appl Physiol. 1996;80(4):1112–7.

91. Davis JM, Burgess WA, Slentz CA, Bartoli WP, Pate RR. Effects of ingesting 6% and 12% glucose-electrolyte beverages during prolonged intermittent cycling in the heat. Eur J Appl Physiol Occup Physiol. 1988;57 (5):563–9.

92. Hubbard RW, Szlyk PC, Armstrong LE. Influence of thirst and fluid palatability on fluid ingestion during exercise. In: Gisolfi CV, Lamb DR, editors. Fluid homeostasis during exercise. Carmel (IN): Benchmark Press; 1990. p. 39–95.

93. Murray R. The effects of consuming carbohydrate-electrolyte beverages on gastric emptying and fluid absorption during and following exercise. Sports Med. 1987;4(5):322–51.

94. Bergeron MF, Waller JL, Marinik EL. Voluntary fluid intake and core temperature responses in adolescent tennis players: sports beverage versus water. Br J Sports Med. 2006;40(5): 406–10.

95. Jeukendrup AE. Nutrition for endurance sports: marathon, triathlon, and road cycling. J Sports Sci. 2011;29(Suppl 1): S91–9.

96. Casa DJ, Armstrong LE, Hillman SK, Montain SJ, Reiff RV, Rich BS, Roberts WO, Stone JA. National Athletic Trainers' Association position statement: fluid replacement for athletes. J Athl Train. 2000;35(2):212–24.

97. Arnaoutis G, Kavouras SA, Angelopoulou A, Skoulariki C, Bismpikou S, Mourtakos S, Sidossis LS. Fluid balance during training in elite young athletes of different sports. J Strength Cond Res. 2015;29(12):3447–52.

98. Kavouras SA, Arnautis G, Makrillos M, Garagouni C, Nikolaou E, Chira O, Ellinikaki E, Sidossis LS. Educational intervention on water intake improves hydration status and enhances exercise performance in athletic youth. Scand J Med Sci Sports. 2012;22(5):684–9.

99. Murray R. Dehydration, hyperthermia, and athletes: science and practice. J Athl Train. 1996;31(3):248–52.

100. Bar-David Y, Urkin J, Landau D, Bar-David Z, Pilpel D. Voluntary dehydration among elementary school children residing in a hot arid environment. J Hum Nutr Diet. 2009;22:455–60.

101. Kenefick RW, Mahood NV, Mattern CO, Kertzer R, Quinn TJ. Hypohydration adversely affects lactate threshold in endurance athletes. J Strength Cond Res. 2002;16:38–43.

102. Naghii M. The significance of water in sport and weight control. Nutr Health. 2000;14:127–32.

103. Casa DJ, DeMartini JK, Berjeron MF, Csillan D, Eichner ER, Lopez RM, Ferrara MS, Miller KC, O'Connor F, Sawka MN, Yeargin SW. National Athletic Trainers' Association position statement: exertional heat illnesses. J Athl Train. 2015; 50(9):986–1000.

104. Bergeron MF. Muscle cramps during exercise—is it fatigue or electrolyte deficit? Curr Sports Med Rep. 2008;7(4):S50–5.

105. Noakes TD. Fluid and electrolyte disturbances in heat illness. Int J Sports Med. 1998;19(2):S146–9.

106. Stofan JR, Zachwieja JJ, Horswill CA, Murray R, Anderson SA, Eichner ER. Sweat and sodium losses in NCAA football players: a precursor to heat cramps? Int J Sport Nutr Exerc Metab. 2005;15:641–52.

107. Bergeron MF. Muscle cramps during exercise-Is it fatigue or electrolyte deficit? Curr Sports Med Rep. 2008. S50–S55 (7:Suppl 4).

108. Bergeron MF. Exertional heat cramps: recovery and return to play. J Sport Rehabil. 2007;16(3):190–6.

109. Hunt AP, Parker AW, Stewart IB. Symptoms of heat illness in surface mine workers. Int Arch Occup Environ Health. 2013;86(5):519–27.

110. Hostler D, Franco V, Martin-Gill C, Roth RN. Recognition and treatment of exertional heat illness at a marathon race. Prehosp Emerg Care. 2014;18:456–9.

111. Poh PYS, Armstrong LE, Casa DJ, Pescatello LS, McDermott BP, Emmanuel H, Maresh CM. Orthostatic hypotension after 10 days of exercise-heat acclimation and 28 hours of sleep loss. Aviat Space Environ Med. 2012;83(4):403–11.

112. Adams WM, Hosokawa Y, Casa DJ. The timing of exertional heat stroke survival starts prior to collapse. Curr Sports Med Rep. 2015;14(4):273–4.

113. Eichner E. Heat stroke in sports: causes, prevention, and treatment. GSSI Sports Sci Exch. 2002;15(3):1–4.

114. Speedy D, Noakes TD, Schneider C. Exercise-associated hyponatremia: a review. Emerg Med (Fremantle). 2001;13:17–27.

115. Hiller WD. Dehydration and hyponatremia during triathlons. Med Sci Sports Exerc. 1989;21(Suppl 5):S219–21.

116. United States Track & Field. USATF announces major change in hydration guidelines (4-19-2003). Accessed 2024 May 22. Available from: https://howtobefit.com/runninghydration-guide.htm

117. Noakes TD. The hyponatremia of exercise. Int J Sport Nutr. 1992;2:205–28.

118. Gisolfi CV. Fluid balance for optimal performance. Nutr Rev. 1996;54:S159–68.

119. Rehrer JN. Fluid and electrolyte balance in ultra-endurance sport. Sports Med. 2001;31:701–15.

120. Mayo Clinic Staff. Low blood sodium in endurance athletes. MayoClinic.com. 2003. Accessed 2028 April 25. Available from: http://www.mayoclinic.com/

121. Adrogué HJ, Tucker BM, Madias NE. Diagnosis and management of hyponatremia: a review. JAMA. 2022;328(3):280–91.

122. Rehrer JN, Beckers E, Brouns F, Ten FH, Saris WH. Exercise and training effects on gastric emptying of carbohydrate beverages. Med Sci Sports Exerc. 1989;21:540–9.

123. Phillips SM, Turner AP, Sanderson MF, Sproule J. Beverage carbohydrate concentration influences the intermittent endurance capacity of adolescent team games players during prolonged intermittent running. Eur J Appl Physiol. 2012;112:1107–16.

124. Nicholas CW, Williams C, Lakomy HK, Phillips G, Nowitz A. Influence of ingesting a carbohydrate-electrolyte solution on endurance capacity during intermittent, high intensity shuttle running. J Sports Sci. 1995;13:283–90.

125. Welsh RS, Davis JM, Burke JR, Williams HG. Carbohydrates and physical/mental performance during intermittent exercise to fatigue. Med Sci Sports Exerc. 2002;34:723–31.

126. Rehrer JN, Brouns F, Beckers EJ, Saris WHM. The influence of beverage composition and gastrointestinal function on fluid and nutrient availability during exercise. Scand J Med Sci Sports. 1994;4:159–72.

127. Triplett D, Doyle JA, Rupp JC, Benardot D. An isocaloric glucose-fructose beverage's effect on simulated 100-km cycling performance compared with a glucose-only beverage. Int J Sport Nutr Exerc Metab. 2010;20(2):122–31.

128. Vist GE, Maughan RJ. Gastric emptying of ingested solutions in man: effect of beverage glucose concentration. Med Scin Sports Exerc. 1994;26(10):1269–73.

129. Currell K, Jeukendrup AE. Superior endurance performance with ingestion of multiple transportable carbohydrates. Med Sci Sports Exerc. 2008;40(2):275–81.

130. Noakes TD, Rehrer NJ, Maughan RJ. The importance of volume-regulating gastric emptying. Med Sci Sports Exerc. 1991;23(3):307–13.

131. Sun WM, Houghton LA, Read NW, Grundy DG, Johnson AG. Effect of meal temperature on gastric emptying of liquids in man. Gut. 1988;29:302–5.

132. Costill DL, Saltin B. Factors limiting gastric emptying during rest and exercise. J Appl Physiol. 1974;37:679–83.

133. Lambert GP, Bleiter TL, Chang RT, Johnson AK, Gisolf CV. Effects of carbonated and noncarbonated beverages at specific intervals during treadmill running in the heat. Int J Sport Nutr. 1993;3(2):177–93.

134. Ryan AJ, Navarne AE, Gisolfi CV. Consumption of carbonated and noncarbonated sports drinks during prolonged treadmill exercise in the heat. Int J Sport Nutr. 1991;1:225–39.

135. Passe DH, Murray R, Horn M. The effects of beverage carbonation on sensory responses and voluntary fluid intake following exercise. Int J Sport Nutr. 1997;7(4):286–97.

136. Wolf, S. The psyche and the stomach. A historical vignette. Gastroenterology. 1981;80(3):605–14.

137. Gisolfi CV, Summers R, Schedl H. Intestinal absorption of fluids during rest and exercise. In: Gisolfi CV, Lamb DR, editors. Fluid homeostasis during exercise. Carmel (IN): Benchmark Press; 1990. p. 39–95.

138. Maughan RJ, Noakes TD. Fluid replacement and exercise stress. A brief review of studies on fluid replacement and some guidelines for the athlete. Sports Med. 1991;12:16–31.

139. Passe DH, Horn M, Stofan J, Murray R. Palatability and voluntary intake of sports beverages, diluted orange juice, and water during exercise. Int J Sport Nutr Exerc Metab. 2004;14:272–84.

140. Burke LM. Rehydration strategies before and after exercise. Austr J Nutr Diet. 1996;53(Suppl 4):S22–6.

141. Hargreaves M. Physiological benefits of fluid and energy replacement during exercise. Austr J Nutr Diet. 1996;53(Suppl 4):S3–7.

142. Luke A, Bergeron MF, Roberts WO. Heat injury prevention practices in high school football. Clin J Sport Med. 2007;17(6):488–93.

143. Maughan RJ, Fenn CE, Leiper JB. Effects of fluid, electrolyte and substrate ingestion on endurance capacity. Eur J Appl Physiol. 1989;58(5):481–6.

144. McConnell G, Burge CM, Skinner SL, Hargreaves M. Ingested fluid volume and physiological responses during prolonged exercise in a mild environment [abstract]. Med Sci Sports Exerc. 1995;27:S19.

145. Walsh RM, Noakes TD, Hawley JA, Dennis SC. Impaired high-intensity cycling performance time at low levels of dehydration. Int J Sports Med. 1994;15(7):392–8.

146. Lyle DM, Lewis PR, Richards DAB, Richards R, Bauman AE, Sutton JR, Cameron ID. Heat exhaustion in The Sun-Herald city to surf fun run. Med J Aust. 1994;161(6):361–5.

147. Cutrufello PT, Dixon CB. The effect of acute fluid consumption following exercise-induced fluid loss on hydration status, percent body fat, and minimum wrestling weight in wrestlers. J Strength Cond Res. 2014;28(7):1928–36.

148. Kristal-Boneh E, Glusman JG, Shitrit R, Chaemovitz C, Cassuto Y. Physical performance and heat tolerance after chronic water loading and heat acclimation. Aviat Space Environ Med. 1995;66:733–8.

149. Nadel ER, Mack GW, Nose H. Influence of fluid replacement beverages on body fluid homeostasis during exercise and recovery. In: Gisolfi, CV, Lamb DR, editors. Fluid homeostasis during exercise. Vol. 3, Perspectives in exercise science and sports medicine. Carmel (IN): Benchmark Press; 1990. p. 181–205.

150. Coombes JS, Hamilton KL. The effectiveness of commercially available sports drinks. Sports Med. 2000;29(3):181–209.

151. Lyons TP, Riedesel ML, Meuli LE, Chick TW. Effects of glycerol-induced hyperhydration prior to exercise in the heat on sweating and core temperatures. Med Sci Sports Exerc. 1990; 22:477–83.

152. Montner P, Stark DM, Riedesel ML, Murata G, Robergs R, Timms M, Chick TW. Pre-exercise glycerol hydration improves cycling endurance time. Int J Sports Med. 1996; 17:27–33.

153. Thevis M, Guddat S, Flenker U, Schänzer W. Quantitative analysis of urinary glycerol levels for doping control purposes using gas chromatography-mass spectrometry. Eur J Mass Spectrom (Chichester). 2008;14:117–25.

154. Coggan AR, Coyle EF. Reversal of fatigue during prolonged exercise by carbohydrate infusion or ingestion. J Appl Physiol (1985). 1987;63:2388–95.

155. Coyle EF, Hagberg JM, Hurley BF, Martin WH, Ehsani AA, Hollöszy JO. Carbohydrate feeding during prolonged strenuous exercise can delay fatigue. J Appl Physiol Envirn Exerc Physiol. 1983;55 (1 Pt 1):230–5.

156. Mitchell JB, Costill DL, Houmard JA, Fink WJ, Pascoe DD, Pearson DR. Influence of carbohydrate dosage on exercise performance and glycogen metabolism. J Appl Physiol (1985). 1989;67:1843–9.

157. Tsintzas OK, Liu R, Williams C, Campbell I, Gaitanos G. The effect of carbohydrate ingestion on performance during a 30-km race. Int J Sport Nutr. 1993;3(2):127–39.

158. Coyle EF, Coggan AR, Hemmert MK, Ivy JL. Muscle glycogen utilization during prolonged, strenuous exercise when fed carbohydrate. J Appl Physiol (1985). 1986;61:165–72.

159. Tsintzas OK, Williams C, Boobis L, Greenhaff P. Carbohydrate ingestion and glycogen utilization in different muscle fiber types in man. J Physiol. 1995;489:243–50.

160. Below PR, Mora-Rodriguez R, Gonzalez-Alonso J, Coyle EF. Fluid and carbohydrate ingestion independently improves performance during one hour of intense exercise. Med Sci Sports Exerc. 1995;27:200–10.

161. Hargreaves M, Costill DL, Coggan A, Fink WJ, Nishibata I. Effect of carbohydrate feedings on muscle glycogen utilization and exercise performance. Med Sci Sports Exerc. 1984;16:219–22.

162. Yaspelkis BB III, Patterson JG, Anderla PA, Ding Z, Ivy JL. Carbohydrate supplementation spares muscle glycogen during variable-intensity exercise. J Appl Physiol (1985). 1993; 75(4):1477–85.

163. Simard C, Tremblay A, Jobin M. Effects of carbohydrate intake before and during an ice hockey match on blood and muscle energy substrates. Res Q Exerc Sport. 1988;59:144–7.

164. Mason WL, McConell GK, Hargreaves M. Carbohydrate ingestion during exercise: liquid vs. solid feedings. Med Sci Sports Exerc. 1993;25(8):966–9.

165. Murray R, Paul GL, Seifert JG, Eddy DE, Halaby GA. The effects of glucose, fructose, and sucrose ingestion during exercise. Med Sci Sports Exerc. 1989;21:275–82.

166. Owen MD, Kregel KC, Wall PT, Gisolfi CV. Effects of ingesting carbohydrate beverages during exercise in the heat. Med Sci Sports Exerc. 1986;18(5):568–75.

167. Bjorkman O, Sahlin K, Hagenfeldt L, Wahren J. Influence of glucose and fructose ingestion on the capacity for long term exercise in well-trained men. Clin Physiol. 1984;4(6):483–94.

168. United States Department of Agriculture Economic Research Service. Sugar and sweeteners: background. 2014 November 14. Available from: https://www.ers.usda.gov/topics/crops/sugar-andsweeteners/

169. Bray GA. How bad is fructose? Am J Clin Nutr. 2007;86(4): 895–6.

170. Coyle EF, Montain SJ. Benefits of fluid replacement with carbohydrate during exercise. Med Sci Sports Exerc. 1992; 24(Suppl 9):S324–30.

171. Wagenmakers AJ, Brouns F, Saris WHM, Halliday D. Oxidation rates of orally ingested carbohydrates during prolonged exercise in men. J Appl Physiol. 1993;75(6):2774–80.

172. Gonzalez-Alonso J, Heaps CL, Coyle EF. Rehydration after exercise with common beverages and water. Int J Sports Med. 1992;3:399–406.

173. Maughan RJ, Leiper JB. Sodium intake and post-exercise rehydration in man. Eur J Appl Physiol Occup Physiol. 1995; 71:311–9.

174. Maughan RJ, Leiper JB, Shirreffs SM. Restoration of fluid balance after exercise-induced dehydration: effects of food and fluid intake. Eur J Appl Physiol. 1996;73(3–4):317–25.

175. Orrù S, Imperiling E, Nigro E, Alfieri A, Cevenini A, Polito R, Daniele A, Buono P, Mancini A. Role of functional beverages on sport performance and recovery. Nutrients. 2018; 10(10):1470.

176. Sherman WM, Peden MC, Wright DA. Carbohydrate feedings 1 h before exercise improves cycling performance. Am J Clinl Nutr. 1991;54(5):866–70.

177. Wright DA, Sherman WM, Dernbach AR. Carbohydrate feedings before, during or in combination improve cycling endurance performance. J Appl Physiol. 1991;71(3):1082–8.

178. Lippincott Professional Development. Philadelphia (PA): LWW; 2014 August.

179. Maughan RJ. Fluid and electrolyte loss and replacement in exercise. In: Harries M, Williams G, Stanish WD, Micheli LL, editors. Oxford textbook of sports medicine. New York (NY): Oxford University Press; 1994. p. 82–93.

Managing Weight and Body Composition in Athletes

CHAPTER OBJECTIVES

- Recognize the different components of body composition and how these components may vary depending on level of fitness.
- Evaluate the different strategies available for assessing body composition, the principles used in each method, and the relative accuracy of each method.
- Describe the hormones that influence weight and body composition and the dietary factors that can have an impact on these hormones.
- Demonstrate an understanding of the health risks associated with obesity and the exercise and dietary strategies that are most likely to lower body fat level.
- Recognize common risks associated with the development of eating disorders in athletes and how best to lower these risks in at-risk sports.

- Evaluate the reasons why weight is not a good metric for determining health risks and performance potential in both athletes and nonathletes.
- Describe how insulin production can be influenced by multiple dietary factors including but not limited to the consumption of sugars.
- Understand the limitations of using body mass index (BMI) as a metric for assessing individual athletes.
- Explain the female athlete triad and how this concept fits into the larger organizational framework of relative energy deficiency in sport (RED-S).

Case Study

Imagine an Olympian who was just behind the best person on the swim team and someone who was willing to do anything to make it to first place. Everyone has an inherited physique, and this powerhouse clearly had inherited all the qualities (mainly good and some bad) of her genetic donors. She was on the short side of small and had a "blockhouse" figure. Nevertheless, while swimming her laps, there was no one better to look at great strokes, perfect flip turns, powerful starts off the blocks, a rocket finish—and it all came together to make her one of the best. Despite her national and international competitive successes, she still was not considered the best this country had to offer, and this ate away at her psyche like nothing else could. To improve, she spent more hours practicing, became more careful about what she ate, and began bugging her coach for more ideas on how to improve every part of the stroke, even if the resultant improvement would be minuscule.

She became so unhappy with herself that she found fault with her appearance. "If only I were leaner" and "If only I had less fat" were common interjections in her conversations. But when you have someone who, for her sport, is already in the 10th percentile for body fat percent (BF%), it is hard to imagine that having less fat would cause a competitive improvement. Nevertheless, she began seeing herself as fat and took the only action she could think of—dieting to the point of starvation in an attempt to lower body fat.

During the regularly scheduled evaluations of the national team swimmers, it was noticed that all of the swimmers were comfortably walking around in their gym shorts and T-shirts—all of them except the swimmer in question. She had on two sweatshirts, gym pants, and a jacket and was still shivering. It was obvious to all the sports medicine staff that there was a problem, so a body composition assessment was performed to document the changes. As suspected, she

(continued)

not only had lost weight but had lost more weight from her fat-free mass (FFM) (muscle) than from her fat mass (FM), so she was less able to move her body weight than before. Her coach expressed concern that she had become impossible to work with. Her starts were poor, her turns had deteriorated, and she no longer had a killer finish. All the strength and skills that were at the core of her successes had disappeared. Her coach was ready to increase her training schedule (even though she was already spending more hours in the pool and weight room than anyone else) because he could not see how she could compete in the next big competition given her poor state of readiness.

When her diet was reviewed, it became clear that she was trying to cover up an eating disorder. It would have been impossible for her to have eaten what she reported she ate and to have lost so much weight. It was decided that, for her to return to the team, she would be required to present a letter from a psychiatrist trained to work with eating disorders, clearly stating that her continued participation in competitive swimming would not place her at risk for an eating disorder. In other words, if she wanted to come back, she had to change what she was doing and she had

to convince an appropriate medical professional that this change would not be altered if she returned to swimming.

Fortunately, this story has a happy ending. She did it. She went home, went to counseling, learned what she needed to do, accepted her physique as it was, ate better, trained smarter, got OK letters from both her psychiatrist and family physician, and became a star.

CASE STUDY DISCUSSION QUESTIONS

If you were working with competitive athletes who believed that achieving a certain weight would make them perform better, and the way in which they were trying to achieve the desired weight was through restrictive eating:

1. What would you tell them?
2. Would you discuss this issue with others who work with the team (coaches, dietitians, exercise physiologists, etc.) or would you try to go it alone?
3. Would you see if there are policies about the appropriateness of talking to an athlete about their weight?
4. If you believed an athlete had an eating disorder, what would you do to help this athlete?

INTRODUCTION

There is a clear interaction between physical activity and nutrition, with an increased requirement for energy that results from the higher rate of energy expenditure during physical activity. Despite this exercise-associated requirement, surveys assessing food and fluid intakes of physically active people have found that they often fail to satisfy the increased energy requirement (1–3). To make this problem worse, it appears that physically active people often supply the needed energy *after* it is most needed (referred to as postloading), which can negatively affect performance and also result in an unwanted **body composition** change (4,5). Athletes have different body types, and often the body type influences the sport they pursue, with strong, small individuals migrating to sports like gymnastics, while taller individuals migrate to sports like basketball. Depending on the environment and the perception of what is perceived to be the most important for the competing athlete, body composition assessments may include selected measures that include body shape, body weight, bone mineral density (BMD), body fat percent (BF%), fat mass (FM), fat-free mass (FFM), muscle mass, and lean soft tissue mass (LSTM) (6). What measure can be obtained is determined

by the history of measurements taken in the past, the available equipment, cost of assessment, and availability of personnel who are capable of taking the measurements. As both coaches and athletes are aware of the importance of the strength-to-weight ratio in achieving competitive excellence, measures of musculature (*e.g.*, skeletal muscle mass, FFM, and LSTM) are a high assessment priority (7).

 Body Composition

Represents the major tissues that compose the human body, including fat mass, lean mass, water, and bones. Techniques for assessing body composition use different assessment models, with a two-compartment model (fat mass and fat-free mass) being the most common and a four-compartment model (fat mass, lean mass, water mass, and skeletal mass) being the most accurate. Assessment strategies range from the most accurate and most expensive (dual-energy X-ray absorptiometry [DXA], multicurrent bioelectrical impedance analysis [BIA], and air displacement plethysmography) to less accurate and less expensive (skinfolds, BMI, and waist circumference).

 Mass

Another word for *weight* that is commonly used in the scientific literature. *Weight of body fat* is equivalent to *body fat mass*, etc.

Much like humans, automobiles have finite storage of fuel. For a car to run, the car fuel tank can never be empty, and it can never be overfilled. Letting the fuel tank go empty causes the car to stop. If you try to overfill an automobile gas tank, the fuel has nowhere to go, but in humans overfilling the tank results in more fuel storage (*i.e.*, an increase in fat mass).

Now imagine that you want to take a car trip from New York to San Francisco, but you are in a hurry and do not want to stop to refuel every 350 miles, so you tell your car: "Please take me to San Francisco, I promise I will give you all the fuel you need for the trip once we get to San Francisco." It should be obvious to anyone that this postloading strategy does not work for your car—and it does not work well for physically active people.

An obvious problem in humans is to allow blood sugar to drop, which can happen quickly with physical activity. Blood sugar is the main fuel for the brain, so the brain increases the production of cortisol, which breaks down muscle for conversion to sugar. Blood sugar is improved but at the cost of losing muscle.

Consumption of inadequate energy may result in multiple problems for the athlete, including the following:

- Poor training benefits
- Difficulties in maintaining fat-free (*i.e.*, lean) mass
- Lowering of metabolic rate
- Increased difficulty with normal eating, leading to even greater reductions in both energy and nutrient intakes that may result in increased risk of disordered eating and/or *eating disorders*
- Increased risk of injury
- Reduction in athletic performance

Consumption of *excess energy* may also result in multiple problems for the athlete, including the following:

- Higher total body mass
- Higher total FM
- Unhealthy ratio of total FM to lean body mass
- Cardiac insufficiency
- Higher risk of **type II diabetes**
- Higher risk of hypertension
- Lower disease resistance
- Dieting-associated adaptations that result in lower energy expenditure
- Increased risk of disordered eating and/or eating disorders
- Increased risk of injury
- Reduction in athletic performance

Type II Diabetes

Associated with obesity, type II diabetes is a condition of excess insulin production but with ineffective insulin (*i.e.*, insulin resistance). Risk factors for **metabolic syndrome** and type II diabetes are related (8). In addition, there is increasing evidence of a strong relationship between type II diabetes and cancer (9). (See Figure 8.1.)

Metabolic Syndrome

Represents a group of factors that elevate risk of developing heart disease, diabetes, and stroke. Factors include high abdominal obesity, high serum triglyceride levels, low high-density lipoprotein cholesterol, and high fasting blood sugar.

Several possibilities exist for why athletes fail to satisfy total energy needs, including a poor understanding of what foods and beverages are best to consume; inadequate availability of foods and beverages before, during, and after exercise; a sport-specific tradition that perpetuates undesirable eating behaviors; and a tendency for athletes to model behavior after those who have excelled in the sport even if their food/beverage consumption behaviors are not

FIGURE 8.1: Relationship between type 2 diabetes, cancer, and obesity. (Based on data from Rahman I, Athar MT, Islam M. Type 2 diabetes, obesity, and cancer share some common and critical pathways. Front Oncol. 2021;10:600824.)

Obesity is associated with altered hormones and higher risk of cardiometabolic disorders.

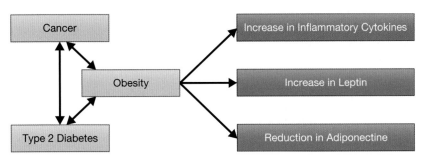

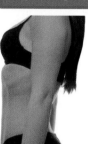
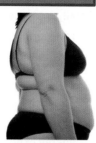

Athletes typically have more muscle (lean mass) weight for height than nonathletes, so may easily be mischaracterized as *overweight* or *obese* using standard BMI or weight for height indices.

Obesity means having too much body fat. It is different from being *overweight*, which means weighing more than the standard weight for a given height.

Weight may come from:
• Lean Mass (more = good)
• Bone Mass (more = good)
• Body Water (more = good)
• Fat Mass (more = bad)

FIGURE 8.2: Obesity is not the same as overweight. BMI, body mass index.

optimal (10). Many athletes also have a level of eating anxiety, with a fear that eating exercise-appropriate foods and beverages, which often contain sugars, will increase body fat and weight (11–13). There may be confusion about what to eat and drink because terms are often misused. For example, high body fat does not mean high body weight, leanness is not the same as thinness, and a higher weight may be desirable if it is the result of more **lean mass** that can improve the strength-to-weight ratio (10) (Figure 8.2).

The coach who insists that an athlete lose 5 lb may be dismayed at the performance outcome if the majority of that weight comes from muscle and not fat. This same athlete who gained 5 lb of muscle and lost 5 lb of fat would have the same weight, but the greater proportion of muscle would serve to improve performance because of an improved strength-to-weight ratio. This more lean athlete would also appear smaller (a clear advantage in certain appearance sports) because **fat-free mass** has a higher density than **fat mass** (*i.e.*, for the same weight, takes up less space) and would likely also have better endurance because there is less nonmuscle tissue to move. See Figure 8.3.

Put simply, the failure of many physically active people to optimally consume energy may be the direct result of using an inappropriate metric, "weight," as the sole measure of performance readiness. It also may be due to a misunderstanding of energy thermodynamics, the factors associated with the utilization of energy, as it relates to humans. Correctly measuring and predicting body composition, therefore, is critically important for helping athletes achieve desired performances, particularly in sports where athletes are judged on both aesthetics and skill (*i.e.*, diving,

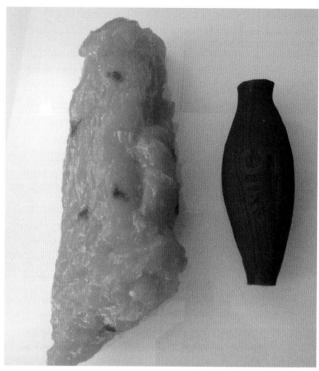

FIGURE 8.3: Different densities of fat tissue and muscle tissue.

gymnastics, figure skating) and in sports driven by weight categories (*i.e.*, wrestling, boxing) (14). Performing body composition assessments requires consideration of multiple associated factors, including (15) the following:

Fat-Free Mass (FFM)

Body tissue that is not fat, including lean mass, skeletal mass, and body water.

Fat Mass (FM)

The total weight of fat that a human has. For instance, if someone weighs 100 lb, and 30 lb is fat, 30% of the weight is fat (body fat percent) and 70 lb (70%) is fat-free weight (FFM).

Subcutaneous Fat Mass

It is typical for 50% of total body fat to express itself under the skin (*i.e.*, subcutaneously). Therefore, as is used with skinfolds, measuring the thickness of subcutaneous fat provides a prediction of total body fat.

Lean Mass

Lean mass represents lean tissue, including skeletal muscle and organ mass, but not including skeletal mass and FM.

Lean Soft Tissue Mass (LSTM)

Represents the lean tissue that does not include skeletal tissue.

- Considering the appropriate reference model for individual or group being assessed;
- Determining the appropriate field or laboratory method to use that will provide the needed information in a minimally invasive, validated, and reliable way;
- Understanding the potential health implications of the results, including both total body fatness and fat distribution;
- Determining how best to make improvements in musculature, body fat, or both.
- Understanding that a failure to track changes over time to determine the trends of body composition changes may result in the wrong conclusions regarding the relative success of an intervention.
- Realizing that different people will have different responses to any intervention that targets modification in body composition.

WEIGHT

Important Factors to Consider

The strategy for losing body fat mass while sustaining body lean mass is different than the strategy to lose weight. It is possible to lose lean body mass and gain fat mass while losing weight. The ideal focus should be on the following:

- Avoiding recommendations that may lower lean mass
- Avoiding recommendations that may increase fat mass

There is no question that weight is an important issue for athletes because it influences the ease with which they can perform required sport-specific skills (16). However, the measurement of weight alone may provide a misleading picture of whether the athlete is in a desirable state (Table 8.1). Athletes may increase the time and/or intensity of a training regimen with the goal of improving performance, but then inappropriately rely on changes in weight as a marker of success. Imagine a football player who comes to training camp at a weight much higher than the coach is accustomed to seeing in this player. It may well be that the athlete worked extremely hard during the off-season to increase muscle mass, and the increase in weight is a result of more muscle. Would the coach be wrong to tell that player that he must lose weight?

Table 8.1	Weight and Body Composition "Realities"
Reality 1	Humans are amazingly effective fat manufacturing machines. Consume too much energy from food and beverages and you make fat. Consume too little energy from food and beverages, you lose body mass—from fat mass and muscle, and in many cases inadequate energy intake results in higher body fat levels (4,17,18).
Reality 2	Humans are always finding ways to become more energy efficient. Exercise more and we eventually find a way to burn less energy to do this exercise (18–22).
Reality 3	For athletes, "weight" is the wrong measure for virtually everything that it is commonly used for. It is all about the ratio of fat mass to lean mass (23–25).
Reality 4	The location and distribution of body fat is also important. For example, central visceral fat deposition is related to higher risk of disease such as metabolic syndrome (26–28).
Reality 5	Low-calorie diets are doomed to fail. Adaptive thermogenesis leads to same weight on lower energy intake, but the resultant weight has relatively higher fat mass (18,29,30).
Reality 6	There are many ways to increase insulin and make more fat besides eating refined carbohydrates (i.e., sugar), including letting yourself get really hungry and/or eating large meals (2,31–36).
Reality 7	The body's reaction to an inadequate energy intake is to lower body weight (mass), including lowering the amount of tissue that needs more energy, resulting in a greater loss of lean mass than fat mass (17,27,37).
Reality 8	A 3,500-calorie energy balance deficit does NOT result in a 1-lb weight loss. This is because there are a number of complex adaptive factors that influence energy balance and body composition. Although 3,500 calories of potential energy as measured by a bomb calorimeter does equal 1 lb of body fat, humans are not bomb calorimeters (38).
Reality 9	The commonly stated calories in, calories out paradigm does not work as commonly applied in 24-hr units. Humans have a physiologic/endocrine system that reacts in "real time" to multiple factors, including blood sugar, stress, rate of energy utilization, and environment (38,39).

Gymnasts often reach their competitive peak during adolescence, a time when fast growth is the normal biologic expectation. Despite this expectation for growth, gymnasts are sometimes weighed weekly to make certain that they are maintaining their current weight. Ideally, the focus should be on a training and nutrition program that will help to enhance the strength-to-weight ratio, which involves improving the lean body mass-to-weight ratio and may involve increasing weight from an enlarged lean body mass. These are examples of how weight is often used arbitrarily and wrongly. Tracking the constituents of weight (fat, bone, muscle, water, etc.) is far more logical and provides athletes with more actionable information on whether the body is changing in a desirable way. Importantly, the strategy for weight is different than the strategy for losing fat while sustaining or increasing muscle. There are long-term health implications for focusing on "weight" in a young, growing athlete, as it may negatively impact skeletal maturation and development (40,41).

Ideal Weight

Ideal weight is considered to be the weight that is associated with good health and is based mainly on height, as adjusted for gender, age, build, and muscularity. As athletes typically have greater muscle mass than nonathletes for any given height, using ideal weight standards for athletes often wrongly places them in an at-risk category because they appear to be excessively heavy for their height. Standard strategies for determining ideal weight for athletes should be used cautiously and should not be the standard for determining if an athlete's weight is desirable.

Therefore, although not ideally used with athletes, the following equations are provided for the reader to understand the strategy used in determining ideal weight. There are several commonly used predictive equations for estimating the ideal body weight. However, these equations are not appropriately used with athletes because of an expected higher weight:height ratio than that for nonathletes. The commonly used formulas for predicting ideal body weight (Box 8.1) include those of Devine (42), Robinson (43), and Miller (44).

Body Mass Index

BMI, also referred to as *Quetelet's Index*, is a calculation of the weight-to-height ratio and may also be a useful tool for categorizing the weight of populations/groups

---

Box 8.1 — Commonly Used Formulas for Predicting "Ideal" Body Weight

Devine Formula

Males: Ideal body weight (in kg) = 50 kg + 2.3 kg/inch over 5 feet
Females: Ideal body weight (in kg) = 45.5 kg + 2.3 kg/inch over 5 feet

Robinson Formula

Males: Ideal body weight (in kg) = 52 kg + 1.9 kg for each inch over 5 feet
Females: Ideal body weight (in kg) = 49 kg + 1.7 kg for each inch over 5 feet

Miller Formula

Males: Ideal body weight (in kg) = 56.2 kg + 1.41 kg for each inch over 5 feet
Females: Ideal body weight (in kg) = 53.1 kg + 1.36 kg for each inch over 5 feet

Source: Pai MP. The origin of the "Ideal" body weight equations. Ann Pharmacother. 2000;34(9):1066–9.

(Table 8.2). However, it is not likely to be as useful for athletes. BMI, while providing a measure of body mass (weight) relative to height, fails to measure individual body fatness, which is the marker of **obesity**. Athletes typically carry more muscle for any given height and, because of this relative increase in body density, may appear to be overweight or obese by BMI standards, but may not be either overweight or obese.

Using BMI on athletes is likely to create false positives, suggesting that they are either overweight or obese. For instance, a large, lean athletic person may have a BMI >30 $kg·m^{-2}$, but has low body fat and so is not obese. It has been found that athletes are often incorrectly classified as obese when based on BMI (45,46). It can also create false negatives. That is, a thin, small person may have a BMI of ~20 $kg·m^{-2}$, but a relatively low lean mass and high body fat, indicating that this person is obese (24). As an illustration of this point, it has been found that BMI fails to identify over a quarter of children with excess body fat levels as obese (23).

The best strategy for BMI is to use it as it was intended, as a measure of characterizing *population* obesity and weight categories that are associated with health problems, and not as a means of identifying *individual* obesity or weight categories.

Table 8.2	Body Mass Index (BMI) Categories	
Classification	BMI Category (kg/m²)	Risk of Developing Health Problems
Underweight	<18.5	Increased
Normal weight	18.5–24.9	Least
Overweight	25.0–29.9	Increased
Obese class I	30.0–34.9	High
Obese class II	35.0–39.9	Very high
Obese class III	≥40.0	Extremely high

BMI, weight in kg/height in m².

Source: National Institutes of Health, National Heart, Lung, and Blood Institute. Clinical guidelines on the identification, evaluation, and treatment of overweight and obesity in adults: the evidence report. Obes Res. 1998;6(Suppl 2):S51–210.

Circumferences

Despite the well-established relationship between higher **visceral fat** (abdominal fat, trunk fat, fat surrounding the organs) and cardiometabolic risk, the traditional measure for assessing obesity risk (BMI) fails to provide a direct estimation of visceral fat (47). There is increasing evidence that taking **waist circumference** is a useful measure for predicting health risks, including hypertension, elevated blood lipids, type II diabetes, and cardiovascular disease. A measure of lower cardiometabolic risk is to have a waist circumference that is less than half your height (48). The waist-to-hip ratio is also a way of estimating if excess body fat is stored in the abdomen in both children and adults. The widest part of the buttocks is used for the hip circumference, and the waist circumference is taken above the hip bone. In both men and women, the circumference of the waist should be smaller than that of the hip. High risk in men is indicated with a waist-to-hip ratio of 1.0+ and in women 0.85+ (49).

Body Mass Index

BMI, also referred to as Quetelet's Index, was developed as a means of predicting *population* obesity. It represents a person's mass in kilograms, divided by their height in meters squared (kg/m²). BMI categorizations include obese (>30 kg/m²), overweight (25–30 kg/m²), normal (18.5–25 kg/m²), and underweight (<18.5 kg/m²). Although often used as an assessment of *individual* obesity, it can create both false positives (*i.e.*, it appears that someone has a high body fat level and is obese, but is not because the extra weight is from high muscle mass rather than high-fat mass) and false negatives (*i.e.*, it appears that someone is not obese because their weight is low, but a high proportion of their weight is fat). BMI is not appropriately used with athletes as a measure of fitness/obesity.

Obesity

An accumulation of body fat that exceeds the threshold for maintaining good health and is associated with higher risk for heart disease, type II diabetes, cancer, osteoarthritis, and sleep apnea. Hyperplastic obesity represents obesity that results from excess fat cell production and is commonly associated with an excess number of fat cells that are produced during a growth phase, such as adolescence. Hyperplastic obesity is one of the dangers of childhood obesity, as it is difficult to lower fat cell numbers to lower obesity risk. Hypertrophic obesity represents obesity that results from excess enlargement of existing fat cells and is the most common form of adult-onset obesity.

Visceral Fat

The fat tissue within the abdominal cavity around the organs (*i.e.*, viscera). This fat protects the organs from sudden concussion and protects the organs from sudden temperature shifts. Also referred to as abdominal fat, excess visceral fat is associated with higher risk of type II diabetes, insulin resistance, and inflammatory diseases that include cancer.

Waist Circumference

As a measure of central obesity (high body fat carried on the trunk), waist circumference (also referred to as waist girth) has been shown to be a good measure of health risks associated with obesity.

Anthropometric Ratios

Especially in children, anthropometric ratios that incorporate height, weight, and age are used for the assessment and prediction of protein-calorie malnutrition and/or failure to thrive. Anthropometric ratios have also been used to identify young athletes who possess good characteristics for specific sports (50). As many young children are increasingly involved in high-level sports, some simple measures that can identify if the child is satisfying energy/nutrition requirements are important to understand.

Weight/Age

This is the most widely used method for assessment of malnutrition in children. Put simply, the ratio intends to assess whether the child's weight for their age is appropriate. A child with a low weight/age may be malnourished and/or have an illness.

Height/Age

Height is a more stable growth parameter than weight because height is irreversible, whereas weight can go up or down. A relatively long period on a deficient diet is needed for height to become sufficiently retarded, and a relatively long time is required for height to return to normal after a period of malnutrition. Therefore, height/age is not considered an indication of the present nutritional status of the child but may be a method for assessing chronic malnutrition or a long-term illness.

Weight/Height

Weight can change rapidly, whereas height is relatively stable. Therefore, this ratio is a measure of the present nutritional status of a child, with low weight/height an indication of acute/short-term/current malnutrition.

Weight/Height/Age

At each age during normal growth and development, a certain amount of weight is associated with any given height. Using standard growth charts, it is relatively easy to determine if a young athlete is deviating from their established percentile in standard growth charts. As an example, rapidly going from the percentile the young athlete is typically near to another lower or higher percentile may be an indication of an energy imbalance and/or illness.

BODY COMPOSITION

Assessment of changes in weight and body composition is not as straightforward as often believed. It is common for people to think that energy restriction (*i.e.*, dieting) is an unpleasant, yet effective, strategy for achieving weight loss and improving body composition (Table 8.3). The

common logic behind dieting suggests that the caloric intake is proportionate to the person's weight, so a 25% reduction in energy intake should result in a 25% reduction in weight. The reality, however, is that energy expenditure following weight loss is lower than would be expected by the amount of weight that was lost (5,38,39,51). This means that the adjustment in energy expenditure to inadequate intake is greater than the mathematical expectation because a higher-than-expected reduction in metabolic mass (*e.g.*, lean mass) occurs, which results in a return to the original weight, but with a lower energy intake. Put simply, low energy intake, relative to energy requirements for energy balance, causes a reduction in FFM that forces an even greater reduction in energy consumption to sustain weight. The body's reaction to an inadequate energy (caloric) intake is to reduce the highly metabolically active tissues like muscle that use energy (calories). This is a perfectly logical survival strategy, as the body attempts to survive the inadequate consumption of energy by lowering the need for energy. Because food is the carrier of more than just energy (calories), the reduction in food intake also diminishes vitamin and mineral exposure, increasing malnutrition risk and related disease risks.

Logic also suggests that, for instance, a 25% increase in energy intake will lead to a proportionate increase in weight. In fact, when people are overfed to gain weight, the amount of weight gain is, at least initially, closely proportionate to the amount of overfeeding (34,52–55). These studies strongly suggest that we have homeostatic mechanisms during periods of energy deficits that help us maintain our weight, which may be a survival-of-the-species mechanism that helps humans survive periods of famine. We also appear able to store energy effectively (as fat) during periods of excess. This may also be a survival-of-the-species mechanism that enables us to store energy when we are lucky enough to have excess food available.

It is increasingly clear that obesity development is complex and associated with numerous factors (56):

- Poor maintenance of energy balance
- Insufficient physical activity
- Living in an environment that fails to support a healthy lifestyle, including
  - Safe places to walk
  - Affordable gyms
  - Exhaustive work schedules
  - Oversized food portions
  - Poor access to or excessively expensive healthy foods, including fresh fruits and vegetables
  - Chronic food advertising that encourages consumption of high-calorie and/or high-sugar foods

Table 8.3	Terms Commonly Associated With Weight and Body Composition
Terms	**Definition**
Static (linear) energy balance	Assumes that a change in one side of the energy balance equation (*e.g.*, energy intake) does not change or influence the other side of the equation (*e.g.*, energy expenditure).
Dynamic (nonlinear) energy balance	Assumes that numerous biologic and behavior factors regulate and influence both sides of the energy balance equation. Thus, a change in factors on one side of the equation (*e.g.*, energy intake) can and does influence factors on the other side of the equation (*e.g.*, energy expenditure).
Dietary energy density	The energy content of food by weight (kcal or kJ/g).
Thermic effect of food	Energy required digesting, metabolizing, or storing energy as fat or glycogen.
Energy flux	The rate of energy conversion after absorption from food into body tissues for use in metabolism or its conversion into energy stores.
PA	Physical activity. Bodily movement that enhances health such as walking, dancing, biking, and yoga.
Exercise	PA that is planned, structured, repetitive, and performed with the goal of improving health or fitness.
Health-related fitness	Cardiovascular or muscular fitness focused on the reduction of chronic disease risk.
Moderate-vigorous PA	Moderate PA is an intensity of exercise similar to walking at 3.0 miles/hr, whereas vigorous PA is an intensity of exercise equivalent to running a 10-min mile.
Weight-bearing PA	PA such as walking, jogging, running, hiking, dancing, stair climbing, lifting weights, jumping, playing tennis, basketball, or soccer.
Body composition	The percentage or amount of fat and fat-free (mineral, protein, and water) in bone, muscle, and other tissues in the body.
Compensatory behavior	Partial or complete compensation, through diet, for the energy expended in exercise (*e.g.*, eating back energy expended during exercise by increasing energy intake), thereby negating body weight loss because of increased PA. Decreasing PA could also be a compensatory behavior.

Source: Manore MM, Larson-Meyer DE, Lindsay AR, Hongu N, Houtkooper L. Dynamic energy balance: an integrated framework for discussing diet and physical activity in obesity prevention–is it more than eating less and exercising more? Nutrients. 2017;9(905).

- Disease states, including conditions that result in low energy metabolism (*e.g.*, hypothyroidism) or loss of metabolic mass (*e.g.*, high cortisol production)
- Use of medications that stimulate weight gain, including corticosteroids and antidepressants
- Emotional factors (*e.g.*, boredom, anger) that may result in overeating
- Age-related loss of muscle
- Poor sleep patterns
- Excess consumption of highly refined/heavily processed foods that result in hyperinsulinemia

Energy Balance

Because major energy balance surpluses and energy balance deficits appear to activate homeostatic mechanisms,

a logical strategy for achieving a desired change in weight and body composition is to avoid major energy balance shifts. Exercise should be at the core of any desired body composition change that increases lean mass and decreases FM. But such a change may be easier to achieve if the energy balance deficits and energy balance surpluses over the course of a day are never too large at any time. It has been suggested that a desired body composition is easier to achieve when energy balance remains within ±300–400 kcal bounds (4,10,57–59). It has also been found that, of female athletes with similar 24-hour energy availability and energy balance, those spending more time in a catabolic state were more likely to develop menstrual dysfunction (60). Eating frequency is likely to play a role in the maintenance of energy balance (4,32). Because the standard three-meal-a-day schedule forces athletes to consume a large amount of food at each meal to obtain the needed energy, this pattern may not be ideal for athletes with large energy requirements (4,10,32,58). It may be far easier, for instance, to stay in a near–energy-balanced state throughout the day on a more frequent pattern that dynamically matches expenditure.

Getting energy balance right is difficult because it is complex. The *energy in* portion of the balance scale involves all the factors associated with the intake of energy, including meal size (*i.e.*, caloric load of the meal), meal frequency, diet quality, and factors that can influence the total absorption and speed of absorption of the consumed foods. The *energy out* portion of the equation involves the metabolism of the individual, the quality of the diet consumed, physical activity, and meal frequency. In addition, the thermic effect of food (*i.e.*, the energy that must be invested to derive energy from the food consumed) may also be influenced by the *energy out* factors. Although seemingly a small influence on total *energy out*, the average thermic effect of food, which averages about 10% of the total calories consumed, can be higher or lower (±2%), depending on diet quality, activity, and meal frequency (Figure 8.4). There is evidence that more frequent eating increases the thermic effect of food (*i.e.*, more calories are burned in the process of deriving energy from food) than eating the same calories in fewer eating opportunities (61–63). In addition, energy balance is influenced by numerous hormones and chemicals that affect appetite, satiety, and metabolic rate (64).

Two common energy balance feedback systems involve the hormones **leptin** and **ghrelin**. As an example of these energy balance feedback mechanisms, which under ideal circumstances serve to sustain the body tissues in a healthy state, see Figure 8.5. These hormones have precisely opposite effects, with leptin decreasing food intake and ghrelin increasing food intake. It should be no surprise that impaired leptin sensitivity and/or production is associated with obesity, and excess ghrelin production is also associated with obesity (65,66).

Traditional View of Energy Balance

The traditional view of energy balance involves a macroeconomic (*i.e.*, daily) view of the human system: A 24-hour energy intake that equals a 24-hour energy expenditure results in perfect energy balance, a state that is associated with weight stability (Figure 8.6).

It is also understood that a *positive* energy balance (*i.e.*, relatively more energy consumed than expended) mandates that the excess energy be stored, resulting in a higher weight, and that a *negative* energy balance (*i.e.*, relatively less energy consumed than expended) mandates that the difference in energy must be provided by body tissues, resulting in lower weight (39,67). This traditional view of energy balance implies that a significant reduction in energy intake (commonly referred to as dieting) results in weight loss that is associated with an improved body profile and body composition. However, there are

Multiple factors are associated with achieving a state of energy balance.

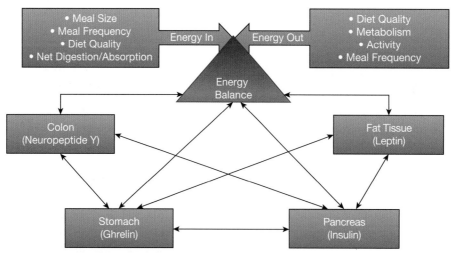

FIGURE 8.4: Energy balance is complex. (Created based on information from Hall KD, Heymsfield SB, Kemnitz JW, Klein S, Schoeller DA, Speakman JR. Energy balance and its components: implications for body weight regulation. Am J Clin Nutr. 2012;95(4):989–94; Loh K, Herzog H, Shi YC. Regulation of energy homeostasis by the NPY system. Trends Endocrinol Metab. 2015;26(3):125–35; Guyenet SJ, Schwartz MW. Regulation of food intake, energy balance, and body fat mass: implications for the pathogenesis and treatment of obesity. J Clin Endocrinol Metab. 2012;97(3):745–55.)

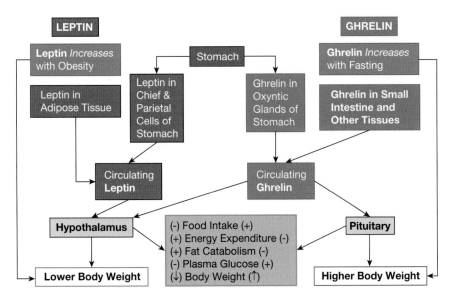

FIGURE 8.5: The energy balance feedback mechanisms of leptin and ghrelin. Leptin and ghrelin have opposing effects on body weight. (From Klok MD, Jakobsdottir S, Drent ML. The role of leptin and ghrelin in the regulation of food intake and body weight in humans. Obes Rev. 2007;8(1):21–34; Shintani M, Ogawa Y, Ebihara K, Aizawa-Abe M, Miyanaga F, Takaya K, Hayashi T, Inoue G, Hosoda K, Kojima M, Kangawa K, Nakao K. Ghrelin, an endogenous growth hormone secretagogue, is a novel orexigenic peptide that antagonizes leptin action through the activation of hypothalamic neuropeptide Y/Y1 receptor pathway. Diabetes. 2001;50(2):227–32.)

complications in determining energy balance that make it difficult to understand whether the expected energy balance outcomes will occur. These issues include the following (38,51,68,69):

📖 Leptin

A *satiety hormone* is produced mainly by adipose (fat) cells to inhibit hunger if fat cell mass becomes enlarged. It has the effect of lowering food intake, increasing energy expenditure, increasing fat catabolism, decreasing plasma glucose, and decreasing body fat mass. Poor leptin production is associated with increased obesity. Ghrelin and leptin have opposing functions.

📖 Ghrelin

The *appetite-stimulating hormone* is produced mainly in the small intestine and increases with fasting and/or low blood sugar. It has the effect of increasing food intake, lowering energy expenditure, lowering fat catabolism, increasing plasma glucose, and increasing body fat mass. Leptin and ghrelin have opposing functions.

- There are few longitudinal studies that help us fully understand the long-term impact of energy balance deviations on body composition and weight.
- Both biologic and psychological factors influence energy balance, but these are rarely studied together to better understand their interactive effects.
- There remain weaknesses in our understanding of how different exercises that vary in amount, intensity, pattern, timing, endurance, and resistance may differentially impact energy balance, body composition, and weight.
- There are large individual differences in how changes in energy balance impact weight and body composition outcomes, making it difficult to know, with certainty, how different individuals will respond to a protocol that was viewed as generally effective for groups of individuals.
- Current strategies for acquiring energy intake and energy expenditure information have a great deal of error associated with them.

A calorie is not necessarily a calorie with proportionally different macronutrient intakes, as macronutrient composition may influence both body fat and body protein mass. The traditional view of energy balance should immediately raise concerns because the human endocrine system does not wait until the end of the day to determine if the energy provided during the previous 24 hours was delivered in a way that satisfied tissue requirements. The endocrine system works in real time, with **insulin**, ghrelin, leptin, and cortisol responses based on the current energy balance state of affairs (38,51).

The often-used mathematical relationship between energy *imbalance* and weight change is 3,500 kcal = 1 lb

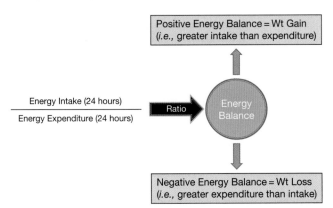

FIGURE 8.6: Traditional view of energy balance.

of body fat (14,644 kJ = 0.454 kg). That is, a negative energy balance resulting in a 3,500 kcal deficit, regardless of the time frame (1 day, 1 week, 1 month, etc.) will result in a 1-lb lowering of fat weight. It is also thought that a positive energy balance resulting in a 3,500 kcal surplus will lead to a 1-lb increase in fat weight. However, there is an increasing body of evidence that these predicted calorie-to-weight outcomes do not stand up to scrutiny. This evidence suggests that anyone failing to adequately satisfy energy needs is most likely to experience a return to the original weight, but the resultant weight will have a lower FFM and higher FM (5,39,70,71).

It is clear that there is a dose–response relationship between levels of physical activity and the amount of weight that is lost. The American College of Sports Medicine's position statement on physical activity and weight loss has concluded that 150 minutes of physical activity per week promotes minimal weight loss and that greater levels of physical activity result in greater levels of weight loss (72). However, the loss of weight, per se, may be misleading, because it fails to differentiate between the loss of FM and FFM (38). In addition, because the currently popular weight control strategy of exercising more and eating less may result in a severe negative energy balance that lowers more lean mass than FM, a leading obesity researcher has said: "Therefore, the mere recommendation to avoid calorically dense foods might be no more effective for the typical patient seeking weight reduction than would be a recommendation to avoid sharp objects for someone bleeding profusely" (30). It has been found that exercise-trained men and women often consume insufficient energy, resulting in negative health consequences (64). Weight cycling, where weight loss is followed by a regaining of weight, is a common feature of low-calorie diets. To make matters even worse, the common weight cycling experienced by people who are on severely energy-deficient diets increases both

cardiovascular disease and renal disease risks (70). Ideally, energy balance should be sustained in a range that helps to sustain or increase lean mass while sustaining or lowering FM (4) (Figure 8.7).

📖 Insulin

A hormone made by the β-cells of the pancreas, which monitor blood glucose. As blood sugar rises, it is detected by the pancreas and results in the production of insulin. The insulin allows body tissues to take up sugar, thus lowering blood sugar and providing an important energy source to the cells. A sudden rise in blood sugar results in excess insulin production (hyperinsulinemia), resulting in excess energy leaving the blood and entering the cells. Hyperinsulinemia is associated with obesity and may also occur from consumption of a high-calorie meal and/or consumption of foods after blood sugar has been allowed to become excessively low. Insulin resistance is likely to occur as a result of excess insulin stimulation of target tissues, including the liver, muscle, and fat tissues. Tissues that are insulin resistant, impairs the movement of glucose from the blood to inside the tissues, resulting in an elevated β-cell insulin production and hyperinsulinemia. The metabolic consequences of insulin resistance typically result in hyperglycemia, hypertension, high blood lipids, elevated body fat levels, and a high level of tissue inflammation (73–75).

An article assessing the metabolic adaptations in "The Biggest Loser" competition, and the subject of a *New York Times* article, illustrates the weight-cycling problems experienced by those who lose weight through low-calorie diets coupled with an increase in physical activity (76,77). The 14 participating contestants lost an average of 128.3 lb (58.3 kg) which was associated with significantly lower average resting metabolic rate (−610 kcal/day). Six years later, the majority (90.2 lb; 41.0 kg) of the weight lost was regained, with a significantly lower resting metabolic rate (−704 kcal/day) and lower energy metabolism

FIGURE 8.7: Weight cycling associated with low-calorie diets increases risks of cardiovascular and renal disease. GFR, glomerular filtration rate. (Reprinted from Montani J-P, Schutz Y, Dulloo AG. Dieting and weight cycling as risk factors for cardiometabolic diseases: who is really at risk? Obes Rev. 2015;16(S1):18.)

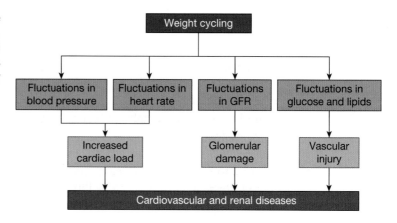

(−499 kcal/day). These findings strongly imply that weight may be an inappropriate marker for understanding the success of a diet, as the loss of weight resulting from inadequate energy provision appears to downregulate metabolic (*i.e.*, lean) mass as the body attempts to adapt to the inadequate energy provision. This **adaptive thermogenesis** appears to make weight gain inevitable, with studies suggesting that the majority of the regained weight is FM (17,18,37). Following a strategy that lowers FM while sustaining or increasing lean mass is likely to be a far healthier long-term strategy for controlling obesity.

The traditional view of energy balance (*i.e.*, energy in; energy out), despite being a standard feature of most books and book chapters that discuss issues related to weight, has never been found to be correct (68,78). It has also been pointed out that it is a fallacy to think that small changes in lifestyle have the capacity to reverse obesity and show that walking to use 100 kcal more each day should result (if using 3,500 kcal = 1 lb fat) in 50 lb of weight loss in 5 years, but the actual loss is typically only ~10 lb (38). An online model presented by the U.S. National Institutes of Health has incorporated this point by including new set point plateau norms (http://bwsimulator.niddk.nih.gov). This system finds that a 40 kcal/day permanent reduction in energy intake should result in ~20 lb of weight loss in 5 years, but the actual predicted weight loss is only 4 lb because the body has a compensatory response that is not considered in the standard (*i.e.*, 3,500 kcal = 1 lb body fat) energy balance prediction. It is important to consider that adaptive thermogenesis is likely to take more than 2 months to occur, yet many studies assessing the efficacy of different "weight loss" strategies often assess change in weight for less than 2 months (27,79). This short assessment period may result in inaccurate effectiveness for the strategy being followed, particularly if only weight is being assessed. (See Figure 8.8.)

Hormonal Response to Energy Balance Shifts

It is important to consider the hormonal alterations that occur in the human system as it attempts to adjust to wide shifts in energy balance. Insulin, through its effect on cell membranes, is a major regulator of blood sugar. When insulin is produced, insulin makes it possible for blood glucose to enter the cell so that the cell has the energy (glucose) to undergo normal metabolic processes. If excess insulin is produced, too much glucose leaves the blood and enters the cell. Because cells have no facility to metabolize this excess energy, the cells create fat from

Adaptive thermogenesis excessively reduces energy expenditure that ultimately leads to higher body weight and body fat, often resulting in an even more severe calorically restrictive diet.

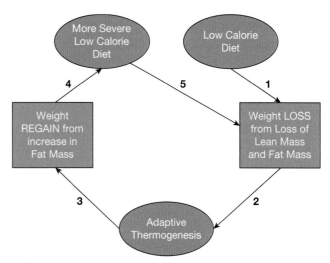

FIGURE 8.8: Low-calorie diets lead to weight gain recidivism that results in lower metabolic (lean) mass and higher fat mass. (Based on data from Montani JP, Schutz Y, Duloo AG. Dieting and weight cycling as risk factors for cardiometabolic diseases: who is really at risk? Obes Rev. 2015;16 (Suppl 1):7–18.)

the glucose and shuttle the fat out of the cell for storage as tissue fat. In simple terms, too much insulin production is associated with greater fat storage (body fat rises).

Relatively large doses of refined/simple carbohydrates may result in *hyperinsulinemia* (excess insulin production), which unlike a normoinsulinemic response (normal insulin production) fails to shut down the appetite-stimulating hormone ghrelin (43,80,81). The continued high presence of ghrelin results in sustained appetite and greater food consumption that could produce a high positive energy balance, which could result in higher weight. Without a stimulus to increase muscle (*i.e.*, appropriate exercise), this excess energy consumption could result in a higher level of stored body fat. It is important to note, however, that the simple/refined carbohydrate explanation for hyperinsulinemia is likely to be incomplete and potentially misleading, as there are multiple causes of hyperinsulinemia in addition to the consumption of high glycemic meals (Table 8.4). For instance, an infrequent eating pattern that allows blood sugar to drop below normal levels may also result in a hyperinsulinemic response at the next eating opportunity (82,83). Insulin is produced exponentially to the caloric load of the food consumed, so eating an excessively large meal (regardless

Table 8.4	Factors That Can Result in Excess Insulin Production
1. A high bolus intake of simple refined carbohydrate and/or sugars	A high consumption of high glycemic foods, including refined/processed grains, sugary beverages, and/or high-sugar foods, are quickly absorbed and induce a fast and high insulin response.
2. Consumption of any large meal	Insulin is produced exponentially to the caloric content of the meal consumed. Therefore, the net insulin production of four 500-kcal meals is lower than the net insulin production of two 1,000-kcal meals, even though the total caloric intake is the same.
3. Consumption of foods/ beverages following a long period without eating that results in low blood sugar	Normal blood sugar ranges from 80 to 120 mg/dL, and if blood sugar is allowed to go below this level (a common occurrence with skipped meals or exercise longer than 30 min that is unsupported with a carbohydrate-containing sports beverage), the next meal is likely to result in a high insulin response regardless of the meal's composition.
4. Having a high body fat level	Individuals with excess fat contributing to total mass are likely to be chronically hyperinsulinemic, making it even more important to avoid points 1–3 above.

Source. Benardot D. Energy thermodynamics revisited: energy intake strategies for optimizing athlete body composition and performance. Pensar en Movimiento: Revista de Ciencias del Ejercicio y la Salud (J Exerc Sci Health). 2013;11(2):1–13.

of its composition) would also result in excess insulin production with the concomitant increase in fat and, because of the associated maintenance of ghrelin, more total energy intake and weight (84,85). Higher total body fat or higher abdominal fat, regardless of the food consumed, is also associated with hyperinsulinemia and all of its sequelae (86,87). Although it is true that refined, high glycemic carbohydrates play a special role in insulin production, there are multiple other causes of hyperinsulinemia that are independent of macronutrient distribution, and these causes cannot be ignored if attempting to understand how energy balance dynamics influence weight and body composition.

Adaptive Thermogenesis

Refers to the decrease in energy expenditure *below* the level that may be predicted from energy expenditure, body weight, and lean mass in response to an inadequate energy intake. In simple terms, someone restricting energy intake by 30% may initially experience a weight loss, but once adaptive thermogenesis occurs the individual becomes overly energy efficient, resulting in rebound weight. It may take several months on a calorically restrictive diet for adaptive thermogenesis to be observed. Many studies that only track the changes in "weight" for 1 or 2 months may be misleading as they fail to track subjects long enough to determine the impact of adaptive thermogenesis (88,89).

An additional potential problem is that the calculation of energy balance using the 24-hour traditional view assumes that the time of day used to assess the prior

24 hours is irrelevant. The typical data collection strategy for such an assessment is to ask a client/athlete for the immediate prior 24-hour energy intake and expenditure regardless of the time of day the client is with you, with the assumption that energy balance at that precise point of time is the same for the entire 24 hours that preceded it. However, the within-day energy balance curve is not flat, so the time of day that the client/athlete is assessed creates differences in the energy balance calculation (Figure 8.9). Also, meals are not always consumed at the same time. A later dinner that is consumed early in the 24-hour assessment period could lead to two dinners being included in the same analysis period, resulting in an apparent large 24-hour energy balance surplus. An early dinner early in

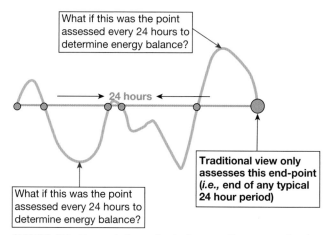

What if this was the point assessed every 24 hours to determine energy balance?

24 hours

What if this was the point assessed every 24 hours to determine energy balance?

Traditional view only assesses this end-point (*i.e.*, end of any typical 24 hour period)

FIGURE 8.9: Energy balance fluctuates over the course of a day. Because of this, the same person, on the same day, would appear as if he or she had an entirely different energy balance depending on the time of day.

the 24-hour assessment period and a late dinner late in the same 24-hour assessment period could exclude both dinners and make it appear as if the client is in a chronic energy balance deficit. The resulting **24-hour energy balance** conclusion would, therefore, be entirely different for the same person, depending on the time of day the evaluation took place.

📖 24-Hour Energy Balance

The ratio of energy consumed over 24 hours versus the energy expended over 24 hours, and represents the traditional way that energy balance has been measured in humans. However, recent studies suggest that wide fluctuations in energy balance during the day (*i.e.*, in real time) may result in the loss of lean tissue or an increase in fat mass, even if 24-hour energy balance appears to be good.

It is possible for a person to appear to be in nearly perfect energy balance at the end of a 24-hour assessment period, but to have arrived at this point with extremely large energy balance surpluses or deficits that could have an impact on body composition. A source of concern with the traditional model for energy balance is the failure to consider that the pattern of energy consumption is an important factor in weight and body composition. This model assumes that a person requiring 2,000 kcal/day (8,368 kJ/day) to satisfy energy requirements could consume that energy

without regard to meal size or eating frequency, and the energy balance influence on weight or body composition would be the same. This person could, for instance, have a 2,000-kcal breakfast and eat nothing else the remainder of the day to satisfy the energy requirement; they could have a 2,000-kcal dinner and eat nothing else prior to that dinner; or they could have four 500-kcal meals during the day. The 24-hour macroeconomic model assumes that the endocrine system only takes action at the point of assessment and that the outcomes in body composition and weight would be the same, but they are not. The large breakfast would cause the person to spend the majority of the day in an energy balance surplus, with excess fat storage the likely outcome; the large dinner would cause the person to spend the majority of the day in an energy balance deficit, with catabolism of lean tissue and a relatively higher fat storage; and the frequent meal eater is more likely to sustain the metabolic mass and the FM.

A study of the association between hourly energy balance and body composition in four different groups of elite athletes illustrates the importance of avoiding wide shifts in energy balance during the day (4). This study found that large within-day energy balance deficits were associated with higher body fat levels (Figure 8.10). An example of this can also be found in an assessment of an elite athlete, whose ending energy balance was very close to perfect, but who achieved a large energy balance deficit while arriving at the end-of-day energy balance

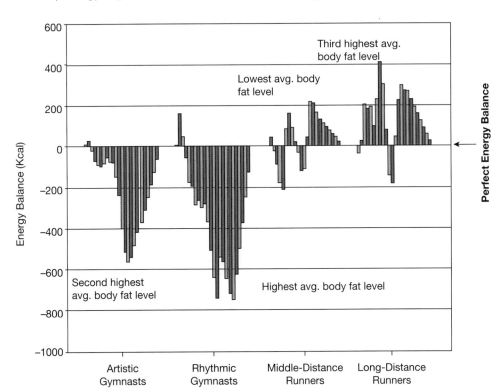

FIGURE 8.10: Large within-day energy balance deficits are associated with higher body fat percent. Athletes who sustained smaller deviations from perfect energy balance over the course of 24 hours had lower body fat levels. (From Deutz R, Benardot D, Martin D, Cody MM. Relationship between energy deficits and body composition in elite female gymnasts and runners. Med Sci Sports Exerc. 2000;32(3):659–68.)

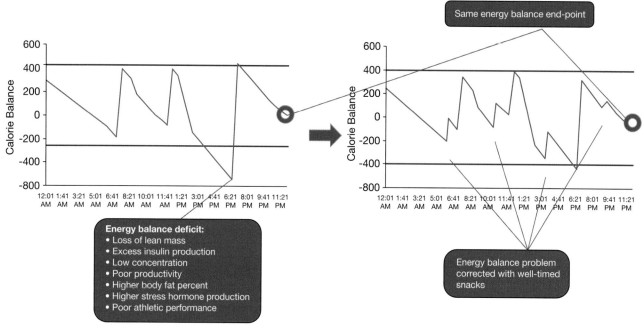

FIGURE 8.11: Maintaining energy balance as a strategy for improving body composition. (From Benardot D. Timing of energy and fluid intake: new concepts for weight control and hydration. ACSM Health Fit J. 2007;11(4):13–9.)

point (Figure 8.11). The corrective action was to adjust the consumed energy during the day to avoid the large energy balance deficit while maintaining total energy intake as it was (10). At no time was the recommendation made to increase or lower total energy intake, but rather to change the timing and caloric content of foods consumed to better sustain energy balance throughout the day and positively influence the hormone/endocrine response.

As demonstrated by several studies, the traditional 24-hour energy balance model is not capable of considering within-day fluctuations in energy balance. It was found that muscle breakdown occurs with inadequate real-time fuel provision as an adaptation to the inadequate energy availability and because of higher cortisol production (32,33). Infrequent eating and large bolus meals result in higher body fat storage, even if total caloric intake is the same, largely because of greater insulin production from the larger meals (4,90). Insulin, blood sugar, and leptin are better controlled with frequent smaller feedings that dynamically match energy requirements (2,34). The exerciser who fails to satisfy the dynamic need for energy and develops low blood sugar will go into a state of gluconeogenesis. This will result in the likely breakdown of lean tissue to release alanine to the liver where the alanine–glucose cycle can manufacture glucose to, among other things, sustain normal brain function. An early study found that after only 40 minutes of strenuous activity,

free serum alanine could increase by 60%–90% or even more if the exercise occurs with low blood sugar (91). Studies have also found that cortisol is elevated if exercise proceeds with a failure to consume a carbohydrate beverage, likely resulting in a negative within-day energy balance and low blood sugar (92). Cortisol is known to be catabolic to both bone and muscle, resulting in higher stress fracture risk and higher BF% (33,93,94). One must ask why an athlete would exercise in a way that breaks down muscle and bone when the goal is to reduce exercise-associated risks and enhance muscle function. Yet, if the traditional 24-hour energy balance view is followed, this is all too possible. As illustrated in Table 8.5, there are multiple hormonal problems that occur when negative energy balance occurs.

Real-Time View of Energy Balance

In studies of both athlete and nonathlete populations, dietary trends that coincide with the steep obesity velocity curve include larger food portion sizes, consumption of fast foods with hidden fats, and decreased meal frequency (32,95). All of these have an influence on ghrelin and leptin. Decreased meal frequency is associated with greater daily energy consumption, possibly from an upregulation of appetite and/or a tendency for greater fat consumption found that visible fats in meals resulted in a lower total energy intake than hidden fats because

Table 8.5	Negative Energy Balance and Hormonal Changes	
Tissue/Organ	**Hormone/Compound**	**Expected Change**
Adipocytes and hypothalamus	Leptin	Decreased
Adrenal	Cortisol	Increased
Gastrointestinal tract	Ghrelin	Increased
Liver	Plasma glucose	Decreased
	IGF-1[a]	Decreased
	IGFBP-1[b]	Increased
Pancreas	Insulin	Decreased (fasting)
		Increased (eating)
Thyroid	Total T3c	Decreased

[a]Insulin-like growth factor-1.

[b]Insulin-like growth factor binding protein-1.

[c]Triiodothyronine.

Sources: Laughlin GA, Yen SSC. Hypoleptinemia in women athletes: absence of a diurnal rhythm with amenorrhea. J Clin Endocrinol Metab. 1997; 82(1): 318–21; Loucks AB, Callister R. Induction and prevention of low-T3 syndrome in exercising women. Am J Physiol. 1993;264(5):R924–30; Loucks AB, Heath EM. Induction of low-T3 syndrome in exercising women occurs at a threshold of energy availability. Am J Physiol. 1994;266(3):R817–23; Loucks AB, Verdun M, Heath EM. Low energy availability, not stress of exercise, alters LH pulsatility in exercising women. J Appl Physiol. 1998;84(1):37–46; Stafford DEJ. Altered hypothalamic-pituitary-ovarian axis function in young female athletes. Treat Endocrinol. 2005;4(3):147–54.

of altered sensory signals (36,96). It was also found that meal skipping has an influence on obesity. They assessed a large sample of people who did not typically skip breakfast as children or adults ($n = 1,359$), those who skipped breakfast only in childhood ($n = 224$), those who skipped breakfast only in adulthood ($n = 515$), or those who skipped breakfast in both childhood and adulthood. Skipping breakfast is associated with a severe energy balance deficit. The chronic breakfast skippers had significantly higher fasting insulin, serum low-density lipoprotein, and waist circumference. Even when adjusting for diet quality, these differences persisted. These data imply that humans do not adapt to poor eating behaviors that fail to sustain energy balance.

It has also been found that the increased energy intake associated with infrequent eating is not matched with higher activity, resulting in a higher body fat level (97,98). Franko et al. (98) found, after studying girls between the ages of 9 and 19 for over 10 years, that the subjects who consumed 3+ meals on more days had lower overweight and obesity rates than girls with lower meal frequency. Berkey et al. (97), studying a cohort of more than 14,000 boys and girls, found that eating breakfast (*i.e.*, increasing eating frequency) was an important strategy for avoiding obesity.

Avoiding hyperinsulinemia, either through preventing hunger (associated with eating when in a severely low–blood-sugar state and a direct result of infrequent eating and poor within-day energy balance) or eluding the consumption of high glycemic foods, is useful in controlling the appetite-stimulating hormone ghrelin. Anderwald et al. (31) found that ghrelin was unchanged in type II diabetics following insulin treatment, but a rise in serum insulin that occurs following a meal had the effect of suppressing ghrelin and reducing appetite in nondiabetics. In an assessment of a small group of young adult males, it was also found that the postmeal drop in ghrelin is likely due to the rise in insulin, but that this relationship does not exist with the hyperinsulinemia associated with insulin resistance (35). In a group of 278 healthy French schoolchildren between the ages of 6 and 8 years, it was found that skipping breakfast and consuming sugar-sweetened beverages while watching television were likely factors in unsuppressed ghrelin, hyperinsulinemia, or both, and that these behaviors were associated with significantly higher BMI, sum of four skinfolds, and waist circumference (99). Put simply, producing excess insulin sustains appetite through sustained ghrelin.

A concern with the macroeconomic view of energy balance is the assumption that an energy balance achieved at the end of a 24-hour period is perfectly sustained for the entire 24 hours that precede it. However, there are natural peaks and valleys in energy balance throughout the day, and it has been found that wide deviations from perfect energy balance during a 24-hour period are associated with higher BF%, even if energy balance is achieved at the end of that 24-hour period. A recent review of studies assessing the relationship between protein intake and sarcopenia found a similar result, with the suggestion that sustaining a steady intake of high-quality protein (between 25 and 35 g/meal) at standard three-meal intervals throughout the day is far more effective at maintaining or increasing muscle mass than the common postloading that many athletes do, resulting in excessively large end-of-day energy and protein intakes (100). A reassessment of athlete protein intakes using this model is warranted, as it appears that many athletes with relatively high protein intakes exceeding 2–3 g/kg/day may actually have inadequate protein intakes when maximal protein utilization rates (~30–35 g protein per meal) are considered. The extremely high single-meal protein and energy intakes seen in some athletes, often at levels exceeding 100 g protein and 4,000 kcal, provide protein and energy at levels that are metabolically inefficient and more likely to increase FM than muscle mass. Once again, the 24-hour model for energy/nutrient intake and expenditure fails to optimally provide actionable information.

Relative Energy Availability in Sport

Energy deficiency has long been reported in athletes, and in particular, it has been widely prevalent in athletes in weight-sensitive sports, including gymnastics, wrestling, diving, and figure skating (101). Energy deficiency can occur as a result of several factors, including intentionally restricting energy intake to make a certain weight class or lean physique, or because of an eating disorder, a sport-associated disordered eating pattern, or from a simple misunderstanding of how a failure to supply the needed energy can compromise health and performance. Sustaining an energy-deficient diet during physical activity may place an athlete in a catabolic state that results in precisely what they wish to avoid: a loss of muscle mass and an increase in FM (4). In 2014, the International Olympic Committee (IOC) introduced a new term to describe this failure of adequately supplying needed energy: **relative energy deficiency in sport** (RED-S), and described problems faced by all physically active people who fail to supply the fuel required for the activity. RED-S includes a broad range of potential health and performance consequences for both males and females who are physically active (101) (Figure 8.12).

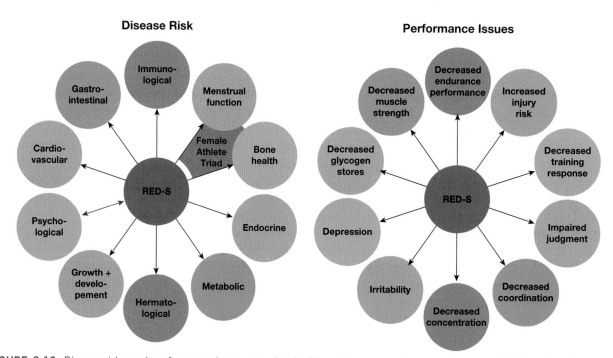

FIGURE 8.12: Disease risks and performance issues associated with relative energy deficiency in sport (RED-S). (Reproduced from Mountjoy M, Sundgot-Borgen J, Burke L, Carter S, Constantini N, Lebrun C, Meyer N, Sherman R, Steffen K, Budgett R, Ljungqvist A. The IOC consensus statement: beyond the Female Athlete Triad—Relative Energy Deficiency in Sport (RED-S). Br J Sports Med. 2014;48:491–97, with permission from BMJ Publishing Group Ltd.)

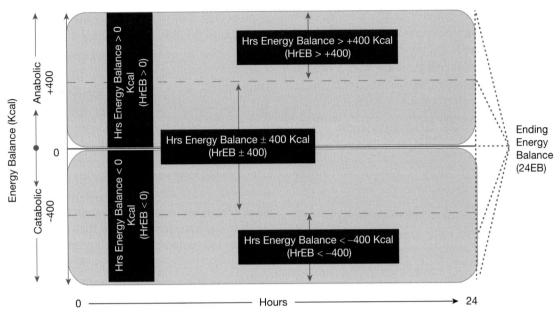

FIGURE 8.13: A new model for energy balance assessment. (From Benardot D. Energy thermodynamics revisited: energy intake strategies for optimizing athlete body composition and performance. Pensar en Movimiento: Revista de Ciencias del Ejercicio y la Salud (J Exerc Sci Health). 2013;11(2):1–13.)

Relative Energy Deficiency in Sport

Also referred to as RED-S, this represents the ratio of energy consumed and expended in real time, to determine if athletes have sufficient energy available to perform a given athletic task. RED-S is associated with poor health, increased injury risk, and poor performance.

Energy deficiency and its consequences have been the focus of numerous studies in recent years, with some studies suggesting that athletes participating in sports with weight classifications or lean physiques are at risk, including female distance runners, figure skaters, gymnasts, divers, and swimmers (102). Studies have found that a surprisingly large cross-section of athletes experience components of RED-S, but these athletes and those who work with them are unaware of the health and performance consequences they may experience (101).

RED-S, besides compromising performance through a reduction in FFM and an increase in FM, may also increase illness frequency and nutrient deficiency, including anemia (101). Failure to adequately supply energy over the long term may affect metabolic rate, immunity, protein synthesis, growth and development, and cardiovascular health while also negatively affecting psychological, endocrine, hematologic, and gastrointestinal well-being. Menstrual dysfunction and lower BMD are well-established negative consequences of poorly satisfying energy needs (103–105). An increase in cortisol, as a result of physiologic and/or psychological stress that is associated with poor energy availability, can also negatively affect BMD (106). Athletes with lower BMD are at greater risk of stress fractures and related musculoskeletal injuries.

The within-day energy balance and within-day energy substrate studies, coupled with the poor predictive ability of the traditional 24-hour energy balance model, suggest that a new within-day energy balance model should be used (Figure 8.13). This model considers both time spent in a catabolic and anabolic energy balance state, and the magnitude of the energy balance surpluses and deficits to predict body composition and weight outcomes. Importantly, by incorporating time spent in different energy balance zones, this model may be more useful in predicting the endocrine response to energy balance inadequacies and surpluses, which may aid in reducing health and performance risks in athletes.

This model also enables the consideration of an important understanding of energy imbalances: *The body's reaction to an inadequate energy intake is to reduce the tissue that needs energy.* Ideally, there should be a dynamic relationship between the need for energy and nutrients, and the provision of energy and nutrients to optimize body composition, weight, and performance. Athletes who spend the majority of time in a near-energy–balanced state are likely to reduce energy balance–related problems described in RED-S, with the suggestion that athletes address how energy is provided over the day and around exercise sessions (4,60,101). Those who spend more time in a large energy balance surplus are likely to increase body fat levels, and those who spend more time in a large energy balance deficit are likely to have difficulty sustaining muscle and could be at risk for more RED-S health- and performance-related problems.

Assessment of Body Composition

Important Factors to Consider

- There are many methods available for the assessment of body composition but all of these methods have some errors associated with them, with some methods having lower error than others, and some methods are more portable and less expensive than others.

- It is important to find a method that can be used with your population repeatedly so that a trend of change can be assessed. For instance, skinfolds do not provide as accurate a prediction of body fat percent as DXA, but skinfold calipers are portable, and with time and training, a practitioner can take skinfolds on a subject repeatedly to obtain a valuable assessment of how body fat is changing. Ultimately, this may be more valuable information to a practitioner than a single measure that cannot be taken more than once or twice a year because of cost or the inability of the athlete to go to the lab or clinic.

The body is composed of different components (water, muscle, fat, bone, nerve tissue, tendons, etc.), and each has a different density (107) (Table 8.6). From a functional standpoint, tissues are grouped together into those that are mainly fat (FM), which has little water associated with it, and those that have little fat (FFM), which has a great deal of water associated with it. The FFM is also commonly but inaccurately referred to as lean mass (108). More recently, because of new techniques and improvements in estimating body composition, BMD (skeletal mass) has been included as a third commonly assessed component of body composition. But for the purpose of this book, the components of body composition generally are referred to as *FM* (the amount of mass in the body that is mainly fat) and *FFM* (the amount of mass in the body that is mainly free of fat).

The FM is composed of essential fat and storage fat. The essential fat is a required component of the brain, nerves, bone marrow, heart tissue, and cell walls that we cannot live without. Storage fat, on the other hand, is an energy reserve that builds up in fat (adipose) cells underneath the skin (**subcutaneous fat**) and around the organs (visceral or interabdominal fat). Average healthy men and women do have ~11%–15% of total body weight from storage fat. Combining the essential fat and storage fat compartments, normal BF% for males is ~15% (3% essential; 12% storage), whereas normal BF% for females is 26% (15% essential; 11% storage) (109,110). (Please note that different methods for assessing body composition have method-specific standards. The values listed here are to provide the relative differences of body fat distributions in males and females.)

There is historical evidence that a BF% of 17%–22% is needed to maintain a normal menstrual cycle in most women (111). There is also evidence that physiologic and/or psychological stress is a trigger for disrupting the reproductive system (112). However, a closer look at both the body fat and stress hypotheses for disturbing normal menstrual function is not likely to be correct. There is strong evidence to suggest that energy availability, not body fatness or stress, is the primary regulator of female reproductive function. Women falling below an energy balance that ranges from 20 to 30 calories of lean body mass per day (*i.e.*, if energy consumption minus energy expenditure falls below 20–30 calories of lean mass per day) are at significantly higher risk of menstrual dysfunction (113,114). In addition, these data strongly suggest that women consuming 45 calories/kg of lean body mass are resistant to developing menstrual dysfunction regardless of body fat level or physical stress. Given the large number of normally menstruating athletic females who are lean (*i.e.*, who have relatively low body fat levels), the energy availability hypothesis is more logical.

Females with an **eating disorder**, dysmenorrhea (abnormal menses), and low bone density have a condition referred to as the **female athlete triad** (115). These are related conditions, as inadequate energy intake (typical of eating disorders) is associated with both abnormal menstrual function and low bone density. Inadequate energy intake results in lower estrogen, and estrogen suppresses osteoclasts, cells that break down bone. Without this suppression, it is difficult to increase BMD. The IOC consensus statement on RED-S described earlier refers to multiple physiologic problems that occur in all athletes who fail to satisfy, in real time, the dietary energy required for health, daily activity, growth, and sporting activities (116). These include problems with metabolic rate, menstrual function, bone health, immunity, protein synthesis, and cardiovascular health, all of which are caused by RED. Importantly, athletes who fail to adequately satisfy

Table 8.6	Important Terms for Body Composition Assessment
Fat mass	Also referred to as body fat, adipose tissue, or stored fat. This represents the total weight of fat that contributes to total body weight.
Lean mass	This refers to *all* of the bodyweight that is not fat mass. Fat-free mass is defined as lean body mass minus the bone mass.
Percent body fat	This represents the total fat mass (*i.e.*, total weight of fat) of a person divided by the person's total body mass (*i.e.*, total weight).
Obesity	Defined as having too much body fat. The common determination for obesity is through calculation of BMI (*i.e.*, a BMI of 30 or greater is considered "obese"). However, this may be misleading because it fails to differentiate between fat and muscle weight. Therefore, a highly muscled person may be defined as overweight (high weight for height), but would not be unhealthy.
Overweight	Defined as weighing too much for your height. This is often based on height/weight tables but may be misleading because it fails to differentiate between fat and muscle weight. Therefore, a highly muscled person may be defined as overweight (high weight for height), but would not be unhealthy.
Body fat distribution or fat patterning	Body fat that is distributed around the abdomen poses greater health risks than fat stored in other areas.
Android-type obesity	This refers to excess fat primarily in the abdomen and surrounding the organs (*i.e.*, apple-shaped obesity). It is associated with glucose intolerance, diabetes, and higher cardiovascular risk and is considered to have higher health risk than gynoid-type obesity.
Gynoid-type obesity	This refers to excess fat around the hips and thighs (*i.e.*, pear-shaped obesity) and is associated with lower disease risk than android-type obesity.
Anthropometry	Refers to the scientific study of measurements and proportion of the human body. Common anthropometric measures taken for the assessment of body composition include height, weight, and circumference. These are often converted to ratios (*e.g.*, BMI) as a predictor of body composition and obesity risk.

BMI, body mass index.

energy requirements are likely to lose FFM and experience a relative increase in FM, which requires body composition assessment to discern. Monitoring weight alone will miss these important changes in body composition.

Eating Disorder

A general term for a psychometric disorder that is associated with abnormal eating behavior, often associated with loss of mass. These disorders include anorexia nervosa, anorexia athletica, and binge eating disorder. Athletes in aesthetic sports or sports where "making weight" is a traditional component of a sport are considered at high risk.

Female Athlete Triad

A triad of conditions exist simultaneously, including an eating disorder, dysmenorrhea (amenorrhea or oligomenorrhea), and low bone mineral density (osteoporosis or osteopenia). Females competing in aesthetic sports or sports where "making weight" is a traditional component of a sport are considered at risk.

There are multiple means for assessing body composition. Commonly used methods, discussed in this chapter, include the following:

- *Multiple skinfolds:* Using a skinfold caliper, a double thickness (derived from pinching and measuring the subcutaneous fat) of different areas of the body is measured. The skinfold values are included in a prediction equation with weight, age, and gender to predict percent body fat.
- *Densitometry (underwater or hydrostatic weighing):* FM is less dense than lean mass, and a lower density will make a person more buoyant in water and weigh

less in water than when compared with their out-of-water weight. The difference between out-of-water weight and in-water weight is a function of body density and has been used to predict body composition.

- *Air displacement plethysmography:* Similar to hydrostatic weighing principle, a less dense person (*i.e.,* someone with a greater proportion of body fat) will displace more air than someone of the same weight with a higher density. The measurement of displacement of air can be used to predict body composition.

- *Ultrasound:* Using an ultrasound wave, this system measures the thickness of different tissues by assessing the time it takes for sound to bounce back from the interface between the subcutaneous fat layer and the muscle layer, and the muscle layer and bone. The thickness of these tissue layers can be used to predict body composition.

- *Bioelectrical Impedance Analysis (BIA):* Electrical current(s) pass through different segments of the body. The difference between the original electrical energy and the ending electrical energy, after it has passed through a body segment, is a measure of how much the electrical current has been impeded. Fat tissue has almost no water, so is a poor conductor of electrical current (*i.e.,* it has high impedance), whereas fat-free tissue has a great deal of water and so is an excellent conductor of electrical current. Therefore, measuring bioelectrical impedance has been used to predict body composition. Early versions of BIA

- *Dual Energy X-Ray Absorptiometry (DXA):* A lower-energy and higher-energy X-ray pass through the body, and the amount of X-ray energy that has passed is read by a detector. Higher tissue densities (bone density is greater than muscle density; muscle density is greater than fat density) absorb relatively more of the low-energy X-ray than the high-energy X-ray. The difference in X-ray absorption is a function of the tissue density and has been used to predict body composition relatively accurately.

Other methods for assessing body composition include the following:

- *Total body water (D$_2$O):* Total body water in humans on average is ~65% of body weight and varies by age, gender, and body fatness. Individuals with relatively higher FFM have more body water than individuals with relatively higher FM. Total body water can be estimated by providing a known dose of water that is made from deuterium rather than hydrogen (D$_2$O vs. H$_2$O). The deuterated water evenly distributes itself throughout the entire body water, and then a sample of body water is analyzed to determine the ratio of D$_2$O to H$_2$O. Higher relative D$_2$O (*i.e.,* a higher concentration) suggests lower total body water, which is associated with lower FFM and has been used to predict body composition.

- *Total body potassium (K^{40}):* Potassium^{40} is a naturally occurring isotope of potassium and represents 0.012% of total body potassium. This isotope gives off a unique γ-radiation wave that is readable and can be differentiated from other isotope waves. The concentration of potassium (the primary intercellular electrolyte) in FFM is known, so by measuring K^{40} by using a whole-body γ-radiation counter, it is possible to predict total body potassium, which can be used to predict FFM. By knowing total mass and FFM, body FM can be predicted using a two-component model of body composition.

- *Infrared interactance:* This method is based on the principle that tissues of different density will absorb and/or reflect infrared light differently. Higher-density tissues (*i.e.,* FFM) absorb less light and reflect more light than lower-density tissues (*i.e.,* FM). The difference in light absorption/reflection can be measured and has been used to predict body composition.

- *Creatinine excretion:* For a given height there is an expectation that humans excrete creatinine, which is a normal nitrogenous metabolic by-product of FFM respiration. Therefore, assuming normal kidney function, the amount of urinary creatinine excreted in a 24-hour period is a measure of FFM, with higher creatinine levels associated with higher FFM. By knowing total mass, creatinine excretion can be used to predict body composition.

- *3-Methylhistidine excretion:* This method is similar to creatinine excretion, except that 3-methylhistidine excretion is specific to skeletal muscle respiration. That is, greater amounts of urinary 3-methylhistidine excretion are associated with higher skeletal muscle mass.

- *Total body electrical conductivity:* This method is based on the fact that water is a conductor of electricity and FFM contains more water than FM. A body is inserted into a tube that has a measured electromagnetic field. The amount of disruption in the electromagnetic field is a function of how much FM the person has. Higher FM creates a greater measured reduction in the electromagnetic field than lower FM, and this measurement has been used to predict body composition.

- *Computed tomography (CT scan):* Using X-rays, the CT scan produces sectional scans (slices) of the body.

The images can be assessed for different densities and can also provide information on fatty infusion in lean tissue. However, this method is limited by cost and by high exposure to X-ray radiation.

- *Magnetic resonance imaging:* A magnetic field passing through the body produces an image of the relative conductance/resistance to the electrical field created by different tissues. The resultant images allow differentiation on FM and FFM, providing information on body composition.

Each method has a different cost and a different standard error of measurement. Some methods are appropriate for laboratory/clinical assessment, whereas others can be used in the field. Regardless of the method, each method attempts to measure relative body fatness (*i.e.,* how much body fat a person has) and relative body FFM (the difference between the FM and all the body mass). Some methods can provide information on where the FM and FFM are held in different amounts, and some methods can also provide information on bone density and total body water. (See Table 8.7 for the theoretical contributors to mass in a relatively lean man and a relatively lean woman.)

Lean mass is mainly water and protein, but also includes minerals and stored carbohydrates (glycogen). The main constituents of the FFM include soft tissues muscle, the heart, and other organs but do not include skeletal (bone) tissue (117). The water content of the FM is below 10% (111,118). Athletes typically have a larger lean mass and a lower FM than nonathletes do, so well-hydrated athletes have a higher proportion of total weight that comes from water.

Using the two-component FM to lean body mass model of body composition, the combined weight of FM and lean mass equals total body weight. Because weight by itself fails to discriminate between the two components, it is considered to be an inappropriate measure of body composition. Therefore, the statement "My weight is increasing, so I must be getting fat" is common but incorrect. It is possible for an athlete to increase the fat-free (*i.e.,* muscle) mass without increasing the FM. Clearly, there would be an increase in weight, but not fat weight. It is also possible for an athlete to maintain weight but experience changes in fat or lean mass. This could be either desirable or undesirable depending on which element is increasing. A high strength-to-weight ratio shows an increase in lean mass (strength) with a maintenance or lowering of FM (weight) equaling total weight. This scenario is obviously desirable. However, should an athlete increase the FM while lowering the lean mass, strength is lost and the strength-to-weight ratio decreases or is low. Assessing these aspects of body composition has become a standard tool for the evaluation of body changes that occur as a result of time, training, and nutritional factors.

Body composition assessment generally results in obtaining a value referred to as BF%, or the proportion of total weight that is made up by the FM. Assuming an athlete weighs 150 lb and has a BF% of 20%, it means that 30 lb (150 × 0.20 = 30) is fat weight and 120 lb is lean weight. If this athlete experiences a reduction in BF% to 15% while maintaining weight, this would mean that 22.5 lb (150 × 0.15 = 22.5) is fat weight and 127.5 lb is lean weight. This increase of 7.5 lb in lean weight and reduction in fat weight means the athlete is now smaller (pound-for-pound, lean mass takes up less space than FM because it has a higher density), which should enable the athlete to move more quickly and more efficiently than before. However, if this 150-lb athlete were to maintain weight but increase FM while reducing the FFM, potential speed and efficiency of movement would be reduced. For all of these reasons, weight is a poor measure for predicting athletic success. This example also emphasizes the importance of assessing changes that occur in both the fat-free and FM, because understanding changes in both compartments is necessary for understanding the potential impact on performance.

Because reporting on FM (*i.e.,* BF%) may be considered undesirable by many athletes, practitioners should consider emphasizing the positive. For instance, an athlete with a BF% of 25% may wish to lower this value to 20%. As a sports medicine practitioner, you should consider asking them to *increase FFM* from 75% to 80%. All too often athletes who are told to lower BF% resort to calorie-restricted diets to achieve the fat loss. This is typically counterproductive, as more lean mass is lost than FM. Therefore, changing the focus to increasing FFM rather than lowering FM could help athletes strategize on how to best satisfy the energy needs of an ever larger FFM, with the side benefit of reducing the risk of the athlete developing one of the RED-S health/performance risks.

Table 8.7	Theoretical Contributors to Total Body Mass	
Body Component	Lean Man (%)	Lean Woman (%)
Water	62	59
Fat	16	22
Protein	16	14
Minerals	5–6	4–5
Carbohydrate	<1	<1

Purpose of Body Composition Assessment

A high fat-free-mass-to-fat-mass ratio is often synonymous with a high strength-to-weight ratio, which is typically associated with athletic success. However, there is no single ideal body composition for all athletes in all sports. Each sport has a range of FFM and FM associated with it, and each athlete in a sport has an individual range that is best for him or her. Athletes who try to achieve an arbitrary body composition that is not right for them are likely to increase health risks and will not achieve the performance benefits they seek. Therefore, the key to body composition assessment is the establishment of an acceptable range of lean and FM for the individual athlete, as well as the monitoring of lean and FM over regular time intervals to ensure the stability or growth of the lean mass and a proportional maintenance or reduction of the FM. As indicated earlier, there should be just as much attention given to changes in lean mass (both in weight of lean mass and proportion of lean mass) as the attention traditionally given to BF%.

Athletes wishing to lower body fat levels should also be aware of the best physical activities to achieve this goal. "Aerobic" or low-intensity training, which is so often used as a fat-loss exercise regimen, may not be the most effective means of achieving this goal. It has been found that high-intensity exercise training was significantly more effective at reducing total abdominal fat and abdominal subcutaneous fat than low-intensity exercise training (119). High-intensity winter sports, for instance, are associated with lower BF% and higher lean mass than less intense activities (120). Care must be taken, however, to avoid low blood sugar during high-intensity exercise, as low blood sugar is a predictor of high cortisol production, which is associated with a loss of FFM, a loss of bone mass, and higher BF% (44). Whatever dietary and exercise strategy is used, periodic assessment of body composition will help an athlete understand if the desired goal is being achieved.

Importance of Body Composition to Performance

Athletic performance is, to a large degree, dependent on the athlete's ability to sustain power (both anaerobically and aerobically) and the athlete's ability to overcome resistance or drag (121). Both of these factors are interrelated with the athlete's body composition. Coupled with the common perception of many athletes who compete in sports where appearance is a concern (swimming, diving, gymnastics, skating, etc.), attainment of an "ideal" body composition often becomes a central theme of training. Besides the aesthetic and performance reasons for wanting to achieve an optimal body composition, there may also be safety reasons. An athlete who is carrying excess weight may be more prone to injury when performing difficult skills than an athlete with a more optimal body composition. However, the means athletes sometimes use in an attempt to achieve an optimal body composition are often counterproductive.

Low-calorie diets and excessive training often result in such a severe energy deficit that, while total weight may be reduced, the constituents of weight also change, commonly with a lower muscle mass and a relatively higher FM. The resulting higher BF% and lower muscle mass inevitably result in a performance reduction that motivates the athlete to follow regimens that produce even greater energy deficits. This downward energy intake spiral may be the precursor to eating disorders that place the athlete at serious health risk. Therefore, although achieving an optimal body composition is useful for high-level athletic performance, the processes athletes often use to attain a desirable body composition may reduce athletic performance, place them at a higher injury risk, and increase health risks.

The mindset that many people have that food, regardless of the amount and type, produces fat is unhealthy. A much healthier (and from the point of view of an athlete, more appropriate) mindset is that food is the provider of energy and the nutrients associated with burning energy. Athletes would not think of trying to run their automobile without fuel, as they are certain it would not run. Athletes should also imagine that putting fuel (food) in their bodies to make their muscles run is normal and desirable.

Within reasonable bounds, having a relatively low BF% may aid athletic performance. It occurs by improving the strength-to-weight ratio: for a given weight, more of it is represented by lean mass that is power-producing and less of it by FM that represents stored fuel. It also helps by lowering the resistance or drag, an athlete has as she or he is going through the air, swimming in water, or skating on ice; the smaller the body profile, the less resistance it is likely to produce.

Less resistance or drag, is so important for some sports (typically the faster you go the greater the importance of drag reduction) that performance techniques are based on reducing drag. Speed skaters, for instance, spend the entire race bent over to reduce wind resistance. Cyclists wear special streamlined helmets and clothing, position their bodies on the bicycle to reduce drag, and even strategize about the best time to sprint ahead of the cycle in front of them. Going too soon can lead to premature exhaustion because it takes a great deal more energy to go the same speed if you are the one facing wind resistance. A gymnast who weighs 110 lb and is 5 feet tall with a BF% of 15% will have a lower wind resistance (*i.e.*, less drag) tumbling through the air than a gymnast with the same weight and height but with a BF% of 20%. For some sports, however, this may make little or no difference. It is hard to imagine how a powerlifter would have a problem with wind resistance, and linemen on football teams are more interested in moving mass than going fast over a distance (although quickness helps). In sports where being aerodynamic helps, body composition could make a big difference. The reason for this is something many of us have already experienced: pound-for-pound, FM takes up more space than FFM because it is less dense than FFM.

How Body Composition Is Estimated

You cannot tell about a person's body composition by weighing or simply observing the person. There are many thin people who have lost so much lean mass that they actually have a relatively high BF%. (They are not lean.) There are also many large people whom you might assume are obese but who are actually relatively lean. Even with modern equipment and sophisticated equations, it is extremely difficult (if not impossible) to accurately measure BF% and to accurately repeat that measure. It is important to consider that all the techniques available for measuring/estimating body composition are estimates of what the body contains. Because each technique uses a different means of estimating body composition, cross-comparisons between techniques should not be made. For instance, an athlete with an initial body composition assessed using skinfold calipers last year should not have that value compared with the body composition assessed using BIA today. It would be misleading to use these values as a means of determining how this athlete's body composition has changed over time.

Ideally, athletes should be assessed several times over equal time periods and at the same time of day to obtain a trend line for how body composition is changing, because the trend is likely to be more important than the absolute value (122,123). Imagine measuring an athlete whose body composition looks fine, so you have no reason to intervene. What if, however, high body fat level was lower on the previous measure and even lower on the measure before that, and this athlete has also lost some lean mass over the same time period? As another example, an

athlete appears to have a high level of body fat, initiating a counseling session to help the athlete lower the FM. What if, however, the athlete had a higher body fat level several months earlier that was reduced still further 1 month before the current measure? This athlete is obviously doing something right, and it would be a pity to intervene in a strategy that is already working. By taking several measures, the health professional has a much better idea of how the athlete is changing and whether an intervention is warranted.

It may be useful to assess the predominant *location* of body fat, as fat stored in different areas is associated with differential health risks. For instance, abdominal body fat poses greater health risks than fat stored in other areas. If health risk assessment, rather than performance, is the focus of the body composition assessment, then a method should be selected that can identify where the preponderance of fat is stored.

The ultimate purpose of body composition assessment is to determine the ratio of FM to FFM. This is referred to as a two-compartment model (1. FM; 2. FFM). However, some methods of body composition assessment have the capacity to provide more information on what constitutes the FFM. For instance, in a three-compartment model body composition assessment, the information includes FM, and the FFM is divided into the protein mass and bone (skeletal) mass. A four-compartment model provides even more information on the FFM, with information on FM, water mass, protein mass, and skeletal (bone mineral) mass (Figures 8.14 and 8.15).

Methods for Predicting Body Composition

Skinfolds

Skinfold calipers, which vary in cost from free to $500, are used to measure a double thickness of skin and the fat layer under the skin (Figure 8.16). This fat layer (called subcutaneous fat) represents ~50% of a person's total body fat. Therefore, measuring the subcutaneous fat layer provides a measurement that can be used to predict total body fat level.

The basic rules for taking skinfold measures are as follows:

- Take skinfold measurements on the right side of the body (most skinfold equations were developed from measurements on the right side).
- Do not take measurements when the subject's skin is moist (ensure that the skin is dry and has no lotion). Also, do not take measurements immediately after

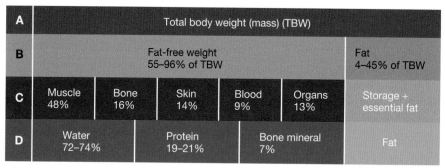

A	Total body weight (mass) (TBW)					
B	Fat-free weight 55–96% of TBW					Fat 4–45% of TBW
C	Muscle 48%	Bone 16%	Skin 14%	Blood 9%	Organs 13%	Storage + essential fat
D	Water 72–74%		Protein 19–21%		Bone mineral 7%	Fat

FIGURE 8.14: Two- and four-compartment body composition assessment models. **A:** Weight alone (one-compartment model; often used). **B:** Fat weight and fat-free weight (two-compartment model; often used). **C:** Muscle, bone, skin, blood, organ, and fat weight (six-compartment model; rarely used with hard-to-obtain technology). **D:** Water, protein, bone mineral, and fat weight (four-compartment model; preferred strategy with available technology). (From Lohman TG. Applicability of body composition techniques and constants for children and youths. Exerc Sport Sci Rev. 1986;14:325–57.)

exercise or when the person being measured is overheated because the shift of body fluid to the skin will inflate normal skinfold size.

■ To reduce error during the learning phase, skinfold sites should be precisely determined, marked, and verified by a trained instructor. The largest source of error in skinfold testing is inaccurate site selection.

■ Firmly grasp the skinfold with the thumb and index finger of the left hand and pull away.

■ Hold the caliper in the right hand, perpendicular to the skinfold and with the skinfold dial facing up and easily readable. Place the caliper heads ¼–½ inch away from the fingers holding the skinfold. Try to visualize where a true double-fold of skin thickness is and place the caliper heads there.

■ Read the caliper dial to the nearest 1 mm within 4 seconds. During the measurement, ensure that the left thumb and forefinger maintain the shape of the skinfold.

Different body mass and body composition assessment strategies have different capabilities for assessing body tissue components.

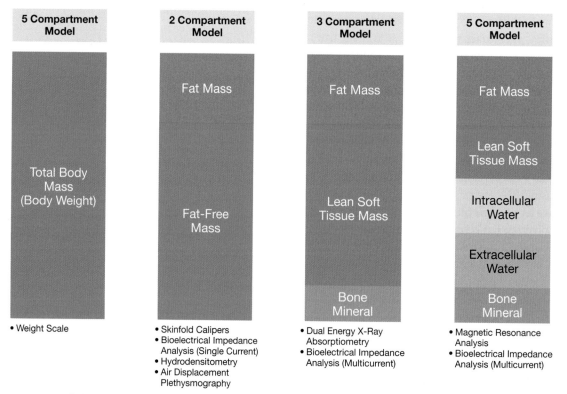

FIGURE 8.15: Common body composition assessment models with assessment strategies.

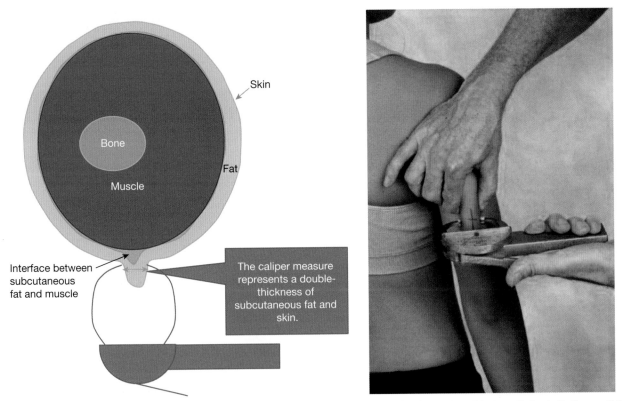

FIGURE 8.16: Basic skinfold technique. (From Thompson WR. ACSM's resources for the personal trainer. 3rd ed. Baltimore (MD): Lippincott Williams & Wilkins; 2010. 286 p.)

Take a minimum of two measurements at each site (at least 15 seconds apart). If the two values are within 10% of each other, take the average. Multiple different body composition prediction equations are available for the general population, and there are also several equations available for athletes. Using an equation that is specific to the person you are measuring (*i.e.*, male, female, athlete, nonathlete) yields more accurate results. Also, equations using a greater number of skinfold measurements are more accurate. For instance, an equation may require height, weight, age, triceps skinfold, and abdomen skinfold, whereas another equation may require height, weight, age, and skinfolds at the triceps, subscapular, midaxillary, suprailiac, abdomen, and midthigh sites (Table 8.8).

Commonly used BF% prediction equations for use with skinfolds are found in Box 8.2.

A new equation for predicting body composition from skinfolds for men has been validated using DXA (124). The new equation produces a relatively low standard error (2.72%) and is strongly correlated with DXA when used with a generally fit male population. No similar DXA-validated skinfold equations are currently available for women. This DXA criterion equation uses seven skinfold sites, including chest, midaxillary, triceps, thigh,

subscapular, suprailiac, and abdomen, with the following formula:

$$\%BF = 0.465 + 0.185 \text{ (sum of seven skinfolds)}$$
$$- 0.0002406 \text{ (sum of seven skinfolds)}^2$$
$$+ 0.06619 \text{ (age)}$$

It is important to mention the values that are derived from skinfold equations and used to predict BF%. Many equations used with athletes are intended to be used with the general nonathlete population. Because athletes are considerably leaner than the average nonathlete, the body fat results derived from skinfold equations are unrealistically low and, therefore, not accurate. However, the derived value can be used as a baseline to determine change over time if the same technique and same equation are used to follow-up values. It is inappropriate to compare the first value with one that was obtained using a different set of skinfolds and a different equation or to compare the skinfold-derived body composition value with values derived from other methods.

Ultrasound

The principle of ultrasound is based on the reflection of sound from the skin to the interface between muscle

Table 8.8 — Skinfold Sites and Measurement Procedures

Site	Procedure
Abdominal	Vertical fold; 2 cm to the right side of the umbilicus
Triceps	Vertical fold; on the posterior midline of the upper arm, halfway between the acromion and olecranon processes, with the arm held freely to the side of the body
Biceps	Vertical fold; on the anterior aspect of the arm over the belly of the biceps muscle, 1 cm above the level used to mark the triceps site
Chest/pectoral	Diagonal fold; one-half the distance between the anterior axillary line and the nipple (men), or one-third of the distance between the anterior axillary line and the nipple (women)
Medial calf	Vertical fold; at the maximum circumference of the calf on the midline of its medial border
Midaxillary	Vertical fold; on the midaxillary line at the level of the xiphoid process of the sternum. An alternate method is a horizontal fold taken at the level of the xiphoid/sternal border on the midaxillary line
Subscapular	Diagonal fold (45-degree angle); 1–2 cm below the inferior angle of the scapula
Suprailiac	Diagonal fold; in line with the natural angle of the iliac crest taken in the anterior axillary line immediately superior to the iliac crest
Thigh	Vertical fold; on the anterior midline of the thigh, midway between the proximal border of the patella and the inguinal crease (hip)

Procedure
- All measurements should be made on the right side of the body with the subject standing upright.
- Caliper should be placed directly on the skin surface, 1 cm away from the thumb and finger, perpendicular to the skinfold, and halfway between the crest and the base of the fold.
- Pinch should be maintained while reading the caliper.
- Wait 1–2 s before reading caliper.
- Take duplicate measures at each site and retest if duplicate measurements are not within 1–2 mm.
- Rotate through measurement sites or allow time for skin to regain normal texture and thickness.

Source: American College of Sports Medicine. Exercise prescription for individuals with metabolic disease risk factors. In: ACSM's guidelines for exercise testing and prescription. 10th ed. Philadelphia (PA): Wolters Kluwer; 2017.

Box 8.2 — Commonly Used Skinfold Equations for Predicting Body Density

Men

- **Seven-Site Formula** (chest, midaxillary, triceps, subscapular, abdomen, suprailiac, thigh)
  Body density = $1.112 - 0.00043499$ (sum of seven skinfolds) $+ 0.00000055$ (sum of seven skinfolds)^2 $- 0.00028826$ (age) (SEE 0.008 or ~3.5% fat)
- **Three-Site Formula** (chest, abdomen, thigh)
  Body density = $1.10938 - 0.0008267$ (sum of three skinfolds) $+ 0.0000016$ (sum of three skinfolds)^2 $- 0.0002574$ (age) (SEE 0.008 or ~3.4% fat)
- **Three-Site Formula** (chest, triceps, subscapular)
  Body density = $1.1125025 - 0.0013125$ (sum of three skinfolds) $+ 0.0000055$ (sum of three skinfolds)^2 $- 0.000244$ (age) (SEE 0.008 or ~3.6% fat)

Women

- **Seven-Site Formula** (chest, midaxillary, triceps, subscapular, abdomen, suprailiac, thigh)
  Body density = $1.097 - 0.00046971$ (sum of seven skinfolds) $+ 0.00000056$ (sum of seven skinfolds)^2 $- 0.00012828$ (age) (SEE 0.008 or ~3.8% fat)

Box 8.2   Commonly Used Skinfold Equations for Predicting Body Density (Continued)

- **Three-Site Formula** (triceps, suprailiac, thigh)
  Body density = 1.0994921 − 0.0009929 (sum of three skinfolds) + 0.0000023 (sum of three skinfolds)^2
  − 0.0001329 (age) (SEE 0.009 or ~3.9% fat)
- **Three-Site Formula** (triceps, suprailiac, abdominal)
  Body density = 1.089733 − 0.0009245 (sum of three skinfolds) + 0.0000025 (sum of three skinfolds)^2
  − 0.0000979 (age) (SEE 0.009 or ~3.9% fat)

SEE, standard error of estimation.

Sources: Reprinted from American College of Sports Medicine. Exercise prescription for individuals with metabolic disease risk factors. In: ACSM's guidelines for exercise testing and prescription. 1st ed. Wolters Kluwer; 2018; Based on data from Jackson AW, Pollock ML. Practical assessment of body composition. Phys Sports Med. 1985;13(5):76,80,82–90; Pollack ML, Schmidt DH, Jackson AS. Measurement of cardiorespiratory fitness and body composition in the clinical setting. Compr Ther.1980;6(9):12–27.

---

and fat. As the ultrasound passes through different tissue densities, a portion of the sound wave is reflected back. The time it takes for the sound to reflect back is a function of the thickness of the tissue it has passed through (Figure 8.17). This technique provides a tissue depth of the subcutaneous fat layer and the underlying muscle layer, thereby providing a measure of relative body fatness. Assuming the operator is experienced and skilled,

studies have found that ultrasound is a reliable, accurate, and safe method for the measurement of subcutaneous fat and muscle thickness (125). Knowing the optimal sites to measure, as determined by fat patterning, is important for obtaining reliable results using ultrasound (126). A recent study applying a standardized ultrasound technique for measuring subcutaneous fat used eight measurement sites and produced high measurement accuracy and reliability in groups ranging from lean to obese (127). The ultrasound device is relatively inexpensive and does not induce any electrical and radiation waves that could be considered potentially unsafe.

Hydrostatic Weighing (Hydrodensitometry)

This is the classic means for determining body composition and applies what is known as Archimedes principle. Archimedes was a Greek mathematician, engineer, and physicist who discovered formulas for determining the area and volume of different shapes and the principle of buoyancy. In essence, this principle states that, for an equal weight, lower-density objects have a larger surface area and displace more water than higher-density objects (Figure 8.18).

From a body composition standpoint, this principle is applied in the following way:

1. The subject is weighed on a standard scale to get a "land" weight.
2. Using specialized equipment, the subject's lung volume is estimated (the subject blows into a tube).
3. The subject sits on a chair that is attached to a weight scale.
4. The chair and weight scale are positioned over water and the chair is slowly lowered into the water.

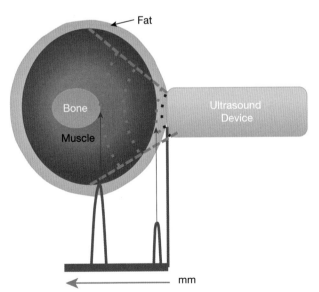

FIGURE 8.17: Ultrasound. The ultrasound device both emits and receives ultrasound signals. A portion of the emitted signal "bounces" off the interface of fat and muscle, and off the interface of muscle and bone. The device analyzes the time it takes for the signal to "bounce" back from each tissue interface, which is a measure of tissue thickness (*i.e.*, the longer it takes, the thicker the tissue). Note: As ultrasound cannot pass through air and bone has air, ultrasound used for body composition assessment cannot be used as a measure of bone thickness/size.

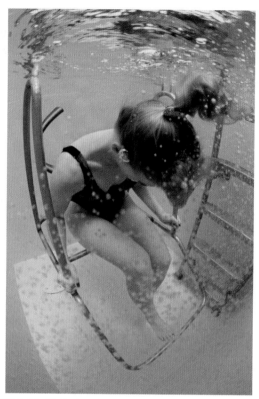

FIGURE 8.18: Hydrodensitometry represents underwater weighing of a subject following Archimedes principle: The weight of a subject is equal to the weight of the fluid that the subject's body displaces. As fat mass has a lower density than lean mass, a subject with greater fat mass will displace more water because the subject is "larger" than a leaner person of the same weight. In practice, out-of-water weight is compared to in-water weight. The greater the difference in weight, the greater the body fat level. (From Plowman S, Smith D. Exercise physiology for health fitness and performance. 5th ed. Philadelphia (PA): LWW (PE); 2017.)

5. When the subject is lowered into the water just below the chin, they are asked to fully exhale and completely lower their head into the water to be completely immersed.

6. While immersed, "underwater weight" is read off the scale that is attached to the chair the subject is sitting on.

Subjects weigh less in water than out of water because body fat (regardless of the amount present) makes the subject more buoyant. The difference between in-water weight and out-of-water weight is a function of how much body fat the subject has. A very obese subject with a high level of body fat would appear light in water relative to land weight. Because lung volume is measured prior to taking the water weight, there is an adjustment for the buoyancy that can be attributed to the air in the lungs. To minimize the lung-air effect, the subject is asked to exhale prior to full submersion, but there is always some

air remaining in the lungs that is referred to as residual volume.

The potential for error using hydrodensitometry is great. The percent of water in FFM is assumed to be 73.2%, but studies indicate that it varies between 60% and 92%. This creates a potential error in estimating percent body fat of between 4% and 22% (128). There is also an assumption that the density of FM is fixed at 0.90 g/cm^3 and the density of FFM is fixed at 1.10 g/cm^3, but it is established that the densities of body fat and FFM vary between individuals. Other potential sources of error include the following:

- Athletes have higher bone densities than nonathletes, potentially causing an underestimation of body fat.
- Older people have lower bone densities than younger people, potentially causing an overestimation of body fat.
- The trapped gas in the gastrointestinal tract can only be estimated.

Nevertheless, this technique is useful for determining the change in body composition over time if the technicians performing the measurements are effective at replicating the measurement procedure. It is also a useful means of determining the body composition of a population because the errors associated with the technique will average themselves out over many measurements.

Air Displacement Plethysmography

The BOD POD Gold Standard Body Composition Tracking System (COSMED) is used to determine body composition via air displacement body density. Because FM is less dense than lean mass, fat displaces more air for the same weight as lean mass. This is the same principle of measurement as underwater weighing (hydrodensitometry), but with air displacement instead of water displacement, the BOD POD measures a subject's mass and air volume, from which their whole-body density is determined. The measure involves assessment of pressure changes with injection of a known volume of air into a closed chamber, with a larger body volume displacing greater air volume and resulting in a greater increase in pressure. Using these data, body fat and lean muscle mass can then be calculated. There are clear advantages over hydrodensitometry measurements, providing higher subject acceptability, greater precision, and eliminating residual long volume as an issue (Figure 8.19).

This technique has been found to be valid and reliable for body composition determination, correlating well with DXA. However, it has been found that results

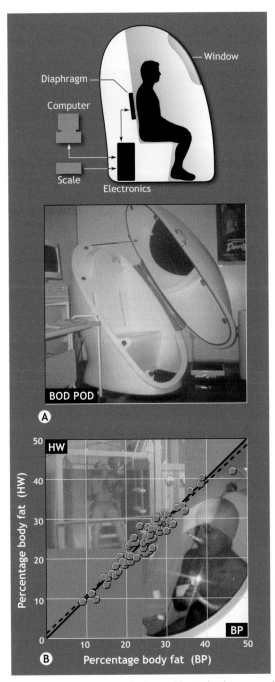

FIGURE 8.19: A: In a Bod Pod a subject sits in an enclosed container. Body composition is assessed by measuring the amount of air that has been displaced by the subject. **B:** BOD POD. Similar to the strategy for assessing body composition using hydrodensitometry, the BOD POD assesses air displacement versus water displacement as a measure of relative body fatness. (Photo courtesy of Dr. Megan McCrory, Boston University College of Health & Rehabilitation Sciences, Boston, MA; Regression of percentage body fat by hydrostatic weighing (HW) versus percentage body fat by BOD POD (BP); From McArdle WD, Katch FI, Katch VL. Exercise physiology. 8th ed. Philadelphia (PA): Lippincott Williams & Wilkins; 2014; Data from McCrory MA, Gomez TD, Bernauer EM, Molé PA. Evaluation of a new air displacement plethysmograph for measuring human body composition. Med Sci Sports Exerc. 1995;27:1686.)

consistently overestimate FFM and underestimate FM (72,129). In a study of test–retest reliability of 283 women, there was no significant mean difference between the first and second tests, suggesting that the BOD POD would be an excellent device for determining body composition change over time (130).

Bioelectrical Impedance Analysis

Water is a good conductor of electricity, and most body water is found in the lean mass. Fat, which is essentially anhydrous (has almost no water in it), impedes the electrical flow, hence the name "BIA." The greater the impedance of electrical current, the greater the amount of fat the electrical current has confronted. Regardless of the BIA equipment used, the principle behind the technique is the same. If you know the beginning level of energy (electricity) that enters the system and you can measure the level of energy that exits the system, you know how much of the energy has been impeded in the system. Muscle, because of the water and electrolytes it contains, is an efficient conductor of electricity. By contrast, because fat is anhydrous it is an efficient insulator (therefore it impedes) of electricity. Therefore, the greater the impedance, the greater the level of fat. If you start with 100 units of electricity going into your system and 80 units of electricity coming out of the system, you have more water and muscle than someone who has 100 units going in and 60 units coming out.

There are several types of BIA equipment, ranging from simple to highly sophisticated. On the simple end of the spectrum, BIA scales have the subject stand on an electronic weight scale, and an electrical current runs from the right foot, up the right leg, down the left leg, and out the left foot. There is also a handheld device that runs a current from one hand to the other (Figure 8.20). The measured impedance (*i.e.*, the difference between the beginning and ending electrical current) is used to predict FM. The least expensive devices use a single electrical current, making these systems highly susceptible to differences in hydration state. For instance, if a relatively lean person is dehydrated at the time of the measurement, the electrical current will not be as efficiently conducted (*i.e.*, there will be greater impedance) because of lower body water and the person will appear to have a higher FM than they actually have. More sophisticated devices use multiple electrical currents that traverse all parts of the body. The equipment compares the relative conductance and impedance of each current to obtain a more accurate assessment of body composition. These multicurrent BIA systems, now referred to as bioelectrical

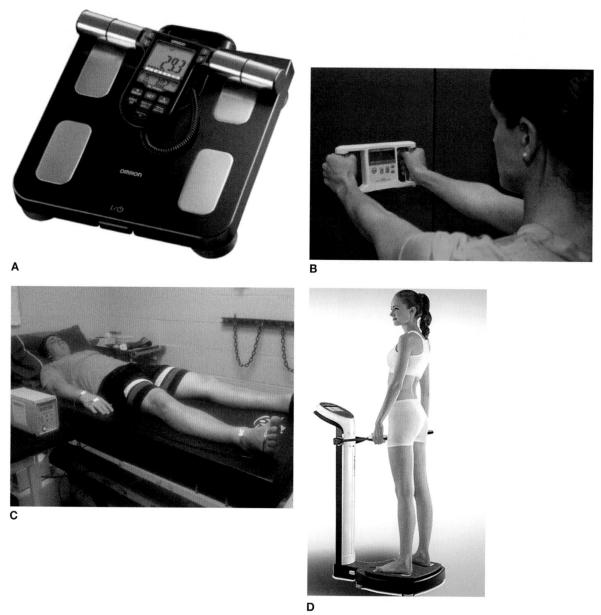

FIGURE 8.20: Different bioelectrical impedance analysis (BIA) devices measure different parts of the body. The portion of the body the current passes through determines the portion of the body that is assessed. **A:** With the BIA scale, the current passes from one foot to the other, so the body composition of both legs and lower pelvis is measured. **B:** With the handheld BIA device, the current passes from one hand to the other, so the body composition of both arms and upper chest is measured. **C:** With the hand-to-foot BIA device, the current passes from one hand to the foot on the same side of the body, so the body composition of one entire side of the body below the neck is measured. **D:** With the BIA device connected to both feet and hands, the current traverses the entire body, enabling a body composition measure of the whole body below the neck. (**A**, from Omron, 2024. Accessed 2024 May 22. Available from: https://www.premiumvials.com/omron-body-composition-monitor-with-scale-7-fitness-indicators-90-day-memory-1702144709/?setCurrencyId=1&sku=B0020MMCDE%201&gad_source=1&gclid=CjwKCAjwr7ayBhAPEiwA6EIGxG7s2-Rz7TC-GQv_Sc4XFhejt7PrdWq4Tv7wC4TSI7KWdmvX7CzoBBoChyMQAvD_BwE; **B**, from Plowman S, Smith D. Exercise physiology for health fitness and performance. 5th ed. Philadelphia (PA): LWW (PE); 2017; **C**, from Kraemer WJ, Fleck SJ, Deschenes MR. Exercise physiology. Philadelphia (PA): LWW (PE); 2011; **D**, from Premier Integrative Health Center for Personalized Medicine. Inbody scale. Accessed 2018 May 4. Available from: http://www.premierintegrativehealthkc.com/inbody-scale/)

vector analysis (BIVA) systems offer promise in assessing body segments to determine differences in, for instance, lean and fat tissue in the left versus right leg, or left versus right arm, etc. (6,123). An obvious weakness of devices that do not measure the entire body is that the prediction of total body fatness is based on the portion of the body assessed, which may not be representative of the body fat level of other parts of the body.

Some newer and more expensive ($5,000–$25,000) BIA models are capable of providing segmental body composition (arms, legs, abdomen) that is useful for determining muscular symmetry and determining the location of fat storage. These models also use multiple current technologies that create far less error with different hydration states than single-current models. A validation study comparing a newer eight-mode multicurrent BIA device (*i.e.*, a device that measures the entire body by running currents between each hand, between each foot, and between each hand and foot) found that there were no significant differences between DXA and the BIA device for FM, percent body fat, and total FFM (131). It is important to note that the BIA device used induces multiple currents, making it more accurate with different degrees of dehydration. With less expensive devices that induce a single current, the state of hydration may pose a significant error in the derived values. With these devices, it is critically important that the person having a BIA measurement taken be in a well-hydrated state, and anything that can compromise hydration should be avoided 24 hours prior to an assessment (drinking alcohol, exercising, consuming large amounts of coffee, and spending time outside in hot and humid weather). It has been noted that there are no athlete-specific BIA-associated equations currently available for predicting body composition in this population (132). Although newer multicurrent BIA systems are likely to produce results similar to those observed with DXA, there are likely to be differences in athletes than in the general population that have not yet been fully addressed with BIA.

Dual-Energy X-Ray Absorptiometry

DXA is widely considered to be the most accurate means of predicting body composition, and it is generally considered the current gold standard for this purpose. It does have certain limitations, however, in that it is not portable and the cost is in excess of $100,000. The information you can derive from a full-body scan on an athlete is invaluable, including bone density, BF%, lean body mass, FM, and the distribution of fat and lean mass in the arms, body trunk, and legs. The standard error of estimation for soft tissue (muscle and fat) is <1.5%, and for bone, it is <0.5%, providing highly reliable and repeatable results (133) (Figure 8.21).

The DXA procedure was originally developed to determine the bone mineral content and density of bone. The subject lies on the DXA table for ~20 minutes, and the pencil-beam X-rays pass through the subject and are measured by the analyzer and interpreted by a technician using device-specific software programs. Because metal

has such a high density, the subject is asked to remove all jewelry and must wear clothing that contains no metal. The resultant value is translated into a density value for bone, lean, and fat tissue.

DXA works by passing two X-ray beams through the subject and measuring the amount of X-ray that has been absorbed by the tissue it has passed through. One beam is a high-intensity beam and the other one is a low-intensity beam, so the relative absorbance of each beam is an indication of the density of the tissue it has passed through. The higher the tissue density, the greater the reduction in X-ray intensity. DXA systems filter the X-ray so that only a very small proportion of the original X-ray passes through the subject. Depending on body thickness, a subject having a DXA scan will receive between 0.02 and 0.05 mREM of radiation. By comparison, typical background nonmedical radiation that most people receive ranges between 0.5 and 0.75 mREM. The induced radiation is so low that a person would require ~800 full-body DXA scans before receiving the same level of radiation received from a single standard chest X-ray. Because of the low radiation induction, DXA is approved by the Food and Drug Administration as a nonmedical screening device to predict body composition. X-ray devices are typically reserved as medically related diagnostic instruments because of the amount of radiation they impart, but not so for DXA. Because DXA is widely considered to be the gold standard for body composition assessment, other methods (skinfolds, BIA, BOD POD, etc.) are validated based on DXA findings (134).

Why Body Composition Changes

Body composition changes, and this change is by altering what and when food is consumed and the amount and intensity of the exercise performed. Because energy is considered precious by the human system, a failure to use energy-requiring tissues causes them to be lost. The general rule for FFM that illustrates this adaptation, including bone mass, is "use it or lose it." An example of this adaptation is what happened to early astronauts (before preactivated vitamin D was developed) when in outer space. They quickly demineralized their bones and lost muscle because the gravity-free environment of outer space eliminates the need for strong gravity-resisting muscle and bone. The same outcome can be seen when people are bedridden because of illness or injury. Both bone mass and muscle mass are rapidly reduced because they "cost calories" and are not required when lying in bed. It is important to consider that body tissues are alive and attempt to adapt to the current situation. If you exercise in a way that requires more muscle to make that

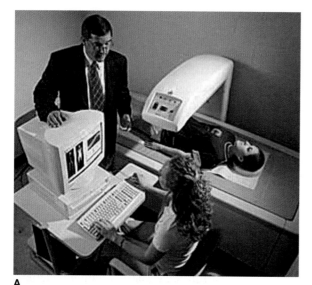

A

FIGURE 8.21: Dual-energy X-ray absorptiometry is capable of assessing both whole body and regional body composition and bone mineral density. **A:** Dual-Energy X-Ray Absorptiometry involves having the subject lie on a table. Low-level X-rays of known intensity pass through the subject and the remaining X-rays not absorbed by body tissues are read by the arm above the subject. Higher tissue densities absorb greater amounts of X-ray, allowing for accurate assessment of body composition. **B:** The results of a DXA scan can display both skeletal tissue and soft tissue (muscle and fat), and compare densities against established standards. **C:** Different parts of the skeleton known to be at higher risk of low bone density can also be assessed, including the femoral neck (sight of osteoporotic hip fractures), and the lower spine (sight of osteoporotic compression fractures). (**A**, from Kraemer WJ, Fleck SJ, Deschenes MR. Exercise physiology. Philadelphia (PA): LWW (PE); 2011; **B** and **C**, from Aktolun C, Goldsmith S. Nuclear oncology. Philadelphia (PA): LWW (PE); 2015.)

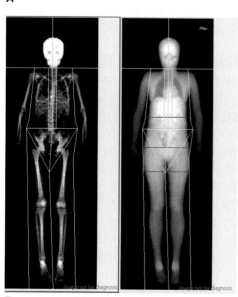

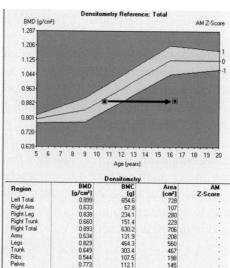

Densitometry Reference: Total

Region	BMD (g/cm²)	BMC (g)	Area (cm²)	AM Z-Score
Left Total	0.899	654.6	728	.
Right Arm	0.633	67.8	107	.
Right Leg	0.838	234.1	280	.
Right Trunk	0.660	151.4	229	.
Right Total	0.893	630.2	706	.
Arms	0.634	131.9	208	.
Legs	0.829	464.3	560	.
Trunk	0.649	303.4	467	.
Ribs	0.544	107.5	198	.
Pelvis	0.773	112.1	145	.
Spine	0.673	83.8	125	.
Total	0.896	1,284.8	1,434	-2.9

B

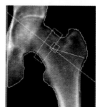

125 × 149
NECK: 49 × 15

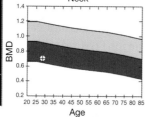

Neck

BMD / Age

T-score versus white male; Z-score versus white male.
Source:BMDCS/NHANES

DXA results summary:

Region	BMD (g/cm²)	T - score	Z - score
Neck	0.703	−1.7	−1.6
Total	0.879	−1.0	−1.0

Total BMD CV 1.0%
WHO classification: Osteopenia
Fracture risk: Increased

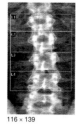

116 × 139

C

L1–L4

BMD / Age

Region	BMD (g/cm²)	T - score	Z - score
L1–L4	0.807	−2.6	−2.6

Total BMD CV 1.0%
WHO classification: Osteoporosis
Fracture risk: High

exercise easier, then the body adaptation is to increase musculature. If you put less stress on muscles by exercising less, then the muscle is lost.

Influences on body composition relate to genetic predisposition, age, gender, type of activity, amount of activity, nutrition, and the gut microbiome.

Genetic Predisposition

People have different inherited body types, and each type has a different predisposition toward accumulating more or less fat (135). Different body types (*i.e.*, somatotypes) have different body compositions. Endomorphs (large trunk, short fingers, shorter legs) have a predisposition toward higher BF%, and ectomorphs (long legs, long fingers, shorter trunk) have a predisposition toward a slender build with less body fat (136,137). There are clear differences in the susceptibility individuals have in becoming obese, even when living in the same environment, strongly suggesting that genetic predisposition plays an important role (138). Because the genetic composition cannot change, the most people can hope to do is to optimize what nature has provided.

Age

People generally develop a lower lean mass and higher FM after the age of 30. Older men were found to weigh 8.2 kg *less* than middle-aged men, mainly from having lower lean tissue (139). The age-related drop in lean mass is even larger when older individuals are compared with younger individuals. By age 65–70 the average male has lost 12 kg of lean mass when compared with age 25, and the average female has 5 kg less (140). Because energy metabolism drops about 2% for each decade after age 30, it gets progressively more difficult to maintain a desirable weight and body composition. However, although this age-related change in body composition is normal, it is not a mandate. It has been clearly shown that a good diet and regular physical activity can keep you lean (141).

Gender

All other things being equal (*i.e.*, equal weight-to-height ratios), women have a higher BF% and lower lean mass than men (142). This gender difference is primarily a manifestation of the different biologic functions of men and women. Because women convert some of the testosterone they produce to develop a uterus, less testosterone is available to develop muscles (143). Despite this difference, it is certainly possible for women to enlarge their muscle mass through regular resistance activity and proper eating.

Type of Activity

Different types of activities place different stresses on the system and, as you would expect, the body responds differently to these stresses. The standard exercise for reducing BF% is aerobic exercise, but there is good evidence that any type of activity (including anaerobic activity) will reduce the BF% and improve exercise capacity (144,145). High-intensity activity may result in a greater increase in lean body mass while reducing body FM, resulting in lower health risks and better body composition with a minimal impact on weight (146). Nevertheless, this shift in body composition is still likely to make the person appear slightly smaller, because, pound-for-pound, fat weight takes up more space than lean mass weight. Low-intensity activity, on the other hand, appears to reduce BF% with minimal impact on lean body mass, resulting in weight reduction. When energy expenditure (calories burned) is equivalent, both anaerobic and aerobic activity appear to equally lower body fat.

Amount of Activity

The greater the volume of exercise, the greater the potential benefits in desirably altering body composition and reducing health risks. There are, of course, limits to training. Excess training may result in overtraining syndrome, which negatively affects both body composition and health. In all training protocols, activity must be supported by an adequate intake of energy. Increasing the time of activity without also increasing the amount of energy intake causes a breakdown of muscle mass to support energy needs and may have multiple negative outcomes (101). In addition, overtraining, although it will not necessarily lead to a reduction in lean body mass, causes an increase in muscle soreness and reduces muscular power and endurance. Therefore, the amount of activity should be carefully balanced with adequate energy intake and adequate rest to ensure maintenance of muscle mass and athletic performance (147).

Nutrition

Numerous nutritional factors can have an impact on body composition, including consumption of too much energy (the FM will enlarge), too little energy (the lean mass will become smaller), or at the wrong times (FM may enlarge and/or lean mass becomes smaller, depending on how the energy is delivered) (101,115). A failure to consume an adequate level of these nutrients (B vitamins, zinc, iron, etc.) may also reduce an athlete's ability to properly burn fuel, thereby limiting the capacity to use fat during exercise.

Gut Microbiome

New data strongly imply that the gut microbiome (*i.e.*, the volume and makeup of the bacteria in the gastrointestinal tract) has an impact on the acquisition of nutrient and energy metabolic pathways (148). These findings demonstrate how important it is to have a healthy gut for lowering obesity risk and related disorders. Early results suggest that microbiota transplantation in males with obesity-related metabolic syndrome lowers obesity and improves insulin sensitivity to lower health risks (149).

Common Issues With Body Composition Assessment

Body composition assessment has become an important part of athlete assessment. The amount of muscle and fat that an athlete has can be predictive of performance, and bone mass assessment is important for understanding if developmental problems exist or if the athlete is at risk for stress fracture. A periodic assessment of body composition also helps the athlete understand if the training regimen is causing the kinds of physical changes that are being sought. However, there are important considerations when assessing body composition.

Desirable Body Composition Change Is Possible

Body composition may change through changes in diet and exercise, but diet and exercise should be considered together when making changes. Changing an exercise protocol without making appropriate changes in food/beverage intake is likely to cause unpredictable problems in achieving the desired body composition. If an athlete is increasing training in a training regimen, it is necessary to increase energy intake to support the increase in energy expenditure. Athletes putting themselves in a severe energy-deficit state by increasing exercise and maintaining or lowering energy intake are likely to lower metabolic rate, increase fat storage, and cause a breakdown of muscle to support energy needs. Eating too much is also likely to increase fat storage. It is best to maintain energy intake throughout the day, so athletes should be careful about consuming enough energy to support exercise, rather than making up for an energy deficit at the end of the day.

Keeping Information Private

Athletes often compare body composition values with other athletes, but this comparison is not meaningful and may drive an athlete to change body composition in a way that negatively affects both performance and health. Health professionals involved in obtaining body composition data should be sensitive to the confidentiality of this information. They should also explain to each athlete that differences in height, age, and gender are likely to result in differences in body composition, without necessarily any differences in performance. Strategies for achieving privacy and helping the athlete put the information in the proper context include the following:

- Obtain body composition values with only one athlete at a time, to limit the chance that the data will be shared.
- Give athletes information on body composition using phrases such as "within the desirable range" rather than a raw value, such as saying, "your body fat level is 18%."
- Provide athletes with information on how they have changed between assessments, rather than offering the current value.
- Increase the focus on muscle mass and decrease the focus on body fat.
- Use body composition values as a means of helping to explain changes in objectively measured performance outcomes.

Comparing Body Composition Results Using Different Methods

Different methods for assessing body composition produce different standard results. Therefore, it is inappropriate to compare the results from one method with the results of another. If athletes are being evaluated to determine body composition change over time (an appropriate use of body composition assessment), this comparison should only be made if the same method has been used for the entire assessment period. For instance, the difference in two DXA scans taken several months apart provides valuable information on how body composition has changed in an individual, as does the difference in two skinfold assessments. However, the difference between body composition values from a DXA scan and skinfold equation is not useful in determining change. Even within methods, the same prediction equations should be used to determine if an athlete's body composition has changed between measurements.

Seeking an Arbitrarily Low Level of Body Fat

Most athletes would like their body fat level to be as low as possible. However, athletes often try to seek a body fat level that is arbitrarily low (so low that it has nothing to do with the norms in the sport or their own body fat predisposition), and this can increase the frequency of illness, increase the risk of injury, lengthen the time the athlete needs before returning to training following an injury, reduce performance, and increase the risk of an eating disorder. Body composition values should be thought of as numbers on a continuum that are usual for a sport. If an athlete falls anywhere on that continuum, it is likely that factors other than body composition (training, skills acquisition, etc.) will be the major predictors of performance success. Seeking arbitrarily low body fat levels and/or weight is a particular problem for athletes in sports where making weight is a common expectation. Wrestlers, in particular, make dangerous efforts—sometimes leading to death—to lower body fat levels and weight in order to be more competitive.

Excessive Frequency of Body Composition Assessment

Athletes who are assessed frequently (frequent weight and/or skinfolds taken) are fearful of the outcome, because the results are often (and inappropriately) used punitively. Real changes in body composition occur slowly, so there is little need to assess athletes weekly, biweekly, or even monthly. Assessing body composition two to four times each year is an appropriate frequency to determine and monitor body composition change. In some isolated circumstances when an athlete has been injured or is suffering from a disease, such as malabsorption, fever, diarrhea, or anorexia, it is reasonable for a physician to recommend a more frequent assessment rate to control for changes in lean mass. Coaches who have traditionally obtained weight and/or body composition values weekly, biweekly, or monthly should shift their focus to a more frequent assessment of objective performance-related measures.

SUMMARY

The assessment of body composition can be a useful tool in helping the athlete and coach understand the changes that are occurring as a result of training and nutritional factors. Health professionals involved in obtaining body composition data should focus on using the same technique with the same prediction equations to derive valid comparative data over time. Care should be taken that body composition values are used constructively as part of the athlete's total training plan. Ideally, the emphasis should be on a periodic monitoring of the athlete's body composition to determine change in both the lean and FM. Many athletes are sensitive about body fat, so care should be taken to use body composition values in a way that enables their constructive use in the athlete's general training plan.

Be cautious about making recommendations that are based on a single body composition measurement. It is possible that a single measurement may suggest that an athlete is overfat. However, if that athlete had an even higher body fat level 1 or 2 months earlier, they are already doing something that is making a desirable change in body composition. Were an intervention to occur it could inadvertently change that successful strategy. The same might be true for an athlete who, on a single measure, appears to be relatively lean, causing no intervention to occur. But what if that athlete has been experiencing a steady increase in body fat levels? This would never be known if only a single measure was taken. Therefore, the key to successful body composition measures is to take several measures at the same time intervals, perhaps monthly, each time using the same equipment to determine an accurate trajectory of change before any intervention takes place.

The Position Statement of the American College of Sports Medicine, The Academy of Nutrition and Dietetics, and the Dietitians of Canada on Nutrition and Athletic Performance makes some important points related to weight and body composition for athletes, including the following (150):

- In three out of six studies of male and female athletes, negative energy balance (losses of 0.02%–5.8% body mass; over five 30-day periods) was not associated with decreased performance. In the remaining three studies where decrements in both anaerobic and aerobic performance were observed, slow rates of weight loss (0.7% reduction in body mass) were more beneficial to performance compared to fast rates (1.4% reduction in body mass), and one study showed that self-selected energy restriction resulted in decreased hormone levels.

- Although it is clear that the assessment and manipulation of body composition may assist in the progression of an athletic career, athletes, coaches, and trainers should be reminded that athletic performance cannot be accurately predicted solely based on body weight and composition. A single and rigid optimal body composition should not be recommended for any event or group of athletes.

- Nutrition goals and requirements are not static. Athletes undertake a periodized program in which preparation for peak performance in targeted events is achieved by integrating different types of workouts in the various cycles of the training calendar. Nutrition support also needs to be periodized, taking into account the needs of daily training sessions (which can range from minor in the case of "easy" workouts to substantial in the case of high-quality sessions [*e.g.*, high-intensity, strenuous, or highly skilled workouts]) and overall nutritional goals.

- Nutrition plans need to be personalized to the individual athlete to take into account the specificity and uniqueness of the event, performance goals, practical challenges, food preferences, and responses to various strategies.

- The achievement of the body composition associated with optimal performance is now recognized as an important but challenging goal that needs to be individualized and periodized. Care should be taken to preserve health and long-term performance by avoiding practices that create unacceptably low energy availability and psychological stress.

- Some nutrients (*e.g.*, energy, carbohydrate, and protein) should be expressed using guidelines per kilogram of body mass to allow recommendations to be scaled to the large range in the body sizes of athletes. Sports nutrition guidelines should also consider the importance of the timing of nutrient intake and nutritional support over the day and in relation to sport rather than general daily targets.

- There is ample evidence in weight-sensitive and weight-making sports that athletes frequently undertake rapid weight-loss strategies to gain a competitive advantage. However, the resultant hypohydration (body water deficit), loss of glycogen stores and lean mass, and other outcomes of pathologic behaviors (*e.g.*, purging, excessive training, starving) can impair health and performance.

- An individualized diet and training prescription for weight/fat loss should be based on assessment of goals, present training and nutrition practices, past experiences, and trial and error. Nevertheless, for most athletes, the practical approach of decreasing energy intake by ~250–500 kcal/day from their periodized energy needs, while either maintaining or slightly increasing energy expenditure, can achieve progress toward short-term body composition goals over ~3–6 weeks.

- Athletes may choose to excessively restrict their fat intake in an effort to lose body weight or improve body composition. Athletes should be discouraged from chronic implementation of fat intakes below 20% of energy intake because the reduction in dietary variety often associated with such restrictions is likely to reduce the intake of a variety of nutrients such as fat-soluble vitamins and essential fatty acids, especially n-3 fatty acids.

- Athletes who frequently restrict energy intake, rely on extreme weight loss practices, eliminate one or more food groups from their diet, or consume poorly chosen diets may consume suboptimal amounts of micronutrients and benefit from micronutrient supplementation. This occurs most frequently in the case of calcium, vitamin D, iron, and some antioxidants. Single-micronutrient supplements are generally only appropriate for correction of a clinically defined medical reason (*e.g.*, iron supplements for iron deficiency anemia).

- Where significant manipulation of body composition is required, it should ideally take place well before the competitive season to minimize the impact on event performance or reliance on rapid weight loss techniques.

- Among other responsibilities, it is the role of the sports dietitian to provide assessment of nutrition needs and current dietary practices, including the following:
  - Energy intake, nutrients, and fluids before, during, and after training and competitions
  - Nutrition-related health concerns (eating disorders, food allergies or intolerances, gastrointestinal disturbances, injury management, muscle cramps, hypoglycemia, etc.) and body composition goals
  - Food and fluid intake as well as estimated energy expenditure during rest, taper, and travel days
  - Nutritional needs during extreme conditions (*e.g.*, high-altitude training, environmental concerns)
    - Adequacy of athlete's body weight and metabolic risk factors associated with low body weight
    - Supplementation practices
    - Basic measures of height, body weight, etc., with possible assessment of body composition

Practical Application Activity

There is a common myth that going on an energy-restricted diet will help you achieve a more desirable weight, but if this energy restriction results in large energy balance deviations during the day (*i.e.*, a large number of hours in a RED), then this strategy is likely to be counterproductive. Assess your own diet to assess energy balance as follows:

1. Predict your hourly resting energy expenditure (REE) using the Harris–Benedict equation, modified by Mifflin et al. (151) for your gender:

Men	Hourly REE = ((10 × weight in kg) + (6.25 × height in cm) – (5 × age in years) + 5)/24
Women	Hourly REE = ((10 × weight in kg) + (6.25 × height in cm) – (5 × age in years) – 161)/24

Source: Mifflin MD, St Jeor ST, Hill LA, Scott BJ, Daugherty SA, Koh YO. A new predictive equation for resting energy expenditure in healthy individuals. Am J Clin Nutr. 1990;51(2):241–7.

2. Using the relative energy expenditure (MET value) scale below, predict your hourly and total daily energy expenditure. (Take the hourly REE and multiply it by the activity factor that comes closest to your activity for each hour of the day.) Using this strategy will give you the hourly energy intake (food/beverage consumed) and hourly energy expenditure (activity intensity).

Factor	Description
1	**Resting, Reclining:** Sleeping, reclining, relaxing
1.5	**Rest +:** Normal, average sitting, standing, daytime activity
2.0	**Very Light:** More movement, mainly with upper body. Equivalent to tying shoes, typing, brushing teeth
2.5	**Very Light +:** Working harder than 2.0
3.0	**Light:** Movement with upper and lower body. Equivalent to household chores
3.5	**Light +:** Working harder than 3.0; Heart rate faster, but can do this all day without difficulty
4.0	**Moderate:** Walking briskly, etc. Heart rate faster, sweating lightly, etc., but comfortable
4.5	**Moderate +:** Working harder than 4.0. Heart rate noticeably faster, breathing faster
5.0	**Vigorous:** Breathing clearly faster and deeper, heart rate faster, must take occasional deep breaths during sentence to carry on conversation
5.5	**Vigorous 1:** Working harder than 5.0. Breathing noticeably faster and deeper, and must breathe deeply more often to carry on conversation
6.0	**Heavy:** You can still talk, but breathing is so hard and deep you would prefer not to. Sweating profusely. Heart rate is very high
6.5	**Heavy 1:** Working harder than 6.0. You can barely talk but would prefer not to. This is about as hard as you can go, but not for long
7.0	**Exhaustive:** Cannot continue this intensity long, as you are on the verge of collapse and are gasping for air. Heart rate is pounding

Begin Hour	End Hour	Activity Factor	Activity Description	Food/Drink Description	Food/Drink Amount
			****Begin Example****		
12 AM	7 AM	1.0	Sleep		
7 AM	8 AM	1.5	Nothing special	Whole wheat waffles (frozen Kellogg)	3
				Maple syrup	2 tablespoons
				1% milk	1 cup

Begin Hour	End Hour	Activity Factor	Activity Description	Food/Drink Description	Food/Drink Amount
				Orange juice (from concentrate)	1.5 cups
				Coffee	2 cups
				1% milk for coffee	2 tablespoons
10 AM	11 AM	5.0	Jog 30 min	Gatorade	16 oz
12 noon	1 PM	1.5	Nothing special	Medium size beef sandwich white bread, mayonnaise, lettuce, and tomato	1 sandwich
				Coffee	2 cups
				Artificial coffee creamer	2 packets
				Apple pie	1 slice (small)
5 PM	6 PM	4.0	Walk 1 hr	Water	16 oz
7 PM	8 PM	1.5	Nothing special	Lasagna with ground beef and cheese	Large plate
				Lettuce salad with tomatoes and cucumbers	Medium size salad
				Blue cheese salad dressing	1 tablespoon
				Red wine	1 medium glass
10 PM	11 PM	1.5	Nothing special	Popcorn (air popped; no butter)	100 calorie pack
			End Example		

3. Determine if your total daily energy consumption closely satisfies your total daily energy expenditure.
4. Using this strategy and a spreadsheet (assess energy balance for each hour of the day), you can also determine the within-day energy balance deviations that you experience, following the strategies of Deutz et al. (4), Fahrenholtz et al. (60), and Torstveit et al. (152).
5. See if you can find a way to distribute your food/beverage consumption so you can maintain an hourly energy balance that maintains shifts that do not exceed ±400 calories of energy balance.

CHAPTER QUESTIONS

1. Low energy availability is defined as a(n):
   a. Energy expenditure that routinely exceeds energy intake in real time
   b. Low energy intake caused by an eating disorder
   c. Hormonal disruption that results in the delayed uptake of glucose
   d. Reduced metabolic rate because of self-imposed starvation

2. When comparing energy inadequacy and energy excess, both have all of these problems except:
   a. Increased injury risk
   b. Reduced athletic performance
   c. Increased risk of disordered eating
   d. Higher risk of type II diabetes

3. Of the following, which is associated with lower food intake, higher energy expenditure, and higher fat catabolism?
   a. Leptin
   b. Insulin
   c. Ghrelin
   d. a and c

4. Of the following, which is most likely to lower ghrelin?
   a. A large breakfast about 2 hours after waking up
   b. A moderately sized meal before blood sugar is allowed to go below normal
   c. A good breakfast, lunch, and dinner

d. A large meal to ensure blood sugar is sufficient to satisfy tissue requirements plus enough to stimulate a high insulin response

5. Decreased meal frequency is associated with:
   a. Lower total daily energy consumption
   b. Higher total daily energy consumption
   c. No difference in total daily energy consumption
   d. Reduced appetite

6. The current method of body composition assessment with the lowest standard error is:
   a. BIA
   b. Hydrostatic weighing
   c. DXA
   d. BOD POD

7. Meal skipping is an effective weight loss strategy.
   a. True
   b. False

8. Studies suggest that a 40 kcal/day permanent reduction in energy intake results in about a _____ lb weight loss in 5 years.
   a. 20
   b. 10
   c. 4
   d. 0

9. Humans are extremely effective at storing fat.
   a. True
   b. False

10. An expectation of exercise is that:
    a. Doing the same exercise at the same intensity and duration will continually improve fitness
    b. Humans adapt to the same activity and will increase energy efficiency doing that activity
    c. The weight and body composition outcomes of exercise are unpredictable
    d. It will always result in a muscle mass increase

ANSWERS TO CHAPTER QUESTIONS

1. a
2. d
3. a
4. b
5. b

6. c
7. b
8. c
9. a
10. b

Case Study Considerations

1. **Case Study Answer 1:** It is important for the athlete to understand that the issue is not about "weight," but about the important constituents of weight: muscle, fat, bone, and water. In addition, it would be important for the athlete to understand how inadequate energy consumption (*i.e.*, low-calorie diets in whatever form they come in) is likely to lower the wrong constituent of weight, leaving the athlete with relatively less muscle and more body fat with a lower "weight." An important consideration is that metabolically active tissue (*i.e.*, muscle and organ mass) requires energy to sustain itself, and muscle requires even more energy to enlarge. However, as a perfectly logical adaptation to an inadequate energy intake that is typical of weight loss diets, metabolically active tissue is reduced to adapt to the poor energy availability. This is not what the athlete is seeking, as they commonly *believe* that the low-calorie diet will only lower fat mass. The goal, therefore, is to sustain a reasonably good energy-balanced state throughout the day to sustain muscle mass. Staying in a good energy-balanced state throughout the day also limits excess energy consumption in a large meal, which is stored as fat. Sustaining a good energy-balanced state throughout the day typically involves eating more often with smaller meals and well-timed snacks. Doing this typically requires the assistance of a Registered Dietitian who can assess energy expenditure during the day, while matching that expenditure will appropriate foods. It also involves assuring that meals and snacks are well planned to avoid leaving eating to chance.

2. **Case Study Answer 2:** It would be helpful to discuss this issue with those who work closely with the athlete. However, discussing private matters with others requires the permission of the individual being discussed, so the first step would be to ask the athlete if it would be OK to discuss this issue with others, including coaches, athletic trainers, and health professionals who can help to resolve this issue. Importantly, working together as a team so that everyone who interacts with the athlete is participating in the same agreed-upon exercise and eating strategy is important for helping the athlete succeed.

3. **Case Study Answer 3:** It is important to fully understand any policies regarding talking to an athlete about any matters that have health implications, including weight. Policies vary widely between groups/organizations, and it is important to make certain existing policies are followed. A best-case scenario is that there is an existing sports medicine team that is tasked with pursuing all weight/health-related issues.

4. **Case Study Answer 4:** Eating disorders are serious clinical conditions that should be treated by medical professionals who are well trained to help resolve the disorder, ideally with an early intervention. Typically, eating disorder treatment requires the lead of a psychiatrist (MD), who may bring other health professionals, including Registered Dietitians and Certified Athletic Trainers, under the psychiatrist's supervision to assist in treating the individual with the eating disorder.

REFERENCES

1. Burke LM. Energy needs of athletes. Can J Appl Physiol. 2001; 26:S202–19.
2. Hawley JA, Burke LM. Effect of meal frequency and timing on physical performance. Br J Nutr. 1997;77(Suppl 1):S91–103.
3. Hubbard RW, Szlyk PC, Armstrong LE. Influence of thirst and fluid palatability on fluid ingestion during exercise. In: Gisolfi CV, Lamb DR, editors. Perspectives in exercise science and sports medicine: fluid homeostasis during exercise. Vol. 3. Carmel, IN: Benchmark Press; 1990. p. 39–95.
4. Deutz RC, Benardot D, Martin DE, Cody MM. Relationship between energy deficits and body composition in elite female gymnasts and runners. Med Sci Sports Exerc. 2000;32(3):659–68.
5. Saltzman E, Roberts SB. The role of energy expenditure in energy regulation: findings of a decade of research. Nutr Rev. 1995;53(8):209–20.
6. Lukaski HC, Raymond-Pope CJ. New frontiers of body composition in sport. Int J Sports Med. 2021;42(7):588–601.
7. Meyer NL, Sundgot-Borgen J, Lohman TG, Ackland TR, Stewart AD, Maughan RJ, Smith S, and Müller W. Body composition for health and performance: a survey of body composition assessment practice carried out by the Ad Hoc Research Working Group on Body Composition, Health and Performance under the auspices of the IOC Medical Commission. Br J Sports Med. 2013;47:1044–53.
8. Baumgartner RN, Heymsfield SB, Roche AF. Human body composition and the epidemiology of chronic disease. Obesity. 1995;3(1):73–95.
9. Rahman I, Athar MT, Islam M. Type 2 diabetes, obesity, and cancer share some common and critical pathways. Front Oncol. 2021;10:600824.
10. Benardot D. Timing of energy and fluid intake: new concepts for weight control and hydration. ACSM Health Fit J. 2007; 11(4):13–9.
11. Haase AM, Prapavessis H, Owens RG. Perfectionism, social physique anxiety and disordered eating: a comparison of male and female elite athletes. Psychol Sport Exerc. 2002;3(3): 209–22.
12. Krane V, Waldron J, Stiles-Shipley JA, Michalenok J. Relationships among body satisfaction, social physique anxiety, and eating behaviors in female athletes and exercisers. J Sport Behav. 2001;24(3):247–64.
13. Vardar E, Vardar SA, Kurt C. Anxiety of young female athletes with disordered eating behaviors. Eat Behav. 2007;8(2): 143–47.
14. Ackland TR, Lohman TG, Sundgot-Borgen J, Maughan RJ, Meyer NL, Stewart AD, Müller W. Current status of body composition assessment in sport: review and position statement on behalf of the ad hoc research working group in body composition health and performance, under the auspices of the I.O.C Medical Commission. Sports Med. 2012;42:227–49.
15. Going S, Lee V, Blew R, Laddu D, Hetherington-Rauth M. Top 10 research questions related to body composition. Res Q Exerc Sport. 2014;85:38–48.
16. Garthe I, Raastad T, Refsnes PE, Koivisto A, Sundgot-Borgen J. Effect of two different weight-loss rates on body composition and strength and power-related performance in elite athletes. Int J Sport Nutr Exerc Metab. 2011;21(2):97–104.
17. Dulloo AG, Miles-Chan JL, Montani J-P. Nutrition, movement and sleep behaviors: their interactions in pathways to obesity and cardiometabolic diseases. Obes Rev. 2017; 18(Suppl 1): 3–6.
18. Dulloo AG, Schutz Y. Adaptive thermogenesis in resistance to obesity therapies: issues in quantifying thrift energy expenditure phenotypes in humans. Curr Obes Rep. 2015; 4(2):230–40.
19. Bangsbo J. Physiological factors associated with efficiency in high intensity exercise. Sports Med. 1996;22(5):299–305.
20. Banks L, Thompson S, Lewis EJH. Efficiency of energy transfer during exercise: what are the limiting factors? J Physiol. 2015;593:2113–4.
21. Broskey NT, Boss A, Fares E-J, Greggio C, Gremion G, Schlüter L, Hans D, Kreis R, Boesch C, Amati F. Exercise efficiency relates with mitochondrial content and function in older adults. Physiol Rep. 2015;3(6):e12418.
22. Morgan DW, Martin PE, Krahenbuhl GS. Factors affecting running economy. Sports Med. 1989;7:310–30.

23. Javed A, Jumean M, Murad MH, Okorodudu D, Kumar S, Somers VK, Sochor O, Lopez-Jimenez F. Diagnostic performance of body mass index to identify obesity as defined by body adiposity in children and adolescents: a systematic review and meta-analysis. Pediatr Obes. 2015;10(3):234–44.

24. Mridha S, Barman P. Comparison of health of height-weight matched young-adult female athletes of hilly and plane regions in selected anthropometric measurements. Int J Sci Res. 2014;3(1):265–8.

25. Svetky LP, Stevens VJ, Brantley PJ. Comparison of strategies for sustaining weight loss: the weight loss maintenance randomized controlled trial. JAMA. 2008;299(10):1139–48.

26. McLaughlin T, Lamendola C, Coghlan N, Liu TC, Lerner K, Sherman A, Cushman SW. Subcutaneous adipose cell size and distribution: relationship to insulin resistance and body fat. Obesity. 2014;22(3):673–80.

27. Montani JP, Schutz Y, Dulloo AG. Dieting and weight cycling as risk factors for cardiometabolic diseases: who is really at risk? Obes Rev. 2015;16(Suppl 1):7–18.

28. Patel P, Abate N. Body fat distribution and insulin resistance. Nutrients. 2013;5(6):2019–27.

29. Benardot D, Thompson WR. Energy from food for physical activity: enough and on time. ACSM Health Fit J. 1999;3(4):14–8.

30. Ochner CN, Tsai AG, Kushner RF, Wadden TA. Treating obesity seriously: when recommendations for lifestyle change confront biological adaptations. Lancet Diabetes Endocrinol. 2015;3(4):232–4.

31. Anderwald C, Brabant G, Bernroider E, Horn R, Brehm A, Waldhäusl W, Roden M. Insulin-dependent modulation of plasma ghrelin and leptin concentrations is less pronounced in type 2 diabetic patients. Diabetes. 2003;52(7):1792–8.

32. Iwao S, Mori K, Sato Y. Effects of meal frequency on body composition during weight control in boxers. Scand J Med Sci Sports. 1996;6(5):265–72.

33. Jenkins DJ, Wolever TM, Vuksan V, Brighenti F, Cunnane SC, Rao AV, Jenkins AL, Buckley G, Patten R, Singer W, Corey P, Josse RG. Nibbling versus gorging: metabolic advantages of increased meal frequency. N Engl J Med. 1989;321(14):929–34.

34. Leibel RL, Rosenbaum M, Hirsch J. Changes in energy expenditure resulting from altered body weight. N Engl J Med. 1995;332:621–8.

35. Solomon TPJ, Chambers E, Jeukendrup AE, Toogood AA, Blannin AK. The effect of feeding frequency on insulin and ghrelin responses in human subjects. Br J Nutr. 2008;100(4):810–9.

36. Dongen MV-V, de Graaf C, Siebelink E, Kok FJ. Hidden fat facilitates passive overconsumption. J Nutr. 2009;139(2):394–9.

37. Dulloo AG, Jacquet J, Miles-Chan JL, Schutz Y. Passive and active roles of fat-free mass in the control of energy intake and body composition regulation. Eur J Clin Nutr. 2017;71(3):353–7.

38. Hall KD, Heymsfield SB, Kemnitz JW, Klein S, Schoeller DA, Speakman JR. Energy balance and its components: implications for body weight regulation. Am J Clin Nutr. 2012;95(4):989–94.

39. Manore MM, Brown K, Houtkooper L, Jakicic J, Peters JC, Edge MS, Steiber A, Going S, Gable LG, Krautheim AM. Energy balance at a crossroads: translating the science into action. Med Sci Sports Exerc. 2014;46(7):1466–73.

40. Georgopoulos NA, Markou KB, Theodoropoulou A, Benardot D, Leglise M, Vagenakis AG. Growth retardation in artistic compared with rhythmic elite female gymnasts. J Clin Endocrinol Metab. 2002;87(7):3169–73.

41. Georgopoulos NA, Markou KB, Theodoropoulou A, Vagenakis GA, Benardot D, Leglise M, Dimopoulos JCA, Vagenakis AG. Height velocity and skeletal maturation in elite female rhythmic gymnasts. J Clin Endocrinol Metab. 2001;86(11):5159–64.

42. Devine BJ, McCarron MM. Clinical pharmacy: case studies: case number 25: gentamicin therapy. Drug Intell Clin Pharm. 1974;8(11):650–5.

43. Robinson JD, Lupkiewicz SM, Palenik L, Lopez LM, Ariet M. Determination of ideal body weight for drug dosage calculations. Am J Hosp Pharm. 1983;40(6):1016–9.

44. Miller DR, Carlson JD, Loyd BJ, Day BJ. Determining ideal body weight (and mass). Am J Health Syst Pharm. 1983;40:1622.

45. Etchison WC, Bloodwood EA, Minton CP, Thompson NJ, Collins MA, Hunter SC, Hongying D. Body mass index and percentage of body fat as indicators for obesity in an adolescent athletic population. Sports Health. 2011;3(3):249–52.

46. Mascherini G, Petri C, Ermini E, Bini V, Calá P, Galanti G, Modesti PA. Overweight in young athletes: new predictive model of overfat condition. Int J Environ Res Public Health. 2019;16(24):5128.

47. Nazare J-A, Smith J, Borel A-L, Aschner P, Barter P, Van Gaal L, Tan CE, Wittchen H-U, Matsuzawa Y, Kadowaki T, Ross R, Brulle-Wohlhueter C, Alméras N, Haffner SM, Balkau B, Després J-P; INSPIRE ME IAA Investigators. Usefulness of measuring both body mass index and waist circumference for the estimation of visceral adiposity and related cardiometabolic risk profile (from the INSPIRE ME IAA Study). Am J Cardiol. 2015;115(3):307–15.

48. Ashwell M, Gibson S. A proposal for a primary screening tool: 'keep your waist circumference to less than half your height'. BMC Med. 2014;12:207.

49. Taylor RW, Jones IE, Williams SM, Goulding A. Evaluation of waist circumference, waist-to-hip ratio, and the conicity index as screening tools for high trunk fat mass, as measured by dual-energy X-ray absorptiometry, in children aged 3–19 y. Am J Clin Nutr. 2000;72(2):490–5.

50. Aitken DA, Jenkins DG. Anthropometric-based selection and sprint kayak training in children. J Sports Sci. 1998;16(6):539–43.

51. Raynor HA, Champagne CM. Position of the Academy of Nutrition and Dietetics: interventions for the treatment of overweight and obesity in adults. J Acad Nutr Diet. 2016;116:129–47.

52. Diaz EO, Prentice AM, Goldberg GR, Murgatroyd PR, Coward WA. Metabolic response to experimental overfeeding in lean and overweight healthy volunteers. Am J Clin Nutr. 1992;56(4):641–55.

53. Forbes GF, Brown MR, Welle SL, Lipinski BA. Deliberate overfeeding in women and men: energy cost and composition of the weight gain. Br J Nutr. 1986;56:1–9.

54. Katan MB, Ludwig DS. Extra calories cause weight gain, but how much? JAMA. 2010;303(1):65–6.

55. Roberts SB, Young VR, Fuss P, Fiatarone MA, Richard B, Rasmussen H, Wagner D, Joseph L, Holehouse E, Evans WJ. Energy expenditure and subsequent nutrient intakes in overfed young men. Am J Clin Nutr. 1990;259(3 Pt 2):R461–9.

56. National Institutes of Health, National Heart, Lung, and Blood Institute. NHLBI health topics [Internet]: overweight and obesity. 2024. [Accessed 2024 May 22]. Available from: https://www.nhlbi.nih.gov/health/overweightand-obesity

57. Bellissimo MP, Benardot D, Thompson W, Nucci A. Relationship between within-day energy balance on body composition in professional cheerleaders. FASEB J. 2017;31(Suppl 1):795.2.

58. Benardot D. Energy thermodynamics revisited: energy intake strategies for optimizing athlete body composition and performance. J Exerc Sci Health. 2013;11(2):1–13.

59. Cole CL, Brandon LJ, Benardot D, Thompson W. Relationships among energy balance, time of day, and obesity prevalence. Med Sci Sports Exerc. 2015;47(5S):637–41.

60. Fahrenholtz IL, Sjödin A, Benardot D, Tornberg ÅB, Skouby S, Faber J, Sundgot-Borgen JK, Melin AK. Within-day energy deficiency and reproductive function in female endurance athletes. Scand J Med Sci Sports. 2018;28(3):1139–46.

61. Farshchi HR, Taylor MA, Macdonald IA. Beneficial metabolic effects of regular meal frequency on dietary thermogenesis, insulin sensitivity, and fasting lipid profiles in healthy obese women. Am J Clin Nutr. 2005;81(1):16–24.

62. Granata GP, Brandon LJ. The thermic effect of food and obesity: discrepant results and methodological variations. Nutr Rev. 2002;60(8):223–33.

63. Timlin MT, Pereira MA. Breakfast frequency and quality in the etiology of adult obesity and chronic diseases. Nutr Rev. 2007;65(6):268–81.

64. Howe SM, Hand TM, Manore MM. Exercise-trained men and women: role of exercise and diet on appetite and energy intake. Nutrients. 2014;6(11):4935–60.

65. Saad MF, Bernaba B, Hwu C-M, Jinagouda S, Fahmi S, Kogosov E, Boyadjian R. Insulin regulates plasma ghrelin concentration. J Clin Endocrinol Metab. 2002;87(8):3997–4000.

66. Zigman JM, Bouret SG, Andrews ZB. Obesity impairs the action of the neuroendocrine ghrelin system. Trends Endocrinol Metab. 2016;27(1):54–63.

67. Melby CM, Hickey M. Energy balance and body weight regulation. Sports Sci Exchange. 2005;18(4):1–6.

68. Hall KD, Guo J. Obesity energetics: body weight regulation and the effects of diet composition. Gastroenterology. 2017;152:1718–27.

69. Manore MM, Larson-Meyer DE, Lindsay AR, Hongu N, Houtkooper L. Dynamic energy balance: an integrated framework for discussing diet and physical activity in obesity prevention—is it more than eating less and exercising more? Nutrients. 2017;9(8):905.

70. Dulloo AG, Montani JP, Schutz Y. Dieting and weight cycling as risk factors for cardiometabolic diseases: who is really at risk? Obes Rev. 2015;16(Suppl 1):7–18.

71. Wing RR, Phelan S. Long-term weight loss maintenance. Am J Clin Nutr. 2005;82(Suppl 1):S222–5.

72. Bushman BA. Physical activity guidelines for Americans: The relationship between physical activity and health. ACSM's Health & Fitness Journal. 2019;23(3):5–9. DOI: 10.1249/FIT.0000000000000472

73. Seong J, Kang JY, Sun JS, Kim KW. Hypothalamic inflammation and obesity: a mechanistic review. Arch Pharm Res. 2019;42(5):383–92.

74. Brown JC, Harhay MO, Harhay MN. The value of anthropometric measures in nutrition and metabolism: comment on anthropometrically predicted visceral adipose tissue and blood-based biomarkers: a cross-sectional analysis. Nutr Metab Insights. 2019;12:1178638819831712.

75. Deacon CF. Physiology and pharmacology of DPP-4 in glucose homeostasis and the treatment of Type 2 Diabetes. Front Endocrinol (Lausanne). 2019;10:80.

76. Fothergill E, Guo J, Howard L, Kerns JC, Knuth ND, Brychta R, Chen KY, Skarulis MC, Walter M, Walter PJ, Hall KD. Persistent metabolic adaptation 6 years after "The Biggest Loser" competition. Obesity. 2016;24(8):1612–9.

77. Kolata G. The science of fat: after 'the biggest loser,' their bodies fought to regain weight. The New York Times. 2016. Accessed 2018 May 4. Available from: http://www.nytimes.com/2016/05/02/health/biggest-loser-weight-loss.html?comments#permid=18394598:18401417

78. Loucks AB, Verdun M, Heath EM. Low energy availability, not stress of exercise, alters LH pulsatility in exercising women. J Appl Physiol. 1998;84(1):37–46.

79. Svetkey LP, Stevens VJ, Brantley PJ, Appel LJ, Hollis JF, Loria CM, Vollmer WM, Gullion CM, Funk K, Smith P, Samuel-Hodge C, Myers V, Lien LF, Laferriere D, Kennedy B, Jerome GJ, Heinith F, Harsha DW, Evans P, Erlinger TP, Dalcin AT, Caughlin J, Charleston J, Champagie CM, Bauck A, Ard JD, Aicher K. Comparison of strategies for sustaining weight loss: the weight loss maintenance randomized controlled trial. JAMA. 2008;299(10):1139–48.

80. Blom WAM, Stafleu A, de Graaf C, Kok FJ, Schaafsma G, Hendriks HFJ. Ghrelin response to carbohydrate-enriched breakfast is related to insulin. Am J Clin Nutr. 2005;81(2):367–75.

81. Knerr I, Gröschl M, Rascher W, Rauh M. Endocrine effects of food intake: insulin, ghrelin, and leptin responses to a single bolus of essential amino acids in humans. Ann Nutr Metab. 2003;47(6):312–8.

82. Bertelsen J, Christiansen C, Thomsen C, Poulsen PL, Vestergaard S, Steinov A, Rasmussen LH, Rasmussen O, Hermansen K. Effect of meal frequency on blood glucose, insulin, and free fatty acids in NIDDM subjects. Diabetes Care. 1993;16(1):4–7.

83. Fábry P, Tepperman J. Meal frequency—a possible factor in human pathology. Am J Clin Nutr. 1970;23(8):1059–68.

84. Cohn C, Berger S, Norton M. Relationship between meal size and frequency and plasma insulin response in man. Diabetes. 1968;17(2):72–5.

85. Toshinai K, Mondal MS, Nakazato M, Date Y, Murakami N, Kojima M, Kangawa K, Matsukura S. Upregulation of ghrelin expression in the stomach upon fasting, insulin- induced hypoglycemia, and leptin administration. Biochem Biophys Res Commun. 2001;281(5):1220–5.

86. Evans DJ, Hoffman RG, Kalkhoff RK, Kissebah AH. Relationship of body fat topography to insulin sensitivity and metabolic profiles in premenopausal women. Metabolism. 1984;33(1):68–75.

87. Peiris AN, Mueller RA, Smith GA, Struve MF, Kissebah AH. Splanchnic insulin metabolism in obesity. Influence of body fat distribution. J Clin Invest. 1986;78(6):1648–57.

88. Rosenbaum M, Leibel RL. Adaptive thermogenesis in humans. Int J Obes (Lond). 2010;34:547–55.

89. Chouchani ET, Kazak L, Spiegelman BM. New advances in adaptive thermogenesis: UCP1 and beyond. Cell Metab. 2019; 29(1):27–37.

90. Fogteloo AJ, Pijl H, Roelfsema F, Frölich M, Meinders AE. Impact of meal time and frequency on the twenty-four-hour leptin rhythm. Horm Res. 2004;62:71–8.

91. Felig P, Wahren J. Amino acid metabolism in exercising man. J Clin Invest. 1971;50(12):2703–14.

92. Nieman DC, Henson DA, Smith LL, Utter AC, Vinci DM, Davis JM, Shute M. Cytokine changes after a marathon race. J Appl Physiol. 2001;91(1):109–14.

93. Canalis E, Mazziotti G, Giustina A, Bilezikian JP. Glucocorticoid-induced osteoporosis: pathophysiology and therapy. Osteoporos Int. 2007;18(10):1319–28.

94. Dimitriou T, Maser-Gluth C, Remer T. Adrenocortical activity in healthy children is associated with fat mass. Am J Clin Nutr. 2003;77(3):731–6.

95. Koletzko B, Toschke AM. Meal patterns and frequencies: do they affect body weight in children and adolescents? Crit Rev Food Sci. 2010;50(2):100–5.

96. Smith K, Gall S, McNaughton SA, Blizzard L, Dwyer T, Venn AJ. Skipping breakfast: longitudinal associations with cardiometabolic risk factors in the Childhood Determinants of Adult Health Study. Am J Clin Nutr. 2010;92:1316–25.

97. Berkey CS, Rockett HRH, Gillman MW, Field AE, Colditz GA. Longitudinal study of skipping breakfast and weight change in adolescents. Int J Obes Relat Metab Disord. 2003; 27:1258–66.

98. Franko DL, Striegel-Moore RH, Thompson D, Affenito SG, Schreiber GB, Daniels SR, Crawford PB. The relationship between meal frequency and body mass index in black and white adolescent girls: more is less. Int J Obes. 2008;32:23–9.

99. Isacco L, Lazaar N, Ratel S, Thivel D, Aucouturier J, Doré E, Meyer M, Duché P. The impact of eating habits on anthropometric characteristics in French primary school children. Child Care Health Dev. 2010;36(6):835–42.

100. Paddon-Jones D, Rasmussen BB. Dietary protein recommendations and the prevention of sarcopenia. Curr Opin Clin Nutr Metab Care. 2009;12(1):86–90.

101. Mountjoy M, Sundgot-Borgen J, Burke L, Carter S, Constantini N, Lebrun C, Meyer N, Sherman R, Steffen K, Budgett R, Ljungqvist A. The IOC consensus statement: beyond the Female Athlete Triad—Relative Energy Deficiency in Sport (RED-S). Br J Sports Med. 2014;48(7):491–7.

102. Day J, Wengreen H, Heath EM, Brown K. Prevalence of low energy availability in collegiate female runners and implementation of nutrition education intervention. Sports Nutr Ther. 2015;1:101.

103. Drinkwater BL, Nilson K, Ott S, Chesnut CH. Bone mineral density after resumption of menses in amenorrheic athletes. JAMA. 1986;256(3):380–2.

104. Seifert-Klauss V, Schmidmayr M, Hobmaier E, Wimmer T. Progesterone and bone: a closer link than previously realized. Climacteric. 2012;15(Suppl 1):26–31.

105. Sonntag B, Ludwig M. An integrated view on the luteal phase: diagnosis and treatment in subfertility. Clin Endocrinol. 2012;77(4):500–7.

106. Fuqua JS, Rogol AD. Neuroendocrine alterations in the exercising human: implications for energy homeostasis. Metabolism. 2013;62(7):911–21.

107. Bolanowski M, Nilsson BE. Assessment of human body composition using dual-energy x-ray absorptiometry and bioelectrical impedance analysis. Med Sci Monit. 2001;7(5):1029–33.

108. Panorchan K, Nongnuch A, El-Kateb S, Goodly C, Davenport A. Changes in muscle and fat mass with hemodialysis detected by multi-frequency bioelectrical impedance analysis. Eur J Clin Nutr. 2015;69(10):1109–12.

109. Katch VL, Campaigne B, Freedson P, Sady S, Katch FI, Behnke AR. Contribution of breast volume and weight to body fat distribution in females. Am J Phys Anthropol. 1980; 53(1):93–100.

110. Williams MH. Nutrition for fitness and sport. Dubuque (IO): William C. Brown Publishers; 1992. p. 224–5.

111. Katch FI, McArdle WD. Introduction to nutrition, exercise, and health. 4th ed. Philadelphia (PA): Lea & Febinger; 1993.

112. Rivier C, Rivest S. Effect of stress on the activity of the hypothalamic-pituitary- gonadal axis: peripheral and central mechanisms. Biol Reprod. 1991;45:523–32.

113. Hilton LK, Loucks AB. Low energy availability, not exercise stress, suppresses the diurnal rhythm of leptin in healthy young women. Am J Physiol Endocrinol Metab. 2000;278:E43–9.

114. Loucks AB. Energy availability, not body fatness, regulates reproductive function in women. Exerc Sport Sci Rev. 2003; 31(3):144–8.

115. Nattiv A, Loucks AB, Manore MM, Sanborn CF, Sundgot-Borgen J, Warren MP; American College of Sports Medicine. American College of Sports Medicine position stand: the female athlete triad. Med Sci Sports Exerc. 2007;39(10):1867–82.

116. Stafford DEJ. Altered hypothalamic-pituitary-ovarian axis function in young female athletes. Treat Endocrinol. 2005; 4(3):147–54.

117. Going SB. Hydrodensitometry and air displacement plethysmography. In: Heymsfield SB, Lohman TG, Wang Z, Going SB, editors. Human body composition. 2nd ed. Champaign (IL): Human Kinetics; 2005. 18 p.

118. Williams MH. Nutrition for health, fitness, and sport. New York (NY): WCB McGraw-Hill; 1999. p. 317–8.

119. Irving BA, Davis CK, Brock DW, Weltman JY, Swift D, Barrett EJ, Gaesser GA, Weltman A. Effect of exercise training intensity on abdominal visceral fat and body composition. Med Sci Sports Exerc. 2008;40(11):1863–72.

120. Meyer NL, Shaw JM, Manore MM, Dolan SH, Subudhi AW, Shultz BB, Walker JA. Bone mineral density of Olympic-level female winter sport athletes. Med Sci Sports Exerc. 2004; 36(9):1594–601.

121. Lamb DR. Basic principles for improving sport performance. GSSI Sports Sci Exch. 1995;55(8):2.

122. Risoul-Salas V, Reguant-Closa A, Sardinha LB, Harris M, Lohman TG, Kirihennedige N, Meyer NL. Body composition applications. In: Lohman TG, Milliken LA, editors. ACSM's Body composition assessment. © 2020 Human Kinetics. p. 135–51.

123. Campa F, Toselli S, Mazzilli M, Gobbo LA, Coratella G. Assessment of body composition in athletes: a narrative review of available methods with special reference to quantitative and qualitative bio impedance analysis. Nutrients. 2021;13(5):1620.

124. Ball S, Cowan C, Thyfault J, LaFontaine T. Validation of a new skinfold prediction equation based on dual-energy x-ray absorptiometry. Meas Phys Educ Exerc Sci. 2014;18(3):198–208.

125. Wagner DR. Ultrasound as a tool to assess body fat. J Obesity. 2013;2013:280713.

126. Müller W, Lohman TG, Stewart AD, Maughan RJ, Meyer NL, Sardinha LB, Kirihennedige N, Reguant-Closa A, Risoul-Salas V, Sundgot-Borgen J, Ahammer H, Anderhuber F, Fürhapter-Rieger A, Kainz P, Materna W, Pilsl U, Pirstinger W, Ackland TR. Subcutaneous fat patterning in athletes: selection of appropriate sites and standardisation of a novel ultrasound measurement technique: ad hoc working group on body composition, health and performance, under the auspices of the IOC Medical Commission. Br J Sports Med. 2015;50:45–54.

127. Störchle P, Müller W, Sengeis M, Ahammer H, Fürhapter-Rieger A, Bachl N, Lackner S, Mörkl S, Holasek S. Standardized ultrasound measurement of subcutaneous fat patterning: high reliability and accuracy in groups ranging from lean to obese. Ultrasound Med Biol. 2017;43(2):427–38.

128. Van Itallie TB, Segal KR, Yang MU, Funk RC. Clinical assessments of body fat content in adults: potential role of electrical impedance methods. In: Roche AF, editor. Body composition assessment in youth and adults. Report of the Sixth Ross Conference on Medical Research. Columbus (OH): Ross Laboratories; 1985.

129. Muntean P, Miclos-Balica M, Popa A, Neagu A, Neagu M. Reliability of repeated trials protocols for body composition assessment by air displacement plethysmography. Int J Environ Res Public Health. 2021;18:10693. https:// doi.org/ 10.3390/ijerph182010693

130. Tucker LA, Lecheminant JD, Bailey BW. Test-retest reliability of the Bod Pod: the effect of multiple assessments. Percept Mot Skills. 2014;118(2):563–70.

131. Karelis AD, Chamberland G, Aubertin-Leheudre M, Duval C; Ecological Mobility in Aging and Parkinson group. Validation of a portable bioelectrical impedance analyzer for the assessment of body composition. Appl Physiol Nutr Metab. 2013;38(1):27–32.

132. Moon JR. Body composition in athletes and sports nutrition: an examination of the bioimpedance analysis technique. Eur J Clin Nutr. 2013;67:S54–9.

133. Toombs RJ, Ducher G, Shepherd A, De Souza MJ. The impact of recent technological advances on the trueness and precision of DXA to assess body composition. Obesity. 2012;20(1):30–9.

134. Kuriyan R, Thomas T, Ashok S, Jayakumar J, Kurpad AV. A 4-compartment model based validation of air displacement plethysmography, dual energy X-ray absorptiometry, skinfold technique & bio-electrical impedance for measuring body fat in Indian adults. Indian J Med Res. 2014;139(5):700–7.

135. Schleinitz D, Böttcher Y, Blüher M, Kovacs P. The genetics of fat distribution. Diabetologia. 2014;57(7):1276–86.

136. Nikolaidis PT, Afonso J, Busko K. Differences in anthropometry, somatotype, body composition and physiological characteristics of female volleyball players by competition level. Sport Sci Health. 2015;11:29–35.

137. Slaughter MH, Lohman TG, Misner JE. Relationship of somatotype and body composition to physical performance in 7- to 12-year-old boys. Res Q. 1977;48(1):159–68.

138. El-Sayed Moustafa JS, Froguel P. From obesity genetics to the future of personalized obesity therapy. Nat Rev Endocrinol. 2013;9(7):402–13.

139. Borkan GA, Hults De, Gerzof SG, Robbins AH, Silbert CK. Age changes in body composition revealed by computed tomography. J Gerontol. 1983;38(6):673–7.

140. Forbes GB, Reina JC. Adult lean body mass declines with age: some longitudinal observations. Metabolism. 1970;19(9): 653–63.

141. Geirsdottir OG, Arnarson A, Rame A, Briem K, Jonsson PV, Thorsdottir I. Muscular strength and physical function in elderly adults 6–18 months after a 12-week resistance exercise program. Scand J Public Health. 2015;43(1):76–82.

142. Geer EB, Shen W. Gender differences in insulin resistance, body composition, and energy balance. Gender Med. 2009; 6(Suppl 1):60–75.

143. Fahey TD, Rolph R, Moungmee P, Nagel J, Mortara S. Serum testosterone, body composition, and strength of young adults. Med Sci Sports. 1976;8(1):31–4.

144. Brach JS, Simonsick EM, Kritchevsky S, Yaffe K, Newman AB; Health, Aging and Body Composition Study Research Group. The association between physical function and lifestyle activity and exercise in the health, aging and body composition study. J Am Geriatr Soc. 2004;52(4):502–9.

145. Grediagin MA, Cody M, Rupp J, Benardot D, Shern R. Exercise intensity does not effect body composition change in untrained moderately overfat women. J Am Diet Assoc. 1995;5(6):661–5.

146. Parizková J. Body fat and physical fitness: body composition and lipid metabolism in different regimes of physical activity. Martinus Nijhoff B.V. Medical Division; 1977.

147. Maffetone PB, Laursen PB. Athletes: fit but unhealthy? Sports Med. 2016;2:24.

148. Devaraj S, Hemarajata P, Versalovic J. The human gut microbiome and body metabolism: implications for obesity and diabetes. Clin Chem. 2013;59(4):617–28.

149. Hartstra AV, Bouter KEC, Bäckhed F, Nieuwdorp M. Insights into the role of the microbiome in obesity and type 2 Diabetes. Diabetes Care. 2015;38(1):159–65.

150. Thomas DT, Erdman KA, Burke LM. American College of Sports medicine joint position statement. Nutrition and athletic performance. Med Sci Sports Exerc. 2016;48(3):543–68.

151. Mifflin MD, St Jeor ST, Hill LA, Scott BJ, Daugherty SA, Koh YO. A new predictive equation for resting energy expenditure in healthy individuals. Am J Clin Nutr. 1990;51(2):241–7.

152. Torstveit MK, Fahrenholtz I, Stenqvist TB, Sylta Ø, Melin A. Within-day energy deficiency and metabolic perturbations in male endurance athletes. Int J Sport Nutr Exerc Metab. 2018;28(4):419–27.

CHAPTER 9

Nutrition Issues Related to Oxygen Transport and Utilization, Reducing Muscle Soreness, and Improving Muscle Recovery

CHAPTER OBJECTIVES

- Comprehend the importance of delivering oxygen to cells for optimal cellular respiration and athletic performance.
- Identify the nutrients closely associated with manufacturing red blood cells (RBCs).
- Recognize the substances associated with iron storage and delivery.
- List the nutrients associated with protecting cells from oxidation reactions and how they function as antioxidants.
- Analyze the relationship between oxygen uptake and VO_{2max} as it relates to exercise intensity.
- Recall the molecules that form reactive oxygen species (ROS) and are potentially damaging to cells.

- Know the diseases associated with insufficient iron and excess iron.
- To understand the importance of diet in the production of nitric oxide (NO).
- Identify the possible causes of iron deficiency in athletes and nutritional strategies that could help to resolve the deficiency.
- Identify the causes of ROS-related oxidative stress and the nutritional countermeasures that can be followed to minimize the stress.
- Understand reduction–oxidation (REDOX) reactions and how they are involved in normal metabolic functions.

Case Study

John was an elite swimmer who made the decision to start competing in triathlons. In his first triathlon, John predictably came in first after the swim portion, but lagged terribly behind in the bike and running portions of the race. He was not dissuaded, however, from continuing to pursue becoming an elite triathlete. John did everything imaginable to improve the running and biking portions of the race, including investing in a top-notch racing bike and hiring coaches who showed him how to train, improve his form, and strategize each portion of the race. All of these, coupled with a superb training program, helped him improve with each race, and he slowly moved up in the rankings. He did so well that the time on his last triathlon qualified him to enter the biggest race of the year. He had 2 months to prepare, and he was leaving no stone unturned in getting ready for the most important competition in his career.

Of course, he was also looking at optimal nutrition strategies for fueling/hydration and had developed some excellent pre-, during-, and postevent strategies to make sure his muscles were ready going into the race, stayed in an optimal state during the race, and recovered well after the race.

There were many choices of what to do, but he found a talented sports dietitian who provided him with the perfect nutritional strategy. Because this was a really important race and John wanted every imaginable edge, he kept an open mind to other options. He read an article about how physical activity increases muscle soreness because of oxidative stress, and that taking a combination of the fat-soluble vitamin E and the water-soluble vitamin C supplements, both powerful antioxidants, would reduce exercise-associated muscle soreness and improve performance. He thought there could be no harm in taking these benign

(continued)

vitamin supplements, and that they could only help his athletic mission, so he started taking daily supplemental doses of the vitamins a couple of months before this important race. Of course, he was also training harder and longer at the same time he was taking the supplements, so he was convinced that the increased muscle soreness he felt was surely attributable to the training—thank goodness he was taking the supplements, because the muscle soreness would have been bad without them.

Race day arrived and John raced pretty well, but not as well as he had hoped. So, he kept up his training and nutrition regimen (including the supplements) to do better next time. Then he saw the summary results of a research study that took place at the very race in which he had hoped to excel. The study found that taking antioxidant

supplements actually *increased* markers of oxidative stress and muscle soreness! He remembered what his sports dietitian told him: "More than enough is not better than enough." This was good advice that he is now following.

CASE STUDY DISCUSSION QUESTIONS

1. Why do you believe so many athletes are predisposed to taking supplements?
2. What messages would you give them to help them understand that "more than enough is not better than enough?"
3. Why would taking high doses of antioxidant vitamins actually make muscle soreness worse than if they were not taken?

INTRODUCTION

There are three bioenergetic pathways that produce energy. These systems can all provide energy during physical activity, with a different system providing the dominant source of adenosine triphosphate (ATP) depending on the duration and intensity of the activity.

- **Phosphagen:** The phosphagen system uses creatine phosphate (CP) for the rapid production of ATP without oxygen (*i.e.*, anaerobic). However, because humans have a limited store of preformed CP, the phosphagen system is only able to provide instantly available energy for, typically, less than 10 seconds for maximal intensity activities, such as the 100-meter sprint, and is also a critically important source of energy for other high-intensity activities, such as ball throwing, jumping, and weightlifting.
- **Anaerobic Glycolysis:** This pathway produces ATP without oxygen (*i.e.*, anaerobic), principally from the conversion of within-cell glucose to pyruvic acid. This system can rapidly produce ATP, mainly for activities that require repeated large bursts of activity, such as a soccer player repeatedly sprinting toward a ball. The anaerobic glycolysis system can typically produce ATP for periods between 30 and 180 seconds, which is longer than the phosphagen system. This system is considered the intermediate energy-producing system between the phosphagen system and aerobic glycolysis.
- **Aerobic Glycolysis:** This energy metabolic pathway requires oxygen to produce ATP (*i.e.*, aerobic),

from the metabolism of both carbohydrate and fat. While the ATP production per unit of time is lower than either the phosphagen or anaerobic glycolysis systems, there is no inherent limitation to the aerobic glycolysis production of ATP provided sufficient oxygen can be delivered to cells. Aerobic glycolysis is the predominant source of ATP for longer duration and lower intensity activities and is the predominant energy metabolic pathway for most daily activities.

Example: Imagine a 100-m sprinter who stores 8 seconds worth of preformed CP and runs the 100-m sprint in approximately 10 seconds. Because the CP system produces the highest level of ATP per unit of time, the first 8 seconds of the race is his fastest. Once the preformed CP runs out, the last 2 seconds of the race is dependent on ATP production from anaerobic glycolysis. Since anaerobic glycolysis does not produce as much ATP per unit of time as CP, the last 2 seconds of the race is a little slower than the first 8 seconds. Once the race is finished and the runner catches his breath (*i.e.*, brings in sufficient oxygen for aerobic glycolysis), he satisfies energy needs aerobically. If the runner waits to run again for 10–15 minutes, much of the CP will be replaced and the lactic acid that was produced from anaerobic glycolysis will be converted back to pyruvic acid, enabling the runner to sprint at a high speed again. There are other examples in sports that emphasize the time limitations of the phosphagen and anaerobic glycolysis systems. Boxing, which is a high-intensity activity, has a series of breaks (rounds) that allow the boxer to recover the phosphagen and anaerobic glycolysis potential. Gymnasts do a series of maximal intensity events (vault, floor routine, rings, beam), and there is always a time interval between each event, both in practice and in competition, to allow the gymnast to regain the phosphagen and anaerobic glycolysis potential.

Acquiring oxygen through pulmonary ventilation (breathing) is an important first step in the transportation of oxygen from inspired air to the delivery of oxygen into body cells. The next step is the exchange of oxygen and carbon dioxide between the lungs and blood, which is followed by the transportation of oxygen and carbon dioxide bound to hemoglobin in RBCs. Finally, there is an exchange of oxygen and carbon dioxide between the RBCs in capillaries and tissue cells (1).

Athletes can only be successful if their body systems are fully capable of capturing sufficient oxygen, moving oxygen through the blood to tissues, and efficiently using the oxygen by having sufficient oxidative enzymes in mitochondria. They must also have efficient excretion of carbon dioxide, a by-product of oxygen utilization, and must also have sufficient antioxidants available in tissues to deal with the potentially negative side effects of excess oxygen exposure. Each function just mentioned has a nutritional component, including:

- *Sufficient protein and energy*, so that the tissues can store iron (ferritin) and deliver iron (transferrin) for the formation of hemoglobin.
- *Vitamins B$_{12}$ and folic acid*, which are involved in RBC formation. RBCs contain hemoglobin, which is the iron-containing and oxygen/carbon dioxide–carrying protein.
- *Iron* has a critical role as part of hemoglobin (in RBCs) and myoglobin (in tissues). Hemoglobin is the iron-containing protein in RBCs responsible for delivering oxygen from the lungs to tissues and removing carbon dioxide from tissues. Myoglobin is an iron-containing protein used for storing iron in tissues. Approximately 70% of iron is found in hemoglobin and myoglobin. A large number of enzymes, including cytochrome enzymes, contain iron primarily for oxidative phosphorylation (the process of obtaining energy from energy substrates). Iron is stored in the protein complex *ferritin*. The protein *transferrin* carries iron in the blood for storage, mainly in the liver, skeletal muscle, and reticuloendothelial cells that line the liver, spleen, and bone marrow. Exceeding the storage capacity for iron results in the formation and deposit of hemosiderin, which is not functionally available to cells. Iron overload disorder results from excess hemosiderin, which is associated with tissue damage. An associated disorder, *hemochromatosis*, results from excess iron absorption, which may also be associated with tissue damage.

- *Copper*, as part of the protein ceruloplasmin, which is involved in transferring iron from the transport protein transferrin to the RBC oxygen-carrying protein hemoglobin.
- *β-Carotene, vitamin C, vitamin E*, and *selenium*, which are *antioxidant* nutrients needed for protecting cells from oxidation reactions.

Physical activity may increase the rate of energy utilization by 20–100 times, depending on intensity, above the energy expended in a resting state, creating an enormous demand for oxygen in metabolically active tissues (2). This chapter reviews the nutrient relationships associated with the utilization of oxygen, the potential tissue-damaging effects from ROS that are associated with physical activity, and the role that oxygen delivery has on human performance.

OXYGEN UPTAKE

Every body cell requires oxygen to survive, and it is through the air we breathe that oxygen and other gases are supplied. Inspired air is composed of 20.95% oxygen and other gases (Table 9.1). Gas exchange in the lungs occurs

Table 9.1	Altitude Adjustments to Measured Hemoglobin Concentrations
Altitude (Meters Above Sea Level)	**Measured Hemoglobin Adjustment (g/dL)**
<1,000	0
1,000	−0.2
1,500	−0.5
2,000	−0.8
2,500	−1.3
3,000	−1.9
3,500	−2.7
4,000	−3.5
4,500	−4.5

Source: World Health Organization. Haemoglobin concentrations for the diagnosis of anaemia and assessment of severity. Vitamin and mineral nutrition information system. World Health Organization, 2011. (WHO/NMH/NHD/MNM/11.1). Accessed 2017 August 6. Available from: http://www.who.int/vmnis/indicators/haemoglobin.pdf

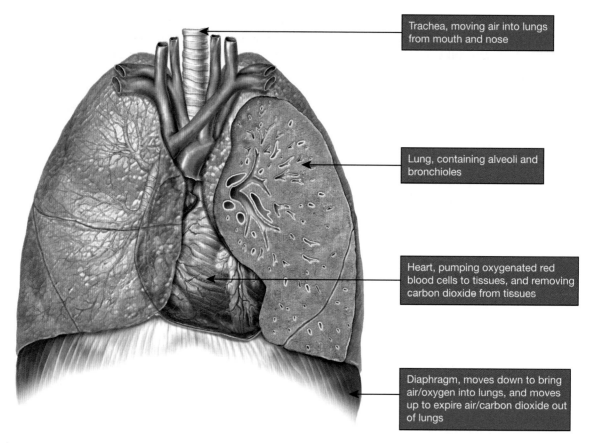

FIGURE 9.1: The diaphragm moves down to pull air into the lungs and pushes up to push air out of the lungs. Lung alveoli capture the oxygen in air and transport the oxygen to the hemoglobin in red blood cells. (From Anatomical Chart Company. Anatomy of the heart anatomical chart. 2nd ed. Philadelphia (PA): Lippincott Williams & Wilkins; 2005.)

in the 150 million alveoli humans have in each bronchi (3). The inspiratory capacity, or the maximal amount of air that can be breathed in through normal expiration, is ~3.6 L (3.8 quarts) for the average adult male, and ~2.4 L (2.5 quarts) for the average adult female (Figure 9.1).

The oxygen diffused into the lung *alveoli* passes into the blood through capillaries and enters the iron-containing hemoglobin in RBCs. RBCs then carry the oxygen to tissues. At the same time that oxygen is being delivered through the alveoli, *carbon dioxide* in the blood (a by-product of energy metabolism) passes to the alveoli and is exhaled (Box 9.1).

The oxygen content of air is ~20.95%, and the oxygen content of the expired air after exercise is 13.6%–16%, suggesting that a relatively small proportion of inspired oxygen is captured by the lungs (4). The typical water content of air is 0.5%, whereas the water content of expired air is ~6%, illustrating why the more rapid respiration during physical activity is a major route of water loss in athletes.

Important Factors to Consider

- The oxygen content of dry air is ~21% atmospheric pressure.
- Inspired oxygen pressure is ~50% *lower* at an altitude of 5,500 m (the height of Mount Blanc) and 30% of that at sea level at an altitude of 8,900 m (the height of Mount Everest) (5).

Athletic performance is affected by how well the heart and lungs can provide an adequate supply of oxygen to working muscles. This is demonstrated by the following (6,7):

- Greater oxygen delivery capacity improves VO_{2max}, whereas lower oxygen delivery capacity lowers VO_{2max}.
- The improvements seen in VO_{2max} from athletic training result from enhanced cardiac output, which is associated with improved oxygen delivery.

Box 9.1 The Contents of the Air We Breathe

Nitrogen—78.09%

Oxygen—20.95% (lower than this amount at high altitudes)

Argon—0.93%

Carbon dioxide—0.039%

Water vapor—1% at sea level; 0.4% average

Source: Republished with permission from Cotes JE, Chinn DJ, Miller MR. Lung function: physiology, measurement and application in medicine. 6th ed. Hoboken (NJ): John Wiley and Sons; 2006.

■ Muscles with enhanced blood flow are able to acquire and use more oxygen, resulting in better muscle function and enhanced performance (Figure 9.2).

As exercise intensity increases, so does the rate of cellular respiration. High-intensity exercise may cause a 25-fold increase in the demand for oxygen in working muscles, which is satisfied through the increase in the rate and depth of respiration. Interestingly, a lower blood pH is associated with a rise in carbon dioxide, rather than the higher need for oxygen that is the trigger for the higher respiration rate. Chemoreceptors in the medulla oblongata of the brain detect the lower pH when carbon dioxide is elevated, which stimulates the motor nerves controlling the intercostal and diaphragm muscles to increase their activity (7). When lactate (*i.e.*, lactic acid) begins to accumulate in the blood at a faster rate than can be removed (typically the result of intense exercise), the blood pH begins to decrease (*i.e.*, it becomes more acidic), and this also results in faster respiration (8). Diseases affecting the lungs, such as pneumonia, asthma, emphysema, bronchitis, chronic obstructive pulmonary disease, and lung cancer, compromise an individual's ability to obtain sufficient oxygen and excrete sufficient carbon dioxide (9). (Exercise-induced asthma [EIA] is discussed later in this chapter.)

Nutrients Associated With Oxygen Delivery

A number of minerals, vitamins, and protein carriers provide for the delivery and cellular utilization of oxygen. These nutrients work together as a team to capture oxygen from the environment, transport oxygen through the blood, transport oxygen from the blood to the cells for metabolic actions, and remove the metabolic by-products of oxygen-related metabolic activities. One of the primary energy metabolic by-products removed is *carbon dioxide*:

Fuel (carbohydrate, protein, or fat) + Oxygen ===>
Energy + Water + *Carbon dioxide*

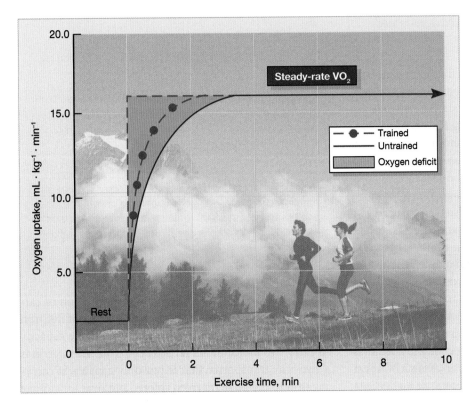

FIGURE 9.2: Greater oxygen using capacity is seen in highly trained versus nontrained subjects. During submaximal cycle ergometer exercise, trained subjects reach a steady-state VO_2 faster than untrained subjects, reducing the oxygen deficit and, therefore, reducing lactate production. (From Katch VL, McArdle WD, Katch FI. *Essentials of Exercise Physiology.* 5th ed. Lippincott Williams & Wilkins; 2015.)

Iron

Iron is a critical element in the delivery of oxygen to working tissues. It is part of RBC *hemoglobin*, muscle *myoglobin*, and enzymes involved in electron transfer for energy metabolism. (See Chapters 2, 3, and 4 for more information on energy metabolism, oxidative phosphorylation, and the electron transport chain, respectively.) Iron exists in two oxidation states: ferrous (Fe^{2+}) or ferric (Fe^{3+}). In a neutral pH (*i.e.*, neutral acidity), iron is typically found in the ferric (Fe^{3+}) form, whereas in an acidic environment, iron is found in the ferrous (Fe^{2+}) form. Aside from transporting oxygen in hemoglobin, iron is also found in cytochromes and iron–sulfur-containing proteins as part of *oxidative phosphorylation*, which is the enzyme-based metabolic pathway cells use to oxidize nutrients and form ATP energy. Excess iron (*i.e.*, iron not part of hemoglobin, myoglobin, or enzymes) is toxic and can increase the risk of liver and colon disease. Severe toxicity of iron causes ferrous iron to generate hydroxyl free radical from hydrogen peroxide, resulting in **ROS** tissue damage and related muscle soreness.

Reactive Oxygen Species

Commonly abbreviated as ROS, these are chemically reactive molecules that contain oxygen and may result in tissue damage if tissues are not adequately protected with antioxidants. Examples include hydrogen peroxide, superoxide, hydroxyl radical, and singlet oxygen. Although ROS are naturally formed by-products of oxygen-related metabolism, excess formation of ROS is tissue damaging.

Hemoglobin is a high priority for the human system. Should low iron availability cause hemoglobin to drop, the iron in myoglobin and iron-containing enzymes are scavenged with the goal of maintaining RBC hemoglobin. Because of this, it is possible for athletes to experience a performance reduction even if measured hemoglobin and hematocrit (the two most common measures of iron status) appear to be in the normal range. It is important, therefore, that ferritin (stored iron) also be measured as a normal component of a blood test intended to screen for iron status (Table 9.1). It is important to note that there is no universally accepted minimum value on the serum ferritin level associated with iron deficiency or iron depletion. The generally used minimum values for serum ferritin that are associated with iron deficiency/depletion range from <10.0 ng/mL to <35 ng/mL (10,11).

Should an iron deficiency **anemia** occur, the anemia is characterized by small RBCs (*microcytic* cells), RBCs that are light in color (*hypochromic cells*), and an inadequate

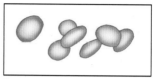
A Iron deficiency anemia

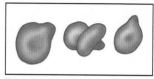
B Megaloblastic anemia

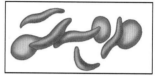
C Sickle cell disease

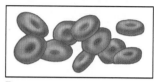
D Normal

FIGURE 9.3: Iron deficiency anemia is characterized by smaller, lighter in color, and fewer in number RBCs. **A:** Iron deficiency anemia is characterized by an insufficient number of red cells (anemia) that are small (microcytic) and low in color (hypochromic) from low hemoglobin concentration. **B:** Megaloblastic anemia is characterized by an insufficient number of red cells (anemia) that are large (macrocytic) and low in color (hypochromic) from dilution of hemoglobin in the cells. The cause is vitamin B_{12} and/or folic acid deficiency. **C:** Sickle cell disease is characterized by an insufficient number of red cells (anemia) that are misshapen (sickle cell). This is a genetic/inherited condition. **D:** Normal RBCs are normally concentrated (*i.e.*, normal hematocrit), normally shaped (normocytic), and have a normal bright red color (normochromic). RBCs, red blood cells. (From Porth C. Essentials of pathophysiology. 3rd ed. Philadelphia (PA): Lippincott Williams & Wilkins; 2011.)

number of RBCs. This condition is referred to as a *microcytic hypochromic anemia* (Figure 9.3).

Anemia

A general term to describe insufficient RBCs with limited hemoglobin, resulting in reduced oxygen-carrying capacity. The common dietary cause is insufficient iron consumption, but anemia may also be the result of insufficient vitamin B_{12}, folate, or protein. It may also be caused by loss of blood as is typical in a woman's menstrual period, but may occur with any chronic bleeding from the gastrointestinal (GI) tract or loss of iron in the urine. Additional anemia risks that athletes face are associated with foot strike and other sources of intravascular hemolysis, periods of rapid growth (*i.e.*, the adolescent growth spurt), training at high altitudes, and increased iron losses via sweat, urine, and feces (12).

Transferrin

Transferrin is a blood glycoprotein (combination of carbohydrate and protein) that is the main carrier of free iron in the blood. Each transferrin molecule has the capacity to carry two molecules of ferric (Fe^{3+}) iron. Transferrin is a two-way transporter that is not only capable of carrying iron to the bone marrow, spleen, and liver for storage but also capable of carrying iron to form hemoglobin in new RBCs (13). It is a molecule with a relatively short half-life that can be measured as an indicator of recent protein status. Low blood transferrin may indicate protein or energy malnutrition, which results in inadequate synthesis of transferrin by the liver. It should be noted that transferrin can also be synthesized by the brain (14). Low blood transferrin may also result from excess protein loss through the kidneys (proteinuria), an infection, or cancer. A high blood transferrin level is an indicator of iron deficiency. Athletes with low blood transferrin may have impaired production of hemoglobin that can lead to anemia, even with ample iron body stores, whereas high transferrin may be an indicator of iron deficiency anemia. In addition to its iron-carrying capacity, transferrin is associated with body immunity by limiting the amount of free iron and ROS creation, which is associated with tissue inflammation, and lowering the amount of free iron required by bacteria for survival (15).

Ceruloplasmin

Ceruloplasmin, which represents 90% of the total plasma copper, is a copper-containing protein involved in transferring iron from transferrin to hemoglobin in the formation of new RBCs, and in transferring iron from deteriorated RBCs for inclusion into newly formed RBCs (16). Copper deficiency results in low ceruloplasmin that can result in low RBC anemia (microcytic hypochromic anemia), because of an inability to transfer iron for the formation of hemoglobin. This poor transfer capacity may result in iron overload disease, referred to as hemochromatosis, with iron accumulating in the pancreas, liver, and brain, resulting in neurologic disorders (17). It is important to note that copper deficiency is a relatively uncommon clinical disorder, with those most at risk of deficiency including premature infants, children recovering from malnutrition, people with any malabsorption syndrome (*i.e.*, celiac disease, sprue, and any surgical shortening of the small intestine), and cystic fibrosis (18,19). There is also some indication that, because of competitive absorption, excess zinc consumption may result in copper deficiency (20,21). Although athletes have a greater requirement for iron and associated nutrients to increase the manufacture of healthy RBCs, there are no data to suggest that the athletic endeavor increases the risk of copper deficiency.

Vitamin B₁₂ (Cobalamin)

Vitamin B₁₂ is a cobalt-containing vitamin that, as a result, is also referred to as *cobalamin*. Two primary functions of vitamin B₁₂ are the formation of new RBCs and the preservation of a healthy nervous system. Although a deficiency is uncommon in adults, deficiencies are seen in people over the age of 60, or in any condition that impairs the gastric production of intrinsic factor, which is needed for vitamin B₁₂ absorption (22). Pure vegans and vegetarians who consume few animal products are considered at higher risk of vitamin B₁₂ deficiency because the vitamin is more easily obtained from animal products (23). The vegetarian athlete is at even greater risk of anemia because of the combination of marginal vitamin B₁₂ status (vegetables are a poor source, and meats are a good source of B₁₂) coupled with the faster exercise-associated RBC breakdown experienced by athletes (24,25). Poor vitamin B₁₂ availability when RBCs are being formed results in cells with weak membranes. These poorly formed cells, called megaloblasts, are fragile and live approximately half as long as a normal RBC (60 days vs. 120 days) (26). The shortened life of these cells requires a constantly faster production of red cells to maintain normal oxygen-carrying capacity (Figure 9.4).

However, this faster-required level of RBC production cannot be maintained, eventually resulting in anemia. The anemia resulting from vitamin B₁₂ deficiency is referred to as *pernicious anemia* because it develops slowly over several years (27). Pernicious anemia is a megaloblastic, hypochromic anemia, with RBCs that are large, misshapen because of a poorly formed membrane, and low in color (the hemoglobin is spread out over a larger cell area, diluting the color) (28).

Folate

The vitamin **folate** refers to both the naturally occurring folates in food and also folic acid, which is the synthetic form used in supplements and in fortified foods. Folate, vitamin B₁₂, and vitamin C are all vitamins involved in protein metabolism, so are important in hemoglobin and RBC synthesis and protein carrier (*i.e.*, transferrin) synthesis. Importantly, folate, in conjunction with vitamin B₁₂, is required for the production of RBCs (28). Folate is also involved in nerve tissue development and, in pregnant females with good folate status, is known to nearly eliminate the risk of neural tube defects in newborns (29,30). The anemia associated with inadequate folate is similar to that produced by a deficiency of vitamin B₁₂ (megaloblastic, hypochromic anemia), and the resulting reduced oxygen-carrying capacity is equally severe. Although vitamin B₁₂ is obtained primarily from animal sources, folic acid can be obtained from folate-fortified foods, fresh fruits, fresh vegetables, and

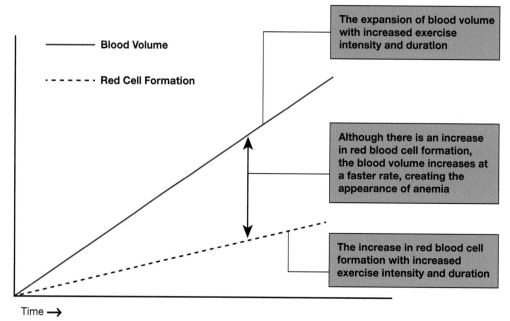

FIGURE 9.4: Sports anemia/dilutional pseudoanemia. The differential in blood volume and red cell concentration becomes noticeable after 3–5 days of an increase in exercise duration/intensity. After some time, blood volume ceases to increase and red cell production catches up, to remove the appearance of anemia.

legumes. Folate has been fortified in the food supply, primarily cereal grain products, since 1998, dramatically reducing the risk of developing folate deficiency as a factor in reduced oxygen delivery (29).

Vitamin B₁₂

Also referred to as cobalamin, a cobalt-containing water-soluble vitamin, it is involved in the formation of RBCs. It not only is derived in the diet from animal-based foods, but can also be obtained from fermented foods (soy tofu, etc.). Insufficient B_{12} results in megaloblastic anemia because of large, fragile RBCs with a shorter life span. The large cells also make it difficult to oxygenate peripheral tissues, including the brain.

Folate

Folate is the generic term used to refer to both naturally occurring folates in food and *folic acid*, which is the synthetic form of the vitamin used in fortified foods and supplements. It is also referred to as vitamin B_9. Where a distinction is necessary, *folates* is used to refer to the forms found in foods and the body tissues, whereas *folic acid* is used to refer to the form in supplements or fortified foods. Where no distinction is needed, the term folate is used. Folates are mainly derived from fresh fruits and vegetables. When consumed, it works with vitamin B_{12} to form new RBCs, without which the red cells are large and fragile (megaloblasts). Deficiency results in megaloblastic anemia, and women who initiate a pregnancy without sufficient folate are at risk of having a baby with a neural

tube defect (anencephaly or spina bifida). To lower this risk, the United States has been fortifying the food supply with folic acid. (For more information, see Chapter 5 on vitamins.)

Oxygen–Nutrient Performance Relationship, Causes of Anemia, and Related Disorders

Iron deficiency and/or iron deficiency anemia impairs muscle function and diminishes muscular work capacity (31,32). There is also no question that physical activity can alter blood-iron status and that blood-iron status can also alter physical activity performance. A number of studies have found that athletes, regardless of sport, are at higher risk of anemia than the nonathlete population (33). Those athletes most at risk for iron deficiency appear to be distance runners, vegetarians, and regular blood donors (11,34). One study assessing 747 athletes and 104 untrained controls found that endurance athletes had lower hemoglobin and hematocrit levels, perhaps from a greater degree of foot-strike hemolysis (35). A study of female volleyball players also found that a high proportion were at risk from inadequate dietary intake of iron, with 13% of the players diagnosed with iron deficiency anemia (36). Virtually all studies show a greater incidence of iron deficiency and iron deficiency anemia in athletes compared with nonathletes, suggesting that a significant proportion of athletes are performance compromised (37). There are a number of possibilities related to iron deficiency in athletes.

Sports Anemia (Dilutional Pseudoanemia)

When athletes begin an intensive exercise program, they experience a rise in both blood volume and RBCs. However, because the blood volume increases at a faster rate than the RBCs, it appears that the athletes have anemia (38). Because this condition is transient (eventually the concentration of red cells becomes normal), it is referred to as a dilutional pseudoanemia, **sports anemia**, or athletic anemia (39). Although it is common for athletes to have hemoglobin concentrations that are ~1 g/dL below normal, the athletes still typically experience an increase in RBCs that is associated with an increase in oxygen-carrying capacity (40). It is for this reason that this condition is referred to as a *pseudo*anemia (*i.e.*, not a true anemia). In fact, athletes do better as a result of the increased plasma volume and red cells because of a more efficient cardiac stroke volume and greater oxygen delivery to working muscles (41).

It is most often seen in endurance athletes, but can be observed in any athletes experiencing increases in training intensity. It is the most common anemia in male athletes (38). When it occurs, hemoglobin concentration appears to be reduced by 1.0–1.5 g/dL, but this reduction is dilutional and occurs despite an increase in RBCs. It is actually a beneficial adaptation to training because the expanded plasma volume helps to maintain sweat rates while lowering cardiac stress (38) (Figure 9.5).

Foot-Strike Hemolysis or Exertional Hemolysis

Anemia has many causes including **hemolysis**, or the abnormal breakdown of RBCs either in the blood vessels (intravascular hemolysis) or in the tissues (extravascular hemolysis). There are multiple causes of hemolysis, including the sudden compression of RBCs caused by foot strike or compressed muscles experienced by athletes. With foot-strike or exertional hemolysis, red cells circulating in capillaries through the bottom of the feet or from compressed muscles are crushed (42). It is important to note that exertional hemolysis may occur in all athletes, including swimmers, and cyclists, suggesting that foot-strike hemolysis commonly experienced by runners is only one of the mechanisms associated with faster red cell breakdown (43,44). The faster RBC breakdown from hemolysis may make it more difficult for athletes to maintain a normal concentration of RBCs, which may increase anemia risk. However, the iron released from hemolyzed RBCs is normally rebound to hemoglobin to produce new red cells, so although the risk of anemia is greater, exertional hemolysis should be considered an *additional* risk factor in the development of anemia, as it would rarely result in anemia by itself (45).

> ### Sports Anemia
>
> A dilutional pseudoanemia that occurs when the intensity of an exercise program is increased. As an adaptation to the exercise, blood volume is increased at a rate faster

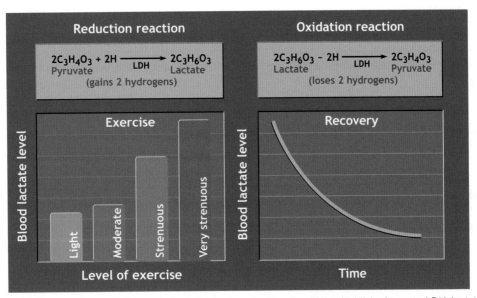

FIGURE 9.5: Redox reactions—relationship between donor (reducing agent) and receiving (oxidizing) agents. LDH, lactate dehydrogenase. (From McArdle WD, Katch FI, Katch VL. *Exercise Physiology.* 9th ed. LWW (PE); 2023.)

than RBCs can be increased, resulting in what appears to be anemia.

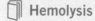 **Hemolysis**

Hemolysis is the rupturing of RBCs from bacteria, sickle cell disease, parasites, and external pressure on tissues (*i.e.*, foot-strike hemolysis). The greater breakdown of RBCs, regardless of the cause, may result in anemia.

Loss of Iron in Urine

A chronic loss of RBCs in the urine (**hematuria**), a condition brought on by frequent high-intensity and long-duration practice sessions, may contribute to anemia, a problem that would clearly lower athletic performance. Athletes should be careful, therefore, to take in sufficient nutrients though consumption of good-quality foods to replace lost nutrients. Luckily, the process of producing new RBCs (erythropoiesis) appears to be remarkably resilient in the face of exercise stress. Assuming sufficient nutrient availability that includes iron, folate, and vitamin B_{12}, humans are capable of producing a large number of new RBCs (46). Some athletes try to enhance erythropoiesis by taking the drug erythropoietin, but this blood-doping technique is *illegal* and has the potential for increasing blood viscosity, with subsequent thrombosis and potentially fatal results (38).

Hematuria

Blood (heme) in the urine (uria), which is seen in athletes but is not common. Hematuria may be the result of vigorous exercise, but is also associated with infection of the urinary tract and other more serious diseases. Hematuria increases the risk of anemia.

Data from past studies indicate that the higher prevalence of hematuria in athletes has multiple causes, including (47,48):

- Foot-strike hemolysis
- Renal ischemia (restriction of blood supply to the kidney, often caused by dehydration in athletes)
- Hypoxic kidney damage
- Release of a hemolyzing factor
- Bladder or kidney trauma
- Nonsteroidal anti-inflammatory drug (NSAID) intake (common NSAIDs include aspirin, Tylenol, etc.)
- Dehydration
- Increased circulation rate
- Myoglobinuria release
- Peroxidation of RBCs
- Sickle cell anemia

Ferritin

Ferritin is an intracellular protein that stores and releases iron and is referred to as "storage iron" (49). Athletes with higher exercise durations and workloads appear to have a lower level of ferritin, suggesting that athletes are at higher risk of compromised iron status than nonathletes and that higher exercise durations may be associated with even greater iron status risk. Endurance athletes who put in large numbers of training hours (and miles) are therefore at the highest risk of poor iron status even though they rely most on aerobic metabolic processes to achieve their endurance (43,44). A multistudy comparison of serum ferritin values in female athletes involved in different sports has found that between 18% and 57% of the measured athletes had values suggesting iron depletion (50). It has been suggested that iron requirements for all female athletes maybe 70% higher, or 13.8 mg/day, than the estimated average requirement (for adult females = 8.1 mg/day) (51).

Diet

Restrictive food intakes, which are commonly observed among athletes involved in weight classification or aesthetic sports, typically fail to adequately supply vitamins and minerals. There is real risk, therefore, that athletes in "make-weight" or "appearance" sports may be at higher risk for developing performance deficits associated with lower oxygen delivery. Iron deficiency, even without anemia, reduces muscle work potential, and iron deficiency anemia makes matters worse because of a further reduction in oxygen-carrying capacity. It should be clear that a failure to supply nutrients, in addition to iron, may also compromise oxygen delivery. Magnesium deficiency increases the oxygen requirements needed to perform submaximal exercise, thereby reducing endurance performance (32). The only reasonable and appropriate way for weight-conscious athletes to ensure adequate nutrient exposure to avoid nutrient deficiencies that could compromise oxygen delivery and performance is to eat foods with a high nutrient density (*i.e.*, more nutrients per calories delivered). It is also important that these athletes have iron status regularly monitored (52).

Gender

Female athletes are at greater risk of poor iron status that may result in iron deficiency from insufficient dietary iron intake, menstruation, increased iron losses associated with hemolysis, sweating, GI bleeding, and exercise-induced acute inflammation (53,54). The effects include reduced athletic performance and impaired immune function. Female athletes should consider either consuming more iron-rich foods (including red meats) or taking iron supplements under the supervision of a physician. Importantly, female athletes should have regular annual screening for iron status that includes hemoglobin, hematocrit, and ferritin. The goal of the screening is to intervene prior to the development of a frank iron deficiency anemia, which can have profoundly negative effects on health and performance (50).

Exercise-Induced Asthma

Oxygen delivery to working tissues is critically important for athlete performance, so any condition that compromises breathing and limits the oxygen that can be brought into the body is an important consideration. An area of particular interest for athletes is *EIA*, which affects a significant proportion of the athlete population (55,56). EIA is an airway obstruction that occurs as a result of exercise (either during or after) and may occur in people who do not suffer from chronic asthma (57). The prevalence of EIA in athletes is not fully established, but there are published reports of a 42.5% prevalence in collegiate athletes, a 55% prevalence in cross-country skiers, and a 12% prevalence in basketball players (58–60). Symptoms may begin within 5–20 minutes after the initiation of exercise and include:

- Coughing and wheezing
- Tight chest with some chest pain
- Shortness of breath
- Early and severe fatigue

These symptoms are most obvious immediately after stopping exercise and usually dissipate within an hour.

Causes of Exercise-Induced Asthma

The causes of asthma-related chronic lung inflammation are not well established, but there appears to be a genetic component, suggesting that some people are born with a predisposition to having asthma. A trigger is required to cause asthma, and in EIA the trigger appears to be a large volume of cold and dry air that is moved into lungs (57). EIA may also be associated with "mouth breathing" when exercising in cold and dry environments, and the chlorine in pools may also serve as a trigger for EIA. Because of this, sports requiring continuous activity with faster breathing, particularly in cold weather, are most likely to induce EIA (55,56). The sports commonly associated with EIA include:

- Long-distance running
- Soccer
- Hockey
- Cross-country skiing
- Downhill skiing
- Hiking
- Swimming
- Figure skating

Studies suggest that the highest population prevalence of EIA appears to be in skiers (55%), competitive figure skaters (30%–55%), swimmers (48%), cross-country skiers (50%), and Canadian professional football players (56%) (59,61–65).

Recommended Treatment for Exercise-Induced Asthma

Recommended nonpharmacologic treatment for EIA includes the following (57,66,67):

1. Understand that EIA is a chronic condition, so knowing the triggers may help in avoiding a severe EIA response.
2. Become well conditioned for the activity that induces EIA. Athletes who are well conditioned and acclimated to the environment can exercise at lower breathing rates at any given work intensity and, therefore, are less likely to suffer from EIA.
3. If possible, avoid exercising in cold and dry air. If the sport mandates exercising outside in these conditions (as, for instance, in cross-country skiing), athletes can try covering the mouth and nose with a scarf or ski mask to warm and humidify the breathed air.
4. A warm-up period is important, with the intensity of the warm-up dependent on how each athlete responds to EIA.
5. A well-planned cool-down period may diminish the severity of EIA by slowing airway changes.
6. Avoid exercise on days when asthma symptoms from other conditions, such as hay fever or food allergies, are present.

It is possible for athletes to use drugs to treat EIA during a sanctioned competition, but they must first obtain permission to do so from the World Anti-Doping Association (WADA, https://www.wada-ama.org) for internationally sanctioned events, or the International Olympic Committee (IOC, https://www.olympic.org/fight-against-doping) Medical Commission for Olympic games. In general, athletes must meet specific criteria that are established as the result of standardized exercise challenge tests from certified laboratories to be given permission to use drugs for the control of EIA (56). Because the drugs used for asthma are constantly being developed and are changing, athletes and physicians must be aware of the current regulations published by WADA and the IOC. The regulations for treating EIA with drugs may change, so the athlete and those involved in treating the athlete should stay abreast of the current regulations through referring to the WADA and IOC websites. *Athletes taking drugs to resolve asthma symptoms who have not followed the proper certification procedures may be sanctioned for doping and removed from competition.*

OXIDATIVE STRESS

Cells are constantly manufacturing free radicals, which are molecules with one or more unpaired electrons, and nonradical derivatives of oxygen, such as hydrogen peroxide, as part of normal metabolic processes. These free radicals and the nonradical derivatives of oxygen are referred to as ROS, which can increase dramatically with higher-energy metabolism associated with exercise (68). **Oxidative stress** occurs when the production of ROS exceeds the body tissue capacity to neutralize them (69,70). ROS causes damage to cells because their radical movement inside cells destroys them, producing "clinkers" (dead cells). The major ROS in humans include superoxide and NO. Both are highly reactive and can initiate reactions to form other ROS. Superoxide rapidly forms hydrogen peroxide, which is responsible for most hydrogen peroxide in cells, and superoxide and NO both also rapidly form other ROS (71) (Box 9.2).

Oxidative Stress

A system imbalance between ROS and the tissue ability to minimize the tissue-damaging effects of ROS. A balance of antioxidants is an important strategy for reducing oxidative stress.

The body inhibits ROS production through **antioxidant** vitamins and minerals (Box 9.3). The minerals work to regulate enzyme activity so as to diminish ROS production, whereas vitamins accept ROS to remove them from the cellular environment, thereby limiting their potential hazards inside the cell. Early studies of vitamin E, a fat-soluble antioxidant vitamin found mainly in vegetable oils, initially showed promise in reducing ROS (96). However, athletes should be cautious about thinking that a greater than normal amount of a vitamin is better than *normal* amount in diminishing the effects of ROS. There has been a recent concern that vitamin E and vitamin C

supplementation, by itself, may place the pool of antioxidants out of balance, thereby diminishing the overall defenses humans have to prevent ROS (97). A reasonable strategy is to avoid this imbalance by regularly consuming foods that contain a variety of antioxidants rather than taking a single antioxidant vitamin supplement. In doing so, the sensitive balance between the antioxidants can remain intact while increasing the antioxidant presence to provide an improved defense against ROS (Table 9.2).

Antioxidant

Common nutrient antioxidants include β-carotene, vitamin C, vitamin E, and selenium. Antioxidant phytochemicals showing preventive and/or therapeutic effects in humans include lycopene, allicin, flavonols, curcumin, resveratrol, flavonoids, and quercetin (98). Other endogenous antioxidants present in tissues include glutathione (GSH) and superoxide dismutase (SOD). They function to inhibit the damaging oxidation of ROS.

REDOX reactions include reactions involving the transfer of electrons between different chemicals. The chemical from which the electron is stripped is oxidized, whereas the chemical to which the electron is added is reduced. An easy way to remember REDOX is the term OIL RIG, where Oxidation Is Loss of electrons; Reduction Is Gain of electrons. REDOX reactions are important to many life functions, including photosynthesis and respiration (99) (Figure 9.5).

The relative balance between the volume of oxidants and the volume of antioxidants is the determinant of REDOX balance. A higher level of oxidants relative to antioxidants leads to oxidative stress. However, it is important to consider that an overabundance of antioxidants relative to oxidants also results in cellular stress. A balance between the two is key to sustaining muscle function and reducing muscle soreness. Because ROS production is likely to occur as a result of exercise, cellular antioxidant defenses are produced to inhibit ROS overproduction, which occurs mainly inside cell mitochondria and cytosol (100). These cellular antioxidant defenses are produced by tissues, but they may also be provided through the diet. Together, these dietary and cellular defenses work to suppress excess ROS.

Small amounts of the free radical *superoxide* are produced during the formation of ATP, resulting in some ROS (101). Because there is a significant increase in the metabolic rate of exercising humans, it is expected that ROS would rise proportionally to the increase in energy metabolism and the formation of ATP. Interestingly, the

Box 9.2 Nitric Oxide

In humans, nitric oxide (NO) functions as a vasodilator and signaling molecule that influences skeletal muscle function through regulation of blood flow, muscle contractility, glucose homeostasis, calcium homeostasis, and mitochondrial respiration and biogenesis (72). It plays key roles in cardiovascular, gastrointestinal, and endothelial systems. NO is known to lower blood pressure, reduces the oxygen cost of exercise, increases time to fatigue, and improves gastric mucosal defenses. It was originally believed that NO was only generated through the oxidation of the amino acid l-arginine in a reaction catalyzed by nitric oxide synthase (73). It is now known that NO can also be produced through the reduction of nitrate to nitrite, and then nitrite to nitric oxide (74). This pathway is important in conditions of low oxygen availability, as occurs during exercise. Dark green leafy vegetables are good sources of nitrate, which can be reduced to nitrite by oral bacteria. The resultant higher nitrite concentration serves as a reservoir for NO production (75). Therefore, consumption of natural food-derived nitrate as a means of enhancing NO production is important for lowering the risk of multiple cardiometabolic disorders and is also important for enhancing fatigue resistance in athletes. While most vegetables contain nitrate, very high food sources of nitrate include beetroot, spinach, lettuce, rocket, celery, water cress, chervil, celeriac, fennel, leek, endive, and parsley.

Studies assessing the physiologic response to exercise have found that consumption of high-nitrate foods, such as beetroot juice, prior to exercise results in a reduction of resting blood pressure, lower the oxygen cost of submaximal exercise by 5%, and extends the time to exhaustion during high-intensity cycling (76,77). There is a positive effect of consuming high-nitrate foods prior to exercise, and this positive effect does not appear to diminish if the foods are repeatedly consumed (78,79). There is also evidence that dietary nitrate consumption can increase time to fatigue through attenuation of through a reduction in leg muscle pain during exercise (80)

The enterosalivary nitrate → nitrite → NO pathway that is initiated in the oral cavity is a crucial step in the process of converting dietary inorganic nitrate to nitrite. It is important to consider the factors that can enhance or diminish the production of NO via the enterosalivary pathway.

Enhancers of Nitric Oxide Formation:

- Consumption of grapefruit juice in conjunction with beetroot juice or other high-nitrate foods was found to enhance the lowering of systolic blood pressure and pulse rate (81). A similar positive effect was found with consumption of other foods high in vitamin C (82)
- Consumption of foods high in polyphenols (*e.g.*, fruits and vegetables) and flavanols (*e.g.*, cocoa) were found to significantly increase plasma nitrite concentration for at least 12 hours postingestion in healthy male athletes, resulting in improved physical endurance (83–85)
- Tongue brushing appears to enhance the bacterial community involved in converting nitrate to nitrite (86)

Inhibitors of Nitric Oxide Formation:

- A high-level consumption of foods high in fructose interferes with the conversion of dietary nitrate to nitric oxide (87,88). This is an important reason for athletes to avoid sports beverages and other foods/drinks that use high-fructose corn syrup as sweetener.
- Simultaneous consumption of cruciferous vegetables with high-nitrate foods/drinks. While these vegetables are known for their anti-inflammatory and anticancerous effects, they are rich in glucosinolate, which impairs nitric oxide formation in the enterosalivary nitrate–nitrite–nitric oxide pathway (89)
- Conjugated linoleic acid (the isomer of the essential fatty acid linoleic acid), when consumed in high amounts via supplementation has been shown to inhibit the vasodilatory benefit derived from nitric oxide (90)
- Smokers have been found to have reduced nitrate-reductase activity resulting in lower nitric oxide formation because of the smoke-associated bromine gas in the oral cavity (91)
- Antiseptic mouthwash eliminates the oral bacteria critical for the conversion of dietary nitrate to nitrite (92). It has been found that twice daily or more frequent use of antiseptic mouthwash is associated with an 85% elevated risk of hypertension (93)
- Regular consumption of organic nitrate salts, commonly available in capsule form and also found in preserved meats, may result in diminishing benefits with potentially negative side effects (94,95).

Box 9.3   Iron-Associated Terminology

Ferritin

Ferritin is an iron-storage protein found in the liver, spleen, and bone marrow, with only a small amount in the blood. The amount in the blood is thought to be proportionate to the amount stored in the liver, spleen, and bone marrow, so a blood ferritin test is an indicator of the amount of stored iron. The lower the ferritin level, even within the "normal" range, the more likely a client is iron deficient.

Normal ferritin values:

- Adult males: Min: >10–35 ng/mL; up to 300 ng/mL
- Adult females: Min: >10–35 ng/mL; up to 120 ng/mL

Note: ng/mL = nanograms per milliliter

Hematocrit

Hematocrit is the proportion of whole blood that is composed of RBCs and is often referred to as the number of RBCs per unit of blood.

Normal hematocrit values:

- Adult males: 42%–52%
- Adult females: 36%–48%

Hemochromatosis

Hemochromatosis is an iron overload disease caused by uninhibited iron absorption. It can result in liver damage if the iron concentration is not lowered.

Hemoglobin

Hemoglobin is the iron-containing, oxygen-carrying protein in RBCs.

Normal hemoglobin values:

- Adult males: 13.8–17.2 g/dL
- Adult females: 12.1–15.1 g/dL

Note: Initial exposure to higher altitude results in a lowering of plasma volume with a related increase in hemoglobin concentration. Remaining at a higher altitude results in a gradual increase in both hemoglobin and blood volume that results in greater oxygen-carrying capacity (11). It is important to have sufficient iron stores (ferritin) for these adaptive changes to occur. See Table 9.1 for altitude-associated adjustments to measured hemoglobin concentrations.

Hemosiderosis

Hemosiderosis is a disease condition that results from excess iron in the body, often from blood transfusions. It is often seen in individuals with thalassemia.

Serum Iron

Serum iron represents the total amount of iron in the blood serum.

Normal serum iron values:

- Adult males: 75–175 mcg/dL
- Adult females: 65–165 mcg/dL

Total Iron Binding Capacity

The total iron binding capacity (TIBC) test measures the amount of iron the blood could carry if transferrin were fully saturated with iron molecules. Because transferrin is produced by the liver, the TIBC can be used to monitor liver function and protein status nutrition.

Transferrin

The transferrin test is a direct measurement of the protein transferrin (also called siderophilin) in the blood. The saturation level of transferrin can be calculated by dividing the serum iron level by TIBC.

Normal transferrin values:

- Adult males: 200–400 mg/dL
- Adult females: 200–400 mg/dL

Note: Normal transferrin saturation values are between 30% and 40%.

---

exercise-associated rise in ROS production appears related to exercise intensity but not to total energy expenditure associated with exercise, suggesting that the mitochondria may not be the only important source of ROS (102). It was found that markers of oxidative damage were highest following maximal intensity activity, and lower intensity activity had lower oxidative damage markers (103).

Nutrient imbalances can also cause difficulties with immune function. Excess vitamin E negatively affects the immune system, but inadequate levels of this vitamin, iron, selenium, zinc, calcium, and magnesium can also create immune deficiencies (13,104–106). All this information points to the importance of maintaining a *balance* of all the nutrients rather than consuming high levels of one or two with the hope of inducing a desirable cellular protective effect.

It is important to consider that oxidative metabolic processes are constantly working, even during events that

Table 9.2		**The Antioxidant Nutrients**	
Nutrient	Recommended Intake for Men	Recommended Intake for Women	Functions
Vitamin C	90 mg/day	75 mg/day	Vitamin C scavenges reactive oxidants in leukocytes and in lung and gastric mucosa, and it reduces lipid peroxidation in cells.
Vitamin E	15 mg/day	15 mg/day	Vitamin E mainly prevents the peroxidation of lipids.
Selenium	55 mcg/day	55 mcg/day	Selenium functions through selenoproteins, which form oxidant defense enzymes. The dietary reference intake is based on the amount needed to synthesize selenoprotein glutathione peroxidase.
β-Carotene[a]	(900 mcg/d)	(700 mcg/d)	12 mcg of β-carotene can form 1 mcg of retinol (vitamin A). The human nutrient requirement is for vitamin A, not β-carotene. However, β-carotene is more than just a precursor to the production of vitamin A. Besides being an important biomarker for the intake of fresh fruits and vegetables, it also has important antioxidant properties.

[a]Represents the generally recommended intake level, but is not the recommended dietary allowance.

are primarily anaerobic. The anaerobic athlete who just completed a 10-second high-intensity sprint has something in common with a gymnast who just completed a 90-second floor routine: the need to breathe a large volume of air (oxygen) to recharge the fuels they will need for the next bout of high-intensity exercise (107). Iron is a primary element for transporting oxygen to working tissues and carbon dioxide away from working tissues, making it a critically important nutrient for athletes. Despite this, iron is the most common nutrient deficiency, and athletes may be at even greater risk for iron deficiency than the general public because of multiple reasons, including foot-strike hemolysis, intravascular hemolysis, and increased iron loss in sweat, urine, and feces (11).

REACTIVE OXYGEN SPECIES IN CELLS

Enzyme Antioxidants

Enzymes within skeletal muscles contain antioxidants, including the following:

- *SOD*: Converts superoxide (a highly reactive ROS) to the less reactive ROS, hydrogen peroxide. Mitochondria contain manganese-containing SOD, whereas the cell cytosol contains a copper- and zinc-containing SOD.

- *Catalase (CAT)*: Once ROS are converted to hydrogen peroxide, CAT works to further neutralize hydrogen peroxide to water.
- *Glutathione peroxidase*: Works with CAT to help neutralize hydrogen peroxide to water.

See Table 9.3 for a more comprehensive list of antioxidant defenses both inside and outside cells.

Nonenzyme Antioxidants (Nutrients)

There are a number of nutrients that function as antioxidants, both in the lipid membrane of cells and in the water-based cytosol of cells. These include GSH, uric acid, vitamin C (ascorbic acid), vitamin E (α-tocopherol), ubiquinone (coenzyme Q10), carotenoids (β-carotene), and flavonoids.

Glutathione

GSH is found in the water-based interior of cells with the capacity to neutralize several ROS. Once used to scavenge ROS, the GSH is recycled by GSH reductase to renew its capacity to continue neutralizing ROS. Additional recycling occurs when it comes in contact with the nutrient antioxidants vitamins C and E. It is this capacity to scavenge ROS and interact with other antioxidants in both lipid- and water-based environments to sustain its scavenging capacity that makes GSH a highly valuable antioxidant. The anti-inflammatory action of GSH, through

Table 9.3	Internal and External Cellular Antioxidant Defenses Against ROS			
Antioxidant		**Form**	**Type**	**Location**
Enzymatic				
Superoxide dismutase (SOD)		I	A	C, E, M
Glutathione peroxidase (GPx)		I	A	C, M
Catalase (CAT)		I	A	C, M
Nonenzymatic (Nutrient) Antioxidants				
Glutathione (GSH) Food sources include asparagus, potatoes, carrots, onion, bell peppers, broccoli, avocados, tomatoes, grapefruit, apples, oranges, peaches, bananas, and melon		I	A	C
Vitamin E Food sources include almonds, spinach, sweet potato, avocado, sunflower seeds, butternut squash, and vegetable oils		D	L	C, E
Vitamin C Food sources include citrus fruits and other fresh fruits and vegetables		D	A	C, E
Carotenoids (β-carotene, etc.) Food sources include red, orange, green, and yellow foods, including tomatoes, carrots, apricots, spinach, and kale		D	L	C, E
Uric acid Food sources include sources of purines, which are converted to uric acid, including organ meats, meats, fish, shellfish, and beer		I	A	C, E
Flavonoids Food sources include tea, citrus fruit, berries, red wine, apples, and legumes		D	A, L	C, E, M
Ubiquinones Food sources include pork heart and liver, beef heart and liver, chicken heart and liver, and red meat		D, I	L	C, M
α-Lipoic acid Food sources include spinach, broccoli, yams, potatoes, yeast, tomatoes, Brussels sprouts, carrots, beets, rice bran, and red meat		I	A	C, E

I, manufactured internally; D, dietary; A, aqueous (water based); L, lipid (lipid based); C, cellular (inside the cell); E, extracellular (outside the cell); M, mitochondrial (inside the mitochondria).

Source: Quindry JC, Kavazis AN, Powers SK. Exercise-induced oxidative stress: are supplemental antioxidants warranted? In: Maughan R, editor. Sports nutrition. Vol. XIX of encyclopedia of sports medicine. International Olympic Committee Medical Commission, Hoboken (NJ): John Wiley & Sons Ltd.; 2014. p. 263–276.

its neutralizing of inflammatory ROS, may also cause it to serve as an anticarcinogenic substance (108). Fruits and vegetables have been found to contribute over 50% of the typical dietary GSH consumption (37). Supplemental consumption of GSH is not likely to be successful, as it is digested in the small intestine and fails to become absorbed as an intact molecule. It has been found, however, that consumption of N-acetylcysteine (NAC), which also functions as an antioxidant, enables GSH resynthesis (109). Nonhuman studies found that providing moderate doses of NAC improved muscle function. However, supplemental NAC consumption in humans results in severe GI effects that make it impossible to use as a supplement to derive an ergogenic benefit (110).

Uric Acid

Uric acid functions as an antioxidant in the blood and in cells (111). A deficiency of the mineral, molybdenum, which is found predominantly in grains and nuts, may inhibit uric acid production and result in higher disease risks (112). Exercise elevates ROS, which may result in higher uric acid as an adaptation to greater antioxidant requirements. However, some attribute the uric acid increase as a result of increased metabolism of a major uric acid precursor, dietary purines. Lowering plasma uric acid using pharmacologic agents does not appear, however, to increase markers of oxidative damage (113). A chronic elevation of uric acid is associated with gout and associated joint pain, making uric acid a poor choice for supplementation with the aim of lowering oxidative stress. Vitamin C, an antioxidant vitamin, has been found to suppress excess plasma uric acid, demonstrating once again that nutrients work together to create a state of cellular/physiologic balance (114).

Vitamin C (Ascorbic Acid)

Vitamin C, a water-soluble vitamin, is an effective antioxidant scavenger of ROS. A useful function of vitamin C is to acquire ROS from both water- and lipid-soluble antioxidants. These ROS "handoffs" to vitamin C enable the water- and lipid-soluble antioxidants to retain their function and scavenge more ROS (115). However, there should be some caution to providing high supplemental doses of vitamin C because when iron and copper are present, vitamin C functions as a *pro*-oxidant rather than as an *anti*oxidant, resulting in a higher rate of lipid oxidative damage (116). Once again, more than enough is not better than enough for producing the desired physiologic outcomes.

Vitamin E (α-Tocopherol)

Vitamin E and related compounds (other tocopherols and tocotrienols) are found in the lipid membranes of cells. Vitamin E is an effective antioxidant that can scavenge and neutralize several ROS forms; it is recycled by transferring the scavenged ROS to water-borne antioxidants such as vitamin C (117,118). Vitamin E is the most abundant lipid-based antioxidant in the human skin and is present in all underlying layers of skin (119). Despite its multiple forms (α-, β-, γ-tocopherol, etc.), only α-tocopherol can reverse a deficiency (120). Although it is a potent antioxidant, athletes should be cautious about taking supplemental doses of vitamin E for the purpose of reducing oxidative damage. A comparison of athletes receiving 800 IU vitamin E daily for 2 months with athletes receiving a placebo prior to competing in the Kona triathlon world championship found that those taking the vitamin E had greater lipid peroxidation and inflammation, as determined by plasma levels of IL-6, IL-1ra, and IL-8, during exercise (106).

Ubiquinone (Coenzyme Q10)

Ubiquinone is a fat-soluble compound that is synthesized by the body but can also be derived from the diet, mainly from soybean oil, meats, fish, nuts, wheat germ, and some vegetables (121). Although a limited amount of Q10 appears in the plasma, most Q10 is found in mitochondria, where it is involved in mitochondrial ATP synthesis and also functions as an antioxidant. Because it is mainly found in the mitochondria and therefore is related to energy metabolism, it is thought that assuring good Q10 status may reduce the oxidative stress and muscle damage associated with heavy exercise. However, in a test of marathoners, it was found that providing excess Q10 reduced neither oxidative stress nor muscle damage (122). A study assessing the combined effects of zinc and Q10 on soccer players found that this antioxidant combination was effective in enhancing the metabolism of thyroid hormone, which is an energy metabolic regulating hormone (123).

Carotenoids (β-Carotene)

The carotenoids are found in the highest concentration in dark green, orange, and yellow-colored fruits and vegetables, directly contributing to their color. They are lipid-soluble compounds, typically found in the membranes of cells, with antioxidant properties making them capable of scavenging ROS. Because they are found in lipids, they limit the formation of peroxides. The most common of the dietary carotenoids are (124):

- *α-carotene* (provitamin A, with 1/24th the activity of vitamin A). Dietary sources include pumpkin, carrots, winter squash, tomatoes, chard, collard greens, green beans, and sweet bell peppers.
- *β-carotene* (provitamin A, with 1/12th the activity of vitamin A). Dietary sources include sweet potato, carrots, dark green leafy vegetables, romaine lettuce, butternut squash, cantaloupe melon, sweet red peppers, dried apricots, peas, and broccoli.
- *β-cryptoxanthin* (provitamin A, with 1/24th the activity of vitamin A). Dietary sources include sweet red peppers, pumpkin, butternut squash, paprika (spice), persimmons, tangerines, papayas, coriander, and carrots.
- *Lutein* (efficient absorber of blue light that helps protect eyes from light-induced oxidative damage) (125). Dietary sources include dark leafy greens, salad greens, summer squash, broccoli, basil, Brussels sprouts, asparagus, green beans, leeks, and green peas.
- *Zeaxanthin* (efficient absorber of blue light that helps protect eyes from light-induced oxidative damage) (125). Dietary sources are the same as for lutein.

- *Lycopene* (powerful anti-inflammatory/antioxidant agent found in red-colored fruits and vegetables, particularly tomatoes, that may reduce prostate and other cancer risk) (126). Dietary sources include watermelon, tomato, pink grapefruit, pink guava, papaya, goji berry, rosehip, asparagus, and red cabbage.

α- and β-carotene and β-cryptoxanthin are all provitamin A substances, meaning that they can be converted by tissues to active vitamin A (retinol). Lutein, zeaxanthin, and lycopene cannot be converted to active vitamin A.

Flavonoids

Flavonoids are found in fruits, vegetables, chocolate, tea, and wine and have important antioxidant and ROS scavenging properties that are health promoting. Although these antioxidant properties are important, their concentrations are 100–1,000 times lower than other antioxidants including vitamin C, uric acid, and GSH (127). Importantly, flavonoids have a risk reduction effect on stroke and cardiovascular disease (128,129). To a large degree, the benefits derived from the consumption of a diet rich in fruits and vegetables are from the high concentration of flavonoids in these foods. The six subclasses of flavonoids include:

- *anthocyanidins* (found in red, blue, and purple berries; red and purple grapes, and red wine)
- *flavan-3-ols* (found in black, green, and oolong tea, cocoa, grapes, berries, red wine, and apples)
- *flavonols* (found in onions, scallions, kale, broccoli, apples, berries, and teas)
- *flavanons* (found in citrus fruit)
- *flavones* (found in parsley, thyme, celery, and hot peppers)
- *isoflavones* (found in soybeans and other legumes)

Measures of Reactive Oxygen Species and Oxidative Damage

It is now well established that physical activity results in ROS production that results in oxidative damage and reduced muscle function. There is also evidence that ROS may result in premature fatigue (130). Further, higher-intensity activities are associated with even greater levels of oxidative damage (71). Taken together, the reduced muscle function and premature fatigue associated with elevated ROS production may have a negative impact on athletic performance. Oxidative stress occurs in specific compartments, including the blood plasma, skeletal muscle, organs, and other tissues. The measure of oxidative stress is complicated because the right compartment(s) must be measured at the right times to detect stress markers. For stress to occur, the antioxidants resident in the measured tissues must be depleted for the markers of oxidative stress to appear (131). The oxidative stress associated with exercise is typically measured through an analysis of metabolites of the ROS reaction(s) that are stable relative to the ROS that created them. (ROS are highly unstable.)

- *DNA oxidation products* are measured via free radical modifications to *guanine*, which can be measured in tissue samples, blood plasma, and urine. Because of the instability of blood and urine samples, direct measurement of muscle tissues is usually preferred (100). A common molecule measured is *8-hydroxydeoxyguanosine*.
- *Protein oxidation* is measured through the presence of carbonyl formation, typically through spectrophotometry or antibody assessment. These assessments can be made from muscle tissue samples and also from blood plasma samples (132).
- *Lipid oxidation* biomarkers are assessed through multiple techniques. Polyunsaturated fatty acids, when affected by ROS, form malondialdehydes, which is a common target for assessment of oxidized lipids (133). Other commonly measured biomarkers of lipid oxidation include lipid hydroperoxides (LOOH) and F_2-isoprostanes. Both biomarkers are derived from lipids in cellular membranes, but the F_2-isoprostanes are considered the superior measure of lipid peroxidation (134).

FINDING A BALANCE BETWEEN MUSCULAR PERFORMANCE AND ANTIOXIDANT INTAKE

It is well established that ROS and their antioxidant countermeasures influence skeletal muscle function (110). A failure to have sufficient antioxidants present in tissues and plasma (*i.e.*, antioxidant deficiencies) to counteract the potentially damaging effects of ROS will increase tissue damage and associated muscle soreness. To a large extent, consumption of antioxidant supplements is thought to be an *easy* strategy for ensuring that tissue defense mechanism is satisfactory. However, there is little evidence to suggest that athletes experiencing frequent high-intensity activity actually benefit from consumption of antioxidant supplements, including vitamins C and E. Moderately low tissue levels of vitamin C and E do not appear to negatively affect exercise capacity or increase muscle weakness (116). Although there are laboratory studies suggesting that providing antioxidants before and during exercise may blunt ROS-related fatigue, there are also studies that antioxidant supplementation may be detrimental (68,135). Importantly, although the consumption of antioxidants may blunt exercise-induced ROS, they may also blunt cellular antioxidant defenses, heat-shock protein, and mitochondrial biogenesis (136–138).

SUMMARY

- The ability of an athlete to obtain and use oxygen is a major factor in athletic performance, regardless of athlete age, gender, or sport.
- Iron is the essential element required in transferring oxygen from the environment and carrying carbon dioxide so it can be expelled via the lungs. Despite these critically important functions, iron deficiency is the most common nutrient deficiency in the general population and in athletes.
- Regardless of the cause of iron deficiency, compromised iron status may have a negative impact on health, mental performance, and athletic performance (11). It is important, therefore, that iron status in athletes be regularly monitored, perhaps yearly, to ensure assessed iron values are within the normal range and to enable an intervention before frank iron deficiency anemia occurs.
- Such a screening should include measures of functional and storage iron, including hemoglobin, hematocrit, and ferritin. Information from such a test will help athletes and those who work with them understand if the foods consumed provide sufficient sources of well-absorbed iron and will help drive dietary changes to help ensure that oxygen uptake is not a limiting factor in athletic performance.
- Surveys have found that normally menstruating female athletes of childbearing age and vegans are at highest risk of developing iron deficiency. However, normal athletic activities can also increase iron deficiency risk through faster RBC destruction and loss via urine and sweat.
- It has been recommended that athletes with iron deficiency anemia seek clinical help to improve iron intake, including from oral iron supplements, and reduce activities that increase iron loss, including a reduction in weight-bearing activity to lower hemolysis, and cessation of blood donations (11).
- Other nutrients, including vitamins B_{12} and folate, are also important in the formation of RBCs, deficiencies of which may lead to macrocytic anemia and lower oxygen delivery to tissues.
- Regardless of the cause, athletes with blood tests indicating iron, folate, or B_{12} deficiency should seek the advice of a physician and registered dietitian to determine the best strategy for corrective action.
- It is well established that physical activity, particularly if it is intense and/or of high duration, will place athletes at higher oxidative stress than nonathletes, suggesting that it is important to consume foods containing adequate amounts of the antioxidant vitamins and minerals.
- Athletes should be cautious, however, of overconsuming these antioxidant nutrients as excess intakes may inhibit normal antioxidant processes.
- Some athletes may suffer from EIA, a condition that limits oxygen uptake and, therefore, performance. There are drugs that are useful in ameliorating EIA, but athletes should be clinically diagnosed as having the condition prior to consuming these prescribed medications to avoid being sanctioned.

Practical Application Activity

Take a survey of friends and family and ask them what supplements they are taking and how often they are taking them. Also, ask what kinds of foods they tend to eat every day. From this survey, do the following:

1. Estimate the antioxidant intake from the supplements.
2. Estimate the antioxidant intake (vitamin C, vitamin E, β-carotene) from the consumed foods. Use the strategy for assessing the nutrient content of foods presented in earlier chapters by accessing the online USDA Food Composition Database (https://fdc.nal.usda.gov).
3. Calculate the percent of the dietary reference intakes (recommended dietary allowance) being consumed by those taking supplements and those not taking supplements, remembering that excessively high intakes may create problems.

CHAPTER QUESTIONS

1. Of the following nutrients, which is involved in delivering oxygen to tissues?
   a. Thiamin
   b. Pyridoxine
   c. Iron
   d. Cobalamin

2. Which of the following nutrients have antioxidant properties that protect cells from oxidation reactions?
   a. Iron, vitamin B_{12}, folic acid, and copper
   b. β-Carotene, vitamin E, vitamin C, and selenium
   c. Vitamin B_1, vitamin B_2, vitamin B_3, and vitamin B_6
   d. Protein and pantothenic acid

3. An iron-containing protein (hemoglobin) in RBCs both picks up oxygen of the lungs and releases carbon dioxide to the lungs.
   a. True
   b. False

4. The air we breathe is ~ ____% oxygen.
   a. 80
   b. 50
   c. 20
   d. 5

5. High-intensity exercise may increase the muscle oxygen requirement by ____ times over a state of rest.
   a. 5
   b. 10
   c. 25
   d. 50

6. Athletes with EIA have no problem bringing sufficient oxygen to cells when exercising.
   a. True
   b. False

7. Transferrin is
   a. Storage iron
   b. The molecule that transfers consumed iron to make new RBCs
   c. The blood protein that transports iron to form hemoglobin
   d. The liver enzyme that oxidizes fatty acids

8. Ceruloplasmin is a _____-containing protein.
   a. Copper
   b. Manganese
   c. Magnesium
   d. Molybdenum

9. Dilutional pseudoanemia occurs because
   a. Iron losses are higher in athletes.
   b. Blood volume increases faster than red blood cells in athletes who initiate an intensive exercise program.
   c. Vitamin B_{12} and folic acid are deficient
   d. Vitamin E deficiency results in faster red blood cell breakdown

10. Foot-strike hemolysis describes a faster breakdown of RBCs because they are "crushed" in the capillaries at the bottom of the feet in a hard running athlete.
    a. True
    b. False

ANSWERS TO CHAPTER QUESTIONS

1. c
2. b
3. a
4. c
5. c

6. b
7. c
8. a
9. b
10. a

Case Study Considerations

1. **Case Study Answer 1:** Athletes have busy schedules, making it difficult to eat right as often as they should, so they often take supplements to help overcome potential nutritional weaknesses in their diet. In a way this can be seen as a "security blanket", but far too often athletes may believe that, since

they are taking nutritional supplements, it is not as important to consider what foods they consume. This leads to a diet that is worse because they feel their nutritional needs are satisfied with the supplements they are consuming. In addition, there is a great deal of "false" information that targets athletes related to the potential benefits of taking the supplements.

2. **Case Study Answer 2**: Supplements often provide an extremely high dose, often greater than the Recommended Dietary Allowances for the nutrients contained in the supplement. This high single dose is likely to exceed the tissue capacity for the nutrient. As a means of self-protection, tissues often reduce their uptake of nutrients provided in large amounts as a means of self-protection. This may result in a down-regulation of the normal tissue adaptation that takes place when athletes change exercise protocols, and the failure of this tissue adaptation leads to more problems related to inflammation and poor recovery. The goal is to "never overfill the tank" and to "never let the tank go to empty." A frequent eating pattern with a wide variety of foods is likely to enhance tissue function by providing nutrients in a manner that the tissues can deal with them. This will lower the risk of nutrient deficiencies, lower the risk of nutrient toxicities, and enable tissue adaptation to the physical demands of exercise.

3. **Case Study Answer 3**: Chronic high doses of antioxidant vitamins may result in tissue rejection of the vitamins and increase the risk that the tissues will be exposed to more ROS that are largely responsible for muscle soreness and a poor muscle recovery. Tissues that are working hard will make adaptations that respond to the activity, but chronically providing extremely high and excessive doses of antioxidant vitamins has the effect of down-regulating absorption and putting the tissues at greater risk because of an inability to make the appropriate adaptations.

REFERENCES

1. Kenney WL, Murray R. Exercise physiology. In: Maughan RJ, editor. Sports nutrition: the encyclopaedia of sports medicine—An IOC publication. Hoboken (NJ): Wiley Blackwell; 2014:20–35.
2. Calbet JAL, González-Alonzo J, Helge JW, Søndergaard H, Munch-Andersen T, Saltin B, Boushel R. Central and peripheral hemodynamics in exercising humans: leg vs arm exercise. Scand J Med Sci Sports. 2015;25(Suppl S4):144–57.
3. Petersson J, Glenny RW. Gas exchange and ventilation-perfusion relationships in the lung. Eur Respir J. 2014;44:1023–41.
4. Raven P, Johnson G, Mason K, Losos J, Singer S. The capture of oxygen: respiration. Biology. 8th ed. New York: McGraw-Hill Education; 2007.
5. Peacock AJ. ABC of oxygen: oxygen at high altitude. BMJ. 1998;317(7165):1063–6.
6. Bassett DR, Howley ET. Limiting factors for maximum oxygen uptake and determinants of endurance performance. Med Sci Sports Exerc. 2000;32(1):70–84.
7. Cotes JE, Chinn DJ, Miller MR. Lung Function: Physiology, Measurement and Application in Medicine. 6th ed. Malden (Mass.): Blackwell Publishing; 2006.
8. Faude O, Kindermann W, Meyer T. Lactate threshold concepts; how valid are they? Sports Med. 2009;39(6):469–90.
9. Vogelmeier CF, Criner GJ, Martinez FJ, Anzueto A, Barnes PJ, Bourbeau J, Celli BR, Chen R, Decramer M, Fabbri LM, Frith P, Halpin DMG, Varela MVL, Nishimura M, Roche N, Rodriguez-Roisin R, Sin DD, Singh D, Stockley R, Vestbo J, Wedzicha JA, Agusti A. Global strategy for diagnosis, management and prevention of chronic obstructive lung disease 2017 report: GOLD executive summary. Respirology. 2017; 22:575–601.
10. Peeling P, Dawson B, Goodman C, Landers G, Trinder D. Athletic induced iron deficiency: new insights into the role of inflammation, cytokines and hormones. Eur J Appl Physiol. 2008;103(4):381–91.
11. Thomas DT, Erdman KA, Burke LM. American College of Sports Medicine Joint Position Statement. Nutrition and athletic performance. Med Sci Sports Exerc. 2016:543–68.
12. Dewoolkar A, Patel ND, Dodich C. Iron deficiency and iron deficiency anemia in adolescent athletes. A systematic review. Int J Child Health Hum Dev. 2014;7(1):11–9.
13. Lee EC, Fragala MS, Kavouras SA, Queen RM, Pryor JL, Casa DJ. Biomarkers in sports and exercise: tracking health, performance, and recovery in athletes. J Strength Cond Res. 2017;31(10):2920–37.
14. Cheng Y, Zak O, Aisen P, Harrison SC, Walz T. Structure of the human transferrin receptor-transferrin complex. Cell. 2004; 116(4):565–76.
15. Barber MF, Elde NC. Escape from bacterial iron piracy through rapid evolution of transferrin. Science. 2014; 346(6215):1362–6.
16. Vashchenko G, MacGillivray RTA. Multi-copper oxidases and human iron metabolism. Nutrients. 2013;5(7):2289–313.
17. Helenius IJ, Tikkanen HO, Haahtela T. Occurrence of exercise induced bronchospasm in elite runners: dependence on atopy and exposure to cold air and pollen. Br J Sports Med. 1998;32:125–9.
18. Best K, McCoy K, Gemma S, Disilvestro RA. Copper enzyme activities in cystic fibrosis before and after copper supplementation plus or minus zinc. Metabolism. 2004;53(1):37–41.
19. Blackmer AB, Bailey E. Management of copper deficiency in cholestatic infants: review of the literature and a case series. Nutr Clin Pract. 2013;28(1):75–86.
20. Nations SP, Boyer PJ, Love LA, Burritt MF, Butz JA, Wolfe GI, Hynan LS, Reisch J, Trivedi JR. Denture cream: an unusual source of excess zinc, leading to hypocupremia and neurologic disease. Neurology. 2008;71(9):639–43.

21. Rowin J, Lewis SL. Copper deficiency myeloneuropathy and pancytopenia secondary to overuse of zinc supplementation. J Neurol Neurosurg Psychiatry. 2005;76(5):750–1.

22. Carmel R. How I treat cobalamin (vitamin B12) deficiency. Blood. 2008;112(6):2214–21.

23. Pawlak R, Parrott SJ, Raj S, Cullum-Dugan D, Lucus D. How prevalent is vitamin B(12) deficiency among vegetarians? Nutr Rev. 2013;71(2):110–7.

24. Barr SI, Rideout CA. Nutritional considerations for vegetarian athletes. Nutrition. 2004;20(7–8):696–703.

25. Stabler SP, Allen RH. Vitamin B12 deficiency as a worldwide problem. Annu Rev Nutr. 2004;24:299–326.

26. Franco RS. The measurement and importance of red cell survival. Am J Hematol. 2009;84(2):109–14.

27. Baik HW, Russell RM. Vitamin B12 deficiency in the elderly. Annu Rev Nutr. 1999;19:357–77.

28. Hernandez CMR, Oo TH. Advances in mechanisms, diagnosis, and treatment of pernicious anemia. Discov Med. 2015; 19(104):59–68.

29. Crider KS, Bailey LB, Berry RJ. Folic acid food fortification-its history, effect, concerns, and future directions. Nutrients. 2011;3(3):370–84.

30. Williams J, Mai CT, Mulinare J, Isenburg J, Flood TJ, Ethen M, Frohnert B, Kirby RS; Centers for Disease Control and Prevention. Updated estimates of neural tube defects prevented by mandatory folic acid fortification—United States, 1995–2011. MMWR Morb Mortal Wkly Rep. 2015;64(1):1–5.

31. Haymes E. Iron. In: Driskell J, Wolinsky I, editors. Sports Nutrition: Vitamins and Trace Elements. Boca Raton: CRC/Taylor & Francis; 2006. p. 203–16.

32. Lukaski HC. Vitamin and mineral status: effects on physical performance. Nutrition. 2004;20(7/8):632–44.

33. Hinton PS. Iron and the endurance athlete. Appl Physiol Nutr Metab. 2014;39(9):1012–8.

34. Portal S, Epstein M, Dubnov G. [Iron deficiency and anemia in female athletes: causes and risks.] Harefuah. 2003;142(10): 698–703, 717.

35. Schumacher YO, Schmid A, Grathwohl D, Bültermann D, Berg A. Hematological indices and iron status in athletes of various sports and performances. Med Sci Sports Exerc. 2002;34(5):869–75.

36. Beals KA. Eating behaviors, nutritional status, and menstrual function in elite female adolescent volleyball players. J Am Diet Assoc. 2002;102(9):1293–6.

37. Jones DP, Coates RJ, Flagg EW, Eley JW, Block G, Greenberg RS, Gunter EW, Jackson B. Glutathione in foods listed in the national cancer institute's health habits and history food frequency questionnaire. Nutr Cancer. 1992;17(1):57–75.

38. Shaskey DJ, Green GA. Sports haematology. Sports Med. 2000;29(1):27–38.

39. Fujii T, Okumura Y, Maeshima E, Okamura K. Dietary iron intake and hemoglobin concentration in college athletes in different sports. Int J Sports Exerc Med. 2015;1(029):1–5.

40. Eichner ER. The anemias of athletes. Phys Sportsmed. 1986; 14(9):122–30.

41. Guy JH, Deakin GB, Edwards AM, Miller CM, Pyne DB. Adaptation to hot environmental conditions: an exploration of the performance basis, procedures and future directions to optimize opportunities for elite athletes. Sports Med. 2015;45(3):303–11.

42. Eichner ER. Fatigue of anemia. Nutr Rev. 2001;59:S17–9.

43. Robinson Y, Cristancho E, Böning D. Intravascular hemolysis and mean RBC age in athletes. Med Sci Sports Exerc. 2006; 38:480–3.

44. Telford RD, Sly GJ, Hahn AG, Cunningham RB, Bryant C, Smith JA. Footstrike is the major cause of hemolysis during running. J Appl Physiol (1985). 2003;94:38–42.

45. Yuka Y, Masaru K, Ayako N, Noriko M. Anemia in female collegiate athletes: association with hematological variables, physical activity and nutrition. Br J Med Med Res. 2015; 7(10):801–8.

46. Fallon KE, Bishop G. Changes in erythropoiesis assessed by reticulocyte parameters during ultralong distance running. Clin J Sport Med. 2002;12(3):172–8.

47. Alhazmi HH. Microscopic hematuria in athletes: a review of the literature. Saudi Sports Med. 2015;15(2):131–6.

48. Jones GR, Newhouse I. Sport-related hematuria: a review. Clin J Sport Med. 1997;7(2):119–25.

49. Wang W, Knovich MA, Coffman LG, Torti FM, Torti SV. Serum ferritin: past, present and future. Biochim Biophys Acta. 2010;1800(8):760–9.

50. Alaunyte L, Stojceska V, Plunkett A. Iron and the female athlete: a review of dietary treatment methods for improving iron status and exercise performance. J Int Soc Sports Nutr. 2015;12:38.

51. DellaValle DM. Iron supplementation for female athletes: effects on iron status and performance outcomes. Curr Sports Med Rep. 2013;12(4):234–9.

52. Constantini NW, Eliakim A, Zigel L, Yaaron M, Falk B. Iron status of highly active adolescents: Evidence of depleted iron stores in gymnasts. Int J Sport Nutr Exerc Metab. 2000; 10:62–70.

53. Beard J, Tobin B. Iron status and exercise. Am J Clin Nutr. 2000;72(2):S594–7.

54. McClung JP, Gaffney-Stomberg E, Lee JJ. Female athletes: a population at risk of vitamin and mineral deficiencies affecting health and performance. J Trace Elem Med Biol. 2014; 28(4):388–92.

55. Carlsen KH, Anderson SD, Bjermer L, Bonini S, Brusasco V, Canonica W, Cummiskey J, Delgado L, Del Giacco SR, Drobnic F, Haahtela T, Larsson K, Palange P, Popov T, van Cauwenberge P; European Respiratory Society; European Academy of Allergy and Clinical Immunology. Exercise-induced asthma, respiratory and allergic disorders in elite athletes: epidemiology, mechanisms and diagnosis: part I of the report from the Joint Task Force of the European Respiratory Society (ERS) and the European Academy of Allergy and Clinical Immunology (EAACI) in cooperation with GA2LEN. Allergy. 2008;63(5):387–403.

56. Carlsen KH, Anderson SD, Bjermer L, Bonini S, Brusasco V, Canonica W, Cummiskey J, Delgado L, Del Giacco SR, Drobnic F, Haahtela T, Larsson K, Palange P, Popov T, van Cauwenberge P; European Respiratory Society; European Academy of Allergy and Clinical Immunology; GA(2)LEN. Treatment of exercise-induced asthma, respiratory and allergic disorders in sports and the relationship to doping: part II of the report from the Joint Task Force of European Respiratory Society (ERS) and European Academy of Allergy and Clinical Immunology (EAACI) in cooperation with GA(2)LEN. Allergy. 2008;63(5):492–505.

57. Boulet L-P, O'Byrne PM. Asthma and exercise-induced bronchoconstriction in athletes. N Engl J Med. 2015;372:641–8.
58. Burnett DM, Burns S, Merritt S, Wick J, Sharpe M. Prevalence of exercise-induced bronchoconstriction measured by standardized testing in healthy college athletes. Respir Care. 2016;61(5): 571–6.
59. Larsson K, Ohlsén P, Larsson L, Malmberg P, Rydström PO, Ulriksen H. High prevalence of asthma in cross country skiers. BMJ. 1993;307:1326–9.
60. Weiler JM, Metzger WJ, Donnelly AL, Crowley ET, Sharath MD. Prevalence of bronchial hyperresponsiveness in highly trained athletes. Chest. 1986;90(1):23–8.
61. Hider RC, Kong X. Iron: effect of overload and deficiency. In: Sigel A, Sigel H, Sigel RKO, editors. Interrelations between essential metal ions and human diseases. Vol 13. Dordrecht: Springer Science and Business Media BV; 2013. p. 229–94.
62. Mannix ET, Farber MO, Palange P, Galassetti P, Manfredi F. Exercise-induced asthma in figure skaters. Chest. 1996;109: 312–5.
63. Provost-Craig MA, Arbour KS, Sestili DC, Chabalko JJ, Ekinci E. The incidence of exercise-induced bronchospasm in competitive figure skaters. J Asthma. 1996;33:67–71.
64. Ross RG. The prevalence of reversible airway obstruction in professional football players. Med Sci Sports Exerc. 2000; 32:1985–9.
65. Wilber RL, Rundell KW, Szmedra L, Jenkinson DM, Im J, Drake SD. Incidence of exercise-induced brochospasm in Olympic winter sport athletes. Med Sci Sports Exerc. 2000; 32:732–7.
66. Hansen-Flaschen J, Schotland H. New treatments for exercise-induced asthma. N Engl J Med. 1998;339:192–3.
67. Lacroix VJ. Exercise-induced asthma. Phys Sportsmed. 1999; 27(12):75–92.
68. Reid MB. Invited review: redox modulation of skeletal muscle contraction: what we know and what we don't. J Appl Physiol (1985). 2001;90(2):724–31.
69. Matsuo M, Kaneko T. The chemistry of reactive oxygen species and related free radicals. In: Radaz Z, editor. Free radicals in exercise and aging. Champaign, IL: Human Kinetics; 2000. p. 1–33.
70. Opara EC. Oxidative stress, micronutrients, diabetes mellitus and its complications. J R Soc Promot Health. 2002; 122(1):28–34.
71. Powers SK, Jackson MJ. Exercise-induced oxidative stress: cellular mechanisms and impact on muscle force production. Physiol Rev. 2008;88(4):1243–76.
72. Stamler JS, Meissner G. Physiology of nitric oxide in skeletal muscle. Physiol Rev. 2001;81(1):209–37.
73. Moncada S, Higgs A. The L-arginine-nitric oxide pathway. N Engl J Med. 1993;329:2002–12.
74. Duncan C, Dougall H, Johnston P, Green S, Brogan R, Leifert C, Smith L, Golden M, Benjamin N. Chemical generation of nitric oxide in the mouth from the enterosalivary circulation of dietary nitrate. Nat Med. 1995;1(6):546–51.
75. Lundberg JO, Govoni M. Inorganic nitrate is a possible source for systemic generation of nitric oxide. Free Radic Biol Med. 2004;37(3):395–400.
76. Larsen FJ, Weitzberg E, Lundberg JO, Ekblom B. Effects of dietary nitrate on oxygen cost during exercise. Acta Physiol (Oxf). 2007;191(1):59–66.
77. Bailey SJ, Fulford J, Vanhatalo A, Winyard PG, Blackwell JR, DiMenna FJ, Wilkerson DP, Benjamin N, Jones AM. Dietary nitrate supplementation enhances muscle contractile efficiency during knee-extensor exercise in humans. J Appl Physiol (1985). 2010;109:135–48.
78. Vanhatalo A, Bailey SJ, Blackwell JR, DiMenna FJ, Pavey TG, Wilkerson DP, Benjamin N, Winyard PG, Jones AM. Acute and chronic effects of dietary nitrate supplementation on blood pressure and physiological responses to moderate-intensity and incremental exercise. Am J Physiol Regul Integr Comp Physiol. 2010 299(4):R1121–31.
79. Lansley KE, Wynyard PG, Fulford J, Vanhatalo A, Bailey SJ, Blackwell JR, DiMenna FJ, Gilchrist M, Benjamin N, Jones AM. Dietary nitrate supplementation reduces the O2 cost of walking and running: a placebo-controlled study. J Appl Physiol (1985). 2011;110:591–600.
80. Husmann F, Bruhn S, Mittlmeier T, Zschorlich V, Behrens M. Dietary nitrate supplementation improves exercise tolerance by reducing muscle fatigue and perceptual responses. Front Physiol. 2019;10:404.
81. O'Gallagher K, Borg Cardona S, Hill C, Al-Saedi A, Shahed F, Floyd CN, McNeill K, Mills CM, Webb AJ. Grapefruit juice enhances the systolic blood pressure-lowering effects of dietary nitrate-containing beetroot juice. Br J Clin Pharmacol. 2021;87(2):577–87.
82. Ashor AW, Shannon OM, Werner A-D, Scialo F, Gilliard CM, Cassel KS, Seal CJ, Zheng D, Mathers JC, Siervo M. Effects of inorganic nitrate and vitamin C co-supplementation on blood pressure and vascular function in younger and older healthy adults: a randomised double-blind crossover trial. Clin Nutr. 2020;39(3):708–17.
83. Jacob J, Gopi S, Divya C. A randomized single dose parallel study on enhancement of nitric oxide in serum and saliva with the use of natural sports supplement in healthy adults. J Diet Suppl. 2018;15(2):161–72.
84. Medina-Remón A, Tresserra-Rimbau A, Pons A, Tur JA, Martorell M, Ros E, Buil-Cosiales P, Sacanella E, Covas MI, Corella D, Salas-Salvadó J, Gómez-Gracia E, Ruiz-Gutiérrez V, Ortega-Calvo M, García-Valdueza M, Arós F, Saez GT, Serra-Majem L, Pinto X, Vinyoles E, Estruch R, Lamuela-Raventos RM; PREDIMED Study Investigators. Effects of total dietary polyphenols on plasma nitric oxide and blood pressure in a high cardiovascular risk cohort. The PREDIMED randomized trial. Nutr Metab Cardiovasc Dis. 2015;25(1):60–7.
85. Rodriguez-Mateos A, Hezel M, Aydin H, Kelm M, Lundberg JO, Weitzberg E, Spencer JPE, Heiss C. Interactions between cocoa flavanols and inorganic nitrate: additive effects on endothelial function at achievable dietary amounts. Free Radic Biol Med. 2015;80:121–8.
86. Tribble GD, Angelov N, Weltman R, Wang B-Y, Eswaran SV, Gay IC, Parthasarathy K, Dao D-HV, Richardson KN, Ismail NM, Sharina IG, Hyde ER, Ajami NJ, Petrosino JF, Bryan NS. Frequency of tongue cleaning impacts the human tongue microbiome composition and enterosalivary circulation of nitrate. Front Cell Infect Microbiol. 2019;9:39.
87. Malakul W, Pengnet S, Kumchoom C, Tunsophon S. Naringin ameliorates endothelial dysfunction in fructose-fed rats. Exp Ther Med. 2018;15(3):3140–6.

88. Cai W, Li J, Shi J, Yang B, Tang J, Truby H, Li D. Acute metabolic and endocrine responses induced by glucose and fructose in healthy young subjects: a double-blinded, randomized, crossover trial. Clin Nutr. 2018;37(2):459–70.

89. Dewhurst-Trigg R, Yeates T, Blackwell JR, Thompson C, Linoby A, Morgan PT, Clarke I, Connolly LJ, Wylie LJ, Winyard PG, Jones AM, Bailey SJ. Lowering of blood pressure after nitrate-rich vegetable consumption is abolished with the co-ingestion of thiocyanate-rich vegetables in healthy normotensive males. Nitric Oxide. 2018;74:39–46.

90. Hughan KS, Wendell SG, Delmastro-Greenwood M, Helbling N, Corey C, Bellavia L, Potti G, Grimes G, Goodpaster B, Kim-Shapiro DB, Shiva S, Freeman BA, Gladwin MT. Conjugated linoleic acid modulates clinical responses to oral nitrite and nitrate. Hypertension. 2017;70(3):634–44.

91. Ahmed KA, Nichols AL, Honavar J, Dransfield MT, Matalon S, Patel RP. Measuring nitrate reductase activity from human and rodent tongues. Nitric Oxide. 2017;66:62–70.

92. Bescos R, Ashworth A, Cutler C, Brookes ZL, Belfield L, Rodiles A, Casas-Agustench P, Farnham G, Liddle L, Burleigh M, White D, Easton C, Hickson M. Effects of Chlorhexidine mouthwash on the oral microbiome. Sci Rep. 2020;10:5254.

93. Joshipura K, Muñoz-Torres F, Fernández-Santiago J, Patel RP, Lopez-Candales A. Over-the-counter mouthwash use, nitric oxide, and hypertension risk. Blood Press. 2020;29(2):103–12.

94. Münzel T, Daiber A. Inorganic nitrite and nitrate in cardiovascular therapy: a better alternative to organic nitrates as nitric oxide donors? Vascul Pharmacol. 2018;102:1–10.

95. Omar SA, Artime E, Webb AJ. A comparison of organic and inorganic nitrates/nitrites. Nitric Oxide. 2012;26(4):229–40.

96. Singh U, Devaraj S, Jialal I. Vitamin E, oxidative stress, and inflammation. Annu Rev Nutr. 2005;25:151–74.

97. Paulsen G, Cumming K, Holden G, Hallén J, Rønnestad BR, Sveen O, Skaug A, Paur I, Bastani NE, Østgaard HN, Buer C, Midttun M, Freuchen F, Wiig H, Ulseth ET, Garthe I, Blomhoff R, Benestad HB, Raastad T. Vitamin C and E supplementation hampers cellular adaptation to endurance training in humans: a double-blind, randomized, controlled trial. J Physiol. 2014;592(8):1887–901.

98. Zhang Y-J, Gan R-Y, Zhou Y, Li A-N, Xu D-P, Li H-B. Antioxidant phytochemicals for the prevention and treatment of chronic diseases. Molecules. 2015;20:21138–56.

99. Ray PD, Huang BOW, Tsuji Y. Reactive oxygen species (ROS) homeostasis and redox regulation in cellular signaling. Cell Signal. 2012;24(5):981–90.

100. Halliwell B, Gutteridge JMC. Free radicals in biology and medicine. 5th ed. New York: Oxford University Press; 2015.

101. Li X, Fang P, Yang WY, et al. Mitochondrial ROS, uncoupled from ATP synthesis, determine endothelial activation for both physiological recruitment of patrolling cells and pathological recruitment of inflammatory cells. Can J Physiol Pharmacol. 2017;95(3):247–52.

102. Anderson EJ, Yamazaki H, Neufer PD. Induction of endogenous uncoupling protein 3 suppresses mitochondrial oxidant emission during fatty acid-supported respiration. J Biol Chem. 2007;282:31257–66.

103. Quindry JC, Stone WL, King J, Broeder CE. The effects of acute exercise on neutrophils and plasma oxidative stress. Med Sci Sports Exerc. 2003;35(7):1139–45.

104. Buonocore D, Negro M, Arcelli E, Marzatico F. Anti-inflammatory dietary interventions and supplements to improve performance during athletic training. J Am Coll Nutr. 2015;34(Suppl 1):62–7.

105. Maggini S, Maldonado P, Cardim P, Newball CF, Latino ERS. Vitamins C, D and Zinc: synergistic roles in immune function and infections. Vitamins Minerals. 2017;6(3).

106. Nieman DC, Henson DA, McAnulty SR, McAnulty LS, Morrow JD, Ahmed A, Heward CB. Vitamin E and immunity after the Kona Triathlon World Championship. Med Sci Sports Exerc. 2004;36(8):1328–35.

107. Venkatraman JT, Pendergast DR. Effect of dietary intake on immune function in athletes. Sports Med. 2002;32(5):323–37.

108. Hwang GH, Ryu JM, Jeon YJ, Choi J, Han HJ, Lee Y-M, Lee S, Bae J-S, Jung J-W, Chang W, Kim LK, Jee J-G, Lee MY. The role of thioredoxin reductase and glutathione reductase in plumbagin-induced, reactive oxygen species-mediated apoptosis in cancer cell lines. Eur J Pharmacol. 2015;765:384–93.

109. Reyes RC, Cittolin-Santos GF, Kim J-E, Won SJ, Brennan-Minnella AM, Katz M, Glass GA, Swanson RA. Neuronal glutathione content and antioxidant capacity can be normalized in situ by N-acetyl cysteine concentrations attained in human cerebrospinal fluid. Neurotherapeutics. 2016;13(1):217–25.

110. Reid MB. Free radicals and muscle fatigue: of ROS, canaries, and the IOC. Free Radic Biol Med. 2008;44(2):169–79.

111. Mikami T, Sorimachi M. Uric acid contributes greatly to hepatic antioxidant capacity besides protein. Physiol Res. 2017;66:1001–7.

112. Maiuolo J, Oppedisano F, Gratteri S, Muscoli C, Mollace V. Regulation of uric acid metabolism and excretion. Int J Cardiol. 2016;213:8–14.

113. McAnulty SR, Hosick PA, McAnulty LS, Quindry JC, Still L, Hudson MB, Dibarnardi AN, Milne GL, Morrow JD, Austin MD. Effects of pharmacological lowering of plasma urate on exercise-induced oxidative stress. Appl Physiol Nutr Metab. 2007;32(6):1148–55.

114. Wilson JX. Mechanism of action of vitamin C in sepsis: ascorbate modulates redox signaling in endothelium. Biofactors. 2009;35(1):5–13.

115. Zuo L, Zhou T, Pannell BK, Ziegler AC, Best TM. Biological and physiological role of reactive oxygen species — the good, the bad and the ugly. Acta Physiol (Oxf). 2015;214(3):329–48.

116. Quindry JC, Kavazis AN, Powers SK. Exercise-induced oxidative stress: are supplemental antioxidants warranted? In: Maughan RJ, editor. Sports nutrition. Vol. XIX of the encyclopedia of sports medicine. International Olympic Committee Medical Commission, Hoboken (NJ): John Wiley & Sons Ltd.; 2014. p. 263–76.

117. Pingitore A, Lima GPP, Mastorci F, Quinones A, Iervasi G, Vassalle C. Exercise and oxidative stress: potential effects of antioxidant dietary strategies in sports. Nutrition. 2015; 31(7–8):916–22.

118. Traber MG. Determinants of plasma vitamin E concentrations. Free Radic Biol Med. 1994;16(2):229–39.

119. Thiele JJ, Weber SU, Packer L. Sebaceous gland secretion is a major physiologic route of vitamin E delivery to skin. J Invest Dermatol. 1999;113(6):1006–10.

120. Traber MG. Vitamin E. In: Erdman JWJ, Macdonald IA, Zeisel SH, editors. Present knowledge in nutrition. 10th ed. Ames, Iowa : Wiley-Blackwell; 2012. p. 214–29.

121. Crane FL. Biochemical functions of coenzyme Q10. J Am Coll Nutr. 2001;20(6):591–8.

122. Kaikkonen J, Kosonen L, Nyyssönen K, Porkkala-Sarataho E, Salonen R, Korpela H, Salonen JT. Effect of combined coenzyme Q10 and d-alpha-tocopheryl acetate supplementation on exercise-induced lipid peroxidation and muscular damage: a placebo-controlled double-blind study in marathon runners. Free Radic Res. 1998;29(1):85–92.

123. Polat M, Polat Y, Akbulut T, Cinar V, Marangoz I. The effects of trainings applied with CoQ10 and zinc supplementation on the thyroid hormone metabolism in soccer players. Biomed Res. 2017;28(16):7070–975.

124. Institute of Medicine, Food and Nutrition Board. Beta-carotene and other carotenoids. Dietary reference intakes for vitamin C, vitamin E, selenium, and carotenoids. Washington (DC): National Academies Press; 2000. p. 325–400.

125. Krinsky NI, Landrum JT, Bone RA. Biologic mechanisms of the protective role of lutein and zeaxanthin in the eye. Annu Rev Nutr. 2003;23:171–201.

126. Di Mascio P, Kaiser S, Sies H. Lycopene as the most efficient biological carotenoid singlet oxygen quencher. Arch Biochem Biophys. 1989;274(2):532–8.

127. Lotito SB, Zhang WJ, Yang CS, Crozier A, Frei B. Metabolic conversion of dietary flavonoids alters their anti-inflammatory and antioxidant properties. Free Radic Biol Med. 2011;51(2): 454–63.

128. Wang X, Ouyang YY, Liu J, Zhao G. Flavonoid intake and risk of CVD: a systematic review and meta-analysis of prospective cohort studies. Br J Nutr. 2014;111(1):1–11.

129. Wang Z-M, Zhao D, Nie Z-L, Zhao H, Zhou B, Gao W, Wang L-S, Yang Z-J. Flavonol intake and stroke risk: a meta-analysis of cohort studies. Nutrition. 2014;30(5):518–23.

130. Reid MB. Reactive oxygen species as agents of fatigue. Med Sci Sports Exerc. 2016;48(11):2239–46.

131. Buettner GR. The pecking order of free radicals and antioxidants: lipid peroxidation, alpha-tocopherol, and ascorbate. Arch Biochem Biophys. 1993;300(2):535–43.

132. Quindry J, Miller L, McGinnis G, Irwin M, Dumke C, Magal M, Triplett NT, McBride J, Urbiztondo Z. Muscle-fiber type and blood oxidative stress following eccentric exercise. Int J Sport Nutr Exerc Metab. 2011;21(6):462–70.

133. Fisher G, Schwartz DD, Quindry J, Barberio MD, Foster EB, Jones KW, Pascoe DD. Lymphocyte enzymatic antioxidant responses to oxidative stress following high-intensity interval exercise. J Appl Physiol (1985). 2011;110(3):730–7.

134. Powers SK, Smuder AJ, Kavazis AN, Hudson MB. Experimental guidelines for studies designed to investigate the impact of antioxidant supplementation on exercise performance. Int J Sport Nutr Exerc Metab. 2010;20(1):2–14.

135. Braakhuis AJ, Hopkinis WG. Impact of dietary antioxidants on sport performance: a review. Sports Med. 2015;45(7): 939–55.

136. Gomez-Cabrera M-C, Domenech E, Viña J. Moderate exercise is an antioxidant: upregulation of antioxidant genes by training. Free Radic Biol. 2008;44(2):126–31.

137. Ristow M, Zarse K, Oberback A, Klöting N, Birringer M, Kiehntopf M, Stumvoll M, Kahn CR, Blüher M. Antioxidants prevent health promoting effects of physical exercise in humans. Proc Natl Acad Sci U S A. 2009;106(21): 8665–70.

138. Strobel NA, Peake JM, Matsumoto A, Marsh SA, Coombes JS, Wadley GD. Antioxidant supplementation reduces skeletal muscle mitochondrial biogenesis. Med Sci Sports Exerc. 2011;43(6):1017–24.

Optimizing Nutrition Strategies for Age and Sex

CHAPTER OBJECTIVES

- Understand the major nutritional issues associated with athletes of different ages and sex.
- Discuss the nutritional demands specific to youth and how these are increased with regular exercise.
- List the multiple factors that must occur simultaneously for bone mineral density (BMD) to achieve a desired level.
- Athletes should understand that the nutritional strategies for *pre-exercise, during-exercise,* and *postexercise* are important components of the exercise itself.
- Discuss the reasons why maintaining a normal growth velocity for young athletes is important and the major nutritional factors that help ensure this occurs.

- Describe the available methods and formulae available for predicting energy expenditure and the formulas that are population specific.
- Understand the potential risks faced by athletes participating in "make weight" and "appearance/aesthetic" sports.
- Determine macronutrient (carbohydrate, protein, and fat) requirements for athletes of different ages and sexes who are involved in different sports.
- Understand the dehydration risks of children and adolescence as compared with those of adults.
- Differentiate between the types of eating disorders observed in athletes.
- Know the major physiologic changes experienced by aging and how meeting nutritional needs can minimize potentially negative changes.

Case Study

All his life he was an athlete—a competitive club swimmer in elementary and junior high school, a competitive high school team swimmer, a scholarship swimmer in college, and a university club water polo swimmer while in graduate school. Then he graduated from graduate school to go to work, and the swimming stopped. John was just too busy with other matters—work, family, young daughter—to continue spending 2–3 hours, 3–5 days each week in the pool.

But after several years he started having a bit more time with his daughter in school, his wife working, and his work requirements less stressful—and of course, the thought of getting back in the pool to race reentered his mind. With support from his family, he decided to join a senior-age group swim club involved in regional, state, and national competitions, and after nearly 10 years he found himself

back in the pool doing laps. The first moment he dove in the water he realized how very much he missed it—and he also realized that his body had changed, with higher body fat and less muscle. But he knew he would not get back into competitive shape if he did not push himself.

To his dismay, after the third day back at swimming practice he could hardly move. Every muscle in his body was sore to the point of making normal movement difficult. The pain was severe, and he did not know what to do. Should he admit that his swimming days were over or should he persevere and keep at it, as best he could? He went to bed thinking about his pain and the decision to make and then had a dream. He dreamt he was back in his collegiate pool and he could visualize the people, the place, the sports beverages, and the food. Yes, the *food*. It struck him like a lightning bolt that when he was competitive, the team had a recovery strategy that included an almost immediate consumption of carbohydrate and protein—sometimes a chicken sandwich and Greek yogurt with fruit—and the coach would not let them leave the pool area without seeing them eat the recovery food. The next morning he made a plan to prepare some recovery food for his late afternoon/early evening swim, although dinner would follow with his family about an hour later. After a few days, he could not believe how much better he felt, and a couple of months later he made the age-group cutoff time to compete at regionals. His swimming life had returned—with a smile.

CASE STUDY DISCUSSION QUESTIONS

Regular exercise coupled with good nutrition helps to minimize the effects of sarcopenia.

1. What are the typical body changes that occur with aging?
2. Are males and females similar? If not, what are the differences?
3. What could be done to minimize the age-related body changes?

INTRODUCTION

No athlete, regardless of age and sex, can perform at an optimal level without a good nutrition plan. The basics of all nutrition plans have similar training and competition strategies, including:

- Eat in a way that encourages long-term health, following general age- and sex-specific population guidelines.
- Satisfy energy needs in a way that dynamically supports the energy requirements of training and competition.
- Ensure that optimal energy stores and hydration status are achieved prior to the initiation of training/competition.
- Follow a hydration strategy that minimizes dehydration while supporting maintenance of blood sugar and blood volume.
- Use a training recovery strategy that returns the athlete to a good state of hydration while supporting efficient muscle synthesis and diminishing muscle soreness.
- Use body composition rather than weight as the marker of whether the nutrition strategy during a training period is providing the right level of nutrients and energy training.
- Allow sufficient time to become well adapted to any new nutrition strategy followed during competition by practicing the strategy during training.

There are additional nutritional considerations for female athletes and for younger and older athletes, to ensure that nutrition supports both optimal health and athletic performance, including nutrition knowledge and practice (1). Female athletes have unique physiologic requirements related to normal menstrual function that may be negatively affected by poor nutrient/energy intake. The *female athlete triad*, which includes eating disorders, menstrual dysfunction, and low bone density, particularly affects a large number of females involved in aesthetic sports where appearance is an integral part of the subjective judging system, including gymnastics, figure skating, and diving. Understanding these risks can help minimize the potential that a female athlete will fail to follow a satisfactory nutrition plan.

Young athletes also have unique risks, particularly related to simultaneously satisfying the combined energy/nutrient needs of growth and physical activity (2). Children have fewer sweat glands that produce less sweat per gland than adults, and children are also susceptible to voluntary dehydration (inadequate fluid consumption even when fluids are available) (3). This combination of lower cooling capacity coupled with inadequate fluid consumption places young athletes at high risk for dehydration-related disorders, which must be a consideration in any nutrition strategy. There is also concern that young athletes are prone to obtain nutrition information from other athletes, health food store personnel, coaches, gym owners, and sports-related magazines. Often, these sources of information are unreliable and may be geared toward selling nutritional product(s) that are neither adequately tested nor needed (4).

Older athletes have a different set of concerns, particularly as they relate to increased heat-stress risk, normal changes in body composition, and the rate of recovery from strenuous athletic endeavors. Individuals working with older athletes should be sensitive to age-associated changes in energy expenditure and increased risk of dehydration. There is also evidence that older athletes may be at risk of inadequate nutrient intakes, particularly of riboflavin, vitamin B_6, vitamin B_{12}, vitamin D, and folate (5,6). Athletes of different ages and sexes have different nutritional risks, associated with energy availability, heat illness, impaired growth and development, menstrual dysfunction, eating disorders, low bone density, alterations in body composition, nutrient inadequacy, and injury risk (7). Although there are general nutrition principles that should be followed by all athletes, different groups (males, females, young, and old) have differing physiologic demands that require modifications of these principles to lower health risks and optimize performance. This chapter reviews the specific nutrition needs of athletes based on age and sex.

THE YOUNG ATHLETE

Youth is a period of accelerated growth, representing a period of life with high nutrient and energy needs. Physical activity further increases the need for nutrients and energy, making nutrition planning an essential component of a young athlete's life to encourage both normal growth and development and also a desired benefit from sport-associated training. Optimal nutrition coupled with physical activity during this period of life has the potential for life-long benefits. However, a poor match between nutrition and physical activity may result in poor tissue and bone development that could increase chronic disease risk later in life. An insufficient energy supply may result in a failure to achieve genetically prescribed growth potential, and inadequate nutrient intake may result in poor development of organ systems. Therefore, nutritional recommendations for young athletes should satisfy both the needs of achieving optimal performance but also satisfy the needs of optimal growth and development (8). As an example, insufficient calcium consumption during the adolescent growth spurt results in low **BMD**, with risk of early-onset osteoporosis (a condition of low BMD that places the individual at fracture risk). It has been estimated that 25% of total bone mass is acquired during the adolescent years (9). Although the stimulation imposed on the skeleton through physical activity is important for bone development, adequate exposure to calcium, vitamin D, protein, and energy is also critically important during this period of growth. There is also beginning evidence that young athletes involved in higher-intensity activity help to reduce the risk of early aging

than low and moderate-intensity activities (10). These data should be a strong encouragement for young people to engage in regular vigorous physical activity to lower chronic disease risk. It is important to consider, however, that lower risk can only occur with an adequate nutrition strategy.

Young athletes should be regularly assessed to ensure the maintenance of a healthy state and normal growth velocity. The growth spurt in girls begins around the age of 10 or 11 and reaches its peak by age 12, with a cessation of growth at age 15 or 16. In boys, the adolescent growth spurt begins at age 12 or 13 and reaches its peak by age 14, with a cessation of growth by the age of 19. During the adolescent growth spurt, lean body mass (LBM) can develop at a rate of approximately 2.3 g/day in females, and 3.8 g/day in males. This represents a LBM increase that is three times faster than before the growth spurt (11). It should be noted that *excess* physical activity (*i.e.*, a level of activity that the individual is not sufficiently accustomed to) that fails to allow for sufficient rest and nutrient intake may result in overuse injuries, including tendinitis, Osgood–Schlatter disease, and stress fractures (12). In adolescent female athletes, secondary amenorrhea (*i.e.*, the cessation of normal menses in someone who has experienced menses) may occur during periods of intense training as a result of insufficient energy intake. Amenorrhea is associated with low estrogen production, which is associated with greater risk of stress fractures (13). A stress fracture can occur at any age with repeated mechanical loading on a bone with a BMD that is too low to handle the repeated stress placed on it. Stress fractures are most likely to be observed in the following situations (Figure 10.1) (12,14):

- When an athlete increases activity intensity too quickly to allow bone density to adapt.
- When the playing/running surface that the athlete has become accustomed to changes, causing greater skeletal stress.
- When an athlete wears shoes that fail to properly cushion and protect the skeleton from the stress of a specific activity.

As a strategy for avoiding overtraining of specific muscles or skeletal area, it has been recommended that young children participate in a *variety* of sports, with sport specialization only occurring after puberty (13,15). This strategy helps young athletes perform better, lower injury risk, and maintain participation in the sport for a longer period of time than those who solely participate in a single sport too early (13).

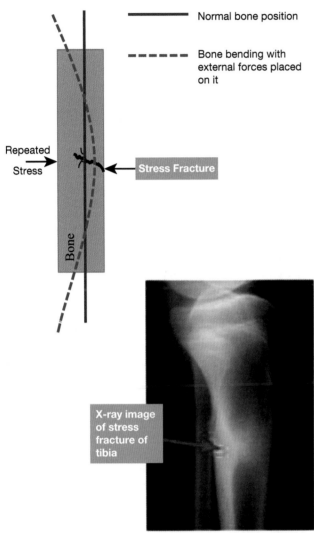

Normal bone position

Bone bending with external forces placed on it

Repeated Stress → ← **Stress Fracture**

Bone

X-ray image of stress fracture of tibia

FIGURE 10.1: What is a stress fracture? (Drawing based on Anderson MW, Greenspan A. Stress fractures. Radiology. 1996; 199:1–12; Bennell KL, Malcolm SA, Wark JD, Brukner PD. Models for the pathogenesis of stress fractures in athletes. Br J Sports Med. 1996;30:200–204; X-ray from Staheli LT. Fundamentals of pediatric orthopedics. 5th ed. Philadelphia (PA): Lippincott Williams & Wilkins; 1996.)

Bone Mineral Density

Cross-sectional area of bone (g/cm^2) and the commonly used measure for determining adequacy of bone strength. Major factors that can affect BMD include race, gender, diet, size, activity amount, activity type, energy availability, cortisol, and estrogen.

ENERGY NEEDS

Consuming sufficient energy is necessary to satisfy the combined needs of growth and development and the demands of training and competition (2). There is difficulty satisfying the nutritional needs during periods of growth because there is a high level of nutritional variability in children of the same age due to sex, size (weight, height), pubertal maturation, genetic history, and growth velocity (7,16). The risk of inadequate energy intake appears to be particularly high in young athletes involved in sports that expend high levels of energy, such as the modern pentathlon, but is also often found to be inadequate in team sports such as soccer (17,18). The relative macronutrient (carbohydrate, protein, and fat) requirement for young athletes is higher than that for an adult involved in the same activity (8,19). To further complicate our understanding of the requirement, the methods available for estimating energy needs in young athletes also have limitations because of their high variability, made worse by the fact that young athletes often report energy consumption patterns that are well below those recommended by predictive equations (20,21). Importantly, the energy needs associated with physical activity induce a higher energy requirement than the energy requirements associated with growth (16). For example, it takes only ~2 kcal/g (or 8.6 kJ/g) of energy for daily weight gain. For a young male athlete, age 15, who is gaining about 13 lb/y (or 6 kg/y), this amounts to an additional growth-related energy requirement of approximately only 33 kcal/day (or 140 kJ/day) (2). Despite this seemingly low requirement for growth, the added requirement of physical activity may place the young athlete in a state of energy intake inadequacy, resulting in compromised growth and development.

One method for considering whether a young athlete has sufficient energy consumption is to use the concept of **energy availability**, which involves asking whether there is sufficient energy available for the activity (22).

Energy Availability

A concept related to having sufficient energy available for physical activity, plus sufficient energy needed to fulfill normal physiologic functions related to growth, the immune system, bone development, muscle development, and muscle repair.

When addressing how much energy is available for the tasks that are done, consider the following equation:

Energy availability = Energy intake − Exercise energy expenditure

[Calculated as: kcal/kg of lean body mass/day]

Failure to supply sufficient energy increases the risk of compromised growth and health, including **delayed**

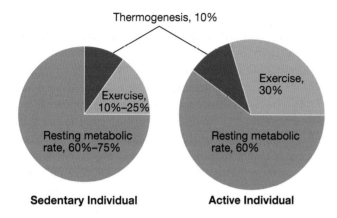

Contributors to total energy expenditure include:
- Resting metabolic rate
- Exercise energy expenditure
- Thermogenesis (Thermic Effect of Food)

FIGURE 10.2: Prediction of total daily energy expenditure. (From Plowman SA, Smith DL. Exercise physiology for health, fitness, and performance. 3rd ed. Philadelphia (PA): LWW (PE); 2010.)

puberty, menstrual dysfunction, low BMD, failure to achieve predicted height, higher injury risk, and higher risk of developing an eating disorder (23,24). Measuring total daily energy expenditure is complex, involving assessment of multiple components with a number of possible strategies for obtaining measures (Figure 10.2).

Total Daily Energy Expenditure

Total (daily) **energy expenditure** (TEE) includes the following components:

- **Resting energy expenditure** *(REE)*: This represents the greatest proportion of energy expended and is either *basal metabolic rate (BMR)*, which is the energy expended by an individual who is at rest and fasting, or the more liberal definition called *resting metabolic rate*, which produces a slightly higher value as the measure is taken when the person may not be in a fasting state or in a complete state of rest. There are common prediction equations for estimating REE, if it cannot be measured via doubly labeled water (DLW) or indirect calorimetry (Box 10.1).
- **Thermic effect of food** *(TEF)*: This represents the energy required to obtain and metabolize the energy in consumed food. TEF accounts for 5%–10% of the total energy consumed, with some foods having a higher TEF than other foods:
  - Carbohydrates: 5%–15% of total energy consumed

Box 10.1 Equations for Predicting BMR

Harris Benedict Equations[a]

BMR calculation for men (metric)

> BMR = 66.47 + (13.75 × weight in kg) + (5.003 × height in cm) − (6.755 × age in y)

BMR calculation for women (metric)

> BMR = 655.1 + (9.563 × weight in kg) + (1.850 × height in cm) − (4.676 × age in y)

Schofield Equations[b]

Age (y): 10–17

Males: BMR = 17.686 × (wt kg) + 658.2
SEE = 105

Females: BMR = 13.384 × (wt kg) + 692.6
SEE = 111

Age (y): 18–29

Males: BMR = 15.057 × (wt kg) + 692.2
SEE = 153

Females: BMR = 14.818 × (wt kg) + 486.6
SEE = 119

Age (y): 30–59

Males: BMR = 11.472 × (wt kg) + 873.1
SEE = 167

Females: BMR = 8.126 × (wt kg) + 845.6
SEE = 111

Age (y): ≥60

Males: BMR = 11.711 × (wt kg) + 587.7
SEE = 164

Females: BMR = 9.082 × (wt kg) + 658.5
SEE: 108

SEE, standard error of estimation.

[a]Source: Harris JA, Benedict FG. A biometric study of human basal metabolism. Proc Natl Acad Sci USA. 1918;4(12):370–3.

[b]Source: Schofield WN. Predicting basal metabolic rate, new standards and review of previous work. Hum Nutr Clin Nutr. 1985:39 Suppl 1):5–41.

- Proteins: 20%–35% of total energy consumed
- Fats: 5%–15% of total energy consumed
  Note: The TEF is also referred to as specific dynamic action and/or thermogenesis.
- **Activity energy expenditure** *(AEE)*: This represents a combination of exercise and nonexercise energy expenditure. There are multiple methods available for predicting AEE (25):
  - *Indirect calorimetry*: Equipment measures inspired and expired air (*i.e.*, oxygen in and carbon dioxide

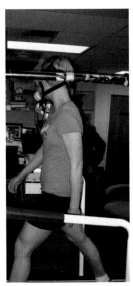

FIGURE 10.3: Subject having energy expenditure measured using indirect calorimetry. A commonly used and relatively accurate measure of energy expenditure at rest and during activity. Device measures oxygen consumed and carbon dioxide expended.

out), providing an excellent prediction of energy expended. The ratio of oxygen in and carbon dioxide out, referred to as the *respiratory quotient*, also provides a good prediction of all components of energy substrate utilization (*i.e.*, of the calories burned, what proportion are from carbohydrate, protein, or fat). Indirect calorimetry equipment is also referred to as a metabolic cart (Figure 10.3).

- *Doubly-Labeled Water (DLW)*: Considered the gold standard, this is capable of assessing all components of energy expenditure. This technique uses isotope tracers to label both the hydrogen and oxygen in water (hence the name "DLW"). By measuring the oxygen tracer (^{18}O) expended in carbon dioxide, it is possible to accurately predict energy expended.
- *Heart rate monitoring*: Heart rate is linearly associated with energy expenditure, so a measure of heart rate provides a prediction of calories burned. A number of wearable activity monitors can predict energy expenditure using heart rate.
- *Accelerometry*: Accelerometers measure movement and thus provide a prediction of energy expenditure. Accelerometry has prediction weaknesses, causing researchers to recommend caution when using accelerometers for predicting energy expended (26,27).
- *Global positioning system (GPS)*: The GPSs have the capacity to monitor movement and speed of movement to predict energy expenditure. Typically, newer GPSs are used in conjunction with accelerometers and heart rate monitors to improve energy expenditure prediction (28).
- *Pedometry*: Although providing a reasonably accurate measure of movement, pedometers fail to provide an accurate means of predicting energy expended across all activity modes. Therefore, they should be used with caution when estimating energy expended (29).

Questionnaires: There are many types of questionnaires available that attempt to predict energy expenditure through a description of activity intensity that is based on a MET-value scale (*i.e.*, multiples of REE). The Ainsworth compendium lists activity codes and associated energy expenditures (Box 10.2) (30).

Box 10.2	**Approximate Energy Expenditure for Various Activities in Relation to Resting Needs for Males and Females of Average Size**

Activity category representative value for activity factor per unit time of activity

Resting, Sleeping, Reclining: REE × 1.0

Very light: REE × 1.5
Seated and standing activities, painting trades, driving, laboratory work, typing, sewing, ironing, cooking, playing cards, and playing a musical instrument.

Light: REE × 2.5
Walking on a level surface at 2.5–3 mph, garage work, electrical trades, carpentry, restaurant trades, house-cleaning, child care, golf, sailing, and table tennis.

Moderate: REE × 5.0
Walking at 3.5–4 mph, weeding and hoeing, carrying a load, cycling, skiing, tennis, and dancing.

Heavy: REE × 7.0
Walking with load uphill, tree felling, heavy manual digging, basketball, climbing, football, and soccer.
When reported as multiples of basal needs, the expenditures of males and females are similar.

Source: Institute of Medicine, Food and Nutrition Board. Recommended dietary allowances. 10th ed. Subcommittee on the Tenth Edition of the RDAs, Food and Nutrition Board, Commission on Life Sciences, National Research Council. Washington (DC): National Academy Press; 1989. Based on values reported by Durnin and Passmore (1967) and WHO (1985).

Delayed Puberty

Puberty is the period of time when a body grows and develops from that of a child to an adult, including maturation of the sex organ, facial hair in males, and conversion of some testosterone to estradiol for the development of the uterus in females. A delay in this biologic clock, often from insufficient energy intake, may have lifelong implications for organ, skeleton, and linear growth development.

Total Energy Expenditure

Represents the combined energy requirements for rest, activity, TEF, and development (if growing, pregnant, or lactating).

Activity Energy Expenditure

Represents the energy needed to satisfy the energy needs for physical activity. This is typically calculated as a multiple of the energy required at rest. Example: If someone requires 50 calories/hour at rest, and this person exercises at an intensity of double that at rest (i.e., walking), the hourly requirement for that hour would be 100 calories. If that person was working at an intensity five times that at rest (i.e., running quickly), the hourly requirement for that hour would be 200 calories.

Thermic Effect of Food

Represents the energy needed to obtain energy from consumed foods. Some foods require more energy investment to derive energy (e.g., protein) than other foods (e.g., carbohydrates). The average for all foods is ~10% of the total energy derived from foods.

TEF and REE can be predicted from indirect calorimetry, whereas TEE can be predicted from DLW (Box 10.3).

Using these methods to predict energy intakes and expenditures is complex, and given the individual variability in methods and individual growth rates, excess reliance on these methods as the sole determinant of whether a young athlete is receiving sufficient energy/nutrients is not advised. There are no commonly available energy expenditure devices/methods/predictive equations that provide sufficiently accurate results to confidently determine whether the nutrients/energy consumed are sufficient to result in desired growth and development. These methods/devices should be considered guides and estimates and, because of the potential inaccuracies, normal indicators of growth and development should be used. In children, the traditional method for assessing the adequacy of energy consumption is through a longitudinal assessment of standard weight-for-age, height-for-age, and weight-for-height percentile tables (Figure 10.4). After the age of 2, there is an expectation that growth percentiles are sustained with increasing age, and a failure to do so may be an indication of inappropriate energy delivery, malnutrition, and/or disease. For instance, a child athlete who is at the 50th percentile in height-for-age at age 12, but at a lower percentile at age 14 would suggest that the athlete has insufficient energy intake, malnutrition, or disease, warranting further investigation to determine the cause

Box 10.3 — Step-by-Step Strategy for Estimating 24-Hr Energy Balance in the Young Athlete

Energy Requirement Prediction

Step 1. Predict REE using the age/sex-appropriate Schofield equation.
Step 2. Calculate the hourly value obtained in step 1, by dividing the REE by 24.
Step 3. Using the obtained REE value, calculate the number of hours spent on different energy expenditures using the information in Table 10.1. Example. Sleeping for 7 hr = 1 × REE × 1; exercising at a light level for 2 hr = 2.5 × REE × 2; etc.
Step 4. Sum the values in step 2 for 24-hr energy expenditure
Step 5. Multiply the value in step 3 by 1.10 to calculate the energy expenditure +10% for the TEF (i.e., the calories required to obtain the energy from the energy consumed). This is the value of the total predicted energy required.

Energy Intake Prediction

Step 1. Write down all the foods/beverages consumed (amounts, preparation, etc.) during the 24-hr period.
Step 2. Using a computerized table of food composition, find the energy (caloric) content of each food/beverage consumed.
Step 3. Sum the values obtained in Step 2.

Calculating Energy Balance

Step 1. Divide predicted energy consumed by predicted energy required to obtain energy balance. Example:

Predicted energy consumed = 2,000 kcal
Predicted energy required = 2,500 kcal
2,000/2,500 = 0.80 (the amount consumed is 80% of the predicted requirements, indicating that the person is in a negative energy balance).

Table 10.1	Internal and External Factors That Can Influence BMD

Internal Factors	External Factors
Sex/race: Women typically have lower BMD than men. However, multiple factors can influence within-sex BMD. ■ Women with menstrual irregularity have lower BMD than women with regular menses. (Estrogen is lower with irregular menses, and estrogen inhibits the activity of osteoclasts, the cells that break down bone.) ■ Population studies suggest that African-American and Hispanic women have *higher* BMD than White and Asian women.	**Diet:** Adequate level of vitamin D, calcium, and energy is associated with higher BMD, whereas an inadequate level of any of these three is associated with lower BMD. Other dietary factors may also influence BMD: ■ High dietary fiber (>30 g/day) may lower calcium absorption; high caffeine intake is associated with high urinary calcium loss; ■ High alcohol consumption alters nutrient absorption and metabolism and is associated with lower BMD.
Age: After peak BMD is reached at around the age of 20, BMD is typically stable with only moderate reductions in BMD until the age of 50. ■ After age 50, BMD decreases more rapidly for both sexes. ■ Women experience a faster decline in BMD following menopause.	**Weight:** Higher weight is associated with higher BMD because of the skeletal adaptation associated with increased loading. ■ However, obesity is associated with higher weight but less physical activity/movement, which can result in a decline in BMD.
Size: Lower size results in less stress on bone, with less adaptive need to increase BMD. ■ With the right nutrient/energy availability, bones respond to increased loading stress from weight or activity with higher BMD.	**Activity:** Mechanical loading on bones is important to derive the adaptive increase in BMD. (Wolff's law of osteology: "Use it or lose it.") ■ When the loading occurs, there is significant skeletal development (youth), bones can achieve a significantly higher BMD that makes the individual more resistant to developing low BMD later in life. ■ However, physical activity during youth that is associated with energy, calcium, or vitamin D deficiency fails to adequately increase BMD, placing the individual at *higher* risk of osteoporosis later in life.

BMD, bone mineral density.

of cessation of linear growth that resulted in the drop in percentile.

Some young athletes may, of course, be overweight, which is commonly addressed through a reduction in energy intake. However, severely restricting energy intake in a growing child has the potential to negatively affecting long-term health (24). Using body composition measures in this population rather than weight may be a useful strategy. Doing so can help to ensure that lean mass is increased, indicating normal growth, while there is a concomitant reduction in fat mass to lower obesity risk. Using weight or body mass index by itself will not provide the information necessary to ensure the athlete is sustaining a normal growth pattern. This is clearly a complicated issue, as insufficient energy consumption may be

associated with lower weight, but the lower weight may be the result of reduced lean mass with a higher body fat percentage (31).

There is a strong connection between sport involvement and positive self-esteem in young athletes (32). However, there is also evidence that *appearance* sports, which are subjectively scored (*i.e.*, figure skating, gymnastics), may increase the risk of eating disorder/disordered eating, resulting in energy intakes that fail to satisfy the combined needs of growth and physical activity (33). There is limited evidence that some athletes with lower-than-expected growth patterns during adolescence may experience catch-up growth after leaving competitive sport (34). This has been seen in former elite gymnasts, suggesting that there may be some potential

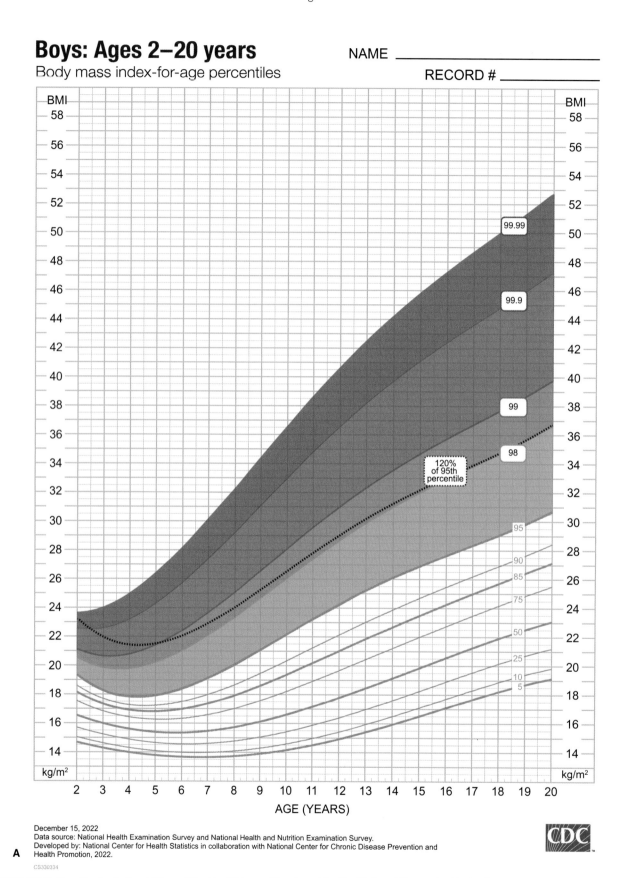

Boys: Ages 2–20 years
Body mass index-for-age percentiles

NAME _____

RECORD # _____

December 15, 2022
Data source: National Health Examination Survey and National Health and Nutrition Examination Survey.
Developed by: National Center for Health Statistics in collaboration with National Center for Chronic Disease Prevention and
Health Promotion, 2022.

A

CS330334

CDC

FIGURE 10.4: Growth charts for children: (**A**) girls (**B**) boys. (Developed by the National Center for Health Statistics in collaboration with the National Center for Chronic Disease Prevention and Health Promotion. Clinical growth charts. 2000. Available from: https://www.cdc.gov/growthcharts/clinical_charts.htm)

Girls: Ages 2–20 years
Body mass index-for-age percentiles

NAME _____

RECORD # _____

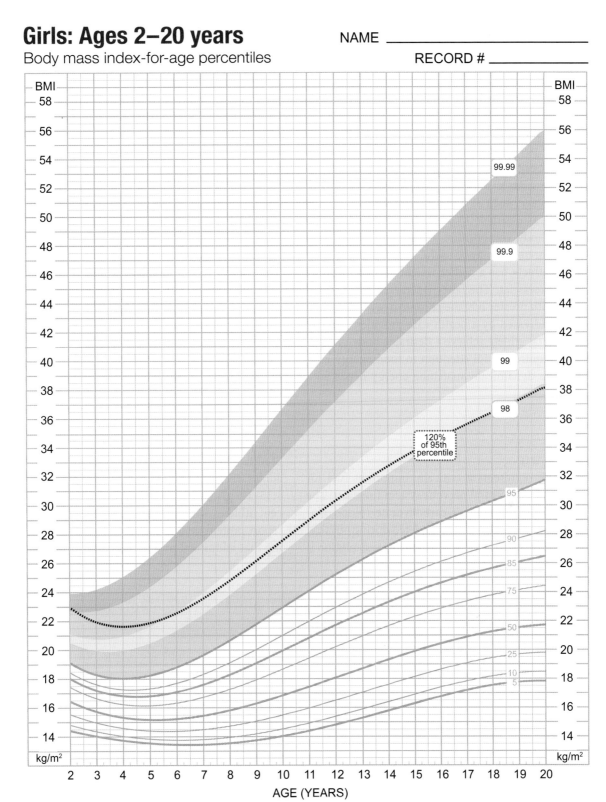

December 15, 2022
Data source: National Health Examination Survey and National Health and Nutrition Examination Survey.
Developed by: National Center for Health Statistics in collaboration with National Center for Chronic Disease Prevention and
Health Promotion, 2022.
CS330334

B

FIGURE 10.4: (*continued*)

to return to the genetically expected weight/height percentile once the energy deficiency associated with sport participation no longer exists (35). However, there is also evidence that athletes with inadequate energy intakes during periods of growth fail to achieve normal developmental expectations (23).

Although not a common occurrence in a physically active young person, there is an ever-increasing rate of childhood obesity across all spectrums of society. In sports where a large mass/size is perceived as providing an advantage, such as a lineman in football, obesity may be seen as desirable (36). This is a prime example of where a body composition assessment, rather than weight measurement, may be useful in determining if the overweight athlete has a higher weight because of more muscle or excess fat. The latter (increased fat mass) is associated with greater lifetime chronic disease risks and should be addressed by a health care provider. Helping a young overfat athlete achieve a desirable body composition will require careful attention to food/energy consumed, while dynamically matching energy needs with expenditure (37).

Energy Substrate Distribution

Carbohydrate

Carbohydrate represents a critically important fuel for both muscular and central nervous system function. The primary fuel for the brain is carbohydrate (blood glucose), which can quickly become depleted during physical activity causing mental fatigue. Carbohydrate depletion is associated with muscular fatigue and poor performance (38). It was found that there is a tendency for young athletes to consume sufficient carbohydrate before and after exercise, but both male and female athletes fail to consume recommended levels of carbohydrate (30–60 g carbohydrate/hour) during practice and/or competition (39). Failure to consume sufficient carbohydrate during exercise, which was found to occur in 82% of young male and 71% of young female athletes, is a contributing factor in failing to satisfy total energy needs. Therefore, care should be taken to ensure that athletes have sufficient carbohydrate availability before, during, and following physical activity. This is particularly important because, unlike fat, humans have limited carbohydrate storage. The current recommended carbohydrate intake strategy for adult athletes with little reason to modify the requirements for young athletes is shown in Box 10.4.

Protein

The general recommendation for adult *athlete* protein intake is 1.2–2.0 g/kg, or approximately doubles that of the adult *nonathlete* population (0.8 g/kg) (40). For nonathlete adolescents experiencing peak growth velocity, protein requirements are higher than for those experiencing steady growth at a slower pace, ranging from ~0.8–1.0 g/kg. Studies have found that the protein requirements for adolescent athletes are nearly double this, or about 1.35–1.6 g/kg (2,20,41). Studies have found that adolescent athletes without disordered eating/eating disorders report protein intakes that tend to satisfy needs, suggesting that additional protein intakes, through either foods

---

Box 10.4	**Current Recommended Carbohydrate Intake Strategy for Adult and Young Athletes**

For immediate recovery after exercise:
- (0–4 hr): 1–1.2 g/kg/hr, then resume daily fuel needs

For daily recovery:
- Low-intensity or skill-based activity: *3–5 g/kg/day*
- Moderate exercise program (*e.g.,* training 1 hr/day): *5–7 g/kg/day*
- Endurance program (*e.g.,* training 1–3 hr/day): *–10 g/kg/day*

- Extreme exercise program (*e.g.,* training 4–5 hr/day): *8–12 g/kg/day*

During sport:
- Short duration exercise (0–75 minutes): *small amount[a]*
- Medium/long duration exercise (75 minutes–2.5 hour): *30–60 g/hr*

[a]The current Joint Position Statement on Nutrition and Athletic Performance recommends small amounts of carbohydrate, including mouth rinse for short-duration exercise lasting 45–75 minutes. However, please note that mouth rinse does not contribute to energy availability.

Sources: Desbrow B, McCormack J, Burke LM, Cox GR, Fallon K, Hislop M, Logan R, Marino N, Sawyer SM, Shaw G, Star A, Vidgen H, Leveritt M. Sports Dietitians Australia Position Statement: sports nutrition for the adolescent athlete. Int J Sport Nutr Exerc Metab. 2014;24: 570–84; Thomas DT, Erdman KA, Burke LM. American College of Sports Medicine Joint Position Statement. Nutrition and athletic performance. Med Sci Sports Exerc. 2016;48(3):543–68.

or supplements, are not necessary (20). However, there is growing evidence that *how* and *when* the protein is consumed makes a difference in whether the protein is optimally utilized by tissues. Studies on adults have found that consumption of relatively small amounts of protein of ~20 g that is distributed throughout the day and also provided immediately after physical activity improves muscle protein synthesis (MPS) (42,43). These findings suggest that creating appropriate environments for young athletes that help to encourage protein consumption at optimal intervals would be a useful strategy. Current protein intake recommendations for optimizing MPS following resistance-type exercise include (44):

- 20 g easily digested protein (*e.g.*, whey protein isolate) postexercise and at rest
- ~40 g of slowly digested protein (*e.g.*, from meals) before a long gap in eating opportunity, such as before evening sleep.
- Frequency and type of intake should be individualized, depending on type and duration of exercise, age, sex, and current body composition.
- Avoiding an energy balance deficiency is critical to ensure protein consumption can be used anabolically to enhance musculature.

Fat

As a concentrated source of energy, sufficient fat intake is necessary to ensure a satisfactory level of energy is consumed. Fat intake is also needed for fat-soluble vitamin intake and the intake of essential fatty acids (7). Stored fat within muscle and fat tissue, even in the leanest athletes, is the primary source of energy for physical activity, with adaptations for improved fat metabolism that occurs as a result of the greater energy needs associated with exercise (45). However, the high energy density of fat also increases the risk of obesity with excess consumption. Currently, the recommended intake of fat as a proportion of total energy intake is 20%–35%. Although there are studies finding that children use more fat and less carbohydrate than adults during endurance activities and more intense activities, the easy availability of high-fat convenience foods may make it too easy for young athletes to exceed the desired level of intake (46,47).

Nutrients

All nutrients are, of course, needed for optimal tissue development and lower disease risk. However, it has been found that three nutrients in particular, including iron, calcium, and vitamin D, may not be obtained in sufficient amounts in young athletes and require special attention. Recent studies have found that many young athletes between the ages of 11 and 17 years take vitamin and mineral supplements, with the belief that these supplements will provide them with the competitive edge they seek, and that a normal diet is simply not enough to attain a performance benefit (46,48,49). There is evidence from these studies that parents (not trainers or coaches) play the major role in young athlete supplement consumption (49). Coaches often provide young athletes with nutrition information, but studies suggest that most coaches have inadequate nutrition knowledge to provide such information (50–52). Although many supplements may neither help nor detract from health and performance, there are known risks associated with excess consumption of some nutrients through supplementation that should encourage those who work with young athletes to be cautious about supplement intake.

Ideally, supplement consumption should be used if and when there is a known nutrient deficiency (*e.g.*, anemia), and consuming foods to correct the problem is not a possible strategy. It is notable that, of the young athletes taking supplements, fewer than 39% had ever met with a dietitian to discuss safe and effective supplementation practices (53).

Iron

Insufficient iron intake is the most common nutrient deficiency worldwide, and iron deficiency anemia has approximately the same prevalence (3%) in the general public as in athletes (54). However, low ferritin levels (*i.e.*, low iron stores) are often observed when young athletes are assessed (55,56). The prevalence of nonanemia iron deficiency ranges from 7% to 57% in female athletes, and from 4% to 31% in male athletes, depending on the criteria used to determine the depletion of iron stores (ferritin) (57). Poor iron storage, even without anemia, is associated with suboptimal adaptation to training and poor athletic performance, both of which appear to be related to poor oxygen delivery and lowered synthesis of adenosine triphosphate (2). The risk of iron deficiency in young athletes is higher than in young nonathletes because of a combination of issues, including a greater rate of red blood cell hemolysis, blood loss in the gastrointestinal (GI) tract, iron losses in sweat, and blood loss through menstruation in female athletes (57).

Studies examining young athletes suggest that males tend to exceed the recommended intake of iron, whereas females have a higher level of variability in iron intake (21). If it is not possible to consume sufficient iron from food, there is clearly an elevated risk of iron deficiency, reduced performance, and impaired immune function. Consumption of iron-rich foods is the best strategy, as food is the carrier of both energy and nutrients, both critically important for ensuring normal growth and development and supporting physical activity (58). A seemingly easy strategy for ensuring adequate iron intake, supplemental iron intake is associated with GI distress and potentially other negative health issues. Therefore, the assumption that a daily iron supplement is an effective strategy for lowering iron deficiency risk requires further investigation. There is evidence, for instance, that a single weekly iron supplement is as effective as a daily iron supplement in reducing iron deficiency, but without the associated negative side effects (59). A good strategy would be for an athlete to seek the advice of a qualified medical professional before self-prescribing iron supplements.

Calcium

Calcium requirements for children and adolescents are higher than those for adults because of the significant bone development that occurs during this period of life. Putting "stress" on the skeleton, which occurs with physical activity, increases calcium acquisition by bones as a logical adaptation to increase the skeletal strength needed for exercise-associated stress (60,61). This increased calcium acquisition by bones requires a higher calcium intake. The recommended calcium intake is 1,300 mg/day for children and adolescents, which is 300 mg/day higher than the adult requirement. Assuming the calcium requirement is satisfied, the combination of higher calcium intake and physical activity will result in significantly higher BMD by the end of adolescence when compared with nonphysically active youth (62). Recent data suggest that endurance athletes may experience skin-related losses of calcium, suggesting that these athletes may consider consuming higher-calcium food or taking a small calcium supplement prior to exercise (63).

Vitamin D

Vitamin D can be obtained from the diet from vitamin D–fortified foods, including milk and orange juice, and several other foods, including egg, beef liver, sardines, margarine, canned tuna, salmon, swordfish, and cod liver oil. With the exception of eggs, milk, and orange juice, which are not always fortified with vitamin D, children and adolescents do not typically consume a significant amount of other foods. As a result, vitamin D status is most likely a function of the vitamin D derived from sunlight exposure (Ultraviolet "B" sunlight converts cholesterol under the skin to inactive vitamin D, which is then converted to the active form by the kidneys and liver.).

Vitamin D is essential for multiple physiologic outcomes, including, calcium absorption, skeletal muscle function, and muscle recovery (64). So the young athlete who consumes ample quantities of calcium, but spends the majority of time in school and training indoors (e.g., basketball, gymnastics, figure skating) may be at risk for inadequate vitamin D status and poor bone development. A study of adolescent female gymnasts found that about 33% had below-optimal serum vitamin D status (65). Poor vitamin D status is also associated with reduced athletic performance and increased musculoskeletal injury risk. There is evidence of widespread vitamin D deficiency in athletes and dancers (mean age 14.7 years), particularly in those who train indoors (66). Improving vitamin D status with regular sunlight exposure or supplementation in athletes with suboptimal serum vitamin D levels helps to correct both performance and injury risk problems (67,68).

Fluids

Children and adolescents have a different physiologic strategy for dissipating exercise-associated heat than adults for several reasons (69–72):

- They have a higher **body surface area (BSA)** (the measured surface of the body) that acquires more heat from the environment on a hot day and loses more heat to the environment on a cold day.
- They produce more heat per unit weight during physical activity.
- They have fewer sweat glands per unit of surface area, and each sweat gland produces less sweat, resulting in a reduced potential to dissipate heat.

Body Surface Area

BSA is the calculated or measured surface area of a human body. The most widely used formula for calculating BSA is the DuBois formula, where: $BSA = 0.007184 \times weight^{0.425} \times height^{0.725}$. Typical BSA for a 12- to 13-year-old is 1.33 m², for an adult woman 1.4 m², and for man 1.9 m². Larger BSAs are associated with higher sweat rates (more sweat glands), resulting in better cooling capacity. The lower BSA of children may increase heat illness risk.

As a result, children and adolescents are more reliant on radiative and conductive cooling through greater peripheral blood flow, rather than through sweating.

In addition, adolescents who exercise regularly appear to adapt to the increased requirement for heat dissipation through greater peripheral vasodilation and blood flow (73).

Regardless of whether cooling occurs primarily through sweating or through greater peripheral blood flow, consumption of adequate fluid of the right composition is necessary to avoid heat illness in young athletes (74). In addition, despite the lower sweat rate, there is strong evidence that physically active adolescents can experience significant fluid loss when training in a hot environment (75). Water consumption is advised for young athletes involved in moderate-intensity activity in thermoneutral environments, but prolonged higher-intensity activity may require the additional carbohydrate and electrolytes offered by sports beverages or, perhaps, milk (76).

Coaches and parents should become fully aware of the mental and physical signs of dehydration and heat-related injuries, with special attention paid to the heat index (see Chapter 7). The voluntary dehydration (*i.e.,* they consume insufficient fluids to maintain hydration state even when fluids are available) seen in young athletes should encourage those who work with them to observe drinking patterns. It is also recommended for these young athletes to have readily available beverages that they are more likely to consume (77). Both parents and coaches should be encouraged to attend nutrition education sessions taught by a qualified sports dietitian, as it has been found that even relatively brief time in these sessions (two for 90 minutes each) significantly improves both the number and accuracy of the nutrition information provided to young athletes (78). There is also good reason to believe that nutrition education programs that target young athletes are successful in helping these athletes understand the nutrition strategies needed for optimizing growth, development, and athletic performance (79).

THE FEMALE ATHLETE

A cursory review of the dietary reference intake (DRI) provides a clear nutritional truth: Males and females have distinctive nutritional needs, which should be addressed through appropriate nutritional intakes that address these differences. Male athletes, for any given sport, have greater relative musculature than females. However, female athletes develop their skeletons sooner than males and, therefore, have nutritional needs specific to this earlier growth pattern. Females have a slightly greater

capacity to "burn" fat as an energy substrate than males, and the larger muscle mass of males represents a larger storage capacity for carbohydrate than females, suggesting that males have a greater potential for power activities, whereas females may be more endurance oriented. Appearance sports, including gymnastics, diving, and figure skating, have female athletes who are more likely than other athletes to restrict energy intake, resulting in a higher risk of eating disorders (80). Similar problems are observed in female athletes participating in weight-category sports, such as judo, taekwondo, wrestling, and lightweight rowing (81). It is important to consider that, when attempting to help these female athletes to improve nutrient/energy intake, appetite and psychological factors should be incorporated into the recommendations (82).

Females, typically between the ages of 11 and 13, have their first menstrual period, which carries with it its own unique set of nutritional requirements (83). These and other sex differences create unique nutritional realities that must be fulfilled to optimally satisfy the health and performance needs of female athletes. It is important that the interpretation of general sport nutrition guidelines, which are often presented as a single set of guidelines that are not sex specific, be interpreted carefully to address the unique requirements of both male and female athletes (84). In particular, there should be some thought to whether the foods/beverages consumed by the female athlete are sufficient to fully support the hormone production required to maintain a normal menstrual cycle; the smaller body size and musculature of females, compared with that of males, should also be a consideration in interpreting general nutrition recommendations. Female athletes in "appearance" sports may be particularly at risk for eating patterns that result in poor energy availability, which can increase health risks and also result in poor training benefits. Nutrition education should be provided to female athletes, as it has been found that higher nutrition knowledge in young female athletes is associated with better dietary quality and improved eating practices (85,86).

ENERGY NEEDS

Energy intakes, regardless of age and sex, are based on total weight, weight of the metabolic mass, growth phase, and duration and intensity of exercise. Surveys of female athletes commonly report an underconsumption of energy, leading many to conclude that female athletes are at an increased risk of developing eating disorders regardless of the type of sport in which they

Box 10.5	**Energy Availability Calculation**

1. **Step 1:** Estimate the energy obtained from the diet.
2. **Step 2:** Estimate the energy used during exercise training.
3. **Step 3:** Subtract the energy used during exercise training from the total energy obtained from the diet to obtain remaining energy (kcal).
4. **Step 4:** Estimate the proportion of the body that is FFM (*i.e.,* total mass – fat mass) to obtain kg FFM.
5. **Step 5:** Calculate energy availability = remaining energy (kcal)/kg FFM/day.

participate (87). In addition, the literature suggests that intense exercise has an impact on the female reproductive system, with amenorrhea or oligomenorrhea a common outcome. An increase in energy intake can offset the high energy demand and may be sufficient to reverse the menstrual dysfunction and halt the associated reduction in bone mass (88). Energy availability (Box 10.5) is an important factor in determining whether female athletes meet their energy requirements. By definition, energy availability represents the available energy for supporting body functions after energy is used to satisfy the requirements for exercise training. It is estimated that female athletes who fall below 30 kcal/kg fat-free mass (FFM) are at risk for insufficient energy to support vital body functions. Furthermore, a negative energy balance results in decreased hormone levels, particularly when self-selected/unguided, and may be associated with reduced performance in both anaerobic and aerobic athletic endeavors (40,89).

Female athletes who participate in vigorous exercise training are at risk for low energy availability, which results in irregular menses or a cessation of menses and is associated with poor skeletal development (*i.e.,* low BMD, Table 10.1) (90,91).

Recent evidence suggests that virtually all menstrual disturbances in female athletes are the result of inadequate energy consumption, either from restrictive intakes or from failure to adequately satisfy increased exercise-associated energy requirements (92,93). A significant proportion (39%) of female athletes were found to have low energy availability, with 54% of these presenting with menstrual function abnormalities (94). Female athletes with components of the *female athlete triad* are at increased risk of developing other endocrine, GI, renal,

neuropsychiatric, musculoskeletal, and cardiovascular problems (95).

This is paradoxical in athletes, as with sufficient energy, vitamin D, and calcium availability, weight-bearing physical activity (*i.e.,* running, jumping, weight-lifting) should *increase* BMD. However, in chronically low energy availability, young female athletes may develop osteopenia (*i.e.,* low bone density) and/or osteoporosis (*i.e.,* bone density sufficiently low that has reached the fracture threshold) (24). The American College of Sports Medicine (ACSM) recommends that energy availability should be restored through an increase in energy consumption, a reduction in energy expenditure, or a combination of the two to improve reproductive function and skeletal health in female athletes (Figure 10.5) (24). Health care professionals working with female athletes should assess the common outcomes of low energy availability, including an assessment of menstrual status and BMD (96).

There is also evidence that wide fluctuations in within-day energy balance may also have an impact on menstrual function and bone health in young female athletes. A case study of an elite junior female triathlete suggested that nearly half of the energy consumed was after 6:00 PM, which was associated with low energy balance earlier in the day while the athlete was physically active. This, coupled with a low energy availability, was associated with low tri-iodothyronine (T_3, a thyroid hormone), where low T_3 is a sign that the body is trying to conserve energy by lowering the rate of energy metabolism, poor menstrual function, and poor bone health (97).

Body Image and Eating Disorders

Female athletes are more likely than male athletes to engage in unhealthy weight loss methods, including inappropriate use of laxatives, diet pills, vomiting, and fasting (98). Many of these strategies are aimed at achieving a desired appearance and improved athletic performance, despite the fact that these methods are likely to be counterproductive and may increase health risks (99). It now seems clear that disordered eating behaviors, if they continue, are precursors to subclinical eating disorders that can be life-threatening because of severe energy restriction and pathologic weight loss methods. The high observed risks of female athletes developing eating disorders and associated inappropriate eating behaviors give importance to physicians, dietitians, nurses, psychologists, and coaches to work together in diagnosis

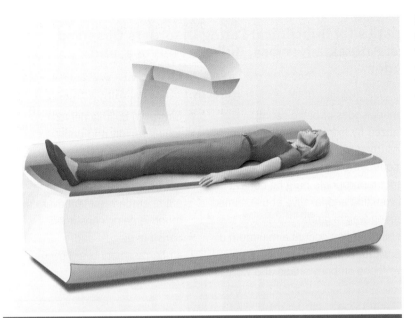

A

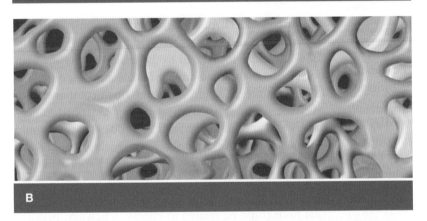

B

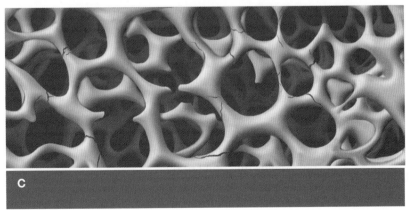

C

FIGURE 10.5: Normal and low bone mineral density (BMD). **A:** The current standard for assessing BMD is dual-energy X-ray absorptiometry. **B:** Normal BMD. **C:** Low BMD characteristic of osteopenia, osteoporosis, and osteomalacia. (From Anatomical Chart Company. Understanding osteoporosis anatomical chart. Philadelphia (PA): LWW (PE); 2003.)

and treatment of female athletes (100). Eating disorders are associated with a distorted perception of body shape (Table 10.2) (101,102).

Health practitioners should use some caution when weighing female athletes or when focusing on athlete weight as a measure of athletic proficiency. It may be counterproductive to have a positive goal (*i.e.*, increased muscle mass) than a negative one (lower weight or lower body fat), as the latter may predispose an athlete to disordered eating behaviors (103).

	General Characteristics for Subclinical Eating Disorders Observed in Female Athletes: Anorexia Nervosa, Bulimia Nervosa, and Binge Eating Disorder	
Table 10.2		

Anorexia Nervosa	Bulimia Nervosa	Binge Eating Disorder
■ Severe restriction of energy intake relative to requirements, resulting in low body weight for age, sex, developmental period, and physical health. ■ Fear of gaining weight or of becoming fat, despite being underweight. ■ Misperception of body weight/shape, with denial of severity of actual low body weight.	■ Recurrent episodes of binge eating characterized by extremely large amount of food consumed within a 2-hr period. ■ Loss of control during binge eating episode. ■ Recurrent inappropriate purging behaviors, such as vomiting and laxative abuse, aimed at preventing weight gain. ■ Average binge eating occurs a minimum of once per wk for 3 mo. ■ Excessive focus on body shape and weight.	■ Similar to bulimia nervosa. ■ Eating rapidly and until uncomfortably full. ■ Eating large amounts even when not hungry, and eating alone out of embarrassment over how much is being consumed. ■ Sense of disgust and embarrassment over how much is being consumed.

Source: American Psychiatric Association. Diagnostic and statistical manual of mental disorders: DSM-V. American Psychiatric Association; 2013.

Female Athlete Triad

The *female athlete triad* (the triad) is a condition characterized by low energy availability, menstrual cycle disturbances, and low BMD. The condition was officially recognized by the ACSM in 1992, after an increase in the number of stress fractures, findings of low BMD, and increased menstrual dysfunction in significant proportions of female athletes (95). The triad commonly begins with inadequate energy consumption, which results in an amenorrhea-associated reduction in estrogen levels and leads to decreased bone development (Box 10.6) (104).

Box 10.6   The Female Athlete Triad

The female athlete triad is a medical condition seen often in physically active girls and women, involving three interrelated factors:

■ Low energy availability that may or may not be associated with disordered eating or an eating disorder.
■ Menstrual dysfunction (typically amenorrhea or oligomenorrhea).
■ Low BMD.

Failure to address this triad with early intervention may result in a progression to a more serious eating disorder and may predispose the athlete to early-onset osteoporosis.

A survey of 191 Australian exercising women between the ages of 18 and 40 years assessed their knowledge, attitude, and behavior related to the triad. Despite the high prevalence of the triad among female athletes, only 10% of those surveyed could name the three components of the triad; 45% did not understand that amenorrhea negatively affects bone health; and 25% indicated they would not take corrective action if experiencing amenorrhea (105). A group of those same lean-build sports participants was also associated with having a history of menstrual dysfunction and stress fractures, despite knowing that both could be related to energy deficiency. In addition, over 33% of the subjects believed that irregular menstrual periods are a "normal" part of being an athlete. Interestingly, a number of the respondents in this study had suffered both amenorrhea and stress fractures, yet did not realize that these are both associated with inadequate energy intake. This study demonstrates the need for educating active females and female athletes about the health risks associated with a failure to consume sufficient energy to support both physical activity and normal physiologic function (105).

Prevalence of the triad may be difficult to estimate because of its multifactorial components and because of poor standardization for determining the presence of each of the triad factors. It is estimated that ~4% of all female athletes meet the criteria for all three components of the triad, with certain sports having a higher prevalence (106). Higher prevalence sports often have an aesthetic component to the competition, including subjectively scored sports (dance, gymnastics, figure skating) and sports where contoured and revealing clothing is required (swimming, diving). Higher prevalence of the triad is also seen in endurance sports (distance, running, and cycling) and weight-category sports (martial arts and wrestling) (24). As an illustration of this higher prevalence, the general female population has a rate of eating disorders in the range of 5%–9%, although studies have found the prevalence of eating disorders in selected female athlete groups to range from 28% to 62%, with menstrual dysfunction as high as 78% in certain sports (24). In a study of high school female athletes, it was found that low energy availability was present in 54% of participants, with a greater prevalence of low BMD in these athletes (94). There is increasing evidence that an effective strategy for reducing the prevalence of the triad is to educate parents, coaches, and athletes on how and why this problem is so pervasive and on nutritional strategies for reducing the risk of relative energy deficiency (107).

The general medical recommendations to decrease the risk of the triad are as follows (108):

- Screen *all* adolescent female athletes for components of the triad as part of the preparticipation examination.
- Perform a BMD scan using dual-energy X-ray absorptiometry (DEXA) on *all* athletes who present with a stress fracture, regardless of whether or not they have reported menstrual dysfunction or disordered eating.

Inadequate Energy Consumption

Energy availability represents the amount of dietary energy required to satisfy all physiologic functions plus the increased energy requirement associated with physical activity. In healthy individuals, it is estimated that an average of 45 kcal/kg FFM/day is sufficient to satisfy needs, whereas intake of <30 kcal/kg FFM/day may result in altered reproductive function and low bone development or decreased BMD as compensation for the inadequate energy availability. Low energy availability is often seen in endurance sports, where the energy expended exceeds the energy consumed. Female athletes in sports that emphasize aesthetics and leanness, including diving, gymnastics, synchronized swimming, and figure skating, are at high risk of having low energy availability (104). A study of eating attitudes, risk for eating disorders, and food intakes of elite figure skaters found that, despite being within a normal weight range for height, 38% thought of themselves as overweight, and 22% were told by others that they were overweight. This resulted in an average daily energy intake that was far below the predicted requirement, increasing risks of menstrual dysfunction and poor bone health (109).

Menstrual Dysfunction

Menstrual dysfunction in female athletes includes a wide array of disorders, including amenorrhea, oligomenorrhea, and anovulation (Box 10.7).

> **Menstrual Dysfunction**
>
> As it relates to female athletes, typically refers to amenorrhea (cessation of the menstrual period) or oligomenorrhea (irregular menstrual period). Both are closely linked to inadequate energy intake. The lower estrogen with either amenorrhea or oligomenorrhea is associated with lower bone density.

Menstrual cycle problems originate from the suppression of the release of gonadotropin-releasing hormone from the hypothalamus. This results in a lowered

---

Box 10.7　Menstrual Function Terms

Menstrual Cycle: A recurring cycle in women of childbearing age that begins at *menarche* and ends at *menopause*. During this cycle, the lining of the uterus prepares for pregnancy, but without pregnancy, the uterus lining is shed (menstruation). The average menstrual cycle is 28 days, with a typical range of between 21 and 35 days.

Eumenorrhea: Normal and regular menstrual cycle (*e.g.*, A eumenorrheic female has a normal and regular menstrual cycle.).

Amenorrhea: Absence of at least three sequential menstrual periods.

- A 15-year-old female who has never had a menstrual period has *primary* amenorrhea.
- A female who has experienced a previous menstrual period, but has missed at least three sequential menstrual periods has *secondary* amenorrhea.

Oligomenorrhea: Infrequent menstrual periods in women of childbearing age. A female who goes longer than 35 days without menstruating and/or only four to nine menstrual periods per year may be diagnosed as having oligomenorrhea.

Anovulation: Failure of the ovaries to release an egg (ova) for over a 3-month period. Typically, ovaries release 1 egg every 25–28 days.

luteinizing hormone and *follicle-stimulating hormone* secretion, both of which are necessary for normal ovarian function. The outcome is decreased *estrogen* and *progesterone* production by the ovaries, resulting in multiple health risks that include a reduced ability to increase BMD (24). Bones are constantly being remodeled through the action of two primary cells, including osteoblasts, which build up bone, and osteoclasts, which break down bone. Estrogen inhibits the activity of osteoclasts, enabling relatively greater osteoblastic activity and, ultimately, higher BMD.

It was initially thought that menstrual dysfunction was the result of an excessively low body fat in female athletes, but this theory has been found to be inaccurate. Energy availability has been found to be the primary regulator of normal ovarian function, and women falling below 30 kcal/kg LBM/day are at risk of abnormal ovarian function (93). It appears that *cortisol*, a stress hormone that is produced with low energy availability, is an inhibitor of estrogen production, while it also is highly catabolic to bone tissue and soft (muscle/fat) tissue (104). Athletes, and the health care providers who work with them, should know that returning an athlete to a state of good energy availability does not immediately result in a return to normal ovarian function, and it may take several months to return to a normally functioning state (110).

Bone Health

Physically active females require good bone health to absorb the additional gravitational and muscular stresses associated with sport. However, bone health is compromised in the triad, predisposing the affected athlete to stress fractures, fractures from increased skeletal fragility, and early-onset osteoporosis (111). On the other hand, female athletes with adequate energy availability experience positive changes in bone development, with higher BMD than nonathletes and lower risk of developing osteoporosis (104).

The reduction in bone mass associated with menstrual dysfunction is clinically relevant for female athletes because it places them at an increased risk for stress fractures and later an increased risk for osteoporosis. In one study of 46 female athletes (31 with multiple stress fractures and 15 without stress fractures), nearly half of all athletes with stress fractures had menstrual irregularities, with a particularly high prevalence observed in endurance runners with high weekly training mileage (112). Although consuming sufficient calories and calcium will not correct the biomechanical factors associated with stress fractures, including a high longitudinal foot arch and leg-length inequality will substantially reduce risk if

this strategy helps females return to normal menstrual function (113).

The prevalence of bone-related problems associated with menstrual dysfunction is high. In runners, it was found that 34.2% were osteopenic (*i.e.,* low BMD) at the lumbar spine and 33% were osteoporotic in the forearm. Of this population, 38% were oligomenorrheic and 25% were amenorrheic, with a significant proportion having low energy availability as a result of disordered eating (114). Low bone density may be used as a primary diagnostic factor associated with low energy availability and/or the triad (115). It has also been found that high dietary fiber intakes and vegetable protein consumption, which are associated with vegetarian diets that often supply insufficient total energy, are associated with low BMD in young female athletes with oligomenorrhea (116). High-fiber diets are associated with high consumption of phytic acid and oxalic acid, both of which have a high binding affinity for bivalent minerals (*e.g.,* calcium, zinc, iron, and magnesium), creating poor absorption for the calcium in food (117,118).

Total Daily Energy Expenditure

Energy Substrates, Vitamins, and Minerals

Carbohydrate

Carbohydrate is a critically important part of the female athlete diet for multiple reasons: (1) it is the primary source of fuel for the central nervous system/brain; (2) it is the primary substrate necessary for glycogen storage in the liver and muscles; (3) it can be metabolized both anaerobically and aerobically, so is important for both endurance and high-intensity activities; and (4) storage of carbohydrate can be easily altered through physical activity (40). Female athletes may put themselves on reduced carbohydrate intake as an ill-founded strategy for lowering body fat and weight, despite current recommendations that carbohydrate should be 50%–60% of total calories consumed (Table 10.3).

A series of studies assessing the carbohydrate consumption pattern of female athletes involved in different sports have indicated a wide range of intakes. Few of the assessed female athlete groups meet the recommended carbohydrate intake of 5–7 g/kg/day for general training and 7–10 g/kg/day for endurance athletes (119). In one study, only 29% of female athletes consumed the recommended carbohydrate during practice and/or competition (39).

Protein

The general (nonathlete) recommendation for protein consumption in adults is 8 g/kg/day. The athlete

Table 10.3	Recommended Carbohydrate Intake for Different Intensities of Activity	
Light activity	Low-intensity or skill-based activity	3–5 g/kg body mass/day
Moderate activity	Moderate exercise program of ~1 hr/day	5–7 g/kg body mass/day
High activity	Endurance program of 1–3 hr/day of moderate- to high-intensity exercise	6–10 g/kg body mass/day
Very high activity	Extreme exercise program of 4–5 hr/day of moderate to high-intensity exercise	8–12 g/kg body mass/day

Source: Burke LM. Chapter 4: nutritional guidelines for female athletes. In: Mountjoy ML, editor. Handbook of sports medicine and science, The female athlete. 1st ed. Philadelphia (PA): Wiley-Blackwell; 2015.

recommendation is approximately double this and ranges between 1.2 and 2.0 g/kg/day, depending on the degree to which the athlete is involved in endurance activity (40,120). It should be noted that no specific protein requirement data are available for female athletes, so these values are derived from mixed-athlete or male studies. Until female-specific protein requirement data are determined, female athletes should aim to consume a protein level within the currently established range. How the protein is consumed is also important, with current recommendations to optimize tissue utilization in the range of 20–25 g protein/meal (40,121,122). As an example, a young female athlete weighing 50 kg (110 lb) would require 50 × 1.5 or 75 g of protein per day. Consumed in 20 g doses, this athlete would require about four meals with 20 g of protein in each meal to satisfy her requirement.

Fat

Fat is a concentrated source of energy, ideally contributing 20%–35% of total energy consumed, and is also needed for providing the essential fatty acids and the fat-soluble vitamins A, D, E, and K (40,123). Although fat restriction is often a component of low-calorie diets aimed at improving appearance, athletes should be discouraged from consuming less than 20% of total energy from dietary fat (40). There has been recent interest in consumption of high-fat/low-carbohydrate diets for the purpose of enhancing fat metabolism, but the results of studies investigating this strategy fail to show that fat metabolism is enhanced, while there is consistent evidence that low-carbohydrate diets may diminish exercise performance (40,124,125).

Nutrients

As food is the carrier of energy and micronutrients, inadequate energy consumption increases the likelihood that micronutrients will also be inadequately consumed. The information on vitamins and minerals that follows

emphasizes the micronutrients that are of the highest concern in female athletes, including calcium, vitamin D, iron, and certain antioxidants.

Iron

It is hard to imagine any athlete performing up to their conditioned capacity with poor iron status. Despite this, young female athletes are at particularly high risk for both iron deficiency and iron deficiency anemia (see Chapter 6). Poor iron status can result in a compromised immune system, extreme fatigue, poor endurance, poor concentration ability, weakness, shortness of breath, and dizziness. A study assessing the prevalence of iron deficiency in young female rhythmic gymnasts found that nearly half (48.3%) had blood values consistent with iron deficiency (126). Similar findings of poor iron status have been found in other female groups, including young ballet dancers, who were found to be at high risk for iron deficiency (127). It was found that the female athletes with iron deficiency had significantly lower energy, protein, and fat intakes than those with normal iron status. Protein intake, in particular, was found to be significantly different among the iron-deficient (protein intake was lower) and normal iron (protein intake was higher) groups. Surveys have found low storage of iron (ferritin) in female runners, and other studies have found that female athletes with anemia can improve aerobic performance through a program of iron supplementation (128,129). However, taking iron supplements in the absence of iron deficiency may cause GI tract and other difficulties, including lower absorption rates of calcium, zinc, and magnesium. In addition, a review has suggested that adequate iron consumption from food in menstruating females may attenuate the risk of poor iron status, eliminating the need for supplementation (130). Given the very real health and performance risks associated with poor iron status, female athletes should have iron status assessed on a yearly basis, with the inclusion of ferritin in the assessment protocol.

Calcium

Adequate calcium consumption is necessary to develop and maintain high-density bones that are resistant to fracture. For athletes concerned about dairy product consumption because of allergies or lactose intolerance, calcium-fortified orange juice is an excellent alternative and per equal volume, has the same calcium concentration as fluid milk. It should be understood, however, that calcium intake alone does not guarantee healthy bones, as vitamin D, estrogen, adequate energy, and physical stress are all needed for bone development.

Despite the difficulties associated with estimating and interpreting dietary adequacy from food intake data in athletes (21), it is especially concerning that the calcium consumption of adolescent athletes may be as low as 50% of the recommended intake level (18,131), with inadequate intakes being much more common in female athletes than in male athletes (132). As amenorrheic adolescent athletes have significantly impaired bone microarchitecture compared with eumenorrheic athletes (those with normal menstrual cycles) and nonathletic controls, it is especially important that all adolescent female athletes, regardless of menstrual function, achieve adequate calcium intakes (Box 10.8) (133).

Vitamin D

There is concern that young female athletes, particularly in sports that involve indoor training and competition, are at risk for low vitamin D status. It has been estimated that in some parts of the world, 32.8% of adolescent females were vitamin D deficient when using plasma concentrations of 25.0 nmol/L; 68.4% were vitamin D deficient when using 37.5 nmol/L; and 89.2% were vitamin D deficient when using 50 nmol/L (134). Poor vitamin D status can negatively affect skeletal development, but may also negatively affect muscle function and athletic performance (see Chapter 5: Vitamin D). This concern is particularly acute in young females involved in indoor

activities because maximal BMD is achieved by the age of 20. Failure to reach a sufficiently high bone density creates a predisposition to early-onset osteoporosis. Seasonal variation also makes a difference in vitamin D status, with winter associated with the lowest serum vitamin D concentrations. Serum vitamin D concentrations are reportedly highest in September, following a period of higher direct sun exposure, and lowest in March, following a period of lower direct sun exposure, with indoor athletes having significantly lower serum vitamin D levels than outdoor athletes regardless of the season (135).

Given the relatively high prevalence of vitamin D deficiency in all populations, including young female athletes, there is good reason to periodically assess athletes for vitamin D status. If it is found to be low, a trained medical professional should recommend appropriate sun exposure for different skin pigmentations (e.g., two times per week between 10 AM and 3 PM with arms and legs exposed for 5–30 minutes), foods, and, if necessary, supplements (136).

THE OLDER ATHLETE

There are far too many examples of older athletes performing well to suggest that there is a maximum age to put away the athletic shoes. The World Masters Athletics Association lists many athletes who are still competing above age 60 in virtually every track and field discipline including steeplechase, pole vault, marathon, and the 10,000-m run. The world record holder for the men's outdoor 100 m in the *100-year-old group* is Russian Philip Rabinowitz with a time of 30.86 seconds, and British Ron Taylor holds the record for 60-year-olds, an impressive 11.70 seconds! Older female athletes also excel. In 1994, Russian Yekaterina Podkopayeva won the world indoor 1,500 m at the age of 42 with a time of 3:59:78. At the age of 80, Johanna Luther from Germany ran the 10,000 m in an impressive time of 58:40:03. Clearly, being older does not mean a mandatory cessation of sport participation. Nevertheless, the aging process does bring with it certain undeniable changes that should be addressed to be certain that exercise remains a healthful activity. Of particular concern are the following health-related issues (5,137,138):

- Age-related changes in body composition and the impact this has on REE;
- Lowered capacity to quickly recover from intensive or long bouts of exercise;
- Gradually diminishing bone mass;

Box 10.8	Good Sources of Calcium in Food

- Milk, 1 cup, 300 mg
- Kale (cooked), 1 cup, 245 mg
- Sardines (with bones), 2 oz, 217 mg
- Canned salmon (with bones), 2 oz, 232 mg
- Cheese, 1 oz, 224 mg
- Almonds, 1 oz, 76 mg
- Broccoli (cooked), 1 cup, 62 mg

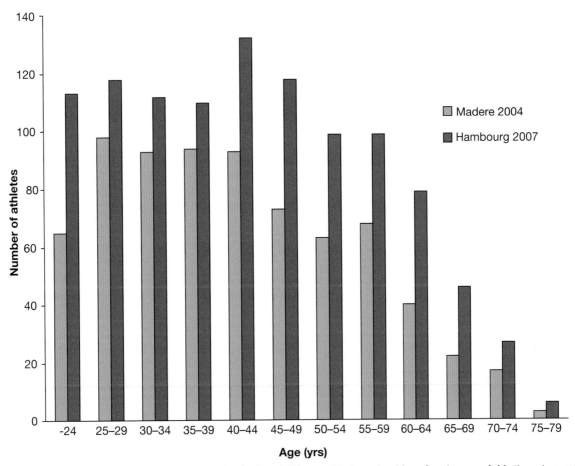

FIGURE 10.6: While there are fewer athletes competing in the triathlon world championships after the age of 44, there is a noticeable increase in the proportion of older athletes competing from 2004 to 2007. (From Bernard T, Sultana F, Lepers R, Haussswirth C, Brisswalter J. Age-related decline in Olympic triathlon performance: effect of locomotion mode. Exp Aging Res. 2010;36(1):64–78.)

- Subtle changes in GI tract function that could influence nutrient absorption;
- Progressively lower heat tolerance;
- Progressive decreases in the glomerular filtration rate and renal blood flow;
- Reduced capacity to concentrating urine, increasing urinary frequency, and, potentially, lowering fluid consumption.

These age-related changes may result in specific performance-related reductions in:

- Aerobic and anaerobic capacity (139,140) (Figure 10.6)
- Exercise efficiency (141)
- Strength (142)
- Power (143)

See Figure 10.6 for age-related reductions in triathlon completion rates.

Despite these changes, appropriate training combined with optimally satisfying nutritional needs can significantly diminish the reduction in performance capabilities (144). It appears that an appropriate nutrition strategy for exercise recovery is an important factor in reducing injuries and benefiting from the exercise bout (145). Included in the postexercise recovery strategy is consumption of carbohydrate and protein to recover glycogen and to stimulate MPS for improved muscle recovery. Postexercise carbohydrate ingestion has been well established as the most important determinant of muscle glycogen resynthesis. In addition, consumption of ~20 g of dietary protein five to six times daily appears to aid MPS rates during the day (146,147). A review of studies investigating protein supplementation providing high levels of protein in conjunction with resistance training, however, found that these high levels fail to increase either muscle mass or strength (148). In a study comparing younger and older athlete rock climbers, it was found that the older athletes had a higher proportion of overuse injuries, suggesting that there is likely a slower recovery in the older athletes, even when appropriate recovery strategies are followed (149).

ENERGY NEEDS

Adulthood is characterized by a decrease in LBM that is associated with a lower metabolic rate and is referred to as **sarcopenia**. Unless accounted for, this lower metabolic rate can be associated with gradually higher body fat levels that predispose adults to type II diabetes, high blood pressure, heart disease, and cancer. The change in body composition is associated with a reduction in energy expenditure, which decreases ~10 calories each year for men and 7 calories each year for women after the age of 20 (5). Active individuals who maintain their lean body (muscle) mass can avoid the conditions associated with sarcopenia. The typical reduction in energy metabolism, therefore, varies greatly with the relative fitness of the older athlete. Interestingly, older male athletes working at near-maximal rates of energy expenditure during a 14-day cycling expedition were unable to consume sufficient energy to fully satisfy tissue needs (150). This inability or unwillingness to consume sufficient energy may be at least partially responsible for the reduction in lean mass commonly seen in aging. It is also recommended that older athletes avoid diets that are high (>35% of total calories) or low (<20% of total calories) in fat, as both extremes are associated with a failure to achieve an appropriate energy intake (40).

Sarcopenia

Age-related degenerative loss of skeletal muscle mass loss of between ½ and 1% for each year after reaching the age of 50. This is also associated with an increase in body fat percentage. The loss of muscle and increase in fat are associated with a progressive increase in weakness, as less muscle is being asked to move relatively more mass. This weakness is associated with less movement, which also results in lower BMD and risk of osteopenia and osteoporosis. Regular exercise coupled with good nutrition practices is a good strategy for limiting the risk of sarcopenia.

Fluids and Heat Stress

Older athletes are more susceptible to dehydration and the problems dehydration creates because of a number of age-associated changes. These include a blunted sensation of thirst, altered kidney function, and slower/lower sweat responses to heat that appear to reduce the older athlete's capacity to drink sufficient fluid to sustain a euhydrated state, resulting in a difficulty to cope with the heat-related stresses of exercise (151). Increased risk of heat stress in older athletes should be seriously considered because the result of heat exhaustion and heatstroke is often death. During periods of high heat and humidity, those most likely to become seriously ill or die are older adults. Although the older adult population should not be confused with the master athlete population, even if they are in the same age group, there may be an age-related drop in the capacity to dissipate heat regardless of fitness level. An important factor in sweat production and cooling capacity is the ability to increase blood flow to the skin. Blood flow to the skin in older, fit athletes is lower than in younger athletes (152,153). In addition, the lower blood flow associated with increasing age appears to be independent of hydration state. It also appears that, although sweat gland recruitment is similar to that of younger athletes, older athletes produce less sweat per gland (154). There is a wide genetically based variability in sweat production, but these studies suggest that older athletes should be vigilant in their capacity to produce sweat. Older athletes and their exercise partners should be cognizant of the symptoms of heat exhaustion and heatstroke. They should also be aware that most heat exhaustion occurs due to poor acclimatization to a hot and humid environment. Therefore, normal exercise intensities and durations should be reduced for the first few days in a new environment until the athlete has adapted.

Bone Mineral Density

Bone density becomes progressively lower with age, and females experience a faster drop in bone density after menopause due to the decrease in the bone-protective action of estrogen. Other factors associated with low bone density include inadequate calcium intakes, lower absorption of calcium, poor vitamin D status, and loss of calcium through sweat. This explains why it is so important to achieve a high bone density by young adulthood so that, even with a progressive loss of density later on, there will be sufficient density to avoid reaching the fracture threshold in older age (155). The rate of change in bone density can be altered through an adequate intake of calcium, periodic and regular exposure to the sun for vitamin D, and regular stress on the skeleton through weight-bearing exercise. In addition, women may choose to take, *through the advice of their physicians*, estrogen/hormone replacement therapy (HRT). HRT may be particularly useful when there is a family history of osteoporosis or a woman has been diagnosed with low bone density (156). Certain cortisone-based drugs taken for the control of pain or osteoarthritis appear to be catabolic to bone; therefore, the regular use of these drugs may place the older athlete at increased risk of low bone density. The fact that older athletes continually stress the skeleton through regular physical activity is a major protective factor in keeping bone density elevated.

Organ Function

It would be expected that older athletes experience some degree of progressive GI dysfunction and changes in nutrient requirements, although no athlete-specific studies confirm that this, indeed, occurs. The typical effects of age on the GI tract include reduced motility; decreased absorption of dietary calcium, vitamin B_6, and vitamin B_{12}; and greater requirement for fluid and fiber to counteract reduced GI motility (5,157). The absorption of iron and zinc may also be a concern, but older individuals appear to have higher iron stores, diminishing the daily requirement for iron (158). Aging is often associated with reduced kidney function, resulting in a loss of nutrients and fluid that may otherwise be retained (151).

Immune Function

Changes in immune function should also be considered, but regular long-term exercise appears to attenuate the changes in the immune system that are typically associated with aging (159). Vitamin D is important for the immune system, but the capability of the older person to synthesize vitamin D from sunlight exposure is reduced, suggesting that vitamin D status may be a concern (160,161). Vitamin and mineral supplementation is common among older athletes, often in an attempt to boost the immune system. However, there is little evidence that this is a useful strategy, but if the supplements target nutrients that are not well absorbed, they may be warranted. It has been suggested that probiotics, vitamin C, and Vitamin D may be useful in enhancing immune function, but further research is needed to determine if such supplements can be taken without blunting desirable training adaptations (162). Attention should be given to older athletes to ensure that nutrition strategies for preventing low BMD and muscle mass are followed. In addition, older athletes should consume foods that lower inflammation and enhance immune function (163). This requires attention to ensure that inflammatory fats (*i.e.*, trans fatty acids) are not consumed, and that the GI tract microbiome is healthy through regular consumption of probiotics and adequate dietary fiber. For older athletes who train primarily indoors, assuring an adequate vitamin D status is important. It is recommended that older

athletes consult with their doctors to determine the best strategy for delivering needed nutrients. In some cases, as in the case of vitamin B_{12}, a periodic injection may be the only strategy that reduces the risk of pernicious anemia (5). Good protein status is an important component of a stable immune function, but there is no evidence that protein intake should in any way be increased beyond the normal values established for athletes (~1.5 g/kg/day). Ideally, protein should be consumed as part of a balanced intake of carbohydrates, protein, and fat to satisfy total energy needs. Aging often brings with it a reduction in kidney function, so increasing protein intake to a level above 2.0 g/kg/day is likely to increase the need to excrete nitrogenous waste, so is not warranted. The current recommendation for protein intake in older adults is at least 1.0–1.2 g protein/kg/day, with a recommendation that daily physical activity or exercise should be undertaken by all older people for as long as possible (164). There is also evidence that calculating the total daily protein requirement and distributing it evenly throughout the day's meals (*e.g.*, 30 g/meal) is a useful strategy for lowering the risk of sarcopenia (122).

SUMMARY

Young Athletes

- Young athletes typically consume sufficient protein, but fail to consume sufficient carbohydrates. As a result, total energy consumption is insufficient to support normal growth and development plus the added energy requirement of physical activity. As a general guide, young athletes should regularly be tracked on growth charts that measure height for age, weight for age, and weight for height (often used by pediatricians). A lowering of the established growth percentile may be a sign of inadequate energy intake, a disease state, or both.
- It is difficult to accurately estimate the energy requirement of physically active young athletes. When making energy requirement predictions it should be considered that all children, but particularly those in a growth spurt, use more energy per unit of body weight than adults performing the same activity. Typically, the added energy need is 20%–25% higher than the adult energy requirement per kg. When estimating energy needs, it is recommended to use prediction equations that have been validated for children (*i.e.*, the Schofield equation). Even when using these equations, it is important to consider that appropriate

growth and development is often the best guide that the young athlete is optimally satisfying energy needs.

- The distribution of energy substrates is important, but parents and coaches should understand that total energy intake adequacy is likely to be more important than the distribution of protein, carbohydrate, or fat in the diet. Fat intake is often a concern because it is easy to access high-fat foods and, as a highly concentrated source of energy, it is easy to consume an excess intake of energy. However, young athletes should be cautious of excessively lowering fat intake, as this can make it far more difficult for them to obtain the energy they require. A good goal is to make sure carbohydrate and protein needs are met, and satisfy the remaining energy requirement with up to 35% of total calories from fat. "Backloading" intake (*i.e.*, consuming most protein and energy at the end of the day) is a common problem in young athletes that detracts both from optimal growth and development and performance.

- Young athletes tend to underconsume fluids, predisposing them to dehydration and increasing the risk of heat illness. There are multiple factors that can increase heat illness risk besides poor hydration, including inadequate cooling between exercise bouts, and poor choice of clothing, but poor hydration is a critical factor (165). Athletes should be encouraged to drink fluids regularly by supervising adults. Voluntary dehydration, or the failure to consume sufficient fluids even when fluids are readily available, is a common problem among young athletes. Resolving a voluntary failure to consume sufficient fluids may require fixed time-schedule drinking opportunities by the "team" that is organized by supervising adults. Young athletes who are in training or competition should have regular opportunities to consume fluids every 10–20 minutes (depending on the heat index), even if that requires periodic stoppage of play. Depending on the duration and intensity of exercise, consumed fluids may require inclusion of electrolytes and carbohydrates.

- Energy-restrictive diets should not be followed by young athletes, as the resulting negative energy balance produced by these diets may likely be counterproductive for the achievement of a desirable weight and body composition while negatively affecting growth and development. Contrary to common beliefs, energy-restrictive diets result in a greater loss of lean (*i.e.*, muscle) mass than fat mass, inhibit skeletal development/growth, and increase long-term chronic disease risk. Strategies for correcting obesity (*i.e.*, lowering the

relative fat mass) should be under the direct supervision of trained medical professionals.

- It is difficult for young athletes, and in particular young *female* athletes, to obtain sufficient iron, and surveys suggest that calcium intake is also marginal. Therefore, the parents of young athletes should consult with the family doctor and a registered dietitian to determine if an altered dietary strategy and/or iron or calcium supplements are warranted. Ideally, a test for iron status that measures hemoglobin, hematocrit, and ferritin performed on a regular yearly basis will help to ensure that the current diet is satisfying iron requirements.

Female Athletes

- Female athletes should be made fully aware of the negative consequences associated with menstrual dysfunction and the role energy inadequacy plays in its development (166). It is important to ensure that female athletes consume sufficient energy to eliminate the risk that menstrual dysfunction results from inadequate energy consumption.

- A preparticipation physical examination should be a standard feature for all athletes involved in all sports. For the female athlete, the screening should include an assessment for the presence of the triad and any of its sequelae, including low BMD and amenorrhea (167).

- Calcium status should be regularly assessed and, if inadequate, corrected through a program of altered food intake (preferred) or through a physician-supervised supplementation program. A reasonable means of assessing calcium status is to periodically assess bone density via DEXA scan. In addition, a dietary intake analysis will determine if consumed foods are providing sufficient calcium.

- Iron status should be assessed yearly, including measures of hemoglobin, hematocrit, and ferritin. In the event of iron deficiency, a dietary modification to increase iron intake and/or a physician-supervised program of iron supplementation with follow-up blood tests should be immediately implemented.

- Female athletes are at higher risk than male athletes for eating disorders, inadequate bone density attainment, and inadequate iron consumption. They also have a unique risk of dysmenorrhea. Most of these difficulties can be controlled through the consumption of a nutritionally balanced diet that delivers an adequate caloric load. To achieve this, female athletes should understand that an underconsumption of calories, while lowering weight, is likely to have a greater catabolic impact on lean mass than on fat mass. This altered body composition, by forcing the athlete to consume a still lower food intake to achieve a desired body profile, will place the athlete at greater future risk of malnutrition and associated diseases.

■ Female athletes may view dieting as a strategy for improving sport performance. However, while they perceive to have a high level of control over their food-eating environment, family, teammates, coaches, and friends all have significant influence over how the athlete actually eats (168). Therefore, nutrition education efforts should target all potential individuals who may have an impact on the female athlete's eating behavior.

Older Athletes

■ Older athletes should take steps to reduce the risk of dehydration and should develop strategies for fluid consumption that they can tolerate. Being aware of the signs of heat stress is important because older athletes are likely to have lower sweat rates than younger athletes involved in the same activity.

■ GI function may require additional vitamin and mineral intake, perhaps through supplements. Older athletes should regularly consult with doctors to determine the biologic need for specific supplements and take them only in reasonable, prescribed doses. Vitamins and minerals of particular concern are calcium, iron, zinc, vitamin B_6, and vitamin B_{12}.

■ Reduced gut motility requires a slight increase in fiber consumption, but this should always take place in conjunction with additional fluid intake. Focusing on fresh fruits and vegetables as well as whole grain products is an excellent means of obtaining additional fiber, plus these foods provide needed carbohydrate energy.

■ Frequent illness may be a sign that immune function is depressed. There is no perfect weapon for combating a reduction in immune function, but exercising reasonably, eating well, and resting well are useful strategies. Older athletes with frequent eating patterns should consult with their physicians.

■ It takes longer for older athletes to adapt to new environments, so reducing exercise intensity and frequency for several days after travel is a logical and useful step to avoid overheating and illness.

■ Older athletes can expect some slowing of the metabolic rate, which makes it more difficult to sustain a desirable body composition and weight without making the appropriate reduction in energy consumption. At the same time, nutrient requirement mandates

the consumption of a diet with a high nutrient density (*i.e.*, a higher nutrient-to-calorie ratio). Avoidance of overtraining is important for injury reduction and sustaining immune function. This is particularly important because healing time for both injury and disease is longer with increasing age. Finally, adequate fluid intake is critically important to avoid dehydration and to sustain gut motility because the frequency of urination associated with advanced age may inhibit fluid consumption.

Practical Application Activity

As a means of assessing the different nutrient requirements of young athletes, female athletes, and older athletes, ask yourself some questions regarding the different issues that are faced by different groups:

1. Do adult male and female athletes face the same nutritional risks? If not, what would you focus on differently if you were working with an adult male and an adult female athlete?

2. How are the DRI/recommended dietary allowances different for different groups:
   a. Do adolescents have the same requirements for calcium as adults? How would you help ensure that the greater adolescent calcium requirement is met without compromising the intake of other nutrients?
   b. Do adult females have the same requirements for protein as adult males? What strategy would you follow for advising adult females and adult males how to optimally satisfy protein intake without providing excess fat or insufficient carbohydrate?
   c. A female of childbearing age has a significantly higher iron requirement than an equivalently aged male. How would you ensure that the female satisfies iron requirements without also providing a level of energy intake that would be considered excessive? Can you think of an appropriate dietary (nonsupplement) strategy for consuming adequate iron in male and female vegan athletes?

3. The focus on weight, particularly in sports that have a subjective scoring scheme, such as figure skating and gymnastics, may predispose the athlete to developing eating disorders. What nutritional strategies could be followed that would diminish the risk of developing an eating disorder?

CHAPTER QUESTIONS

1. In female athletes, amenorrhea is likely to be a sign of:
   a. Poor fluid intake
   b. Inadequate energy consumption
   c. Low calcium intake
   d. Protein being used to satisfy energy needs

2. Heat stress is most likely to be of high concern in:
   a. Younger and older athletes
   b. Male athletes
   c. Female athletes
   d. Power athletes

3. Because children and adolescents have such high appetites, it is easy to satisfy the energy needs of young athletes.
   a. True
   b. False

4. Satisfying calcium needs in young athletes is important because _____% of bone mass is acquired during adolescence.
   a. 10
   b. 25
   c. 50
   d. 75

5. Girls commonly end their adolescent growth spurt by age_____, while boys typically end their growth spurt by age _____.
   a. 16, 19
   b. 13, 20
   c. 18, 18
   d. 15, 21

6. Secondary amenorrhea in female athletes refers to a condition where:
   a. Menses has never been experienced.
   b. The first menses occurred late, but by no later than age 16.
   c. Menses occurs irregularly.
   d. The athlete has experienced a menstrual period, but has not had a period 3 months or more.

7. Eumenorrhea refers to a female of childbearing age who:
   a. Has never had a period.
   b. Has irregular periods.
   c. Has regular periods.
   d. Has missed only 3 or 4 periods in the last year.

8. Young athletes who practice and compete indoors are at risk for poor status for which of the following nutrients?
   a. Calcium
   b. Vitamin A
   c. Vitamin D
   d. β-Carotene

9. Protein consumption exceeding 30 g at a single meal may result in an increase in blood urea nitrogen, which is associated with both dehydration and lower BMD.
   a. True
   b. False

10. Which of the following young athletes is at increased risk for having low BMD?
    a. Long-distance runners
    b. Football players
    c. Swimmers
    d. Tennis players

ANSWERS TO CHAPTER QUESTIONS

1. b
2. a
3. b
4. b
5. a

6. d
7. c
8. a
9. d
10. c

Case Study Considerations

1. **Case Study Answer 1:** Typically, the following changes occur with aging, particularly in people who are inactive:
   - Sarcopenia
     - Muscle weakness and loss of strength and stamina associated with lower muscle mass
     - Greater fracture risk associated with lower BMD
     - Higher body fat which is a contributor to muscle weakness
   - Aging is associated with a significant reduction in whole-body sweating, predisposing older individuals to higher risk of heat stress than younger adults.

2. **Case Study Answer 2:** There are differences in aging between men and women. Typically, the level of estrogen in women drops earlier and more rapidly in women than the drop in testosterone in men. This faster drop in estrogen, which is an inhibitor of osteoclasts (the cells that break down bones), predisposes women to an earlier onset of osteoporosis (low BMD) than men. Despite this difference, men have higher early death rates than women. This higher death rate is associated with higher risks of heart disease, diabetes, stroke, and cancer.

3. **Case Study Answer 3:** Current strategies for minimizing age-related changes include:
   - Taking steps to have a healthy/high BMD as a young adult. This involves placing stress on the bones via regular physical activity, avoiding relative energy deficiency, and consuming a well-balanced diet that contains adequate levels of calcium. Adequate vitamin D is also important for achieving and sustaining a good BMD, and this can be achieved through diet, sunlight exposure, or a combination of the two. Reaching a satisfactory peak BMD as a young adult helps to ensure that an age-related reduction in bone density will not reach the fracture threshold.
   - Developing and sustaining good musculature is critical to avoiding the effects of age-related sarcopenia. This is best done by participating in regular physical activity and avoiding low blood sugar and relative energy deficiency through a regular eating regimen. It is important to consider that older individuals can increase muscle mass just as easily as younger individuals with the right eating and exercise protocols, but older people can lose muscle mass much faster than younger individuals with poor nutrition and/or inactivity.
   - Better musculature is associated with lower body fat, and this combination is associated with better-sustained circulation and sweat rates, making it easier for an older individual to participate in sustained physical activity.

REFERENCES

1. Debnath M, Chatterjee S, Bandyopadhyay A, Datta G, Dey SK. Prediction of athletic performance through nutrition knowledge and practice: a cross-sectional study among young team athletes. Sport Mont J. 2019;17(3):13–20.
2. De Souza MJ, Nattiv A, Joy E, Williams NI, Mallinson RJ, Gibbs JC, Olmsted M, Goolsby M, Matheson G; Expert Panel. Female athlete triad coalition consensus statement on treatment and return to play of the female athlete triad: 1st International Conference held in San Francisco, California, May 2012 and 2nd International Conference held in Indianapolis, Indiana, May 2013. Br J Sports Med. 2014;48(4):289.
3. Unnithan VB, Goulopoulou S. Nutrition for the pediatric athlete. Curr Sports Med Rep. 2004;3(4):206–11.
4. Cotugna N, Vickery CE, McBee S. Sports nutrition for young athletes. J Sch Nurs. 2005;21(6):323–8.
5. Campbell WW, Geik RA. Nutritional considerations for the older athlete. Nutrition. 2004;20(7/8):603–8.
6. Huang YC, Chen W, Evans MA, Mitchell ME, Shultz TD. Vitamin B-6 requirement and status assessment of young women fed a high-protein diet with various levels of vitamin. J Appl Physiol. 1998;67(2):208–20.
7. Petrie HJ, Stover EA, Horswill CA. Nutritional concerns for the child and adolescent competitor. Nutrition. 2004; 20(7/8):620–31.
8. Hannon MP, Close GL, Morton JP. Energy and macronutrient considerations for young athletes. Strength Cond J. 2020; 42(6):109–19.
9. Unnithan VB, Baxter-Jones ADG. The young athlete. In: Maughan RJ, editor. Nutrition in sport. London: Blackwell Science; 2000. p. 429–41.
10. Sellami M, Al-Muraikhy S, Al-Jaber H, Al-Amri H, Al-Mansoori L, Mazloum NA, Donati F, Botre F, Elrayess MA. Age and sport intensity-dependent changes in cytokines and telomere length in elite athletes. Antioxidants. 2021;10:1035.
11. Desbrow B. Youth athlete development and nutrition. Sports Med. 2021;51(Suppl 1):S3–12.
12. Anderson MW, Greenspan A. Stress fractures. Radiology. 1996;199:1–12.
13. American Academy of Pediatrics, Committee on Sports Medicine and Fitness. Intensive training and sports specialization in young athletes. Pediatrics. 2000;106(1):154–7.

14. Bennell KL, Malcolm SA, Wark JD, Brukner PD. Models for the pathogenesis of stress fractures in athletes. Br J Sports Med. 1996;30:200–4.

15. Bompa T. From childhood to champion athlete. Toronto: Veritas;1995.

16. Torun B. Energy requirements of children and adolescents. Public Health Nutr. 2005;8(7A):968–93.

17. Coutinho LAA, Porto CPM, Pierucci APTR. Critical evaluation of food intake and energy balance in young modern pentathlon athletes: a cross-sectional study. J Int Soc Sports Nutr. 2016;13:15.

18. Gibson JC, Stuart-Hill L, Martin S, Gaul C. Nutrition status of junior elite Canadian female soccer athletes. Int J Sport Nutr Exerc Metab. 2011;21(6):507–14.

19. Morgan DW. Locomotor economy. In: Armstrong N, van Mechelen W, editors. Paediatric exercise science and medicine. Oxford, UK: Oxford University Press, 2008. p. 283–95.

20. Aerenhouts D, Deriemaeker P, Hebbelinck M, Clarys P. Energy and macronutrient intake in adolescent sprint athletes: a follow-up study. J Sports Sc. 2011;29(1):73–82.

21. Heaney S, O'Connor H, Gifford J, Naughton G. Comparison of strategies for assessing nutritional adequacy in elite female athletes' dietary intake. Int J Sport Nutr Exerc Metab. 2010;20(3):245–56.

22. Loucks A, Kiens B, Wright H. Energy availability in athletes. J Sports Sci. 2011;29(Suppl 1):S7–15.

23. Bass S, Inge K. Nutrition for special populations: children and young athletes. In: Burke LM, Deakin V, editors. Clinical sports nutrition. 4th ed. Sydney: McGraw Hill; 2010. p. 508–46.

24. Nattiv A, Loucks AB, Manore MM, Sanborn CF, Sundgot-Borgen J, Warren MP. American College of Sports Medicine position stand. The female athlete triad. Med Sci Sports Exerc. 2007;39(10):1867–82.

25. Hills AP, Mikhtar N, Byrne NM. Assessment of physical activity and energy expenditure: an overview of objective measures. Front Nutr. 2014;1:5.

26. Jeran S, Steinbrecher A, Pischon T. Prediction of activity-related energy expenditure using accelerometer-derived physical activity under free-living conditions: a systematic review. Int J Obes (Lond). 2016;40(8):1187–97.

27. Stephens S, Takken T, Esliger DW, Pullenayegum E, Beyene J, Tremblay M, Schneiderman J, Biggar D, Longmuir P, McCrindle B, Abad A, Ignas D, Van Der Net J, Feldman B. Validation of accelerometer prediction equations in children with chronic disease. Pediatr Exerc Sci. 2016;28:117–32.

28. Silvia C, Ogilvie D, Dalton A, Westgate K, Grage S, Panter J. Quantifying the physical activity energy expenditure of commuters using a combination of global positioning system and combined heart rate and movement sensors. Prev Med. 2015; 81:339–44.

29. Nelson BM, Kaminsky LA, Dickin DC, Montoye AHK. Validity of consumer-based physical activity monitors for specific activity types. Med Sci Sports Exerc. 2016;48(8);1619–28.

30. Ainsworth BE, Haskell WL, Whitt MC, Irwin ML, Swartz AM, Strath SJ, O'Brien WL, Bassett DR Jr, Schmitz KH, Emplaincourt PO, Jacobs DR Jr, Leon AS. Compendium of physical activities: an update of activity codes and MET intensities. Med Sci Sports Exerc. 2000;32(9):S498–516.

31. Deutz RC, Benardot D, Martin DE, Cody MM. Relationship between energy deficits and body composition in elite female gymnasts and runners. Med Sci Sports Exerc. 2000; 32(3):659–68.

32. Ekeland E, Heian F, Hagen KB. Can exercise improve self-esteem in children and young people? A systematic review of randomized controlled trials. Br J Sports Med. 2005; 39(11):792–8.

33. Monthuy-Blanc J, Maiano C, Morin AJ, Stephan Y. Physical self-concept and disturbed eating attitudes and behaviors in French athlete and non-athlete adolescent girls: direct and indirect relations. Body Image. 2012;9(3):373–80.

34. Georgopoulos NA, Markou KB, Theodoropoulou A, Vagenakis GA, Benardot D, Leglise M, Dimopoulos JC, Vagenakis AG. Height velocity and skeletal maturation in elite female rhythmic gymnasts. J Clin Endocrinol Metab. 2001;86(11):5159–64.

35. Caine D, Lewis R, O'Connor P, Howe W, Bass S. Does gymnastics training inhibit growth of females? Clin J Sport Med. 2001;11(4):260–70.

36. Chu L, Timmons BW. Nutritional considerations for the overweight young athlete. Pediatr Exerc Sci. 2015;27:463–76.

37. Aull JL, Rowe DA, Hickner RC, Malinauskas BM, Mahar MT. Energy expenditure of obese, overweight, and normal weight females during lifestyle physical activities. Int J Pediatr Obes. 2008;3(3):177–85.

38. David JM, Alderson NL, Welsh RS. Serotonin and central nervous system fatigue: nutritional considerations. Am J Clin Nutr. 2000;72(2):573s–8s.

39. Baker LB, Heaton LE, Nuccio RP, Stein KW. Dietitian-observed macronutrient intakes of young skill and team-sport athletes: adequacy of pre, during, and postexercise nutrition. Int J Sport Nutr Exerc Metab. 2014;24:166–76.

40. Burke LM. Nutritional guidelines for female athletes. In: Mountjoy ML, editor. The female athlete. 1st ed. London: John Wiley & Sons, Inc.; 2015.

41. Boisseau N, Vermorel M, Rance M, Duché P, Patureau-Mirand P. Protein requirements in male adolescent soccer players. Eur J Appl Physiol. 2007;100(1):27–33.

42. Hawley JA, Burke LM, Phillips SM, Spriet LL. Nutritional modulation of training-induced skeletal muscle adaptations. J Appl Physiol. 2011;110(3):834–45.

43. Phillips SM, Van Loon LJ. Dietary protein for athletes: from requirements to optimum adaptation. J Sports Sci. 2011; 29(Suppl 1):S29–38.

44. Trommelen J, Betz MW, van Loon LJC. The muscle protein synthetic response to meal ingestion following resistance-type exercise. Sports Med. 2019;49:185–97.

45. Shaw CS, Clark J, Wagenmakers AJ. The effect of exercise and nutrition on intramuscular fat metabolism and insulin sensitivity. Annu Rev Nutr. 2010;30:13–34.

46. Jeukendrup A, Cronin L. Nutrition and elite young athletes. Med Sport Sci. 2011;56:47–58.

47. Smith JW, Holmes ME, McAllister MJ. Nutritional considerations for performance in young athletes. J Sports Med. 2015; 2015:734649.

48. Maughan RJ, Depiesse F, Geyer H; International Association of Athletics Federations. The use of dietary supplements by athletes. J Sports Sci. 2007;25(Suppl 1):S103–13.

49. Wiens K, Erdman KA, Stadnyk M, Parnell JA. Dietary supplement usage, motivation, and education in young Canadian athletes. Int J Sport Nutr Exerc Metab. 2014; 24: 613–22.

50. Cigrovski V, Malec L, Radman I, Prenda N, Krističević T. Nutritional knowledge and dietary habits of young athletes' advisors. Hrvat Športskomed Vjesn. 2012;27:28–33.

51. Couture S, Lamarche B, Morissette E, Provencher V, Valois P, Goulet C, Drapeau V. Evaluation of sports nutrition knowledge and recommendations among high school coaches. Int J Sport Nutr Exerc Metab. 2015;25:326–34.

52. Torres-McGehee TM, Pritchett KL, Zippel D, Minton DM, Cellamare A, Sibilia M. Sports nutrition knowledge among collegiate athletes, coaches, athletic trainers, and strength and conditioning specialists. J Athl Train. 2012;47(2):205–11.

53. Parnell JA, Wiens K, Erdman KA. Evaluation of congruence among dietary supplement use and motivation for supplementation in young, Canadian athletes. J Int Soc Sports Nutr. 2015;12:49.

54. Shaskey DJ, Green GA. Sports haematology. Sports Med (New Zealand). 2000;29(1) 27–38.

55. Rodenberg RE, Gustafson S. Iron as an ergogenic aid: iron-clad evidence? Curr Sports Med Rep. 2007;6(4):258–64.

56. Sandström G, Börjesson M, Rödjer S. Iron deficiency in adolescent female athletes – is iron status affected by regular sporting activity? Clin J Sport Med. 2012;22(6):495–500.

57. Koehler K, Braun H, Achtzehn S, Hildebrand U, Predel HG, Mester J, Schanzer W. Iron status in elite young athletes: gender-dependent influences of diet and exercise. Eur J Appl Physiol. 2012;112(2):513–23.

58. Beard J, Tobin B. Iron status and exercise. Am J Clin Nutr. 2000;72(2):S594–7.

59. Shaw BK, Gupta P. Weekly vs daily iron and folic acid supplementation in adolescent Nepalese girls. Arch Pediatr Adolesc Med. 2002;156(2):131–5.

60. Stear SJ, Prentice A, Jones SC, Cole TJ. Effect of a calcium and exercise intervention on the bone mineral status of 16–18-y-old adolescent girls. Am J Clin Nutr. 2003;77(4):985–92.

61. Weeks BK, Young CM, Beck BR. Eight months of regular in-school jumping improves indices of bone strength in adolescent boys and girls: the POWER PE study. J Bone Miner Res. 2008;23(7):1002–11.

62. Bailey DA, McKay HA, Mirwald RL, Crocker PRE, Faulkner RA. A six-year longitudinal study of the relationship of physical activity to bone mineral accrual in growing children: the University of Saskatchewan bone mineral accrual study. J Bone Miner Res. 1999;14(10):1672–9.

63. Sale C, Elliott-Sale KJ. Nutrition and athlete bone health. Sports Med. 2019;49(suppl 2):S139–51.

64. Byers AW, Connolly G, Campbell WW. Vitamin D status and supplementation impacts on skeletal muscle function: comparisons between young athletes and older adults. Curr Opin Clin Nutr Metab Care. 2020;23(6):421–7.

65. Lovell G. Vitamin D status of females in an elite gymnastics program. Clin J Sport Med. 2008;18(2):159–61.

66. Constantini N, Arieli R, Chodick G, Dubnov-Raz G. High prevalence of vitamin D insufficiency in athletes and dancers. Clin J Sport Med. 2010;20(5):368–71.

67. Lappe J, Cullen D, Haynatzki G, Recker R, Ahlf R, Thompson K. Calcium and vitamin D supplementation decreases incidence of stress fractures in female navy recruits. J Bone Miner Res. 2008;23(5):741–9.

68. Ward KA, Das G, Berry JL, Roberts SA, Rawer R, Adams JE, Mughal Z. Vitamin D status and muscle function in post-menarchal adolescent girls. J Clin Endocrinol Metab. 2009;94(2):559–63.

69. Astrand P. Experimental studies of working capacity in relation to sex and age. Copenhagen: Munksgaard; 1952.

70. Bar-Or O, Dotan R, Inbar O, Rothstein A, Zonder H. Voluntary hypohydration in 10- to 12-year-old boys. J Appl Physiol. 1980;48:104–8.

71. Drinkwater BL, Kupprat IC, Denton JE, Crist JL, Horvath SM. Response of prepubertal girls and college women to work in the heat. J Appl Physiol Respir Environ Exerc Physiol. 1977; 43(6):1046–53.

72. Shibasaki M, Inoue Y, Kondo N, Iwata A. Thermoregulatory responses of prepubertal boys and young men during moderate exercise. Eur J Appl Physiol Occup Physiol. 1997;75:212–8.

73. Roche D, Rowland T, Garrard M, Marwood S, Unnithan VB. Skin microvascular reactivity in trained adolescents. Eur J Appl Physiol. 2010;108:1201–8.

74. Centers for Disease Control and Prevention. Nonfatal sports and recreation heat illness treated in hospital emergency departments–United States, 2001–2009. MMWR Morb Mortal Wkly Rep. 2011;60(29):977–80.

75. Aragon-Vargas LF, Wilk B, Timmons BW, Bar-Or O. Body weight changes in child and adolescent athletes during a triathlon competition. Eur J Appl Physiol. 2013;113(1):233–9.

76. Volterman K, Obeid J, Wilk B, Timmons BW. Ability of milk to replace fluid losses in children after exercise in the heat. In: Williams CA, Armstrong N, editors. Children and exercise: the proceedings of the XXVII international symposium of the European Group of Pediatric Work Physiology. London and New York: Routledge; 2011. p. 101–5.

77. Bar-Or O. Nutrition for child and adolescent athletes. Sports Sci Exchange. 2000;13(2):77.

78. Jacob R, Lamarche B, Provencher V, Laramée C, Valois P, Goulet C, Drapeau V. Evaluation of a theory-based intervention aimed at improving coaches' recommendations on sports nutrition to their athletes. J Acad Nutr Diet. 2016;16; 1308–15.

79. Márquez S, Molinero O. Energy availability, menstrual dysfunction and bone health in sports; an overview of the female athlete triad. Nutr Hosp. 2013;28(4):1010–7.

80. Gastrich MD, Quick V, Bachmann G, Moriarty AM. Nutritional risks among female athletes. J Women's Health 2020; 29(5):693–702.

81. Langan-Evans C, Reale R, Sullivan J, Martin D. Nutritional considerations for female athletes in weight category sports. Eur J Sport Sci. 2022;22(5):730–2.

82. Black KE, Baker DF, Sims ST. Nutrition needs of the female athlete: risk and prevention of low energy availability. Strength Cond J. 2020;42(4):77–81.

83. Chumlea WC, Schubert CM, Roche AF, Kulin HE, Lee PA, Himes JH, Sun SS. Age at menarche and racial comparisons in US girls. Pediatrics. 2003;111(1):110–3.

84. Tarnopolsky LJ, MacDougall JD, Atkinson SA, Tarnopolsky MA, Sutton JR. Gender differences in substrate for endurance exercise. J Appl Physiol. 1990;68:302–8.

85. Spronk I, Heaney SE, Prvan T, O'Connor HT. Relationship between general nutrition knowledge and dietary quality in elite athletes. Int J Sport Nutr Exerc Metab. 2015;25:243–51.

86. Jürgensen LP, Daniel NVS, Costa Padovani R, Juzwiak CR. Impact of a nutrition education program in gymnasts' perceptions and eating practices. Motriz Rev Educ Fis. 2020;26(1):e10200206.

87. Bass M, Turner L, Hunt S. Counseling female athletes: application of the stages of change model to avoid disordered eating, amenorrhea, and osteoporosis. Psychol Rep. 2001;88(3 Pt 2):1153–60.

88. Warren MP, Perlroth NE. The effects of intense exercise on the female reproductive system. J Endocrinol. 2001;170(1):3–11.

89. Fahrenholtz IL, Sjödin A, Benardot D, Tornberg ÅB, Skouby S, Faber J, Sundgot-Borgen JK, Melin AK. Within-day energy deficiency and reproductive function in female endurance athletes. Scand J Med Sci Sports. 2018;28:1139–46.

90. Gibson JH, Mitchell A, Harries MG, Reeve J. Nutritional and exercise-related determinants of bone density in elite female runners. Osteoporos Int. 2004;15(8):611–8.

91. Rauh MJ, Nichols JF, Barrack MT. Relationships among injury and disordered eating, menstrual dysfunction, and low bone mineral density in high school athletes: a prospective study. J Athl Train. 2010;45(3):243–52.

92. Ihle R, Loucks AB. Dose-response relationships between energy availability and bone turnover in young exercising women. J Bone Miner Res. 2004;19:1231–40.

93. Loucks AB. Energy availability, not body fatness, regulates reproductive function in women. Exerc Sport Sci Rev. 2003;31(3):144–8.

94. Hoch AZ, Pajewski NM, Moraski L, Carrera GF, Wilson CR, Hoffmann RG, Schimke JE, Gutterman DD. Prevalence of the female athlete triad in high school athletes and sedentary students. Clin J Sport Med. 2009;19(5):421–8.

95. Desbrow B, McCormack J, Burke LM, Cox GR, Fallon K, Hislop M, Logan R, Marino N, Sawyer SM, Shaw G, Star A, Vidgen H, Leveritt M. Sports Dietitians Australia Position Statement: sports nutrition for the adolescent athlete. Int J Sport Nutr Exerc Metab. 2014;24:570–84.

96. Tayne S, Hrubes M, Hutchinson MR, Mountjoy M. Female athlete triad and RED-S. In: Piedade SR, Imhoff AB, Clatworthy M, Cohen M, Espreegueira-Mendes J, editors. The sports medicine physician. Springer Publishers; 2019. p. 395–411.

97. Vescovi JD, VanHeest JL. Case study: impact of inter- and intra-day energy parameters on bone health, menstrual function, and hormones in an elite junior female triathlete. Int J Sport Nutr Exerc Metab. 2016;26:363–9.

98. Hudson JI, Hiripi E, Pope HG Jr, Kessler RC. The prevalence and correlates of eating disorders in the national comorbidity survey replication. Biol Psychiatry. 2007;61(3):348–58.

99. Kong P, Harris LM. The sporting body: body image and eating disorder symptomatology among female athletes from leanness focused and nonleanness focused sports. J Psychol. 2015;49(2):141–60.

100. Canbolat E, Çakıroğlu FP. Eating disorders and nutritional habits of female university athletes. Turk J Sports Med. 2020;55(3):231–8.

101. American Psychiatric Association. Diagnostic and statistical manual of mental disorders: DSM-V. Arlington (VA): American Psychiatric Association; 2013.

102. Torstveit MK, Rosenvinge JH, Sundgot-Borgen J. Prevalence of eating disorders and the predictive power of risk models in female elite athletes: a controlled study. Scand J Med Sci Sports. 2008;18(1):108–18.

103. Carrigan KW, Petrie TA, Anderson CM. To weigh or not to weight? Relation to disordered eating attitudes and behaviors among female collegiate athletes. J Sport Exerc Psychol. 2015;37:659–65.

104. Maruyama-Nagao A, Sakuraba K, Suzuki Y. Seasonal variations in vitamin D status in indoor and outdoor female athletes. Biomed Rep. 2016;5:113–7.

105. Miller SM, Kukuljan S, Turner AI, van der Pligt P, Ducher G. Energy deficiency, menstrual disturbances, and low bone mass: what do exercising Australian women know about the female athlete triad? Int J Sport Nutr Exerc Metab. 2012;22(2):131–8.

106. Nazem TG, Ackerman KE. The female athlete triad. Sports Health. 2012 4(4):302–11.

107. Selby CLB, Reel JJ. A coach's guide to identifying and helping athletes with eating disorders. J Sport Psychol Action. 2011;2(2):100–12.

108. Payne JM, Kirchner JT. Should you suspect the female athlete triad? J Fam Pract. 2014;63(4):187–92.

109. Dwyer J, Eisenberg A, Prelack K, Song WO, Sonneville K, Ziegler P. Eating attitudes and food intakes of elite adolescent female figure skaters: a cross sectional study. J Int Soc Sports Nutr. 2012;9(1):53.

110. Łagowska K, Kapczuk K, Friebe Z, Bajerska J. Effects of dietary intervention in young Female athletes with menstrual disorders. J Int Soc Sports Nutr. 2014;11(1):21.

111. Barrack MT, Gibbs JC, Souza MJD, Williams NI, Nichols JF, Rauh MJ, Nattiv A. Higher incidence of bone stress injuries with increasing female athlete triad–related risk factors a prospective multisite study of exercising girls and women. Am J Sports Med. 2014;42(4):949–58.

112. Korpelainen R, Orava S, Karpakka J, Siira P, Hulkko A. Risk factors for recurrent stress fractures in athletes. Am J Sports Med. 2001;29(3):304–10.

113. Nattiv A. Stress fractures and bone health in track and field athletes. J Sci Med Sport. 2000;3(3):268–79.

114. Pollock N, Grogan C, Perry M, Pedlar C, Cooke K, Morrissey D, Dimitriou L. Bone-mineral density and other features of the female athlete triad in elite endurance runners: a longitudinal and cross-sectional observational study. Int J Sport Nutr Exerc Metab. 2010;20:418–26.

115. Kransdorf LN, Vegunta S, Files JA. Everything in moderation: what the female athlete triad teaches us about energy balance. J Womens Health. 2013;22(9):790–2.

116. Barron E, Sokoloff NC, Maffazioli GDN, Ackerman KE, Woolley R, Holmes TM, Anderson EJ, Misra M. Diets high in fiber and vegetable protein are associated with low lumbar bone mineral density in young athletes with oligoamenorrhea. J Acad Nutr Diet. 2016;116:481–9.

117. Mangels AR. Bone nutrients for vegetarians. Am J Clin Nutr. 2014;100(Suppl 1):469S–75S.

118. Oatway L, Vasanthan T, Helm JH. Phytic acid. Food Rev Int. 2001;17(4):419–31.

119. Burke LM, Cox GR, Culmmings NK, Desbrow B. Guidelines for daily carbohydrate intake: do athletes achieve them? Sports Med. 2001;31(4):267–99.

120. Lemon PWR. Do athletes need more dietary protein and amino acids? Int J Sport Nutr. 1995;5:S39–61.

121. Bollwein J, Diekmann R, Kaiser MJ, Bauer JM, Uter W, Seiber CC, Volkert D. Distribution but not amount of protein intake is associated with frailty: S cross-sectional investigation in the region of Nürnberg. Nutr J. 2013;12:109.

122. Paddon-Jones D, Rasmussen BB. Dietary protein recommendations and the prevention of sarcopenia. Curr Opin Clin Nutr Metab Care. 2009;12:86–90.

123. Rodriguez NR, DiMarco NM, Langley S. Position of the American Dietetic Association, Dietitians of Canada, and the American College of Sports Medicine: nutrition and athletic performance. J Am Diet Assoc. 2009;109:509–27.

124. Havemann L, West SJ, Goedecke JH, MacDonald IA, Gibson SC, Noakes TD, Lambert EV. Fat adaptation followed by carbohydrate loading compromises high-intensity sprint performance. J Appl Physiol. 2006;100(1):194–202.

125. Volek JS, Noakes T, Phinney SD. Rethinking fat as a fuel for endurance exercise. Eur J Sport Sci. 2015;15(1):13–20.

126. Kokubo Y, Yokoyama Y, Kisara K, Ohira Y, Sunami A, Yoshizaki T, Tada Y, Ishizaki S, Hida A, Kawano Y. Relationship between dietary factors and bodily iron status among Japanese collegiate elite female rhythmic gymnasts. Int J Sport Nutr Exerc Metab. 2016;26:105–13.

127. Beck KL, Mitchell S, Foskett A, Conlon CA, von Hurst PR. Dietary intake, anthropometric characteristics, and iron and vitamin D status of female adolescent ballet dancers living in New Zealand. Int J Sport Nutr Exerc Metab. 2015;25:335–43.

128. Alaunyte I, Stojceska V, Plunkett A. Iron and the female athlete: a review of dietary treatment methods for improving iron status and exercise performance. J Int Soc Sports Nutr. 2015;12:38.

129. Matsumoto M, Hagio M, Katsumata M, Noguchi T. Combined heme iron supplementation and nutritional counseling improves sports anemia in female athletes. Ann Sports Med Res. 2015;2(6) 1036–42.

130. Badenhorst CE, Goto K, O'Brien WJ, Sims S. Iron status in athletic females, a ship in perspective of an old paradigm. J Sports Sci. 2021;39(14):1565–75.

131. Juzwiak CR, Amancio OMS, Vitalle MSS, Pinheiro MM, Szejnfeld VL. Body composition and nutritional profile of male adolescent tennis players. J Sports Sci. 2008;26(11):1209–17.

132. Martin SA, Tarcea M. Consequences of lack of education regarding nutrition among young athletes. Palestrica of the Third Millennium—Civilization and Sport. 2015;16(3):241–6.

133. Ackerman KE, Misra M. Bone health and the female athlete triad in adolescent athletes. Phys Sports Med. 2011;29(1):131–41.

134. Foo LH, Zhang Q, Zhu K, Ma G, Trube A, Greenfield H, Fraser DR. Relationship between vitamin D status, body composition and physical exercise of adolescent girls in Beijing. Osteoporos Int. 2009;20:417–25.

135. Martínez S, Pasquarelli BN, Romaguera D, Arasi C, Tauler P, Aguiló A. Anthropometric characteristics and nutritional profile of young amateur swimmers. J Strength Cond Res. 2011;25(4):1126–33.

136. Willis KS, Peterson NJ, Larson-Meyer DE. Should we be concerned about the vitamin D status of athletes? Int J Sport Nutr Exerc Metab. 2008;18(2):204–24.

137. Miller KK. Mechanisms by which nutritional disorders cause reduced bone mass in adults. J Womens Health. 2003;12(2):145–50.

138. Weinstein JR, Anderson S. The aging kidney: physiological changes. Adv Chronic Kidney Dis. 2010;17(4):302–7.

139. Neder JA, Jones PW, Nery LE, Whipp BJ. The effect of age on the power/duration relationship and the intensity-domain limits in sedentary men. Eur J Appl Physiol. 2000;82(4):326–32.

140. Vigorito C, Giallauria F. Effects of exercise on cardiovascular performance in the elderly. Front Physiol. 2014;5:51.

141. Woo JS, Derleth C, Stratton JR, Levy WC. The influence of age, gender, and training on exercise efficiency. J Am Coll Cardiol. 2006;47(5):1049–57.

142. Peiffer JJ, Galvao DA, Gibbs Z, Smith K, Turner D, Foster J, Martins R, Newton RU. Strength and functional characteristics of men and women 65 years and older. Rejuvenation Res. 2010;13(1):75–82.

143. Kostka T. Quadriceps maximal power and optimal shortening velocity in 335 men aged 23–88 years. Eur J Appl Physiol. 2005;95(2–3):140–5.

144. Borges N, Reaburn P, Driller M, Argus C. Age-related changes in performance and recovery kinetics in masters athletes: a narrative review. J Aging Phys Act. 2016;24:149–57.

145. Beelen M, Burke LM, Gibala MJ, Van Loon LJC. Nutritional strategies to promote postexercise recovery. Int J Sport Nutr Exerc Metab. 2010;20(6):515–32.

146. Churchward-Venne TA, Holwerda AM, Phillips SM, van Loon LJC. What is the optimal amount of protein to support post-exercise skeletal muscle reconditioning in the older adult? Sports Med. 2016;46:1205–12.

147. Doering TM, Reaburn PR, Phillips SM, Jenkins DG. Postexercise dietary protein strategies to maximize skeletal muscle repair and remodeling in masters endurance athletes: a review. Int J Sport Nutr Exerc Metab. 2016;26:168–78.

148. Finger D, Golz FR, Umpierre D, Meyer E, Rosa LHT, Schneider CD. Effects of protein supplementation in older adults undergoing resistance training: a systematic review and meta-analysis. Sports Med. 2015;45:245–55.

149. Lutter C, Hotfiel T, Tischer T, Lenz R, Schöffl V. Evaluation of rock climbing related injuries in older athletes. Wilderness Environ Med. 2019;30(4):362–8.

150. Rosenkilde M, Morville T, Andersen PR, Kjær K, Rasmusen H, Holst JJ, Dela F, Westerterp K, Sjödin A, Helge JW. Inability to match energy intake with energy expenditure at sustained near-maximal rates of energy expenditure in older men during a 14-d cycling expedition. Am J Clin Nutr. 2015;102:1398–405.

151. Reaburn P. Nutrition and the ageing athlete. In: Burke L, Deakin V, editors. Clinical sports nutrition. Melbourne: McGraw-Hill; 2000. 602 p.

152. Kenney WL, Hodgson JL. Heat tolerance, thermoregulation and aging. Sports Med. 1987;4:446–56.

153. Kenney WL, Tankersley CG, Newswanger DL, Hyde DE, Turner NL. Age and hypohydration independently influence the peripheral vascular response to heat stress. J Appl Physiol. 1990;68:1902–8.

154. Kenney WL, Fowler SR. Methylcholine-activated eccrine sweat gland density and output as a function of age. J Appl Physiol. 1988;65:1082–6.

155. Myburgh KH, Hutchins J, Fataar AB, Hough SF, Noakes TD. Low bone density is an etiologic factor for stress fractures in athletes. Ann Intern Med. 1990;113:754–9.

156. United States Department of Health and Human Welfare, National Institutes of Health. Women's health initiative reaffirms use of short-term hormone replacement therapy for younger women. National Institutes of Health News Release, 2013. Accessed 2018 May 8. Available from: https://www.nih.gov/news-events/news-releases/womens-health-initiative-reaffirms-use-short-term-hormone-replacement-therapy-younger-women

157. Manore MM. Vitamin B6 and exercise. Int J Sport Nutr. 1994; 4:89–103.

158. Casale G, Bonora C, Migliavacca A, Zurita IE, de Nicola P. Serum ferritin and ageing. Age and Ageing. 1981;10: 119–22.

159. Nieman DC. Exercise immunology: future directions for research related to athletes, nutrition, and the elderly. Int J Sports Med. 2000;21(Suppl 1):S61–8.

160. MacLaughlin J, Holick MF. Aging decreases the capacity of human skin to produce vitamin D3. J Clin Invest. 1985; 76:1536–8.

161. Scott D, Ebeling PR, Sanders KM, Aitken D, Winzenberg T, Jones G. Vitamin D and physical activity status: associations with five-year changes in body composition and muscle function in community-dwelling older adults. J Clin Endocrinol Metab. 2015;100(2):670–8.

162. Walsh NP. Nutrition and athlete immune health: new perspectives on an old paradigm. Sports Med. 2019;49(Suppl 2): S153–68.

163. Strasser B, Pesta D, Rittweger J, Burtscher J, Burtscher M. Nutrition for older athletes: focus on sex differences. Nutrients. 2021;13:1409.

164. Deutz NEP, Bauer JM, Barazzoni R, Biolo G, Boirie Y, Bosy-Westphal A, Cederholm T, Cruz-Jentoft A, Krznariç Z, Nair KS, Singer P, Teta D, Tipton K, Calder PC. Protein intake and exercise for optimal muscle function with aging: recommendations from the ESPEN Expert Group. Clin Nutr. 2014;33(6):929–36.

165. Desbrow B, Burd NA, Tarnopolski M, Moore DR, Elliott-Sale KJ. Nutrition for special populations: young, female, and masters athletes. Int J Sport Nutr Exerc Metab. 2019;29:220–7.

166. Dueck CA, Manore MM, Matt KS. Role of energy balance in athletic menstrual dysfunction. Int J Sport Nutr. 1996; 6(2):165–90.

167. Van de Loo DA, Johnson MD. The young female athlete. Clin Sports Med. 1995;14(3):687–707.

168. Karpinski CA, Milliner K. Assessing intentions to eat a healthful diet among national collegiate athletic association division II collegiate athletes. J Athl Train. 2016;51(1):89–96.

CHAPTER 11

Nutrition Strategies for Power, Endurance, and Combined Power/Endurance Sports

CHAPTER OBJECTIVES

- Identify the differences in energy metabolic processes between power, team, and endurance athletes.
- Explain the best dietary strategies for fueling power athletes before, during, and after training/competition.
- Explain the best dietary strategies for fueling endurance athletes before, during, and after training/competition.
- Explain the best dietary strategies for fueling team sport athletes before, during, and after training/competition.
- Discuss the common dietary problems observed in power athletes, endurance athletes, and team sport athletes.

- Identify appropriate foods and beverages that can be consumed during competitions for specific power sports, endurance sports, and team sports.
- Know the different muscle types and their energy utilization characteristics.
- Analyze the different potential outcomes well-nourished and poorly nourished athletes may obtain from consumption of creatine monohydrate supplements.
- Identify the relative energy availability from stored glycogen, fat, and protein.
- Know the primary reason for gluconeogenesis, and the amino acid and nonamino acid substances that can be used to create glucose from noncarbohydrate substances.

Case Study: Lots of Protein—All the Time

Jonathan, a recent college graduate, was deeply saddened by the recent death of his father at age 72 from cardiovascular disease with kidney failure complications. He thought seriously about what he could do to honor his father, a successful businessman and a former competitive weightlifter with a family room full of trophies. He decided that his dad would be greatly pleased to know that his son had taken up weightlifting with an eye toward being competitive. Jonathan's father always wanted his son to take up weightlifting to help build both his muscles and his self-esteem, but Jonathan was a bookworm with only minimal interest in sport. Jonathan joined a weightlifting club, got all the necessary gear and clothes, and met his coach, who instructed him on the weightlifting schedule and the nutritional protocol to follow. Jonathan was seriously committed

to doing this in honor of his dad's memory, so after his first session he immediately went to the neighborhood health food store and picked up large jars of whey protein concentrate, whey protein isolate, and boxes of high-protein bars—his new dietary focus to help his muscles and to develop the weightlifting. He also went to the grocery store and stocked up on meats—steak, chicken, fish. He was told to eat lots of protein all the time, as that was the key to his development as a weightlifter, and that is precisely what he was going to do. Carbohydrates, he was told, were not good for him, so he decided to limit his intake to an occasional baked potato.

After following the weightlifting and high-protein intake protocol for several weeks, Jonathan started noticing some changes. His body was definitely growing muscle, and

(continued)

some of the muscles were starting to peek through this body fat. Despite these changes, he was not feeling as good as he had hoped. The first few weeks were terrible, but he understood that to be a common problem associated with the increased physical activity. But he had hoped that, by now, he could feel better and more vigorous. Instead, he smelled terrible, he was urinating with greater frequency than ever before, and his urine was dark yellow. To make matters worse, he felt tired all the time, as if his brain needed to be purposely jolted to focus. His bookworm days were over, as reading just one page made him lose his concentration.

After a few more weeks of this he decided something was just not right, so he forced himself to look into some recommended nutrition protocols for getting fit. What he found surprised him. All that protein was not the best way to fuel his muscle, plus the volume of protein he was eating was forcing him to excrete a great deal of nitrogenous waste that increased dehydration risk (thus the deep-yellow urine). To make matters worse, the low-carbohydrate intake made it difficult for him to maintain normal central nervous system (*i.e.*, brain) function, which is reliant on blood sugar (carbohydrates) as a primary fuel. Then he learned that much of the protein he was eating was really high in saturated animal fat that, in the long term, would cause the same problems responsible for his dad's death.

He decided to do it right by eating good foods with good-quality protein distributed well throughout the day. The way he felt changed almost immediately, and his time at the gym while weightlifting became an act of pleasure rather than an act of suffering.

CASE STUDY DISCUSSION QUESTIONS

High protein consumption is common among power athletes, as it is commonly believed that only protein will help to increase muscle mass, which is a necessary part of power sports such as weightlifting.

1. What is the maximum protein consumption that an athlete, including a power athlete, should consume daily (in g/kg)?
2. What are the components of eating protein and other nutrients correctly to help ensure that the consumed protein can be used anabolically to help build and maintain muscle tissue?
3. What are the common health problems that can be experienced from a high-protein/low-carbohydrate intake?
4. If you were standing in front of a group of power athletes, what are the three key nutrition messages you would give them to help them achieve their goals?

INTRODUCTION

Following an appropriate nutritional strategy that is well integrated into the athlete's lifestyle and sport-specific demands is a critical component of success in the competitive athlete. Interestingly, many of the general nutrition recommendations for athletes deviate little from the general recommendations for the general public to lower chronic disease risk. Regardless of the sport, poor nutrient exposure through consumption of foods that have low nutrient density, poor hydration, and poor energy balance during the day has a negative impact on athlete health, increases injury risk, and diminishes performance. However, the type of physical activity related to the demands of sport-specific training and competition requires that nutrition recommendations are fine tuned to ensure that the athlete can perform at her or his conditioned capacity.

Ensuring that these specific nutritional requirements are met requires an understanding of the energy metabolic pathways, the desired body composition of the athlete, and the opportunities during the competition (*i.e.*, breaks between quarters, half-time) that provide natural opportunities for supplying needed nutrients and fluids. Importantly, studies of competitive athletes suggest that many have suboptimal dietary intakes that fail to provide the nutrients and fluids that could enable better performance (1). Athletes often consume the same few foods, resulting in a monotonous intake that fails to optimally expose tissues to the wide array of needed nutrients. In addition, they often attempt to "make weight" using strategies that result in poor energy availability, and hydration strategies suggest insufficient consumption of less-than-optimal beverages. A failure to provide sufficient energy in a way that dynamically matches need is likely to result in low blood sugar, which will result in **gluconeogenesis** and diminish the potential muscular benefit an athlete may achieve from exercise. Any of these factors alone can diminish performance, but athletes often fail to satisfy *all* of these nutritional factors (*i.e.*, energy, nutrients, and fluids). This may be due to not only inadequate dietary planning, but also nutrition-related myths and the confusion associated with the availability of a wide array of different products, each with different contents, that is marketed to athletes. As an example, the carbohydrate energy products commercially available to athletes all *appear* to target the same nutritional needs, but they have an enormous variability in energy delivered, carbohydrate content, composition of carbohydrate and free sugar content, and osmolality (2) (Table 11.1).

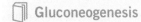 **Gluconeogenesis**

Refers to the metabolic process for producing glucose from noncarbohydrate substances, including lactate, glycerol, and glucogenic amino acids. The primary stimulus for gluconeogenesis is to maintain blood glucose, which is the primary fuel for the brain. As there is no storage depot for proteins, the glucogenic amino acids are obtained from the undesired catabolism of lean mass (muscle and organ mass).

Some sports require quick bursts of activity, some require steady continuous movement with occasional periods of fast activity, and others require that muscles work slowly and continuously for hours. Each type of activity places

Table 11.1	Descriptions of CHO Gels for Parameters Related to Service Size, Energy Density, Energy Content, CHO Content, Free Sugar Content, Fructose Content, and Osmolality			
	Mean ± SD	**Median**	**Range**	**Comments**
Serving size (g)	50 ± 22	45	29–120	20 out of 31 products are offered in packages below 45 g. Only two product ranges are packaged over 100 g.
Energy density (kcal/g)	2.34 ± 0.70	2.60	0.83–3.40	Only one product has an energy density <1 kcal/g. The most popular range of energy densities is 2–3 kcal/g, although a significant number of products (7 out of 31) do offer energy densities >3 kcal/g.
Energy/gel (kcal)	105 ± 24	100	78–204	The most popular energy range is between 100 and 120 kcal/gel. 25/31 products fall within this range, the majority falling within 100–110 kcal/gel.
Total CHO (g)	25.9 ± 6.2	24.6	18–51	The most popular carbohydrate range is 20–30 g/gel. 25/31 products fall into this range, with the majority of those (14 products) containing less than 25 g. Only three products offer less than 20 g, and only three offer more than 30 g.
Free sugars/gel (g)	9.3 ± 7.0	7.9	0.6–26.8	Only one product has free sugars <1 g/gel. Of the remainder, the majority (15 products) provide 5–15 g free sugar/gel. Four products provide >20 g free sugars/gel.
Free sugars/gel (% of total CHO)	35 ± 25	33	3–95	Only two products have free sugars <10% total CHO. 20/31 products have free sugars >20% of total CHO, and of these nearly half (nine products) have free sugars >50% of total CHO.
Fructose content	Unknown	Unknown	0–>20% CHO	Out of 31 products, only 3 do not contain fructose in some form. Exact amounts present cannot be quantified from the ingredient labels.
Osmolality (mmol/kg)	4,424 ± 2,883	4,722	303–10,135	Only one product range is isotonic. 27 out of 31 products have osmolality >1,000 mmol/kg.

CHO, cholesterol.

Source: Reprinted with permission from Zhang X, O'Kennedy N, Morton JP. Extreme variation of nutritional composition and osmolality of commercially available carbohydrate energy gels. Int J Sport Nutr Exer Metab. 2015;25:504–9.

unique demands on the muscles and on the fuels that muscles demand. There are clear metabolic differences in endurance activities and power activities. This chapter reviews the special nutrition requirements for athletes involved in power sports, endurance sports, and team sports.

The type of physical activity being performed influences the demands on how cells will derive the energy they require. Different sports place different demands on the energy system, but it is important to consider that all energy metabolic systems are functioning during **power activities**, including anaerobic metabolism, which includes energy derived from phosphagen breakdown and from anaerobic glycolysis (carbohydrates), and from aerobic metabolism from energy derived from carbohydrates and fats. Power activities mandate that the athlete has the ability to explode off a starting block, jump high distances, moves faster than a competitor to get to the ball or puck, throw a heavy weight, or push someone of equal size backward. The better the power athlete can do the activities associated with the sport they compete in, the more successful the athlete is. Getting power athletes to train muscles for these activities is critical for competitive success, and this training regimen must be supported by proper nutrition, or all that hard work will be fruitless.

Individual amino acids have been widely used by athletes and amino acid mixtures represent a large category of supplements targeting bodybuilders (3,4). There are no convincing studies to show that self-directed consumption of supplements is an effective strategy for performance enhancement. In addition, there are potential health risks associated with taking high-dose supplements (5). However, there are several studies on athletes demonstrating that consumption of milk-based protein following resistance activity effectively increases muscle **strength** and enables favorable changes in body composition (6,7). Good food sources of protein, such as meat, fish, poultry, dairy products, and legumes, in combination with cereals all provide good-quality protein with a desirable distribution of essential amino acids. Because of the scant evidence that consumption of supplementary protein is superior to eating these foods, which also expose athletes to other needed nutrients that include iron and zinc, athletes should take a *food-first* nutritional approach to improving performance (8–10).

📙 Power Activities

The term applied to sports that require the athlete to generate a high level of muscular force to produce fast and powerful movement speeds that are highly reliant on anaerobic metabolic processes. Examples of these

anaerobic sports include sprinting, boxing, weightlifting, baseball, wrestling, speed skating, sprint swimming, gymnastics, and hockey.

📙 Anaerobic Sports

Similar to power activities, anaerobic sports rely heavily, but not exclusively, on anaerobic metabolic processes and are typically sports that involve short duration/short distances with relatively high intensity. Examples are similar to those listed under power activities above, and include sprinting, gymnastics, boxing, wrestling, weightlifting, and bodybuilding.

📙 Strength

Often used synonymously with *power*, strength is a measure of the mass that can be moved (*i.e.*, lifted, pushed) by an athlete and is highly dependent on muscular mass or the muscle-to-weight ratio. For instance, an athlete with a high muscle-to-weight ratio should be able to move more mass for his/her weight than an athlete with a lower muscle-to-weight ratio.

ENERGY DEMANDS

Important Factors to Consider

- Different sports place different demands on energy metabolic systems, but all energy metabolic systems are being used nearly all the time. The difference is the proportion of demand. For instance, long-distance runners may be 10% reliant on anaerobic metabolic systems and 90% reliant on aerobic metabolic systems, whereas a 100-m sprinter may have proportions reversed (after all, the sprinter is still breathing and bringing oxygen into the system).

- Different energy systems draw on different sources of energy, which helps explain why primarily anaerobic activities can only proceed for a relatively short period of time. We have high levels of fat storage, which can be accessed aerobically for energy and allow the aerobic athlete to perform for long periods of time. However, anaerobic fuels, phosphocreatine (PCr) and glycogen, have limited storage that will become depleted quickly with continuous high-intensity activity.

- It is important to consider that athletes in a wide spectrum of sports commonly have dietary intakes that fail to meet recommended energy and carbohydrate recommendations (11). This inadequate intake will compromise training-associated benefits and increase injury risks.

Table 11.2	Muscle Fiber Types and Their Energy Utilization Characteristics		
Muscle Fiber	**Type I (Red)-Slow Twitch (High Fatigue Resistance)**	**Type IIa (Red)-Intermediate Fast Twitch (Moderate Fatigue Resistance)**	**Type IIb (White)-Fast Twitch (Low Fatigue Resistance)**
Ability to store and use glycogen	Low	Moderate	High
Ability to store and use fat	High	Moderate	Low
Ability to store and use phosphocreatine	Moderate	High	High
Ability to use oxygen in energy reactions (oxidative capacity)	High	Moderate	Low
Ability to produce power (contraction speed)	Low	High	Very High
Blood (capillary) supply to muscle fibers	High	Moderate	Low

Sources: Gleeson M. Chapter 3: Biochemistry of exercise. In: Maughan RJ, editor. Sports nutrition: volume XIX of the encyclopaedia of sports medicine—an IOC Medical Commission publication. London (England): Wiley/Blackwell; 2014. p. 36–8; Kenney LW, Wilmore J, Costill D. Physiology of sport and exercise. 6th ed. Champaign (IL): Human Kinetics; 2015. p. 40–1; Kenney LW, Wilmore J, and Costill D. Physiology of sport and exercise. 6th ed. Human Kinetics/Champaign. 2015. p. 40–1.

Power athletes utilize multiple energy-producing pathways that provide energy from phosphagen, carbohydrate, and/or fat. Understanding the different energy systems and the fuels needed for the production of **adenosine triphosphate** (ATP) is necessary when making nutritional recommendations (12). Power activities rely on appropriate conditioning of fast-twitch muscle fibers. Fast-twitch (type IIb) fibers can produce a tremendous amount of power and also have a high capacity to store carbohydrates as glycogen. However, they have a limited capacity to store fats as triglycerides. The different energy fuel storage potential helps to clarify the fuel dependence of each unique muscle fiber type (Table 11.2). At their genetic baseline, the intermediate fast-twitch muscle fibers (type IIa) also produce a high level of power, but these muscle fibers can be trained to behave more like the type I slow-twitch fibers in athletes who spend long hours in endurance activities (13). The type of training that is done is an important factor, therefore, in determining muscle fiber behavior. Power athletes require that the muscle fibers are capable of producing a high level of power. If a significant proportion of the training involves aerobic (*i.e.*, endurance) conditioning, the type IIa fibers may lose some power capacity because they have been conditioned to have more endurance potential. Interestingly, there is evidence that the intermediate fast-twitch fibers will revert to their genetic baseline (more power and less aerobic potential) rather quickly if the aerobic training ceases (14).

High-speed activity of short duration (such as the 100-m sprint) demands fuel that is already in the muscles in a near ready-to-go state. The amount of this ready-to-go fuel, **PCr**, that muscles can hold is limited, creating limits to the maximum duration of maximal speed/power activity. For a well-nourished athlete, the phosphagen system may provide sufficient fuel for the first 5–8 seconds. This is not sufficient for most events, requiring muscles to have the ability to quickly convert stored glycogen into useable fuel that can be metabolized anaerobically.

Adenosine Triphosphate

Abbreviated as ATP, a molecule synthesized by ATP synthase, is made of high-energy bonds that can rapidly release energy for all body processes that include muscle contraction. The storage of preformed ATP is small and can support maximal effort for only 1–2 seconds.

Phosphocreatine

Abbreviated as PCr, it is the main high-energy phosphate found in muscle cells and are a critically important part of the anaerobic PCr energy system. PCr, which is also referred to as *creatine phosphate*, can be used to rapidly replenish ATP. The preformed PCr storage in the body is small (the typical range will allow maximal effort for 2–8 seconds).

More ATP is produced per unit of time from the phosphagen system (*i.e.*, PCr) than from anaerobic glycolysis. As a result, the reduction in energy availability to muscles results in slower contraction and reduced speed. As a result, the speed of a sprinter slows when PCr can no longer provide the necessary ATP (Figure 11.1). Total fatigue occurs when PCr is depleted and blood and muscle lactate

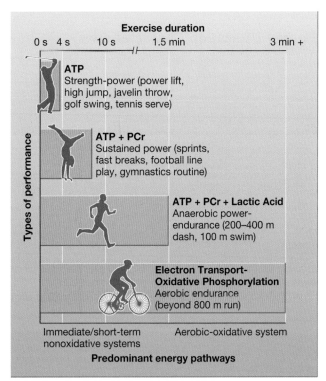

FIGURE 11.1: The predominant energy systems for different activities, ranging from sudden high intensity to endurance. Short-term maximal high-intensity activity is highly reliant on PCr to obtain sufficient ATP. When the limited stores of PCr are exhausted, more energy must be derived from anaerobic glycolysis, which cannot produce ATP at the same high rate as that of PCr. In practical terms, exhausting PCr stores necessarily results in having to "slow down" because of lower ATP production. Complete fatigue occurs when PCr is depleted and blood and muscle lactate are at the maximal level. ATP, adenosine triphosphate; PCr, phosphocreatine. (Illustration from Premkumar K. The massage connection, anatomy and physiology. 2nd ed. Baltimore (MD): Lippincott Williams & Wilkins; 2004. Data from Hirvonen J, Nummela A, Rusko H, Rehunen S, Härkönen M. Fatigue and changes of ATP, creatine phosphate, and lactate during the 400 m sprint. Can J Sport Sci. 1992;17(2):141–4 and Hirvonen J, Rehunen S, Rusko H, Härkönen. Breakdown of high-energy phosphate compounds and lactate accumulation during short supramaximal exercise. Eur J Appl Physiol Occup Physiol. 1987;56(3):253–9.)

are at the maximum level. Most scientists believe that the anaerobic maximum (*i.e.*, the amount of time an athlete can exercise at a maximal level) is ~1.5 minutes, but with wide variability depending on conditioned state (15,16). The combination of both anaerobic systems (phosphagen and anaerobic glycolysis), which are used when an athlete is going as hard and fast as possible, will be depleted in ~1.5 minutes with a concomitant increase in lactate, resulting in athlete fatigue and cessation of high-intensity work. This stoppage of high-intensity work varies widely between athletes, often a function of anaerobic

conditioning, occurs in ~1.5 minutes, and is commonly referred to as the **anaerobic threshold**.

As exercise time increases, power production decreases and a higher proportion of energy is derived from aerobic metabolic processes. **Aerobic metabolism** enables the metabolism of fat as an energy substrate, thereby reducing the reliance on glycogen and PCr, both of which have a limited storage capacity. Faster/harder physical activity results in greater fuel utilization per unit of time, with greater oxygen requirements needed to oxidatively burn the fuel. Muscular work that is sufficiently hard and fast to exceed the capacity to supply sufficient oxygen results in the anaerobic metabolism of PCr and glycogen to provide the needed fuel. However, although fat storage is virtually unlimited for even lean athletes, both PCr and glycogen have limited storage. Well-conditioned athletes have better oxygen delivery to cells, enabling relatively greater reliance on aerobic/oxidative metabolic processes and lower reliance on anaerobic metabolic processes (17). This allows them to go faster longer without achieving the fatigue associated with a buildup of lactate and depletion of PCr and glycogen. However, for fats to burn cleanly, carbohydrates are also necessary. Running out of available carbohydrate fuel diminishes the capacity to burn fats effectively and muscular fatigue sets in.

Anaerobic Threshold

Refers to the intensity of exercise during which lactic acid buildup exceeds the tissue capacity to remove it from working muscles. It is at this point that muscle function quickly degrades and the activity must stop, which is typically about 1.5 minutes after the initiation of the high-intensity activity. It is also referred to as the lactate threshold, the lactate turning point, and the lactate inflection point. In practical terms, the anaerobic threshold is often expressed as 75% of maximal oxygen consumption (*i.e.*, 75% VO_{2max}) or 85% of the maximal predicted heart rate. It is important to note that there and now portable skin-attached devices for detecting the anaerobic threshold by assessing sweat lactate during exercise (18). The primary components of the anaerobic threshold include (19):

- Inadequate oxygen delivery to exercising muscle, which results in…
- Elevated glycolysis, lactic acid, and hydrogen, which results in…
- Lower (*i.e.*, more acidic) blood pH, which results in…
- Increased Hydrogen (H+) buffered by blood, which results in…
- Higher Carbon Dioxide (CO_2) released from blood, which results in…
- More CO_2 released with each breath exhale.

It is important to consider that lactate is not a "waste" product of anaerobic metabolism. Instead, it should be considered an important stress response product that aims to diminish stress. With recovery, lactate is converted to pyruvate and oxidized for energy in working muscles (20).

📖 Aerobic Metabolism

Refers to energy processes that occur with the incorporation of oxygen. These processes include aerobic glycolysis, which is used for high-intensity activities that require a large volume of ATP, but that are within the athlete's capacity to bring sufficient oxygen into the system; and also the metabolism of fats, which is used for low-intensity activities of long duration that can produce a substantial volume of ATP, but without the production of system-limiting by-products such as lactic acid (lactate).

To summarize, energy can be obtained anaerobically (without oxygen) and also aerobically (with oxygen). Proportionately greater anaerobic energy pathways are used with high-intensity activities of shorter duration, whereas proportionately greater aerobic energy pathways are typically used with activities of lower intensity but longer duration (Table 11.3).

Phosphagen System (Creatine Phosphate)

Energy can be released anaerobically from the phosphates in ATP and creatine phosphate (PCr) to support high-intensity exercise for up to ~8 seconds. This system, referred to as the phosphagen system because of the immediate availability of high-energy phosphate, is dependent on PCr to quickly provide a high-energy phosphate molecule to form ATP, which is the ultimate source of energy for all body functions. There are a number of sports that rely heavily (if not exclusively) on this phosphagen system. These sports include shot put, long jump, triple jump, discus, gymnastics vault, and short sprints. In addition, other sports that have quick bursts of activity intermingled in the activity (such as football, volleyball, and hockey) are also reliant on this energy pathway. In some of these sports, the ability to do repeat high-intensity moves often determines the winner. For instance, the high jumper, long jumper, and pole-vaulter all need two or three stellar efforts with the hope that one of them will be good enough to win. These repeated bouts of high-intensity work place a tremendous reliance on the phosphagen system. The athlete who has the ability to store more creatine may be at an advantage in these activities. With improved creatine storage, it is possible that the athlete would retain, because of the capacity to adequately reform PCr, much of the power produced on the first attempt than in the second and third attempts.

Assuming that total energy and protein intake is adequate, athletes can manufacture the creatine needed for multiple quick bursts of high-intensity activity. To improve the storage of ATP-PCr in the muscles, athletes must practice activities that focus on this system (*i.e.*, activities that last no more than 8 seconds, that are high intensity, and that are repeated multiple times during an exercise

Table 11.3	**Energy Metabolic Systems**	
System	**Characteristics**	**Duration**
PCr system	Anaerobic production of ATP from stored PCr.	Used for maximal intensity activities lasting no more than 8 s.
Anaerobic glycolysis (lactic acid system)	Anaerobic production of ATP from the breakdown of glycogen. By-product of this system is the production of lactic acid.	Used for extremely high-intensity activities that exceed the athlete's capacity to bring in sufficient oxygen. Can continue producing ATP with this system no more than 2 min.
Aerobic glycolysis	Aerobic production of large amounts of ATP from the breakdown of glycogen.	Used for high-intensity activities that require a large volume of ATP, but that are within the athlete's capacity to bring sufficient oxygen into the system.
Oxygen system (aerobic metabolism)	Aerobic production of ATP from the breakdown of carbohydrates and fats.	Used for lower-intensity activities on long duration that can produce a substantial volume of ATP, but without the production of system-limiting by-products.

ATP, adenosine triphosphate; PCr, phosphocreatine.

session). This type of training, by itself, is not sufficient to improve short-duration, high-intensity performance. At the same time, consuming sufficient energy and protein, by itself, is also not sufficient to improve short-duration, high-intensity performance. However, when both proper training and proper nutrition are combined, the athlete can experience very real gains in short-duration, high-intensity performance. Even with higher creatine storage, the maximum preformed PCr is sufficient to last up to only 8 seconds of hard physical work. (If humans stored more than 8 seconds worth, we could probably combust from the high heat created with so much energy produced so quickly). Athletes performing maximal exercise for up to 8 seconds (sprint, vault, jumps) must take a break of 2–4 minutes with ample oxygen availability to allow for the regeneration of PCr before undertaking another maximal bout of exercise (21,22). Imagine a 100-m sprinter accelerating over the first 8 seconds of the race, but then PCr runs out and anaerobic glycolysis takes over. Because anaerobic glycolysis cannot produce as much ATP per unit of time as PCr, the person who wins the 100-m dash is typically the person who slows down the least during the last 2 seconds of the race.

In theory, having a higher level of stored creatine in the tissues enables improved PCr availability to form ATP and, therefore, greater capacity to do more extremely high-intensity work. It is for this reason that creatine monohydrate supplementation is popular with athletes who want to find a way to increase power and reduce the onset of fatigue. Although supplementation of creatine, typically in the form of creatine monohydrate, may increase creatine storage, the upper limit for preformed PCr remains about 8 seconds worth of fuel. In addition, the high creatine storage resulting from creatine monohydrate supplementation may result in water retention (23). This elevated body water weight is likely to have adverse performance effects. In athletes who fail to consume sufficient energy and protein, supplementing with creatine may be useful in maximizing PCr potential (24). However, there is evidence that sufficient energy intake may be the key to ensuring that sufficient PCr is stored and remanufactured when required (25). As displayed in Table 11.4, different fuels have different capacities to supply energy. As indicated, we have an enormous capacity to supply fat for energy, whereas the storage of carbohydrate fuels is limited. Although the protein mass has the potential of being broken down as a source of energy, this typically only occurs when carbohydrate fuel becomes depleted.

The glucogenic amino acids can be converted to carbohydrates (glucose) (Box 11.1), but fat cannot be converted to carbohydrates (26). It is important, therefore, for athletes to sustain carbohydrate availability during physical activity to help ensure that the protein mass (*i.e.*, muscles) is not broken down as a source of needed fuel. The protein mass indicated in Table 11.4 is provided as a source of potential energy, but by no means should this protein mass be considered as a desired source of energy for the athlete.

Table 11.4	Energy Stores in an Average Man Weighing 70 kg (154 lb) With 15% Body Fat		
Energy Source	**Mass (kg)**	**Energy (kcal)**	**Exercise (min)**[a]
Liver glycogen	0.08	307	16
Muscle glycogen	0.40	1,530	80
Blood glucose[b]	0.01	38	2
Fat	10.5	92,800	4,856
Protein	12.0	48,725	2,550

Values assume sole energy substrate availability during marathon pace activity or about 20 kcal/min.

[a]Minutes refer to the hypothetic time of exercise if the person were solely reliant on the energy source indicated. The value is provided for comparison purposes, to display relative availability of different fuels.

[b]Value for blood glucose includes the glucose content of extracellular fluid. Not all of this and not more than a very small part of the total protein is available for use during exercise.

Source: Adapted from Gleeson M. Biochemistry of exercise. In: Maughan R, editor. Nutrition in sport: volume VII of the Encyclopedia of Sports Medicine—an IOC Medical Commission publication. London (England): Wiley Blackwell; 2000. p. 29.

Box 11.1 Glucogenic Amino Acids

Amino acids derived from protein tissues, including muscles and organs, that can be converted to glucose are:

- alanine
- threonine
- serine
- glycine
- α-aminobutyrate
- methionine
- tyrosine
- lysine

Anaerobic Metabolism (Glycolysis)

Anaerobic metabolism (glycolysis) is used to provide energy during high-intensity exercise that exceeds the athlete's ability to provide sufficient oxygen to tissues for the work being performed. Intense physical activity is, to a large degree, dependent on the availability of muscle glycogen (the storage form of glucose). Depletion of glycogen during high-intensity activity results, therefore, in rapid fatigue and the cessation of exercise. In normal daily nonintense activity, glycolysis provides only a small proportion of the total energy required by working muscles. A sudden increase in muscle movement and/or continuous high-intensity activity is reliant on glycolysis because it can provide tissue energy quickly and fills the energy gap between the onset of sudden movement and/or intense activity and the time required for aerobic energy metabolism to satisfy energy needs. If someone tries to maintain a high-intensity (*i.e.*, anaerobic) activity, the fuel for this will run out after ~1.5 minutes, and the athlete will become quickly fatigued.

Even predominantly **aerobic sports** may rely on the anaerobic energy pathway to make the difference between winning and losing. The long-distance runner who has run most of the race aerobically and has preserved some muscle glycogen is likely to require the added ATP energy from glycolysis to finish the race with a strong (anaerobic) "kick" (27,28). The athlete who has this energy preserved at the end of the race may be the only difference between first place and those who follow. For runners running short-distance races, for swimmers in short races, and for hockey players skating at full bore at the end of a game to go for a winning score, this anaerobic pathway is an important key to success. Carbohydrate storage is the key to making this happen, and storage occurs best with the consumption of carbohydrate foods/beverages (29).

Anaerobic Metabolism

Refers to energy processes that occur without the need for oxygen. Includes anaerobic glycolysis, which involves cellular metabolic processes that produce energy from glycogen (stored carbohydrate) without the need for oxygen; also includes the phosphagen system, which produces energy from PCr metabolism.

Aerobic Sports

Includes sports that rely heavily, but not exclusively, on aerobic metabolic processes and typically involve long duration/long distances with relatively low intensity. Examples include long-distance running, distance swimming, distance cycling, and speed walking.

NUTRITION STRATEGIES FOR IMPROVING POWER AND SPEED

Depending on the speed and VO_{2max} percent of the activity, the proportion of the energy derived from these different energy metabolic systems varies (12). As indicated in Table 11.5, *quicker* activities are proportionately more reliant on anaerobic energy metabolism, whereas *longer duration* activities are proportionately more reliant on aerobic energy metabolism. However, all metabolic systems are contributors to satisfying the athlete's energy needs.

Power athletes perform power and speed activities that utilize primarily the PCr and glycolytic anaerobic metabolic systems. Glycogen and lipid stores are present in all muscle fiber types, but fast-twitch muscle fibers have a 16%–31% greater level of glycogen storage than slow-twitch fibers (30). During exercise, the glycogen concentration decreases first in slow-twitch fibers, but decreases quickly in fast-twitch fibers thereafter (31). The lower fat

Table 11.5	Proportionate Usage of Energy Metabolic Systems to Satisfy Energy Needs in Power Sports				
Event Time Range		% VO_{2max}	Anaerobic Phosphocreatine	Anaerobic Glycolysis	Aerobic
0.5–1 min, such as 400-m run; 100-m swim		~150	~10	~47–60	~30–43
1.5–2.0 min, such as 800-m run; 200-m swim; 500-m kayak		113–130	~5	~29–45	~50–66
3.0–5.0 min, such as 1,500-m run; 40-m swim; 1,000-m kayak		103–115	~2	~14–18	~70–84
5.0–8.0 min, such as 3,000-m run; 2,000-m rowing		98–102	<1	~10–12	~88–90

Source: Adapted from Stellingwerff T, Maughan RJ, Burke LM. Nutrition for power sports: middle-distance running, track cycling, rowing, canoeing/kayaking, and swimming. J Sports Sci. 2011;29(S1):S79–89.

storage in type IIa and IIb muscle fibers is a result of having limited oxidative capacity because of relatively poor blood supply. This makes it difficult to supply these fibers with energy substrates and to remove metabolic by-products (*i.e.*, lactate) out of the fibers during physical activity. This also helps to explain why high-intensity/power activities rarely go beyond 1.5–2.0 minutes and why athletes require a recovery break of 2–5 minutes to enable muscle recovery of PCr (32).

Important Factors to Consider

Sprinting is used to define brief maximum effort in running, cycling, swimming, canoeing, rowing, field hockey, soccer, and rugby. In general, a sprint is considered brief maximal effort of less than 60 seconds duration, with an exercise intensity of effort well beyond VO_{2max}.

- Elite male sprinters can maintain maximal speed for 20–30 m
- Elite female sprinters can maintain maximal speed for 15–20 m
- Gender differences due to
  - Mechanical factors (foot strike, neuromuscular coordination, air resistance) and
  - Metabolic factors (PCr availability)

The high dependence on fast-twitch muscle fibers needed for high-intensity anaerobic work makes it relatively more difficult for power athletes to metabolize fat as an energy substrate when compared with athletes that perform aerobic activities and are more reliant on oxidative metabolism (33). Power athletes continue to burn limited amounts of fat, but high-intensity anaerobic activity dramatically favors carbohydrates (glycogen) over fat as a fuel because of the kind of muscle fibers that are being used. When power athletes stop their intensive in-season training but maintain their high calorie, relatively high-fat diets, a sufficient difference in energy balance occurs that causes inevitable increase in body fat. This may be at least in part due to fat intakes that often exceed recommended intake levels, perhaps from an emphasis on meat-derived high-protein diets that are naturally high in fat (34). Besides the poor competitive body composition this excessively high-fat intake results in, there is evidence that the weight cycling many power athletes often experience may predispose them to obesity following retirement from the sport, which

increases risk of greater illness frequency and earlier mortality (35,36).

Important Factors to Consider

Air resistance can influence speed and energy utilization in sprint performance:

- Elite 100-m sprinters running 10 m/s would run 0.25–0.5 s faster if they did not have to overcome air resistance (37).
- Air resistance accounts for 16% of total energy expended to run 100 m in 10 s (38).
- Mexico City altitude (less air resistance) provides a 0.07 s advantage over 100 m (39).

Carbohydrate Recommendations for Power/Strength/Speed Athletes

Glycogen is a key source of energy in anaerobic metabolism, and high-carbohydrate diets enhance glycogen stores, resulting in longer time to fatigue when compared with high-protein, low-carbohydrate diets (40). Studies have consistently found that low-carbohydrate diets providing ~3%–15% of total calories from carbohydrate weaken high-intensity performance (41,42). Carbohydrate metabolism provides the majority of ATP during exercise exceeding 75% VO_{2max}. These high intensities mandate consumption of high-carbohydrate diets to avoid glycogen depletion. Even a single bout of high-intensity training can lower glycogen stores by 24%–40%, depending on exercise duration and intensity (43,44).

Current carbohydrate intake guidelines recommend consumption of ~8–12 g/kg/day for power/strength athletes who spend a significant proportion of the day (>4–5 hrs/day) involved in moderate- to high-intensity exercise. For athletes involved in 1–3 hr/day of moderate- to high-intensity activity, the recommended carbohydrate intake is 6–10 g/kg/day (45). Surveys of strength athletes vary widely in the typical consumption of carbohydrate, often suggesting that intakes are far below the recommended level. Lifters and throwers typically report carbohydrate intakes of 3–5 g/kg/day, and bodybuilders report intakes of 4–7 g/kg/day, regardless of gender (33). It is clear that inadequate carbohydrate intake negatively impacts performance, particularly when exercise intensity is high (46). It is also clear that carbohydrate ingestion has an ergogenic benefit on high-intensity resistance exercise by, importantly, increasing time to fatigue (47).

Protein Recommendations

For power/speed athletes, a protein intake of 1.5–1.7 g/kg/day is recommended, or approximately double the requirement for an average healthy nonathlete (0.8 g/kg/day) (48). The recommendation of the American College of Sports Medicine (ACSM) for all athletes is a protein intake that typically ranges from 1.2–2.0 g/kg/day (45). The ACSM now also recommends that the protein be consumed in modest amounts (~0.3 g/kg per meal) of high-quality protein with regular spacing throughout the day to optimize muscle protein synthesis and muscle recovery (see Example 11.1). Optimal utilization of protein only occurs with sufficient energy availability, so ensuring an adequate caloric intake that is dynamically spaced during the day to satisfy energy requirements is an important dietary strategy (49). Taking these factors together strongly implies that athletes should consume good-quality protein in meals and snacks that are distributed throughout the day, with special focus on protein consumption immediately following exercise to encourage muscle protein synthesis (50).

Example 11.1: Calculating Protein Distribution During the Day for Athletes Weighing 110 kg

Calculate total protein requirement:

110 kg × 1.7 g protein/day = 187 g protein/day

Calculate amount per meal:

0.3 g/meal × 110 kg = 33 g protein/meal

Calculate number of meals with recommended protein:

187 g/33 g = 5.7 (rounded to 6)

Interpretation: This athlete requires 33 g of protein ~6×/day to satisfy the protein requirement of 187 g/day

---

Surveys of athletes consuming >3,000 kcal/day suggest that they consume at or above the currently recommended level of protein, but often fail to appropriately distribute the protein consumption in amounts that will result in optimal muscle protein synthesis (33). There is also reason to believe that consumption of greater than the recommended amount of protein, often at the expense of carbohydrates, fails to enhance muscle protein synthesis and muscle recovery and results in catabolizing more protein as a source of energy with no anabolic benefit (51).

Fat Recommendations

Carbohydrate should serve as the primary fuel for power athletes, but fat is also an important fuel that is available for moderate- to high-intensity activity of up to 85% VO_{2max} (52). The generally recommended level of fat intake has been estimated at 2 g/kg/day, as intakes greater than this level may interfere with muscle glycogen recovery and muscle tissue repair through displacement of needed carbohydrate and protein (53). This level of intake should suffice for the delivery of fat-soluble vitamins, essential fatty acids, and synthesis of hormones (12). Surveys of power/strength athletes suggest that fat consumption exceeds currently recommended levels, and the fat is often high in saturated fatty acids (34). It has been suggested that the excessively high intake of fat may be the result of a high consumption of meat, as these athletes try to consume high levels of protein (33). It is important to consider that excess consumption of one energy substrate necessarily results in an inadequate consumption of another energy substrate in athletes who are satisfying total energy requirements.

Building Lean (Muscle) Mass

Building muscle mass has been the tradition for centuries with power athletes, including for the 6th century Greek Olympic wrestling champion, Milo of Croton, who was famous for carrying a growing calf the length of the stadium each day (progressive resistance exercise), and after 4 years of carrying it, he ate the calf (excessively high protein intake) (54,55). Modern power athletes also investigate strategies for enhancing muscle mass to improve both strength and power. There are many techniques employed for increasing muscle mass, including resistance training, consumption of more energy (calories), and consuming products (often illegal) that claim to improve muscle acquisition. Some strategies work, whereas others do not, so power/strength athletes should be careful about the strategies that follow. It may appear that consumption of a substance works to improve musculature, but often this may be because it merely fulfills a dietary weakness that could more easily and less expensively be resolved by following some relatively simple dietary strategies. Excess protein consumption is commonly believed to enhance muscle development, but this strategy may be counterproductive because of the excess nitrogenous excretion and associated dehydration that develops. Excess protein consumption has been reported in several surveys, ranging from 1.9–4.3 g/kg for men and 0.8–2.8 g/kg for women (56,57). Assuming the protein is distributed well throughout the day, there is some evidence that protein intake levels of up to 2.2 g/kg/day may be useful in bodybuilding (58). It appears that the source of protein (animal or plant), when an adequate level of protein is consumed, does not affect changes in lean mass or muscle strength in older adults, but younger adults appear to have greater lean mass and strength benefits from the consumption of similar doses of animal versus plant protein (59). However, while there remain few studies assessing the source of plant protein consumed and the impact lean mass and strength, there is evidence that consuming slightly higher servings of plant protein sources result in similar favorable changes in lean mass and strength (60). It is well established that resistance training stimulates muscle development and that the level of muscle development may be influenced by the circulating level of human growth hormone, insulin, testosterone, and other anabolic hormones (61–64). In as much as nutrition may have an impact on the availability of these substances, it seems reasonable to believe that specific nutrients may play a role in muscle development. However, it is also reasonable to believe that nutrient intake would not influence the body's production of these substances if their levels are already normal. In other words, in the absence of a specific nutrient deficiency it is difficult to believe that taking more of a nutrient would alter the production of muscle-building hormones. Again, more than enough is not better than enough.

NUTRITION STRATEGIES FOR IMPROVING ENDURANCE

Endurance athletes are involved in events with continuous movement for longer than 20 minutes. Typically, endurance sports require continuous movement over long distances or time periods (marathon, cross-country skiing, triathlon, etc.). Premature fatigue most likely occurs from either dehydration or depletion of carbohydrate stores (65). Other problems experienced by endurance athletes, including gastrointestinal (GI) distress and hyponatremia, may also result in performance failure (66). GI distress is most likely to occur in long-distance races, often the result of poor adaptation to the consumption of drinks that contain excessively concentrated electrolytes, energy substrates, or other substances. Hyponatremia is typically seen in events lasting longer than 4 hours in athletes who overconsume fluids with insufficient electrolyte concentrations and, should the associated edema occur in the brain, could be life-threatening (67). The endurance athlete's goal is to establish a strategy, practiced in training, for supplying sufficient fluids and energy of the right types and concentrations to sustain muscular work for a long duration.

As defined earlier in this chapter, aerobic metabolism is the energy system of greatest importance for endurance athletes, with both fat and glycogen serving as critically important fuels. In this energy pathway, oxygen is used to help transfer phosphorus into new ATP molecules. Unlike anaerobic metabolism, this energy pathway can use protein, fat, and carbohydrate for fuel by converting pieces of these energy substrates into a compound called acetyl coenzyme A (acetyl CoA). Glucose is converted to pyruvic acid (an anaerobic, energy-releasing process), and this pyruvic acid can be converted either to acetyl CoA with the help of oxygen or to an energy storage product called lactic acid. Of course, if too much lactic acid builds up, the muscle will fatigue and activity will stop (the problem with doing exclusively anaerobic work). However, the lactic acid can easily be reconverted to pyruvic acid to be used as a fuel aerobically. Aerobic metabolism occurs in the mitochondria of cells, where the vast majority of all ATP is produced from the entering acetyl CoA. Fats can be converted to acetyl CoA through a process called the β-oxidative metabolic pathway. This pathway is very oxygen dependent, which means that fats can only be burned aerobically.

The majority of endurance activity takes place at an intensity that allows fats to contribute a high proportion of the fuel for muscular work (Figure 11.2). Because there is an almost inexhaustible supply of fat in even the leanest athlete, supplying fats before and during physical activity is not a concern and would not be a goal. However, carbohydrate is involved in the complete combustion of

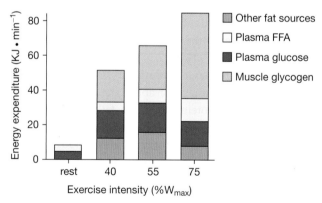

FIGURE 11.2: Energy utilization changes with duration of exercise. During 20 minutes of exercise with increasing intensity, the utilization of carbohydrate and fat changes, with an increasing proportion of muscle glycogen satisfying total energy requirements of higher intensities. FFA, free fatty acids. (Reprinted with permission from Van Loon LJC, Greenhaff PL, Constantin-Teodosiu D, Saris WH, Wagenmakers AJ. The effects of increasing exercise intensity on muscle fuel utilization in humans. J Physiol. 2001;536:301.)

fats, and because the storage capacity for carbohydrates is relatively low and easily depleted, the goal for endurance athletes is to find a way to supply enough carbohydrates to last for the duration of the activity. In prolonged exercise, approximately half the energy is initially derived from carbohydrates and half from fat. However, as muscle glycogen concentration becomes reduced, blood glucose becomes a more important source of muscle energy. After 2 hours of exercise, or sooner depending on conditioning and exercise intensity, carbohydrate intake is required to maintain blood glucose and carbohydrate metabolism (68). Failure to maintain blood glucose results in mental fatigue, which results in muscular fatigue even if there is remaining energy availability in muscles.

An athlete's ability to achieve a steady state of oxygen uptake into the cells is a function of how well an athlete is aerobically conditioned. An athlete that frequently trains aerobically is likely to reach a steady state faster than one who does not train aerobically (69). Well-conditioned athletes may require 5 minutes before sufficient oxygen is available to cells for aerobic metabolism to continue at a steady state. As indicated in Figure 11.3, the first 5 minutes of activity is supported by a combination of anaerobic and aerobic metabolism. The ability to quickly achieve a fast steady state is important because it diminishes the duration of time spent in acquiring energy anaerobically, which places a heavy burden on carbohydrates (muscle and liver glycogen), for which humans have limited storage.

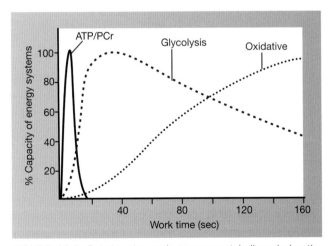

FIGURE 11.3: Relative change in energy metabolism during the initiation of exercise. At the onset of exercise, three energy systems are used continuously, but the contribution of each system to satisfying total energy needs changes as the exercise continues. At the initiation of exercise, the anaerobic PCr system provides the most ATP, following by anaerobic glycolysis, and then followed by aerobic metabolism. ATP, adenosine triphosphate; PCr, phosphocreatine. (From Bandy WD. Therapeutic exercise for physical therapy assistants. 3rd ed. Philadelphia (PA): LWW (PE); 2013.)

Table 11.6	Typical Maximal Oxygen Uptake (mL/kg/min) of Trained Athletes in Selected Sports[a]	
	Males	**Females**
Sport/Activity	**VO_{2Max}**	**VO_{2Max}**
Cross-country skiing	73.4 ± 6.7	68 ± 4.2
Endurance running	69.8 ± 6.3	(No Data)
5-km running	64.0 ± 4.0	53.2 ± 5.5
Cyclists	64.0 ± 5.5	53.5 ± 3.6
Triathlon	61.9 ± 9.6	(No Data)
Soccer	58.3 ± 4.2	(No Data)
Sedentary	51.5 ± 4.40	34.8 ± 5.6

[a]Data for sport specific female athletes provided where available.

Sources: Crisp AH, Verlengia R, Gonsalves Sindorf MA, Germano MD, de Castro Cesar M, Lopes CR. Time to exhaustion at VO_{2max} velocity in basketball and soccer athletes. J Exerc Physiol 2013;16(2):82–5; Marsland F, Mackintosh C, Holmberg H-C, Anson J, Waddington G, Lyons K, and Chapman D. Full course macro-kinematic analysis of a 10km classical cross-country skiing competition. PLoS One. 2017;12(8):e0182262; Sandbakk Ø, Holmberg H-C. A reappraisal of success factors for Olympic Cross-Country Skiing. Int J Sports Physiol Perform. 2014;9:117–21; Nummela AT, Paavolainen LM, Sharwood KA, Lambert MI, Noakes TD, Rusko HK. Neuromuscular factors determining 5 km running performance and running economy in well-trained athletes. Eur J Appl Physiol. 2006;97:1–8; Galbraith A, Hopker J, Cardinale M, Cunniffe B, Passfield L. A 1-year study of endurance runners: training, laboratory tests, and field tests. Int J Sports Physiol Perform. 2014;9:1019–25; Ramsbottom R, Nute MGL, Williams C. Determinants of five kilometer running performance in active men and women. Br J Sports Med. 1987;21(2):9–13; Costa VP, de Matos DG, Pertence LC, Martins JAN, de Lima JRP. Reproducibility of cycling time to exhaustion at VO_{2max} in competitive cyclists. J Exerc Physiol. 2011;14(1):28–34; Vikmoen O, Ellefsen S, Trøen Ø, Hollan I, Hanestadhaugen M, Raastad T, and Rønnestad BR. Strength training improves cycling performance, fractional utilization of VO_{2max} and cycling economy in female cyclists. Scand J Med Sci Sports. 2016;26:384–96; Karlsen A, Racinais S, Jensen MV, Nørgaard SJ, Bonne T, Nybo L. Heat acclimatization does not improve VO_{2max} or cycling performance in a cool climate in trained cyclists. Scand J Med Sci Sports. 2015;25(suppl 1):269–76; Brisswalter J, Wu SSX, Sultana F, Bernard T, Abbiss CR. Age difference in efficiency of locomotion and maximal power output in well-trained triathletes. Eur J Appl Physiol. 2014;114:2579–86; Unal M, Unal DO, Baltaci AK, Mogulkoc R, Kayserilioglu A. Investigation of serum leptin levels in professional male football players and healthy sedentary males. Neuro Endocrinol Lett. 2005;26(2):148–51; Woorons X, Mollard P, Lamberto C, Letournel M, Richalet J-P. Effect of acute hypoxia on maximal exercise in trained and sedentary women. Med Sci Sports Exerc. 2005;37(1):147–54.

Athletes in aerobic sports are better able to use oxygen metabolically than power athletes (Table 11.6). However, because carbohydrates is needed for the complete combustion of fat, carbohydrate remains the limiting energy source for endurance work because, relative to fat storage, the storage of carbohydrates is low. This is clearly demonstrated by findings that athletes consuming a high-fat diet have a maximal endurance time of 57 minutes; on a normal mixed diet their endurance rises to 114 minutes; and on a high-carbohydrate diet, their maximal endurance rises to 167 minutes (70).

Athletes with different levels of conditioning achieve steady state at different levels of exercise intensity. A well-conditioned athlete may be capable of maintaining a steady state at a sufficiently high level of exercise intensity to win a race. For instance, this athlete can perform at a very high pace but is still able to provide enough oxygen to cells to satisfy aerobic requirements. At the London Olympic Games in the summer of 2012, the winner of the marathon ran 26.2 miles at a pace of about 4 minutes 50 seconds per mile! This is an extremely fast pace, but the athlete maintained primarily aerobic metabolism during the race or would not have been able to complete it if a higher proportion of energy was derived anaerobically from carbohydrates. Whatever the athlete's oxidative capacity, exceeding that level causes a greater proportion of the muscular work to rely on anaerobic metabolism, with an associated increase in the reliance on carbohydrate fuel. Because there is a limited storage of carbohydrate fuel, the carbohydrate fuel tank runs out more quickly, and the person becomes exhausted faster.

Important Factors to Consider

Carbohydrate Depletion Causes Activity Cessation in Both Anaerobic and Aerobic Activities

- The primary fuel for anaerobic metabolism is carbohydrates. Power athletes are involved in short-duration, high-intensity activity that is characterized by a high proportion of anaerobic activity that is carbohydrate dependent. Therefore, carbohydrate depletion is an inhibition to the continuation of anaerobic activity.
- The primary fuels for aerobic metabolism are fat and, to a lesser extent, carbohydrates. Endurance athletes are involved in long-duration aerobic activity that is both fat and carbohydrate dependent. Although a smaller proportion of carbohydrate is used in endurance activity, the activity is longer than in anaerobic activity. Therefore, carbohydrate depletion is an inhibition to the continuation of aerobic activity.

Practicing nutrition strategies for the provision of fuel and fluids makes it easier for the athlete to tolerate the strategies during competition. Human systems require time and repetition to adapt to whatever you do, and this adaptation also affects nutritional strategies.

Energy Demands

It has been estimated that cross-country skiers use ~4,000 calories during a 50-km race and may use even more energy (up to 8,000 calories per day) when in intensive training (71). The energy consumption in ultramarathon runners is reported to average 5,530 kcal/day, with average hourly energy expenditures that exceed 333 kcal/day (69). It has been estimated that a 25-year-old female marathoner weighing 125 lb and running 10 miles at a 6-minute-per-mile pace in the morning and 8 miles of interval training in the afternoon would require 3,000 calories for the activity, plus 1,331 calories to cover the needs of "resting energy expenditure," for a total daily energy requirement of more than 4,300 kcal (72). (Resting energy expenditure represents the energy needed to maintain the lean mass and to carry on normal body functions when the body is at rest.) A consistent failure to supply sufficient energy to satisfy both the needs of exercise and resting energy expenditure results in the loss of weight and muscle (73).

Fluid Recommendations

As athletes exercise, there is an inevitable loss of body water through sweat. This cooling system, plus the normal urinary water loss, may amount to over 10 L (about 11 quarts) of daily water loss when exercising in a warm environment (74). In a hot and humid environment, water loss may exceed 3 L/hr but may be less than 0.5 L/hr in cool and dry environments (75). Despite the high rates of sweat loss experienced by athletes, most athletes replace only 50% of the water that is lost, a behavior that inevitably leads to progressive dehydration and a decline in performance (76,77). Research has clearly demonstrated that even a slight dehydration (2% of body weight) causes a measurable decrease in athletic performance (78,79). Therefore, when athletes take steps to satisfy fluid requirements, they are helping to guarantee optimal athletic performance (see Chapter 7, "Hydration Issues in Athletic Performance").

Carbohydrate Recommendations

Because carbohydrate storage is relatively low when compared with fat stores, athletes must make a conscious effort to replace carbohydrate at every opportunity. Having high levels of stored carbohydrates (glycogen) and consuming carbohydrates during activities that last 1 hour or more are well-established techniques for optimizing athletic endurance. It is well documented that consuming carbohydrate during activity helps to maintain blood sugar (glucose) and insulin, which encourages sugar uptake by working muscles (80). An example can be seen in the 100 km ultramarathon world champion winner, who ran for ~6.5 hours. It was necessary for him to consume ~58 g of carbohydrate/hr during the race to avoid glycogen depletion (69). It was found that endurance cyclists who consumed a carbohydrate-containing beverage during the exercise were able to exercise *an additional hour* when compared with cyclists who consumed only water (68). Athletes are encouraged to consume ~9–10 g (35–40 calories) of carbohydrate per kilogram of body weight each day. For a 150 lb athlete, this level of intake amounts to 600 g (2,400 calories) of daily carbohydrates consumption. Expressed as a percent of total calories, this recommendation suggests that ~60% of total calories should be derived from carbohydrates (81).

During competition, the concentration of carbohydrates is an important consideration to avoid GI distress. It has been found that a 5.5% (13 g of carbohydrate per 8 oz of fluid) carbohydrate solution produced almost no GI distress, which was similar to the lack of gastric distress with the consumption of plain water. However, a concentration slightly greater than this level (6.9% carbohydrate, or 16 g of carbohydrate per 8 oz of fluid) appeared to double the incidence of GI distress when athletes were asked to perform the same exercise (82). This finding suggests that endurance athletes should consume appropriate amounts of carbohydrate early in the event with continued regular consumption to obtain the needed amount without inducing GI distress. There were similar results in a study of marathon running performance, which found on three separate tests that consumption of a 5.5% carbohydrate solution produced superior performance results than a 6.9% carbohydrate solution (83). Therefore, the classic nutritional paradigm of *more than enough is not better than enough* appears to be true. Although athletes have a high requirement for carbohydrates, providing excessive amounts too quickly creates difficulties that may detract from performance.

The composition of the carbohydrate provided may also influence endurance performance and GI distress. A study comparing 6% carbohydrate solutions containing a combination of glucose, fructose, and sucrose or fructose alone during 105 minutes of cycling exercise found that the fructose-only beverage resulted in a greater frequency of GI distress, a more significant drop in blood volume, a higher increase in cortisol, angiotensin-I, and adrenocorticotropic hormone (all of which are considered stress hormones), and reduced exercise performance (84). It is generally recommended that for events lasting longer than 2.5 hours, relatively large amounts (up to 90 g/hr) of mixed source carbohydrates (*i.e.*, combinations of glucose, sucrose, maltodextrin) should be consumed during physical activity to avoid glycogen depletion (66,45). For endurance events of between 1 and 2.5 hours, the recommended carbohydrate intake is between 30 and 60 g/hr (45).

Resynthesis of glycogen *following* activity is also important, because glycogen reserves are severely depleted following activity lasting 1 hour or longer. The efficiency of glycogen resynthesis is dependent on several factors (85):

- the timing of the carbohydrates intake,
- the amount of carbohydrates consumed,
- the type of carbohydrates consumed, and
- the degree to which muscle has been damaged during the exercise (damaged muscle is slower to resynthesize glycogen than healthy muscle).

Foods containing carbohydrates that enter the blood quickly (*i.e.*, high glycemic index foods) are better able to resynthesize liver and muscle glycogen than foods low on the glycemic index scale, especially when consumed immediately following exercise. The general recommendation is to consume ~200 calories of carbohydrates every 2 hours following exercise, with the first 200 calories being provided as soon after exercise as possible (86).

Protein Recommendations

Although power/speed athletes, on average, consume more protein, it appears that endurance athletes actually require slightly more protein than power athletes (87,88). The estimated requirement for endurance athletes is approximately double the level recommended for nonathletes (1.5 vs. 0.8 g/kg) (86). With the exception of vegetarians, most endurance athletes appear to consume this level of protein from food alone (55,89). A summary of protein intakes suggests an average intake of 1.8 g/kg for both male and female endurance runners (90). High levels of protein consumption are common for athletes, but there is concern that chronic excess protein consumption may result in progressive renal damage (91). There is also concern that excess protein intakes may compromise bone mineral density, placing the athlete at higher risk of fracture (92). In addition, excess protein may also increase dehydration risk (93). Regardless of the athletic endeavor, therefore, athletes should be cautious about getting sufficient protein to satisfy needs and to consume the protein in a pattern that optimizes utilization but should also be careful that they do not consume levels of protein that far exceed requirements.

Fat Recommendations

High-fat diets are periodically recycled in the literature as being performance enhancing, but there are clear data to suggest that improving fat metabolism occurs best with high-carbohydrate diets in endurance athletes. Therefore, endurance athletes should consume fats at levels that enable satisfaction of total energy requirements when consuming relatively high-carbohydrate and moderate protein diets (45,94).

Vitamin Recommendations

The B-vitamins (thiamin, riboflavin, and niacin) are particularly important for endurance activities, but endurance athletes with carbohydrate intakes that satisfy needs (~60% of total calories) are virtually ensured of satisfying the need for B-vitamins from the foods they consume (95). Despite this, many endurance athletes take vitamin supplements, but these supplements fail to provide any performance benefit. In addition, the excess niacin consumption resulted in the inhibition of fat metabolism with greater reliance on glycogen, resulting in premature fatigue (96). Endurance athletes should consider performing a cost–benefit analysis to determine if the money spent on supplements might be better spent on good-quality foods (45).

Minerals

Ensuring optimal iron status is critically important for endurance performance, which relies heavily on aerobic metabolism (97). Given the importance of iron status in endurance activity, and because iron deficiency is the most common nutrient deficiency in both athletes and nonathletes, endurance athletes should give serious consideration to having iron status (hemoglobin, serum ferritin, hematocrit) assessed at regular yearly intervals. Vegetarian athletes are at higher risk of iron, zinc, and calcium deficiencies, all of which are important for aerobic metabolism and/or athlete health (45). As such, it may be even more important for vegetarian athletes to have regular, objective measures of these nutrients. Should an examination of the blood and/or bone density suggest

a nutritional weakness, a medical professional can then prescribe an appropriate strategy, which may include supplementation, to the athlete.

Endurance athletes should be cautious about excess nutrient consumption. It was found that men who supplemented with an oral dose of 1 g (1,000 mg) of vitamin C per day experienced a significant reduction in endurance capacity, perhaps by preventing key cellular adaptations to exercise that would allow for training improvements (98). On the other hand, getting enough of each nutrient and enough energy is critical to both performance and health. It is clear that restrained eating patterns in elite female endurance runners are the single biggest factor in low bone mass, and that the longer the caloric restriction, the greater the problems associated with recovery of muscle mass and glucose tolerance (99,100). So, although *more than enough is not better than enough*, it is still important to *get enough*. Many endurance athletes fail to consume sufficient nutrients and/or energy to get the most out of their training and reduce injury risk. Studies of athletes participating in the Ironman® triathlon, simulated adventure races, and other ultraendurance cycling events all have found significant nutritional weaknesses in participating athletes (99,101). Ideally, these athletes should obtain all of the needed nutrients through the appropriate consumption of food. Failing that, however, taking low-dose supplements of targeted nutrients that are known to be inadequate through medical tests is a reasonable option. The clear message is *food first*.

Building Energy and Fluid Reserves to Support Endurance Activities

In virtually every study that has examined athletes with high glycogen reserves versus those with lower reserves, those with higher reserves consistently perform better. Endurance athletes who begin competition with more stored carbohydrates (glycogen) have more glycogen available at the end of the competition. This difference alone may be enough to determine the winner (69). In addition, endurance athletes who initiate exercise in a better hydrated state perform better than those who are less well hydrated (65,45). Achieving an optimal carbohydrate and fluid intake does not happen, however, without careful planning for what to consume before, during, and after practice and/or competition.

Before Training and/or Competition

Consumption of between 800 and 1,200 kcal of carbohydrates for the 24 hours prior to exercise results in improved performance (102,103). Current recommendations encourage additional carbohydrate intake (1–4 g/kg) in the period immediately prior to exercise to ensure sustained glycogen availability (45). Ideally, the foods consumed prior to training or competition should be familiar foods that are known to be well tolerated. New foods, gels, or sports beverages consumed prior to a competition have the potential to create unexpected GI distress that inhibits performance at a high level. Ideally, the athlete should practice what they intend to do during competition during training to ensure the body is well adapted to both the type of food/beverage and the amounts that are likely to be consumed. Competition is not the best time for athletes to experiment with any nutrition strategy. Importantly, there is clear evidence that many athletes fail to follow appropriate pretraining nutrition strategies, regardless of age, sex, sport, and competition level (104).

Hydration

Ensuring that the endurance athlete achieves a well-hydrated state prior to exercise is important, as any level of underhydration may have a negative impact on performance (105). The current recommendation is consumption of 5–10 mL/kg during the 2–4 hours before exercise initiation (65). Ideally, the athlete should strive to achieve urine that is light, pale yellow in color, as darker urine color is a sign of underhydration (106). In the past, endurance athletes tried consuming high-sodium foods and beverages to enhance fluid retention, and some consumed glycerol (glycerine) as a means of enlarging the blood volume. Although glycerine consumption has been found to be successful, the use of glycerol and other substances that can be used to superhydrate is specifically banned by the World Anti-Doping Agency, making this strategy one that should not be followed (107).

Fluid loss during physical activity exceeds the rate that fluids can be consumed and absorbed. Therefore, it is impossible to achieve a well-hydrated state during exercise if the athlete initiates exercise already poorly hydrated. Consumption of sports beverages prior to exercise is useful because they provide several things that athletes most require: carbohydrates, fluids, and electrolytes:

- the fluid consumed should be flavored and sweetened to encourage fluid intake,
- to help maintain training intensity, the fluid should contain carbohydrates, and
- to stimulate rapid and complete rehydration, the beverage should contain sodium chloride (salt).

Glycogen Stores

Optimizing glycogen stores can typically occur within 24 hours of training, with consumption of high levels of carbohydrates and cessation of any activity that may be glycogen depleting (108). For ultraendurance events, athletes can maximize glycogen storage through consumption of high levels of carbohydrates for 4–5 days, during which glycogen-depleting exercise is diminished (109). During the period immediately preceding training or competition, athletes can continue to ensure that liver and muscle glycogen remain high through consumption of well-tolerated carbohydrates and beverages at a level of 1–4 g/kg. Ideally, these foods should be relatively low in fiber and fats, and moderate in protein to enable gastric emptying (108,110). (Athletes do best if they initiate exercise with no solids in the stomach.) Carbohydrate-containing liquids consumed prior to exercise may also be useful for athletes who are predisposed to GI distress prior to competition (45). Consuming a small amount of protein, coupled with carbohydrates and fluids, prior to exercise may be useful for synthesizing glycogen and for stimulating muscle protein synthesis (7). However, current studies are mixed regarding whether protein consumed prior to exercise improves endurance performance (111). Consumption of fat is important to ensure adequate energy consumption, typically with a recommended range of 20%–35% of total energy consumed. However, consumption of fat prior to physical activity may delay gastric emptying, thereby limiting the consumption of adequate levels of carbohydrates and fluids, and increasing the risk of GI distress. There are relatively new claims that restricting carbohydrates and replacing carbohydrates with fat is performance enhancing. However, there is no evidence that this high-fat dietary strategy is supported by scientific studies (45).

During Training and/or Competition

In events such as 10-km races and marathons, where fluids are available at regular intervals, the athlete should take full advantage of each fluid station and consume fluids. Because water is constantly being lost, frequent and regular consumption of fluids helps to maintain the body's water level. Because most athletes consume less water than they need, techniques for ensuring hydration during activity have been studied. The following recommendations have been suggested (112):

- Make certain that fluid is always nearby, because accessibility helps to ensure better fluid intake.
- All athletes should have their own bottle from which to drink, and this bottle should be with them whenever they exercise or are at a competition.

- Coaches should design practices that enable athletes to drink frequently.
- The coaching staff should be aware of those athletes with high sweat rates to make certain they consume more fluids than those with lower sweat rates.
- Help athletes learn to drink frequently by considering this to be part of the training regimen.

To understand how much fluid an athlete needs to consume during practice and competition, a log should be maintained with the amount of fluid consumed and the beginning and ending weight of the athletes. If an athlete consumes 32 oz during practice and weighs 2 lb less at the end of practice than at the beginning, this athlete should learn to consume an additional 32 oz of fluid during the practice (1 lb = 16 oz of fluid). Consumption of fluids that contain carbohydrates is important during exercise, and properly designed sports beverages can aid in providing both fluids and carbohydrates quickly. The ideal sports beverage should have the following characteristics:

- Cool beverages are tolerated best.
- A carbohydrate solution of between 6% and 7% delivers both the carbohydrate and the fluid quickly. A higher carbohydrate concentration slows delivery to the muscles by delaying gastric emptying and may increase the risk of gut upset.
- A small amount of sodium helps drive the desire to drink, and in so doing helps to ensure that the athlete stays better hydrated. Sodium may also aid in getting the water and carbohydrates absorbed more quickly and help to maintain blood volume. Maintenance of blood volume is an important predictor of athletic performance. There is some evidence that hyponatremia (low blood sodium), which results from large losses of sodium in sweat that goes unreplaced, occurs in endurance and ultraendurance events (113). This is a rare but serious condition that may result in seizures, coma, or death.
- The beverage should taste good to the athlete. The taste sensation may be altered during exercise, so there is no guarantee that a fluid you enjoy drinking at dinner will taste good to you while exercising. Make sure an athlete tries different flavors during exercise to determine what is best liked.
- The carbohydrate should be from a combination of glucose and sucrose. Beverages containing predominantly fructose increase the risk of creating gut upset.
- Noncarbonated sports drinks are preferred over carbonated drinks during endurance exercise.

Consumption of carbohydrates in both solid and liquid forms results in the same performance outcomes, so athletes in some sports may choose to consume carbohydrate foods rather than carbohydrate beverages (114). Cyclists who go long distances, for instance, often consume bananas and carbohydrate gels to support their carbohydrate requirement. It appears as if the consumption of 45–75 g of carbohydrates per hour (180–300 calories from carbohydrates per hour) helps to improve athletic performance (115). This amount of carbohydrate can be found in approximately one quart of sports beverage with a 6% carbohydrate concentration.

After Training and/or Competition

Although you may think you have done everything you need to do once your exercise is over—except shower—it is clear that drinking more fluids and consuming more carbohydrates after the exercise or competition is important. Doing this will help you replenish your glycogen stores and get you ready for the next day of exercise. The best glycogen replenishment occurs if you consume high glycemic index carbohydrates immediately following exercise and continue consuming carbohydrates (via snacks) until the next meal (86). Dietary protein plays a role. There is increasing evidence strongly suggesting that skeletal muscle breakdown increases with endurance training and/or with a single endurance exercise bout. Athletes who consume foods immediately following endurance activity have a favorable synthesis of skeletal muscle protein (95). The postendurance activity period is critically important for athletes, making it a time for serious planning. Carbohydrates should be consumed during this postexercise period at a rate of 1.2 g of carbohydrate per kilogram of body weight per hour (1.2 g/kg/h) over several hours, and mixing this with some high-quality protein appears to be useful from an exercise recovery standpoint (116). There is also a good deal of beginning evidence to suggest that the amount and timing of protein is important from a tissue utilization standpoint.

General Daily Considerations

The before-, during-, and after-exercise periods are meant to provide carbohydrates and fluids to support the activity, but what you do the rest of the time helps to ensure that the before-, during-, and after-exercise strategies actually work. Obviously, the consumption of carbohydrates and fluids during these periods does not provide all the nutrients and minerals an athlete needs to support health and activity. For this reason, it is imperative that what you eat the rest of the time provides a balance of nutrients that can keep you healthy. It is very true that healthy athletes are better athletes. A good basic strategy to follow is to encourage the consumption of a wide variety of foods that are high in complex carbohydrates, moderate in protein, and low in fats and sugars. This type of food distribution is perfect for athletes and will help to ensure that all necessary nutrients are consumed.

There is nothing an athlete can do just before competition to correct a nutrient deficiency and help performance. If your intake of iron is consistently low, and you develop iron deficiency anemia, it could take 6 months on a good diet and iron supplements to bring your iron level up to a point where performance will not be negatively affected. If you have a nutrient deficiency, doing everything right before, during, and after exercise still will not have you performing up to your conditioned ability. So eat well and eat wisely when you have the chance and, of course, drink plenty of fluids.

Other Nutritional Recommendations

There are several rules of nutrition that apply here. Among them is the idea of the need to consume a wide variety of foods to ensure that the body is exposed to all of the essential nutrients. On the backside of this rule, there is another benefit. By consuming a wide variety of foods, athletes can avoid being exposed to any potentially toxic substances that are more prevalent in some foods. Therefore, eating a wide variety of foods is a good nutritional rule to live by. Another rule is the idea that it is possible to eat too much of something, even if it is believed to be a "good" food. Learning to balance your diet through variety will help ensure your body of both proper maintenance and adequate nutrient intake.

NUTRITION STRATEGIES FOR COMBINED POWER/ ENDURANCE SPORTS

Most team sports (basketball, volleyball, soccer, etc.) have combinations of higher- and lower-intensity activities (**combination aerobic/anaerobic sports**), making them different from purely power activities, such as gymnastics, or purely endurance activities, such as the marathon. Therefore, team athletes must possess both power and endurance characteristics that were described earlier in this chapter. Different team sports have different metabolic requirements. For instance, American football has a greater emphasis on power than soccer (117). Despite these differences, the major characteristic of team sports is that there are periods of relatively low-intensity activity that are interrupted with bursts of high-intensity activity, and this intermittent activity influences nutritional requirements (118,119). The high-intensity bursts of activity, which are dependent on the phosphagen and anaerobic glycolysis systems, place high importance on carbohydrate availability, and the lower-intensity aerobic activity places high importance of carbohydrate and fat availability (120). It makes perfect sense, therefore, that studies have found clear performance benefits from consumption of carbohydrate in intermittent sprint activities, such as those seen in football or basketball (121,122).

Despite the importance of carbohydrate consumption in intermittent-intensity activities, surveys of team sport athletes suggest carbohydrate intake that, on average, are below the recommended level for carbohydrate of 6–10 g/day, with average intakes of both male and female team sport athletes consuming less than 6 g/day (117). Of concern is that the expenditure of energy and carbohydrate on competition days is higher than on training days, yet team sport athletes consume less on these competition days than on training days (120).

Combination Aerobic/Anaerobic Sports

Include sports that have a heavy reliance on both aerobic and anaerobic metabolic processes and are typically sports that involve intermittent activity that varies from slower movement to sprinting. Examples include basketball, hockey, field-hockey, and soccer.

Before Training and/or Competition

It is generally recommended that the pre-exercise or precompetition meal be constituted heavily of starchy, easy-to-digest, high-carbohydrate foods, and consumed ~3–4 hours before exercise (123). Consumption of ample fluids with meals and during the period between the meal and the exercise session or competition is also important (124). It has been reported that teams prefer to add low-fat protein sources to provide more satiety, but high-fiber foods should not be consumed prior to an event to avoid GI distress. It is also recommended that high-fat foods also be limited to avoid delays in gastric emptying (125). Food consumption patterns in team sport players typically occur 2–4 hours prior to training and/or competition (125).

During Training and/or Competition

Consumption of carbohydrate is also important in team sports. Compared with the results of a trial when a placebo (water) was consumed, subjects performed seven additional 1-minute cycling sprints at 120%–130% of VO_{2max} when they consumed a 6% carbohydrate–electrolyte beverage. This is equivalent to making a dramatic improvement in sprint capability during the last 5–10 minutes of a basketball game (126). A similar study found that sports drinks (*i.e.*, carbohydrate–electrolyte beverages) can help maintain high-intensity efforts that consist of intermittent sprinting, running, and jogging (127). The general recommendation is to consume carbohydrate–electrolyte sports beverages at every opportunity the game permits and to take particular advantage of half-time to consume carbohydrates and fluids (117).

After Training and/or Competition

Postexercise or postcompetition is a time to support muscle recovery through appropriate nutritional strategies. Ideally, athletes should immediately consume high-carbohydrate foods/drinks that also contain protein. This strategy enables better glycogen and protein synthesis (128,129). Fluid consumption for rehydration and replenishment of depleted glycogen stores should provide ~24 oz/lb of body weight (1.5 L/kg of body weight) that was lost during the activity (45). Because the enzyme involved in synthesizing glycogen (glycogen synthetase) reaches its peak immediately following physical activity, muscle glycogen stores are efficiently replaced if the athlete consumes carbohydrate immediately following the activity. For the 2 hours immediately following activity, consume high glycemic index foods (*i.e.*, foods high in natural sugars or foods that are quickly and easily digested into sugars) (95). The goal is to consume at least 50 g (200 calories) of carbohydrates every hour until the next meal time. In general, strive to consume ~4 g of carbohydrate per pound of body weight during the 24 hours following exercise or competition.

The two keys to these guidelines are fluids and carbohydrates in the context of a generally varied diet. Athletes should find ways to consume both fluids and carbohydrates at, literally, every opportunity. Recent findings tend to contradict the traditional and commonly followed belief that carbohydrate-containing beverages are useful only for endurance (aerobic) activities that last longer than 60 minutes. The best predictors of athletic performance are maintenance of blood volume and maintenance of glycogen/glucose.

SUMMARY

Nutrition plays an important role in optimizing performance in all sports. Issues that should be considered in determining the optimal nutritional procedures include the following (124):

- Avoiding hydration issues, including dehydration and hyponatremia
- Assuring optimal central nervous system function
- Optimizing muscle and liver glycogen stores
- Repairing muscle soreness and assuring optimal muscle recovery
- Avoiding gut discomfort
- Assuring rapid gastric emptying

Strategies that might be useful for achieving both enhanced hydration and improved maintenance of system carbohydrate in different sports are as follows:

Power/Speed Sports

- Power and speed sports require a high muscle-to-weight ratio. A critically important strategy for achieving greater muscle mass is to stop doing things that *decrease* muscle mass.
- A dietary factor that is associated with a reduced muscle synthesis and loss of muscle is achievement of frequent relative energy deficiency, making avoidance of relative energy deficiency a key component of success in power and speed sports. In addition, relative energy deficiency is also associated with lower glycogen stores (130).
- Energy availability of ~45 kcal/kg fat-free mass (FFM)/day is associated with energy balance, whereas levels below 30 kcal/kg FFM/day are associated with impaired body functions.
- It is also important for the athlete to consume an appropriate level of protein to support lean body mass (typically ~1.7 g/kg/day) and to consume this protein in an evenly distributed pattern during the day (45). Ideally, this protein should be consumed when the athlete is not in a severe relative energy deficiency to help ensure the protein is utilized anabolically to build/repair tissue, rather than used to satisfy the energy requirement. (Humans have *energy-first* systems.)
- Following practice/activity, power and speed athletes should consume ~10 g of high-quality protein with carbohydrates and fluids in the early recovery phase (0–2 hours postexercise) to stimulate muscle

protein synthesis and help recover used glycogen (131). Because anaerobic glycolysis is an important metabolic pathway for power/speed athletes, they should plan on consuming plenty of carbohydrate (typically ~10 g/kg/day) that is evenly distributed throughout the day (45).

Endurance Sports

- In general, endurance athletes should focus on the consumption of diets that are relatively high in carbohydrates before, during, and after exercise, as the limiting energy substrate in endurance events is glycogen (66).
- They should also develop strategies that sustain blood volume to ensure maintenance of sweat rates, delivery of nutrients to working muscles, and removal of metabolic by-products from working muscle.
- Fats, blood, and tissues are the source of most energy for endurance (aerobic) activities, and the storage capacity for fat is relatively high for even lean athletes. The storage capacity for carbohydrates, however, is limited. Because fats require some carbohydrates to be completely burned, the limited storage capacity for carbohydrate can limit the body's ability to burn fat during exercise. To overcome this limitation, athletes should be constantly vigilant to keep body stores of carbohydrate at maximal levels before activity begins and should replace carbohydrates during activity through whatever means are available (132).
- Ideally, athletes should attempt to replace carbohydrates at a rate that is dynamically linked to the proportion of time spent in more intense exercise, as higher intensity will more quickly deplete glycogen stores.
- The best carbohydrates are composed of more than a single carbohydrate molecular type to optimize carbohydrate receptors. As an example, a carbohydrate beverage containing sucrose and free glucose is superior to one containing only glucose (133).
- Failure to supply sufficient carbohydrate before and during endurance activity will significantly reduce athletic performance. Recovery of depleted glycogen requires a relatively high consumption of carbohydrates. Ideally, endurance athletes should consume a mix of protein, carbohydrate, and fluids immediately postexercise, followed by relatively high carbohydrate and moderate protein consumption at other times (134).

Team Sports

- Studies assessing sports that require a combination of power and endurance have found that carbohydrate consumption is useful in enhancing performance even if the activity lasts less than 1 hour (135,136). This is an important finding, because the traditional thought has been that water is an appropriate hydration beverage for activities lasting less than 1 hour, but that carbohydrate-containing sports beverages are important to consume for activities lasting longer than 1 hour. It appears that even in these shorter intermittent-intensity activities, carbohydrate consumption as part of a sports beverage is performance enhancing.
- Because many of these sports (basketball, soccer, tennis) place an enormous caloric drain on the system, athletes should develop eating strategies (*i.e.*, eating enough) that encourage maintenance of muscle mass during long and arduous seasons (137). Team sports often have natural breaks in the event, including halftime. These are opportunities for athletes to replenish carbohydrates and fluids that should be taken advantage of (138).

Practical Application Activity

Using the procedure provided in Chapter 8 for predicting the energy cost of activity, do the following:

1. Ask an endurance athlete what a *nontraining day* looks like in terms of foods consumed and activity, and analyze the energy cost of this day.
2. Then ask an endurance athlete what his or her *typical training schedule* is, including the number of hours and the typical intensity during each hour that the athlete is training, and analyze the energy cost of this day.
3. Determine if the food consumed satisfies energy needs for both the training and nontraining day. If not, try adding or subtracting foods and beverages to/from each day to see what it would take to satisfy energy needs.
4. Repeat steps 1 through 3, but now for a power athlete. It should become quickly clear that even though a power athlete may spend less time in training, the higher intensity of training quickly increases energy needs.

CHAPTER QUESTIONS

1. Commercially available athlete performance gels are different in the following ways:
   a. Serving size, energy density (kcal/g), total energy (kcal), total carbohydrates, free sugars, and osmolality (mmol/kg)
   b. Service size, energy density (kcal/g), and osmolality (mmol/kg)
   c. Serving size and osmolality (mmol/kg)
   d. Flavor

2. Although all energy systems are functioning during power activities, the predominant energy systems are anaerobic
   a. True
   b. False

3. There is convincing evidence that high consumption of amino acid supplements in addition to a well-balanced diet improves power activities and body-building by:
   a. Enhancing fast enlargement of skeletal muscle mass
   b. Improving reaction time
   c. Improving creatine synthesis
   d. All the above
   e. None of the above

4. The nutritional needs of power athletes are so high that it is nearly impossible to obtain all of the needed nutrients from food alone.
   a. True
   b. False

5. The fastest 100-m sprinters use the greatest amount of _____ during the first 80 m of the sprint.
   a. Glycogen
   b. Blood glucose
   c. PCr
   d. Triglyceride

6. Air resistance accounts for ~_____% of total energy expended to run 100 m in ~10 seconds:
   a. 5
   b. 12
   c. 16
   d. 21

7. The *typical* male endurance athlete eating patterns suggest:
   a. Overconsumption of carbohydrate and underconsumption of protein
   b. Underconsumption of carbohydrate and overconsumption of fat
   c. Overconsumption of both carbohydrate and protein
   d. Underconsumption of both protein and carbohydrate

8. The optimal tissue temperature range for muscular enzymes to metabolize energy is _____ °F.
   a. ~98.6
   b. ~102.2
   c. ~100.5
   d. ~104.0

9. The recommended hourly intake of carbohydrates during prolonged endurance activity is:
   a. 10–20 g/hr
   b. 30–60 g/hr
   c. 60–90 g/hr
   d. 90–111 g/hr

10. The recommended hourly intake of carbohydrate during "stop and go" activity (*e.g.*, soccer, basketball) is:
    a. 10–20 g/hr
    b. 30–60 g/hr
    c. 60–90 g/hr
    d. 90–111 g/hr

ANSWERS TO CHAPTER QUESTIONS

1. a
2. a
3. e
4. b
5. c

6. c
7. b
8. b
9. b
10. b

Case Study Considerations

1. **Case Study Answer 1:** The American College of Sports Medicine recommends a range of protein that is between 1.2–2.0 g/kg/day for all athletes. The generally recommended protein intake for power athletes is between 1.5–1.7 g/kg/day. This is approximately double the average protein requirement (0.8 g/kg/day) for a healthy, active, nonathlete adult.

2. **Case Study Answer 2:** Protein can be used optimally for all of its important functions (building and repairing tissues, synthesizing enzymes and hormones, etc.) only if the protein is available when there is sufficient energy availability. Poor energy availability results in the consumed protein to be broken down and used to satisfy the energy requirement, rather than all of its other critically important functions. This requires that athletes have an eating plan that dynamically satisfies energy requirements so that, when the protein is consumed, it results in the desired anabolic outcomes.

3. **Case Study Answer 3:** High protein/low carbohydrate diets result in a significant portion of the protein to be broken down so the glucogenic amino acids satisfy the carbohydrate requirements. This results in elevated blood urea nitrogen, which must be excreted in the urine, elevating the potential for dehydration from the higher urinary output. In addition, the urea being excreted is acidic, so the kidneys retain more blood ironized calcium to buffer (neutralize) the acidity. Because blood pH has a very narrow range, calcium is taken from the bones to replace the calcium that was taken by the kidneys. Doing this repeatedly can lower bone mineral density and predispose an athlete to fracture.

4. **Case Study Answer 4:** The principal aims are as follows:
   a. Make certain glycogen stores are appropriately high for the power event. This requires maintenance of a relatively high carbohydrate intake, provided as small, frequent meals. Prior to an important event it would also be important to diminish glycogen-using high-intensity activity for several days to help assure glycogen store are at the desired level for the event.
   b. Maintain a good state of hydration by drinking plenty of water during meals, and always having a sports beverage easily available during practice. Maintaining blood sugar and blood volume are important factors for assuring that the athlete benefits from training.
   c. Having an eating frequency that is dynamically linked to energy expenditure to avoid the negative aspects of Relative Energy Deficiency in Sport (RED-S). The goal is to assure that fuel is available for muscles during physical activity. Far too often athletes consume fuel *after* the muscles need it, compromising muscle function and increasing the risk of muscle soreness and injury.

REFERENCES

1. Burkhart SJ, Pelly FE. Dietary intake of athletes seeking nutrition advice at a major international competition. Nutrients. 2016;8(10):638.
2. Zhang X, O'Kennedy N, Morton JP. Extreme variation of nutritional composition and osmolality of commercially available carbohydrate energy gels. Int J Sport Nutr Exerc Metab. 2015;25(5):504–9.
3. Goston JL, Correia MITD. Intake of nutritional supplements among people exercising in gyms and influencing factors. Nutrition. 2010;26(6):604–11.
4. Grunewald KK, Bailey RS. Commercially marketed supplements for bodybuilding athletes. Sports Med. 1993; 15(2):90–103.
5. Consumer Lab. Liver injuries linked with dietary supplement use on the rise [Internet]. 2016. [Accessed 2018 May 14]. Available from: https://www.consumerlab.com/m/recall_detail.asp?recallid=14010
6. Josse AR, Tang JE, Tarnopolsky MA, Phillips SM. Body composition and strength changes in women with milk and resistance exercise. Med Sci Sports Exerc. 2010;42(6):1122–30.
7. Tipton KD, Elliott TA, Cree MG, Aarsland AA, Sanford AP, Wolfe RR. Stimulation of net muscle protein synthesis by whey protein ingestion before and after exercise. Am J Physiol Endocrinol Metab. 2007;292(1):E71–6.
8. Mares-Perlman JA, Subar AF, Block G, Greger JL, Luby MH. Zinc intake and sources in the U.S. adult population: 1976–1980. J Am Coll Nutr. 1995;14(4):349–57.
9. Pate RR, Miller BJ, Davis JM, Slentz CA, Klingshirn LA. Iron status of female runners. Int J Sport Nutr. 1993;3(2):222–31.
10. Telford RD, Bunney CJ, Catchpole EA, et al. Plasma ferritin concentration and physical work capacity in athletes. Int J Sport Nutr. 1992;2(4):335–42.
11. Jenner SL, Buckley GL, Belski R, Devlin BL, Forsyth AK. Dietary intake of professional and semi-professional team sport athletes do not meet sport nutrition recommendations-a systematic literature review. Nutrients. 2019;11:1160.

12. Stellingwerff T, Maughan RJ, Burke LM. Nutrition for power sports: middle-distance running, track cycling, rowing, canoeing/kayaking, and swimming. J Sports Sci. 2011; 29(S1):S79–89.

13. Zierath JR, Hawley JA. Skeletal muscle fiber type: influence on contractile and metabolic properties. PLoS Biol. 2004; 2(10):E348.

14. Trappe S, Harber M, Creer A, Gallagher P, Slivka D, Minchev K, Whitsett D. Single muscle fiber adaptations with marathon training. J Appl Physiol. 2006;101(3):721–7.

15. Hirvonen J, Nummela A, Rusko H, Rehunen S, Härkönen M. Fatigue and changes of ATP, creatine phosphate, and lactate during the 400-m sprint. Can J Sport Sci. 1992;17(2): 141–4.

16. Hirvonen J, Rehunen S, Rusko H, Härkönen M. Breakdown of high-energy phosphate compounds and lactate accumulation during short supramaximal exercise. Eur J Appl Physiol Occup Physiol. 1987;56(3):253–9.

17. Sawyer BJ, Stokes DG, Womack CJ, Morton RH, Weltman A, Gaesser GA. Strength training increases endurance time to exhaustion during high-intensity exercise despite no change in critical power. J Strength Cond Res. 2014;28(3):601–9.

18. Seki Y, Nakashima D, Shiraishi Y, Ryuzaki T, Ikura H, Miura K, Suzuki M, Watanabe T, Nagura T, Matsumoto M, Nakamura M, Sato K, Fukuda K, and Katsumata Y. A novel device for detecting anaerobic threshold using sweat lactate during exercise. Sci Rep. 2021;11:4929.

19. Poole DC, Rossiter HB, Brooks GA, Gladden LB. The anaerobic threshold: 50+ years of controversy. J Physiol. 2021; 599(3):737–767.

20. Brooks GA. The "anaerobic threshold" concept in not valid in physiology and medicine. Med Sci Sports Exercise. 2021; 53(5):1093–6.

21. Forbes SC, Paganini AT, Slade JM, Towse TF, Meyer RA. Phosphocreatine recovery kinetics following low- and high-intensity exercise in human triceps surae and rat posterior hindlimb muscles. Am J Physiol Regul Integr Comp Physiol. 2009;296(1):R161–70.

22. Haseler LJ, Hogan MC, Richardson RS. Skeletal muscle phosphocreatine recovery in exercise-trained humans is dependent on O_2 availability J Appl Physiol. 1999;86(6):2013–8.

23. Antonio J, Candow DG, Forbes SC, Gualano B, Jagim AR, Kreider RB, Rawson ES, Smith-Ryan AE, VanDusseldorp TA, Willoughby DS, Ziegenfuss TN. Common questions and misconceptions about creatine supplementation: what does the scientific evidence really show? J Int Soc Sports Nutr. 2021;18(1):13.

24. Patrizia L, Chiara De W, Concetta De M, Elisa T, Francesco Di N, Walter R. Does the use of dietary supplements enhance athlete's sport performances? A systematic review and a meta-analysis. Epidemiol Biostat Public Health. 2015;12(4): e115931–15.

25. Koenig CA, Benardot D, Cody M, Thompson WR. Comparison of creatine monohydrate and carbohydrate supplementation on repeated jump height performance. J Strength Cond Res. 2008;22(4):1081–6.

26. Pozefsky T, Tancredi RG, Moxley RT, Dupre J, Tobin JD. Effects of brief starvation on muscle amino acid metabolism in nonobese man. J Clin Invest. 1976;57(2):444–9.

27. Callow M, Morton A, Guppy M. Marathon fatigue: the role of plasma fatty acids, muscle glycogen and blood glucose. Eur J Appl Physiol Occup Physiol. 1986;55(6):654–61.

28. Murray R, Bartoli WP, Eddy DE, Horn MK. Physiological and performance responses to nicotinic-acid ingestion during exercise. Med Sci Sports Exerc. 1995;27(7):1057–62.

29. Roberts KM, Noble EG, Hayden DB, Taylor AW. Simple and complex carbohydrate-rich diets and muscle glycogen content of marathon runners. Eur J Appl Physiol Occup Physiol. 1988;57(1):70–4.

30. Schiaffino S, Reggiani C. Fiber types in mammalian skeletal muscles. Physiol Rev. 2011;91(4):1447–531.

31. Greenhaff PL, Soderlund K, Ren JM, Hultman E. Energy metabolism in single human muscle fibres during intermittent contraction with occluded circulation. J Physiol. 1993;460:443–53.

32. Kappenstein J, Ferrauti A, Runkel B, Fernandez-Fernandez J, Müller K, Zange J. Changes in phosphocreatine concentration of skeletal muscle during high-intensity intermittent exercise in children and adults. Eur J Appl Physiol. 2013; 113(11):2769–79.

33. Slater G, Phillips SM. Nutrition guidelines for strength sports: sprinting, weightlifting, throwing events, and bodybuilding. J Sports Sci. 2011;29(S1):S67–77.

34. Zello GA. Dietary reference intakes for the macronutrients and energy: considerations for physical activity. Appl Physiol Nutr Metab. 2006;31(1):74–9.

35. Horswill CA. Weight loss and weight cycling in amateur wrestlers: implications for performance and resting metabolic rate. Int J Sport Nutr. 1993;3(3):245–60.

36. Strauss RH, Lanese RR, Leizman DJ. Illness and absence among wrestlers, swimmers, and gymnasts at a large university. Am J Sports Med. 1988;16(6):653–5.

37. Davies CT. Effect of air resistance on the metabolic cost and performance of cycling. Eur J Appl Physiol Occup Physiol. 1980;45(2–3):245–54.

38. Pugh LG. Oxygen intake in track and treadmill running with observations on the effect of air resistance. J Physiol. 1970; 207(3):823–35.

39. Linthorne N. The effect of wind on 100-m sprint times. J Appl Biomech. 1994;10(2):110–31.

40. Burke LM, van Loon LJC, Hawley JA. Postexercise muscle glycogen resynthesis in humans. J Appl Physiol. 2017; 122(5):1055–67.

41. Coggan AR, Coyle EF. Carbohydrate ingestion during prolonged exercise: effects on metabolism and performance. Exerc Sport Sci Rev. 1991;19:1–40.

42. Maughan RJ, Poole DC. The effects of a glycogen-loading regimen on the capacity to perform anaerobic exercise. Eur J Appl Physiol Occup Physiol. 1981;46(3):11–9.

43. Koopman R, Manders RJF, Jonkers RA, Hul GB, Kuipers H, van Loon LJC. Intramyocellular lipid and glycogen content are reduced following resistance exercise in untrained healthy males. Eur J Appl Physiol. 2006;96(5):525–34.

44. Tesch PA, Colliander EB, Kaiser P. Muscle metabolism during intense, heavy-resistance exercise. Eur J Appl Physiol Occup Physiol. 1986;55(4):362–6.

45. Thomas DT, Erdman KA, Burke LM. American College of Sports Medicine Joint Position Statement. Nutrition and athletic performance. Med Sci Sports Exerc. 2016;48(3):543–68.

46. Rebić N, Ilić V, Zlatović I. Effects of a low carbohydrate diet on sports performance. Trends Sport Sci. 2021;28(4):249–58.

47. King A, Helms E, Zinn C, Jukic I. The ergogenic effects of acute carbohydrate feeding on resistance exercise performance: a systematic review and meta-analysis. Sports Med. 2022;52(11):2691–712.

48. Phillips SM. Protein requirements and supplementation in strength sports. Nutrition. 2004;20(7-8):689–95.

49. Tang JE, Phillips SM. Maximizing muscle protein anabolism: the role of protein quality. Curr Opin Clin Nutr Metab Care. 2009; 12(1): 66–71.

50. Phillips SM, Van Loon LJC. Dietary protein for athletes: from requirements to optimum adaptation. J Sports Sci. 2011;29(Suppl 1):S29–38.

51. Moore DR, Robinson MJ, Fry JL, Tang JE, Glover EI, Wilkinson SB, Prior T, Tarnopolsky MA, Phillips SM. Ingested protein dose response of muscle and albumin protein synthesis after resistance exercise in young men. Am J Clin Nutr. 2009;89(1):161–8.

52. Stellingwerff T, Boon H, Jonkers RA, Senden JM, Spriet LL, Koopman R, van Loon LJC. Significant intramyocellular lipid use during prolonged cycling in endurance- trained males as assessed by three different methodologies. Am J Physiol Endocrinol Metab. 2007;292(6):E1715–23.

53. Decombaz J. Nutrition and recovery of muscle energy stores after exercise. Sportmedizin und Sporttraumatologie. 2003;51:31–8.

54. Kleiner SM. The role of meat in an athlete's diet: its effect on key macro- and micronutrients. Sports Sci Exch.1995;8(5). https://www.gssiweb.org/sports-science-exchange/article/sse-58-the-role-of-red-meatin-an-athlete's-diet

55. Ryan AJ. Anabolic steroids are fool's gold. Fed Proc. 1981; 40(12):2682–8.

56. Helms ER, Aragon AA, Fitschen PJ. Evidence-based recommendations for natural bodybuilding contest preparation: nutrition and supplementation. J Int Soc Sports Nutr. 2014; 11: 20.

57. Spendlove J, Mitchell L, Gifford J, Hackett D, Slater G, Cobley S, O'Connor H. Dietary intake of competitive bodybuilders. Sports Med. 2015;45(7):1041–63.

58. Paddon-Jones D. Protein recommendations for bodybuilders: in this case, more may indeed be better. J Nutr. 2017;147(5):723–4.

59. Lim MT, Pan BJ, Toh DWK, Sutanto CN, Kim JE. Animal protein versus plant protein in supporting lean mass and muscle strength: a systematic review and meta-analysis of randomized controlled trials. Nutrients. 2021;13:661.

60. Kerksick CM, Jagim A, Hagele A, Jäger R. Plant proteins and exercise: what role can plant proteins have in promoting adaptations to exercise? Nutrients. 2021;13(6):1962.

61. Binnerts A, Swart GR, Wilson JH, Hoogerbrugge N, Pols H, Birkenhager J, Lamberts SW. The effect of growth hormone administration in growth hormone deficient adults on bone, protein, carbohydrate, and lipid homeostasis, as well as on body composition. Clin Endocrinol. 1992;37(1):79–87.

62. Deyssig R, Frisch H, Blum WF, Waldhör T. Effect of growth hormone treatment on hormonal parameters, body composition, and strength in athletes. Acta Endocrinol. 1993; 128(4):313–8.

63. Gregory JW, Greene SA, Thompson J, Scrimgeour CM, Rennie MJ. Effects of oral testosterone undecanoate on growth, body composition, strength and energy expenditure of adolescent boys. Clin Endocrinol. 1992;37(3):207–13.

64. Yarasheki KE, Campbell JA, Smith K, Rennie MJ, Holloszy JO, Bier DM. Effect of growth hormone and resistance exercise on muscle growth in young men. Am J Physiol. 1992; 262(3 Pt 1):E261–7.

65. Sawka MN, Wenger CB. Physiological responses to acute exercise-heat stress. In: Pandolf KB, Sawka MN, Gonzalez RR, editors. Human performance physiology and environmental medicine at terrestrial extremes. Indianapolis (IN): Benchmark Press; 1988.

66. Jeukendrup AE. Nutrition for endurance sports: marathon, triathlon, and road cycling. J Sports Sci. 2011;29(S1):S91–9.

67. Noakes TD, Norman RJ, Buck RH, Godlonton J, Stevenson K, Pittaway D. The incidence of hyponatremia during prolonged ultraendurance exercise. Med Sci Sports Exerc. 1990;22(2):165–70.

68. Coyle EF, Coggan AR, Hemmert MK, Ivy JL. Muscle glycogen utilization during prolonged strenuous exercise when fed carbohydrate. J Appl Physiol. 1986;61(1):165–72.

69. Stellingwerff T. Competition nutrition practices of elite ultramarathon runners. Int J Sport Nutr Exerc Metab. 2016; 26(1):93–9.

70. Penry JT, Manore MM. Choline: an important micronutrient for maximal endurance-exercise performance? Int J Sport Nutr Exerc Metab. 2008;18(2):191–203.

71. Ekblom B, Bergh U. Physiology and nutrition for cross-country skiing. In: Lamb D, Knuttgen H, Murray R, editors. Perspectives in exercise science and sports medicine: physiology and nutrition for competitive sport. Indianapolis (IN): Benchmark Press; 1994.

72. Murray B, Rosenbloom C. Fundamentals of glycogen metabolism for coaches and athletes. Nutr Rev. 2018;76(4):243–59.

73. Pate RR, Branch JD. Training for endurance sport. Med Sci Sports Exerc. 1992;24:S340–3.

74. Armstrong L. Considerations for replacement beverages: fluid-electrolyte balance and heat illness. In: Marriott B, Rosemont C, editors. Fluid replacement and heat stress. Washington (DC): National Academy Press; 1991.

75. American College of Sports Medicine; Sawka MN, Burke LM, Eichner ER, Maughan RJ, Montain SJ, Stachenfeld NS. American College of Sports Medicine position stand: exercise and fluid replacement. Med Sci Sports Exerc. 2007;39(2): 377–90.

76. Hargreaves M, Dillo P, Angus D, Febbraio M. Effect of fluid ingestion on muscle metabolism during prolonged exercise. J Appl Physiol. 1996;80(1):363–6.

77. Racinais S, Alonso JM, Coutts AJ, Flouris AD, Girard O, González-Alonso J, Hausswirth C, Jay O, Lee JKW, Mitchell N, Nassis GP, Nybo L, Pluim BM, Roelands B, Sawka MN, Wingo JE, Périard JD. Consensus recommendations on training and competing in the heat. Scand J Med Sci Sports. 2015;25(S1):6–19.

78. Armstrong LE, Costill DL, Fink WJ. Influence of diuretic-induced dehydration on competitive running performance. Med Sci Sports Exerc. 1985;17(4):456-61.

79. Walsh RM, Noakes TD, Hawley JA, Dennis SC. Impaired high-intensity cycling performance time at low levels of dehydration. Int J Sport Med. 1994;15(7):392–8.

80. Maughan R. Carbohydrate-electrolyte solutions during prolonged exercise. In: Lamb D, Williams M, editors. Perspectives in exercise science and sports medicine: ergogenics-enhancement of performance in exercise and sport. Indianapolis (IN): Brown and Benchmark; 1991. p. 35–50.

81. Costill DL. Carbohydrates nutrition before, during, and after exercise. Fed Proc. 1985;44(2):364–8.

82. Tsintzas OK, Williams C, Wilson W, Burrin J. Influence of carbohydrate supplementation early in exercise on endurance running capacity. Med Sci Sports Exerc. 1996;28(11):1373–9.

83. Tsintzas OK, Williams C, Singh R, Wilson W, Burrin J. Influence of carbohydrate-electrolyte drinks on marathon running performance. Eur J Appl Physiol Occup Physiol. 1995;70(2):154–60.

84. Davis JM, Cokkinides VE, Burgess WA, Bartoli WP. Effects of a carbohydrate/electrolyte drink or water on the stress hormone response to prolonged intense cycling: Renin, Angiotestin-I, Aldosterone, ACTH, and Cortisol. In: Laron Z, Rogo AD, editors. Hormones and Sport. Vol. 55. New York (NY): Raven Press; 1989. p. 193–204.

85. Costill DL, Hargreaves M. Carbohydrate nutrition and fatigue. Sports Med. 1992;13(2):86–92.

86. Coyle EF, Coyle E. Carbohydrates that speed recovery from training. Phys Sportsmed. 1993;21(2):111–23.

87. Chen JD, Wang JF, Li KJ, Zhao YW, Wang SW, Jiao Y, Hou XY. Nutritional problems and measures in elite and amateur athletes. Am J Clin Nutr. 1989;49(5 Suppl):1084–9.

88. Rodriguez NR, Vislocky LM, Gaine PC. Dietary protein, endurance exercise, and human skeletal-muscle protein turnover. Curr Opin Clin Nutr Metab Care. 2007;10(1):40–5.

89. Tarnopolsky MA. Building muscle: nutrition to maximize bulk and strength adaptations to resistance exercise training. Eur J Sport Sci. 2008;8(2):67–76.

90. Stellingwerff T. Distance running. In: Maughan RJ, editor. Encyclopaedia of sports medicine: sports nutrition. Oxford: Wiley Blackwell Publisher; 2014. p. 576.

91. Abbate M, Zoja C, Remuzzi G. How does proteinuria cause progressive renal damage? J Am Soc Nephrol. 2006;17(11):2974–84.

92. Feskanich D, Willet WC, Stampfer MJ, Colditz GA. Protein consumption and bone fractures in women. Am J Epidemiol. 1996;143(5):472–9.

93. Eisenstein J, Roberts SB, Dallal G, Saltzman E. High-protein weight-loss diets: are they safe and do they work? A review of the experimental and epidemiologic data. Nutr Rev. 2002;60(7):189–200.

94. Volek JS, Noakes T, Phinney SD. Rethinking fat as a fuel for endurance exercise. Eur J Sport Sci. 2015;15(1):13–20.

95. American Dietetic Association; Dietitians of Canada; American College of Sports Medicine; Rodriguez NR, Di Marco NM, Langley S. American College of Sports Medicine position stand. Nutrition and athletic performance. Med Sci Sports Exerc. 2009;41(3):709–31.

96. Murray R, Horswill CA. Nutrient requirements for competitive sports. In: Wolinsky I, editor. Nutrition in exercise and sport. 3rd ed. Boca Raton (FL): CRC Press; 1998. p. 521–58.

97. Dellavalle DM, Haas JD. Iron status is associated with endurance performance and training in female rowers. Med Sci Sports Exerc. 2012;44(8):1552–9.

98. Gomez-Cabrera M-C, Domenech E, Romagnoli M, Arduini A, Borras C, Pallardo FV, Sastre J, Viña J. Oral administration of vitamin C decreases muscle mitochondrial biogenesis and hampers training-induced adaptations in endurance performance. Am J Clin Nutr. 2008;87(1):142–9.

99. Barrack MT, Rauh MJ, Barkai HS, Nichols JF. Dietary restraint and low bone mass in female adolescent endurance runners. Am J Clin Nutr. 2008;87(1):36–43.

100. Fontana L, Klein S, Holloszy JO. Effects of long-term caloric restriction and endurance exercise on glucose tolerance, insulin action, and adipokine production. Age. 2010;32(1):97–108.

101. Zimberg IZ, Crispim CA, Juzwiak CR, Antunes HKM, Edwards B, Waterhouse J, Tufik S, de Mello MT. Nutritional intake during a simulated adventure race. Int J Sport Nutr Exerc Metab. 2008;18(2):152–68.

102. Coggan AR, Swanson SC. Nutritional manipulations before and during endurance exercise: effects on performance. Med Sci Sports Exerc. 1992;24:S331–5.

103. Sherman WM. Metabolism of sugars and physical performance. Am J Clin Nutr. 1995;62:228S–41S.

104. Rothschild JA, Kilding AE, Plews DJ. Pre-exercise nutrition habits and beliefs of endurance athletes vary by sex, competitive level, and diet. J Am Coll Nutr. 2021;40(6):517–28.

105. Shirreffs SM, Sawka MN. Fluid and electrolyte needs for training, competition, and recovery. J Sports Sci. 2011;29(Suppl 1):S39–46.

106. Goulet ED. Dehydration and endurance performance in competitive athletes. Nutr Rev. 2012;70(2):S132–6.

107. Montner P, Stark DM, Riedesel ML, Murata G, Robergs R, Timms M, Chick TW. Pre-exercise glycerol hydration improves cycling endurance time. Int J Sports Med. 1996;17(1):27–33.

108. Burke LM, Kiens B, Ivy JL. Carbohydrates and fat for training and recovery. J Sports Sci. 2004;22(1):15–30.

109. Burke LM, Hawley JA, Wong SH, Jeukendrup AE. Carbohydrates for training and competition. J Sports Sci. 2011;29(Suppl 1):S17–27.

110. Rehrer NJ, van Kemenade M, Meester W, Brouns F, Saris WH. Gastrointestinal complaints in relation to dietary intake in triathletes. Int J Sport Nutr. 1992;2(1):48–59.

111. van Essen M, Gibala MJ. Failure of protein to improve time trial performance when added to a sports drink. Med Sci Sports Exerc. 2006;38(8):1476–83.

112. Broad EM, Burke LM, Cox GR, Heeley P, Riley M. Body weight changes and voluntary fluid intakes during training and competition sessions in team sports. Int J Sport Nutr. 1996;6(3):307–20.

113. Eichner ER, Laird R, Nadel E, Noakes T. Hyponatremia in sport: symptoms and prevention. Sports Sci Exch. 1994;12:5.

114. Lugo M, Sherman WM, Wimer GS, Garleb K. Metabolic responses when different forms of carbohydrate energy are consumed during cycling. Int J Sport Nutr. 1993;3(4):398–407.

115. Sherman WM, Lamb DR. Nutrition and prolonged exercise. In: Lamb DR, Murray R, editors. Perspectives in exercise science and sports medicine: prolonged exercise. Indianapolis (IN): Benchmark Press; 1988.

116. Tarnopolsky MA, MacDugall JD, Atkinson SA. Influence of protein intake and training status on nitrogen balance and lean body mass. J Appl Physiol. 1988;64(1):187–93.

117. Holway FE, Spriet LL. Sport-specific nutrition: practical strategies for team sports. J Sports Sci. 2011;29(S1):S115–25.

118. Gabbett T, King T, Jenkins D. Applied physiology of rugby league. Sports Med. 2008;38(2):119–38.

119. Hoffman JR. The applied physiology of American football. Int J Sports Physiol Perform. 2008;3(3):387–92.

120. Burke LM, Loucks AB, Broad N. Energy and carbohydrate for training and recovery. J Sports Sci. 2006;24(7):675–85.

121. Bishop DJ. Proceedings of the Australian physiological society symposium: Fatigue mechanism limiting exercise performance. Clin Exp Pharmacol Physiol. 2012;39:836–41.

122. Little JP, Chilibeck PD, Ciona D, Forbes S, Rees H, Vandenberg A, Zello GA. Effect of low-and high-glycemic index meals on metabolism and performance during high-intensity, intermittent exercise. Int J Sport Nutr Exerc Metab. 2010;20(6):447–56.

123. Wynne JL, Ehlert AM, Wilson PB. Effects of high-carbohydrate versus mixed-macronutrient meals on female soccer physiology and performance. Eur J Appl Physiol. 2021;121(4):1125–34.

124. Burke L. Practical Sports Nutrition. Chicago (IL): Human Kinetics; 2007.

125. Williams C, Serratosa L. Nutrition on match day. J Sports Sci. 2006;24(7):687–97.

126. Skein M, Duffield R, Kelly BT, Marino FE. The effects of carbohydrate intake and muscle glycogen content on self-paced intermittent-sprint exercise despite no knowledge of carbohydrate manipulation. Eur J Appl Physiol. 2012;112(8):2859–70.

127. Nicholas CW, Williams C, Lakomy HK, Phillips G, Nowitz A. Influence of ingesting a carbohydrate-electrolyte solution on endurance capacity during intermittent, high-intensity shuttle running. J Sports Sci. 1995;13(4):282–90.

128. Beelen M, Burke LM, Gibala MJ, van Loon LJ. Nutritional strategies to promote postexercise recovery. Int J Sport Nutr Exerc Metab. 2010;20(6):515–32.

129. Ryan M. Eating for training and recovery. In: Performance nutrition for team sports. Boulder (CO): VeloPress; 2005. p. 87–103.

130. Mountjoy M, Sundgot-Borgen J, Burke L, Carter S, Constantini N, Lebrun C, Meyer N, Sherman R, Steffen K, Budgett R, Ljungqvist A. The IOC consensus statement: beyond the Female Athlete Triad–Relative Energy Deficiency in Sport (RED-S). Br J Sports Med. 2014;48(7):491–7.

131. Phillips SM. Dietary protein requirements and adaptive advantages in athletes. Br J Nutr. 2012;108(Suppl 2):S158–67.

132. Vergauwen L, Brouns F, Hespel P. Carbohydrate supplementation improves stroke performance in tennis. Med Sci Sports Exerc. 1998;30(8):1289–95.

133. Triplett D, Doyle JA, Rupp JC, Benardot D. An isocaloric glucose-fructose beverage's effect on simulated 100-km cycling performance compared with a glucose-only beverage. Int J Sport Nutr Exerc Metab. 2010;20(2):122–31.

134. Berardi JM, Price TB, Noreen EE, Lemon PWR. Postexercise muscle glycogen recovery enhanced with a carbohydrate-protein supplement. Med Sci Sports Exerc. 2006;38(6):1106–13.

135. Bangsbo J, Norregaard L, Thorsoe F. The effect of carbohydrate diet on intermittent exercise performance. Int J Sports Med. 1992;13(2):152–7.

136. Winnick JJ, Davis JM, Welsh RS, Carmichael MD, Murphy EA, Blackmon JA. Carbohydrate feedings during team sport exercise preserve physical and CNS function. Med Sci Sports Exerc. 2005;37(2):306–15.

137. Nowak RK, Knudsen KS, Schulz LO. Body composition and nutrient intakes of college men and women basketball players. J Am Diet Assoc. 1998;88(5):575–8.

138. Mujika I, Burke LM. Nutrition in team sports. Ann Nutr Metab. 2010;57(Suppl 2):26–35.

139. Van Loon LJC, Greenhaff PL, Constantin-Teodosiu D, Saris WH, Wagenmakers AJ. The effects of increasing exercise intensity on muscle fuel utilization in humans. J Physiol. 2001;536:295–304.

12

Impact of Travel, High Altitude, High Heat, and Humidity on Nutrition

CHAPTER OBJECTIVES

- Recognize the nutritional problems that may occur with travel associated with crossing multiple time zones.
- Identify how circadian rhythm changes can influence dietary requirements and how, unless adjusted, it can influence athletic performance.
- Recall the logical planning strategies that athletes should follow when traveling to unfamiliar locations.
- Know the nutritional strategies associated with minimizing the effects of jet lag.
- List the items that athletes should bring along when traveling to countries that have different cultures than their own.
- Identify the food safety concerns that could create health problems unless appropriate preventative actions are followed.

- Analyze the nutritional issues associated with performance-related athletic endeavors in high altitudes and cold environments.
- List the health and nutrition-associated health conditions (high-altitude sickness) that may occur when exercising in a high-altitude and cold-weather environment.
- Create strategies that athletes can follow to help satisfy fluid, energy, and nutrient needs when exercising in a high-altitude and cold-weather environment.
- Recognize the nutritional issues associated with exercise in a high heat and humid environment, and how to best ameliorate these issues.

Case Study: Traveling to His First International Marathon

John, after several years of trying, finally made the qualifying time to run the Athens (Greece) Marathon, allowing him to run with the best runners in the world at the front of the pack. He could not wait to get on the plane to travel from his home in San Diego, California, to a city he had never before visited: Athens, the original home of the modern Olympic Games. He was even more excited to begin the race from Marathonas, the city for which the marathon is named, to finish in the famous Panathenaic Stadium in Athens, which was originally built as a racecourse in the 6th century BC and reconstructed in 1896 as the primary stadium for the first modern Olympic Games. When he arrived in Athens at 5 PM, 2 days before the marathon, he was more than excited and happy to be there for

two reasons: because of what he had accomplished and also because of the immense history of the city.

He went for dinner to the hotel dining room, only to find a menu filled with unfamiliar dishes. Excellent! he thought and was excited to try the new cuisine. He ordered *barbounia* (small red mullet) sautéed in olive oil, with roasted quartered potatoes covered in delicious spices, and more green vegetables than he had ever eaten in a single meal. Delicious! After dinner, he took a brief tour around the city, and at about 10 PM decided it was time to sleep. He was not certain if the rumblings in his stomach were keeping him up, or if it was due to the difference in time zones (after all, it was only noon in San Diego). After a sleepless night, he got out of bed exhausted and decided to go for his usual

6-mile prebreakfast run at 7 AM. Difficult run, he thought, because he was so exhausted, but then breakfast of some fried eggs with toast, fruit, and feta cheese went down nicely—but he was totally exhausted. He went back to bed and, to his surprise, he slept soundly from 10 AM to 4 PM.

When he awoke, he prepared all of his running gear for the marathon, scheduled to begin at 8 AM the next morning. He was feeling great after that long nap and was excited to go to dinner with a friend from home who was leading a historical tour of the city for his university. His friend knew some great restaurants in the Plaka historical district of Athens, and John was excited to go and see the city with someone familiar with it. It was agreed between them that it would be an early evening so John could get some rest before the marathon. They left the hotel at 7 PM and went to the Plaka, only a 10-minute taxi ride away. Beautiful place, with a full view of the Parthenon, and restaurants and music everywhere. Pure fun. They ate at a traditional Greek restaurant that specialized in lamb dishes, and the restaurant owner made his own retsina (a pine resin–laced wine). The owner insisted that John try a small glass, and John agreed that a small glass of wine could not hurt. At 9 PM they headed back to the hotel, where John went to bed excited for the next day's marathon. He set the alarm for 5 AM to have plenty of time to prepare and take the bus to the city of Marathonas for the start of the race.

John did not sleep much (from the excitement, he thought) and dragged himself to the bus. The race started (it is an uphill run for the first 20 km of the race), and by the time it finished, John had his slowest marathon time in

2 years with terrible gastrointestinal (GI) problems during the last half of the race. This was not what he expected or wanted. John came to the first-hand realization that so many of his fellow runners had warned him about: Travel is exhausting and potentially performance reducing no matter how experienced the athlete is, and it is particularly exhausting for athletes traveling across multiple time zones to unfamiliar countries with unfamiliar food and drink.

CASE STUDY DISCUSSION QUESTIONS

Imagine that you were flying from your current location to an unfamiliar location/country that is at least six time zones away. Consider the following:

1. What nutrition planning would you do prior to your trip to help ensure that you can perform up to your conditioned capacity?
2. What would you bring with you that could help you sustain performance and illness in an unfamiliar location?
3. What would you do on the long flight to reduce the chance that the flight would negatively influence how you feel and your readiness to perform, while also reducing possible feelings of ill health?
4. Once you get to your location, how would you time eating and sleep behavior to help you adjust to your new location?
5. What foods and beverages would you avoid consuming to minimize any potential negative performance and health risks?

INTRODUCTION

Athletes often find themselves having to travel to competitions or to train at a new location with a new coach. Without good planning and a logical strategy, travel itself may be the cause of several problems that have nutritional implications. If the travel location is in an environment that is hotter, colder, or at a higher altitude than the athlete is accustomed to, then the athlete should make plans to arrive at the location sufficiently early to allow time to acclimate to the new environment. If the travel is in a location with an unfamiliar cuisine, there should be planning to see what foods in this new environment are likely to be well tolerated. Athletes with existing food allergies, intolerances, or sensitivities should take no chances when traveling by printing out cards in the native language that clearly spell out what they cannot eat, with the goal of

giving these cards to chefs and servers to limit the chance of eating a poorly tolerated food or food ingredient. In some cases, it is possible that the only logical solution is to bring snacks and other foods to ensure sufficient energy consumption. This chapter reviews the planning steps that should be taken by traveling athletes, and the special considerations to account for when traveling long distances and to environments that are warmer, colder, or at different altitudes than those to which the athlete is accustomed.

TRAVEL

Athletes often find themselves traveling to competitions far from home, where the foods are unfamiliar. To overcome both the exhaustion of travel and the unfamiliar cuisine, planning ahead to be prepared for any contingency is important for the athlete to compete at their conditioned capacity. It is a mistake to believe that a healthy athlete can quickly adapt to a new time zone and new foods, and it is also a mistake to assume that they can sleep and eat in a pattern they have adapted to at home. Although it takes time to adapt to a new location, it also takes time to adjust to different temperatures and altitudes. For instance, in high-heat environments, it may take 1 to 2 weeks to develop the physiologic adjustments necessary to perform at an optimal level (1). The relative humidity of the high-heat environment also makes a difference, as the higher the humidity the less efficient the dissipation of heat through sweat, resulting in greater sweat loss (2). There is also a potential difference in thermoregulation between male and female athletes, as females experiencing the luteal phase of the menstrual cycle may have a disadvantage in controlling core temperature (3). Whether it concerns food or time for adaptation, carefully planning the trip will greatly enhance the probability that the athlete can compete at their conditioned capacity (Figure 12.1).

Travel is associated with unfamiliar stress that affects body function with a potential detrimental effect on

performance. Having an appropriate nutrition strategy can help to moderate the effect of travel-associated changes in **circadian rhythms** that can negatively affect sleep and the GI tract, including alterations in food absorption that can result in sleep disruption and bloating (4–9). There is evidence that how the meals are timed, the content of the foods consumed, and the size of the meals consumed before, during, and after flights can have an impact on how the athlete feels. In general, lower fat and smaller meals are better tolerated before, during, and after travel (10–12). There are also a number of hormones affected by circadian rhythms that show diurnal (during the day) variation and can affect the cardiovascular and other systems. These include arginine vasopressin, corticotropin, endogenous opioids, insulin, melatonin, somatotropin, serotonin, thyrotropin-releasing hormone, and vasoactive intestinal peptide (13–19) (Table 12.1).

Circadian Rhythms

Circadian (circa = approximately; dian = day) rhythms are physical, mental, and behavioral changes that follow a roughly 24-hour cycle, responding primarily to light and

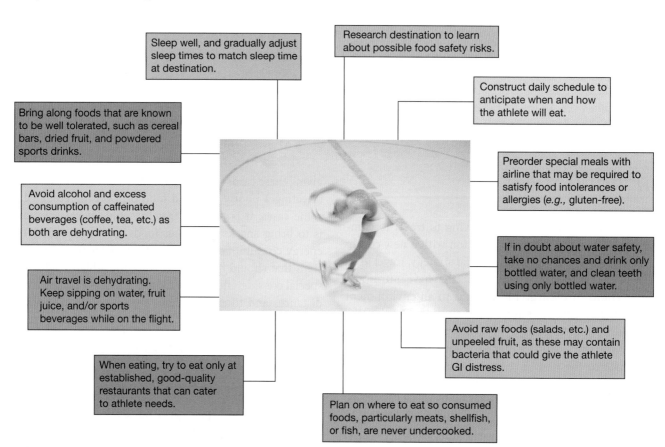

Sleep well, and gradually adjust sleep times to match sleep time at destination.

Research destination to learn about possible food safety risks.

Construct daily schedule to anticipate when and how the athlete will eat.

Bring along foods that are known to be well tolerated, such as cereal bars, dried fruit, and powdered sports drinks.

Preorder special meals with airline that may be required to satisfy food intolerances or allergies (*e.g.*, gluten-free).

Avoid alcohol and excess consumption of caffeinated beverages (coffee, tea, etc.) as both are dehydrating.

If in doubt about water safety, take no chances and drink only bottled water, and clean teeth using only bottled water.

Air travel is dehydrating. Keep sipping on water, fruit juice, and/or sports beverages while on the flight.

Avoid raw foods (salads, etc.) and unpeeled fruit, as these may contain bacteria that could give the athlete GI distress.

When eating, try to eat only at established, good-quality restaurants that can cater to athlete needs.

Plan on where to eat so consumed foods, particularly meats, shellfish, or fish, are never undercooked.

FIGURE 12.1: Planning for the trip is important for an athlete's success. GI, gastrointestinal. (Sapozhnikov-Shoes Georgy/Shutterstock.com with added labels.)

Table 12.1	Major Hormones Affected by Circadian Rhythms That Affect the Cardiovascular and Other Systems
Hormone	**Action**
Arginine vasopressin (AVP)	Also referred to as antidiuretic hormone, AVP mainly acts on the kidney to increase the reabsorption of water to help sustain body water and blood volume. The result is the production of a concentrated urine with a deep-yellow color that is suggestive of dehydration.
Corticotropin	Produced by the anterior pituitary gland, its principal effect is the increased production and release of cortisol (stress hormone) by the adrenal gland.
Endogenous opioids	A group of peptides referred to as "endorphins" that are involved in "built-in" pain relief that are produced by the pituitary gland and the central nervous system. Besides the analgesic (pain relief) effect, endorphins may also result in a state of feeling good.
Insulin	A peptide hormone produced by the β-cells of the pancreas and involved in the regulation and metabolism of energy substrates (particularly blood glucose) through enabling fat, liver, and muscle cells to take up glucose.
Melatonin	A hormone produced by the pineal gland of the brain that is involved in the regulation of sleep and wakefulness and also as a defense against oxidative stress. It is involved in regulation of circadian rhythms, including sleep–wake timing and regulation of blood pressure.
Serotonin (5-hydroxytryptamine [HT])	Also referred to as 5-HT, this neurotransmitter, made from the amino acid L-tryptophan, is found in the gastrointestinal tract, red blood cells, and the central nervous system. It is involved in creating a sense of well-being, a state of relaxation, and memory.
Somatotropin	Also referred to as growth hormone or human growth hormone, it is produced by the anterior pituitary gland and is involved in stimulating growth, cell reproduction, and cell regeneration. It is also involved in the production of insulin-like growth factor 1 (IGF-1), which is necessary for muscle development and repair.
Thyrotropin-releasing hormone	Produced by the hypothalamus, it stimulates the release of thyroid-stimulating hormone, which is involved in the control of energy metabolism.
Vasoactive intestinal peptide	A peptide hormone found in the intestine and stimulates heart contractility, results in vasodilation, increases the breakdown of glycogen (glycogenolysis), lowers blood pressure, and helps to regulate circadian rhythm.

Sources: From Refs. (4–7,9,11,13–20).

darkness in a person's environment. Circadian rhythms affect biologic processes, including sleep, appetite, bowel movements, and optimal alertness that are associated with specific times of the day. Alterations in circadian rhythm may be the result of alterations in sun exposure, weather, and other common stimuli. Travel, as it may result in changes in all of these, may be associated with alterations in circadian rhythm that can influence these timed biologic processes and negatively impact athletic performance.

Jet lag has implications for performance, with Olympic and sport-governing bodies creating training camps near competition sites to enable precompetition adjustments in circadian rhythms and to allow for jet lag recovery (12).

Specific diets have been suggested to help reset the athlete's circadian rhythm. For instance, lower protein and higher carbohydrate diets may improve cellular tryptophan levels, thereby enhancing serotonin to improve a sense of relaxation and well-being and improve sleep (21). It has also been suggested that athletes consume diets higher in protein and lower in carbohydrate to enhance epinephrine production and alertness through a greater cellular uptake of the amino acid tyrosine (22). Consumption of excess energy, particularly through higher fat diets, may cause an athlete to take longer to adapt to the new environment, whereas carefully controlling energy intake to sustain energy availability may improve adaptation to the new environment (23). There is evidence that switching from a high-carbohydrate, low-fat diet to a high-fat, low-carbohydrate diet while keeping total energy intake the same alters the circadian clock in humans, as measured by salivary cortisol and human blood monocytes (24). These findings suggest that adaptation to a new environment may be made more complicated if the composition of the typical diet is also changed.

General Rules for Travel

Satisfying fueling and hydration needs is critically important for athletic success, and these are the primary concerns for the traveling athlete. Thought should be given to ensuring that the traveling athlete will have familiar foods and beverages to consume prior to the competition and that the athlete will adapt well to the available beverages to be consumed during the competition (Competitions are no time to try out new foods/beverages.). Having a checklist well in advance of the trip is a good strategy to make sure the items required by the athlete are readily available. Athletes should make plans to ensure that, while traveling, thirst and/or hunger will never occur because of poor food/beverage availability.

Ideally, the athlete should begin planning for the trip long before the trip begins. This planning involves studying the cuisine, culture, and eating behaviors in the destination (25). It also involves knowing the daily schedule while at the destination to plan for meals, snacks, and drinks. The athlete should know the typical times that meals are consumed and how many meals they can rely on. In some countries, it is typical to have three meals per day (breakfast, lunch, and dinner), whereas in others it is common to have six meals per day (early breakfast, midmorning meal, lunch, midafternoon meal, dinner, and evening meal). It helps for athletes to visit local traditional restaurants serving the cuisine of the country they will be visiting prior to the trip so the athlete knows what they like and tolerate. If visiting a country where the population generally adheres to Ramadan, it is customary to fast between sunrise and sunset. If unaccustomed to this pattern of eating, athletes should make more advanced planning and preparation to find culturally acceptable eating locations and to develop strategies that will enable eating in an accustomed pattern with foods known to be well tolerated, while maintaining sensitivity to those around who are adhering to Ramadan.

Athletes should consider following these tips for travel (25–27):

- Bring snacks that are liked and tolerated. Fresh fruits, fruit juices, crackers, low-fat rice, and low-fat energy bars are nutritious, easy to carry, and have few food safety risks.

- Beware of hidden fats. Creamy soups, bread-type flaky/crispy pastries, mayonnaise-based salad dressings, and sauces in sandwiches add unnecessary fat to the food. Good alternatives to these include clear, broth-based soups instead of creamy soups; lemon juice–based salad dressing rather than mayonnaise-type dressing.

- Grilled, baked, boiled, and broiled foods are better than fried, deep-fried, or sautéed foods. Athletes must learn to be specific about how they would prefer the food to be prepared and should make no assumptions about how it will be prepared by the description on the menu. There is nothing wrong with requesting low-fat dairy products and low-fat salad dressings.

- Athletes should order à la carte to have the food exactly as they want it. Full dinners may have some desired foods, but may also provide foods that are unwanted. As an example, the grilled fish may be precisely what is wanted, but the grilled fish full dinner also comes with gravy-soaked mashed potatoes, broccoli covered with cheese sauce, and apple pie with ice cream. The à la carte order might better request broiled fish, a plain baked potato, broccoli with lemon juice, and fresh fruit for dessert.

- If traveling by air, athletes should give the airlines fair warning of special dietary requirements at least 24 hours in advance of the flight. Vegetarian offerings are often lower in fat and higher in needed carbohydrate than the standard fare.

- Air travel is one of the most dehydrating experiences a person can have. Because of this, passengers often contract sore throats and other upper respiratory illnesses. As a preventative measure, keep sipping on fluids during the flight to keep your mouth and throat moist because there may be a significant delay between the time you take off and when you receive your first drink. Drink bottled water or sports beverages.

- To avoid any delay in available beverages and if traveling by air, athletes should bring something to drink on the plane. Note, however, that liquids and gels brought from home or purchased before going through the security checkpoint in amounts larger than 100 mL (note: 1 cup = 240 mL) are only allowed in checked luggage. Beverages that are purchased after security screening may be brought onto the plane.

- Athletes changing time zones should make every attempt to get on the local schedule as soon as possible. As an example, they should have dinner when

> | Box 12.1 | **Sample Card for Someone With a Gluten Intolerance Who Is Traveling to Norway** |

I have a problem eating gluten, and it makes me ill if I consume any gluten-containing foods. Please make certain that none of the foods you give me to eat contain any of the following:

- Barley
- Bulgur
- Oats (oats themselves do not contain gluten, but are often processed in plants that produce gluten-containing grains and may be contaminated. If you give me oats, they must specifically be gluten-free oats)
- Rye
- Seitan
- Triticale and mir (a cross between wheat and rye)

Gluten may also show up as ingredients in barley malt, chicken broth, malt vinegar, some salad dressings, veggie burgers (if not specified gluten-free), and soy sauce. Gluten may even hide in many common seasonings and spice mixes.

Norwegian Translation

Jeg har et problem å spise gluten, og det gjør meg syk hvis jeg bruker noen glutenholdige matvarer.

Listen av glutenholdig korn slutter ikke på hvete. Andre lovbrytere er:

- bygg
- bulgur
- havre (havre seg selv ikke inneholder gluten, men blir ofte bearbeidet i planter som produserer glutenholdige korn og kan vþre forurenset)
- rug
- seitan
- rughvete og Mir (en krysning mellom hvete og rug)

Gluten kan også dukke opp som ingredienser i byggmalt, kyllingbuljong, malt eddik, noen salatdressinger, veggisburgere (hvis ikke angitt glutenfri), og soyasaus. Gluten kan skjule i mange vanlige krydder og kryddermikser.

the local population is eating rather than at the time dinner would be eaten while at home. This is tiring and disorienting if changing time zones, but making this change as quickly as possible makes it easier for the athlete to perform at their conditioned best. Ideally, the athlete should try to arrive at the competition site early. The general rule is 1 day early for every time zone change.

- Because safety/hygiene standards are not the same worldwide, athletes traveling to other countries increase the risk of developing diarrhea, which can result in dehydration. To lower risk of developing diarrhea and the inevitable dehydration that is associated with it, traveling athletes should take great care to avoid consumption of raw or minimally cooked foods. For instance, it is better to consume fully cooked scrambled eggs than eggs with runny yolks and albumin. When the safety of the water is in doubt, consumption of bottled water is strongly recommended for use with personal hygiene (*i.e.*, brushing teeth). When showering/bathing in water of unknown safety, care should be taken to avoid ingesting the water (21).
- Athletes with food sensitivities, allergies, or intolerances should create 3 × 5 cards in advance of the travel *in the native language of the country of destination.*

These cards should list in clear terms the foods/ingredients that create GI difficulties/allergic responses, and when giving the order at a restaurant, the card should be handed to the waiter. See Box 12.1 for an example of someone with a gluten intolerance. There are a number of excellent online programs for translating into virtually any language.

Minimizing Jet Lag

Even seasoned travelers suffer from **jet lag**, which can make the athlete feel ill, lowers appetite, and keep the athlete from getting a good night's sleep (28). Adjustment to jet lag is important to enable athletes to perform at their conditioned capacity. Jet lag has two primary forms: (i) travel involving small but consecutive trips, causing multiple shifts in usual eating patterns, and (ii) travel involving one large trip that crosses multiple time zones, causing a major change in eating and sleeping behaviors. Traveling across multiple time zones affects the normal circadian rhythms and is associated with sleeplessness, poor concentration, irritability, depression, disorientation, light-headedness, loss of appetite, and GI distress (29). Airline crews have reported sleeplessness in ~60% to 70% of cases after crossing a time zone, with only ~30% of the crews reporting sleeplessness by the third

Travel Fatigue Results in Multiple Problems for the Athlete

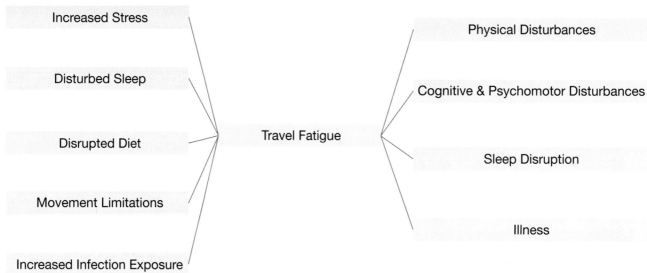

FIGURE 12.2: The effects of long-haul travel result in poor recovery and poor athletic performance. (Based on information from Rossiter A, Warrington GD, Comyns™. Effects of long-haul travel on recovery and performance in elite athletes: a systematic Review. J Strength Cond Res. 2022;36(11):3234–45.)

day following travel (22). The direction of travel also makes a difference in the time it takes to recover from jet lag. While time zone change, regardless of direction, has a negative impact on athletic performance, there is evidence that more time is required to adapt to travel toward the east than traveling toward the west (30,31). Jet lag significantly interferes with performance when traveling across time zones. Often this performance reduction is due to insufficient sleep that, by itself, can result in a 10% reduction in the expected performance (22). The change in location resulting from travel can negatively influence the athlete circadian rhythm, which refers to the daily biologic clock that controls cells through the production of enzymes and hormones (21). (See Figure 12.2.)

📖 Jet Lag

Also referred to as *desynchronosis* and *circadian dysrhythmia*, it is associated with physiologic changes that result because of changes in circadian rhythm. These conditions include loss of sleep, changes in appetite, and severe fatigue, all of which may influence athletic performance. Some of these jet lag–related changes are associated with changes in daylight, while others are related to changes in time-associated habits (32). The severity of jet lag symptoms is typically more severe and lasts longer after a flight going east than a flight going west, and more intense with more time zones that are crossed (31).

A review of the impact of sleep and circadian rhythm on athletic performance suggests the following (33,34):

■ The evidence on the impact of sleep deprivation on athletic performance is mixed. Current findings suggest that exercise requiring a combination of short-term and high-power output appears to be mainly unaffected. However, endurance performance appears to be negatively impacted following sleep deprivation.

■ Travel-associated desynchronization of circadian rhythms resulting from passing multiple time zones may be impacted if the time of the athletic endeavor is different than the athlete is accustomed to, relative to the athlete's "biologic" time.

■ Regardless of sport, athletic performance is likely to be closer to the athlete's norm if it is in the afternoon or evening, rather than in the morning.

■ Sports requiring more technical skills may be better when performed earlier in the day than skills demanding more power. Performing in warmer environments may mediate this effect.

■ The loss of sleep is a risk factor for exercise-related injuries.

Although these factors may seem minor, the margin of athletic prowess between competing athletes is often very small, making it important for athletes to have sufficient time to normalize the circadian clock, an important factor in athletic success. It is also important to consider that sleep loss impacts individuals differently, although most athletes who have been evaluated on this issue report that they feel as if they require more effort to do the same task when sleep deprived than when well rested (35).

As indicated earlier, many athletic endeavors may be negatively affected by alterations in the circadian rhythm, with sport-specific studies suggesting a performance impact in soccer, cycling, and swimming (7,36,37). The alteration in circadian rhythm may affect:

- Leg strength (38)
- Back strength and leg flexor strength (39)
- Jump height and peak power (40)
- Anaerobic (power/speed) tasks (41)
- Aerobic tasks (42)

Suggested changes to adapt to the jet lag associated with crossing time zones include the following (21,43–45):

- In advance of travel, the athlete should try to live on the new time zone schedule through gradual (1 hr/day) shifts in the time of sleep.
- An attempt should be made to mimic light exposure to the light exposure to be experienced at the new destination.
- Arrive at the destination at least 1 day early for each time zone crossed. Athletes should plan on arriving 1 week prior to the event for flights crossing more than six time zones. Where financial limitations and/or scheduling problems keep athletes from arriving sufficiently early, they should try to get on the local schedule quickly, but with as much rest as possible prior to the event.
- Short naps of ~20–30 minutes may be useful in helping athletes recover from the typical sleep deprivation that occurs with travel.
- Eat meals at regular times after arriving at the new destination. This will aid in adjustment to the new time zone.
- Never put off eating when hungry, so have some snacks readily available.
- Drink plenty of liquids. Plane cabins are notoriously dry, and dehydration is the cause of many complaints, including headaches and mild constipation.
- Consume ample fluids to help maintain a good state of hydration (water, sports beverages, fruit juices, etc.). If traveling to a location where the water is of unknown quality, consume only bottled water.
- Food safety is an important issue: Avoid consumption of raw foods or foods that are only minimally cooked (*i.e.*, raw eggs, eggs with soft yolk). Peel fruits and vegetables that have been washed in the local water supply.

- Avoid alcohol during and after the flight. Besides the negative metabolic alterations that alcohol causes, it is also a diuretic that can increase water loss. There is no logical reason for any athlete to consume alcoholic beverages at any time, particularly when traveling or when close to a competition.
- Engage in social activity or exercise after the flight. This will help to reduce the stress associated with travel.
- The sooner the athlete can eat and sleep on the new destination schedule, the more quickly the athlete will feel ready to perform athletically.
- Maintaining a frequent eating and drinking schedule (eating something about every 3 hours) is an important strategy for helping the athlete adjust to the new environment. Bringing snacks to get started is useful to ensure food availability until a good source of snacks can be found after arrival at the new location.

Travel Location

Travel locations in the United States and Western Europe have foods that are familiar to American athletes. American-style breakfast cereals and breads/rolls/crackers are easily found in grocery stores. Food preparation is also likely to be highly familiar but with some variations. Coffee, for instance, has many common variants in virtually every eating establishment (*i.e.*, espresso, Turkish/Greek, café latté, French press, Americano). If accustomed to drinking coffee in the morning, the athlete should become familiar with the terms to ensure receipt of the accustomed coffee style.

When traveling abroad, athletes should have the following items available even if the food and water supply are safe and familiar (25):

- Power cord adapters and converters to fit the power supply of the country you are traveling to
- An in-cup electric heater
- A water-filter pump
- Supply of shelf-stable foods (Table 12.2)
- Powdered sports beverage packets to make 20 quarts of beverage
- Two quarts of bottled water

Food Safety Considerations

The food safety concerns differ with each country and these differences, coupled with the athlete's travel-related stress and fatigue, may predispose the athlete to illness. These illnesses may be due to food/water contamination from bacteria, viruses, parasites, and chemicals (Table 12.3).

Table 12.2 Examples of Shelf-Stable Foods Available for Travel

Carbohydrates	Proteins	Fats	Condiments
Instant rice	Chicken pouch	Olive oil	Jam
Instant mashed potato	Tuna pouch		Honey
Pasta	Salmon pouch		Peanut butter
Couscous	Shelf-stable tofu		Mustard
Quinoa	Soy or whey protein powder		Vegemite
Dry breakfast cereal (granola, etc.)	Powdered and liquid meal replacements		Spices and herbs
Instant oats	Milk powder		Salt and pepper
Dried crackers, rice cakes, biscuits	(Nuts)	(Nuts)	
Whole grain tortillas			
Dehydrated vegetables			
Dried fruit (raisins, etc.)			

Source: Adapted from Parker-Simmons S, Andrew K. Chapter 34: the traveling athlete. In: Maughan RJ, editor. The encyclopaedia of sports medicine: an IOC Medical Commission Publication, sports nutrition. John Wiley & Sons, Ltd; 2014. p. 415–24.

Table 12.3 Common Foodborne Illnesses

Microorganism/Illness	Source	Common Foods Involved	Prevention
Salmonellosis (*Salmonella*)	Intestinal tract of humans and animals	Raw and undercooked eggs, poultry, meat, fish, dressings, pies, cream desserts, dairy products	■ Cook animal foods thoroughly ■ Prevent cross-contamination
Campylobacteriosis (*Campylobacter jejuni*)	Intestinal tract of animals, soil, and water	Undercooked meat, poultry, fish, raw dairy products	■ Cook animal foods thoroughly ■ Prevent cross-contamination
Listeriosis (*Listeria monocytogenes*)	Intestinal tract of animals, soil	Raw milk, cheese made from raw milk, cabbage, undercooked meat and poultry, hot dogs, and smoked fish	■ Good sanitation ■ Use only pasteurized dairy products ■ Cook meat and poultry thoroughly ■ Prevent cross-contamination ■ Limit refrigerator storage—watch "use-by" dates
Vibriosis (*Vibrio* species)	Seawater (especially during warmer months)	Undercooked seafood, including oysters, shrimp, crabs, and clams	■ Cook all seafood thoroughly ■ Prevent cross-contamination ■ Keep cold foods cold (below 40°F)
Hemorrhagic colitis (*Escherichia coli* O157-H7)	Intestinal tract of animals and humans	Undercooked meats and poultry, ground beef, raw milk and cheeses, unpasteurized apple juice and cider	■ Cook meats thoroughly ■ Prevent cross-contamination ■ Keep cold foods cold (below 40°F)
Shigellosis (Bacillary dysentery; *Shigella* species)	Intestinal tract of humans and primates	Salads, seafoods, milk, dairy products, poultry, potato salad, parsley	■ Good sanitation ■ Minimize contact of hands with food ■ Keep cold foods cold (below 40°F)

Table 12.4	Safe Minimum Internal Temperatures (as Measured With a Food Thermometer)
Food Type	**Internal Temperature**
Beef, pork, veal, and lamb (chops, roasts, steaks)	145°F with a 3-min rest time
Ground meat	160°F
Ham, uncooked (fresh or smoked)	145°F with a 3-min rest time
Ham, fully cooked (to reheat)	140°F
Poultry (ground, parts, whole, and stuffing)	165°F
Eggs	Cook until yolk and white are firm
Egg dishes	160°F
Fin fish	145°F or flesh is opaque and separates easily with fork
Shrimp, lobster, and crabs	Flesh pearly and opaque
Clams, oysters, and mussels	Shells open during cooking
Scallops	Flesh is milky white or opaque and firm
Leftovers and casseroles	165°F

Source: U.S. Department of Health and Human Services, U.S. Food and Drug Administration. Safe food handling: what you need to know. Available from: https://www.fda.gov/Food/FoodborneIllnessContaminants/BuyStoreServeSafeFood/ucm255180.htm

Even different levels of bromide or fluoride, purposely added to the water supply to make it safe and/or to enhance health, may result in GI distress. Common health problems that are of food and beverage origin most often result in diarrhea, but infectious hepatitis, typhoid fever, and cholera may also be the result of consuming unsafe foods and beverages. Well-established strategies to lower the risk of developing a food or water-borne illness include (25,46):

- *Fruits and vegetables:* Uncooked fruits and vegetables may be carriers of field manure/sewage used as fertilizer to grow the plants, and water used to wash the fruits and vegetables may also be contaminated. Cutting/peeling contaminated fruits and vegetables may result in the contamination (bacteria, etc.) entering the food. Ideally, vegetables should be fully cooked to resolve any contamination issue, and fresh fruits should be cleaned thoroughly with bottled water and, if available, vegetable wash (soap) prior to peeling, cutting, or eating.
- *Meats, poultry, seafood, dairy:* Animal foods are common carriers of bacteria and, potentially, other contaminating substances. To reduce the possibility of eating these contaminants, all animal foods should be fully cooked to eliminate any possibility of foodborne illness. Many cuisines often serve foods that are uncooked or undercooked (*i.e.*, sushi and other raw seafood, steak tartare), and these should be avoided. Eggs are an ideal medium for bacterial growth, so

should be fully cooked (firm to the touch, with no liquid albumin or yolk). See Table 12.4 for safe minimum internal food temperatures.
- *Environmental temperature and cleanliness:* The athlete should use his or her senses and good logic to determine if the environment where foods are available for purchase is clean, and if foods are appropriately stored in temperature-controlled containers. Foods from street vendors, open buffets, and markets that appear to be and smell unclean have a high risk of providing foods that may induce foodborne illness and should be avoided.
- *Pasteurization:* Pasteurization is a process used with milk, juice, and canned foods to kill bacteria and denaturing enzymes that enable bacterial growth. Consumption of unpasteurized milk and dairy products or juices may dramatically increase risk of developing a foodborne illness, so should be totally avoided. Only a few countries, including the United States and Australia, mandate the pasteurization of dairy foods, requiring that athletes specifically look for the Radura symbol (Figure 12.3) as a sign that the food has been pasteurized.
- *Water:* Unless the water supply has been well established as clean and safe for human consumption, athletes should become accustomed to reliance on bottled water for drinking, brushing teeth, and cleaning fresh fruits. As ice typically comes from the local water supply, which may not be clean, it is also best to skip

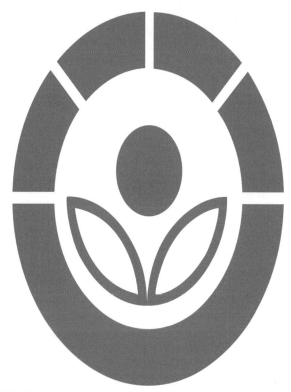

FIGURE 12.3: International Radura symbol of pasteurization.

consumption of beverages that contain ice. Athletes should also be aware of the importance of avoiding the consumption of water that may happen passively, such as while swimming in a pool and/or while showering. Camping stores have small portable water filters that remove both parasites and bacteria. Where bottled water is not available, drinking water that has been filtered is an excellent alternative.

- *Personal hygiene:* Athletes should develop the habit of carefully washing hands with soap and water prior to handling or consuming foods. Where this is not possible, carrying a small bottle of hand sanitizer is an appropriate alternative so that hands can be cleaned regardless of where the food will be consumed.

- *Sharing foods:* Avoid sharing foods where the food the athlete is eating may be touched and contaminated by someone who has not properly washed their hands. For instance, putting shared food into separate bowls rather than consuming food from a shared bag is a safer strategy.

- *Food storage:* When storing foods, keep foods (*i.e.*, meats, dairy) that may become hazardous if kept between 40°F and 140°F (4.4°C to 60°C) out of that temperature zone. The food storage area should be clean and used only for storing foods, and the wrappers/packages of stored foods should be clean and undamaged.

Important Factors to Consider

Special Food Concern

It has been reported that beef tainted with a banned steroid (clenbuterol) and consumed by competing athletes resulted in a large proportion of positive urine tests in tested samples, including in the Tour de France winner, Alberto Contador, who was suspended but insisted that the positive test was the result of unknowingly consuming tainted food (47). Clenbuterol is added to the feed of cattle, poultry, and pigs in some locations to enhance growth of both muscle and fat (48). Although illegal in many countries for this purpose, not all countries have laws banning its use or sufficient testing protocols to determine whether clenbuterol has been used. Professional football players were recently warned that high meat consumption while abroad may result in a positive blood or urine test for clenbuterol, a banned substance. The memo by the National Football League to the players stated: "Players are warned to be aware of this issue when traveling to Mexico and China. Please take caution if you decide to consume meat, and understand that you do so at your own risk" (49).

Eating Locations

Travel inevitably keeps athletes from eating when and where they would like to eat, requiring that sufficient planning take place prior to the trip to ensure that athlete performance is not compromised because of poor food selection or poorly timed meals. On those occasions when even the best planning cannot account for all contingencies, the traveling athlete must be willing to make requests when ordering food.

Airport restaurants have many options, but the foods are often high in fat and/or high in sugar. When possible, athletes should select foods that are not fried and foods high in complex/starchy carbohydrates. For instance, a baked potato would be preferred over French fries. As another example, a hungry athlete may want to order a double-patty hamburger, but would be better to order two regular hamburgers because that would provide twice the carbohydrate (hamburger buns). Pasta, bread, vegetables, and salad are all good sources of carbohydrate that are typically low in fat. Athletes should be willing to ask for a food substitution on plates that include meat/fish, vegetable, and starch. For instance, asking for sautéed fish

Table 12.5	**What to Eat, What Not to Eat; What to Drink, What Not to Drink When Traveling to Other Countries**
Eat	**Do Not Eat**
■ Food that is cooked and served hot	■ Food served at room temperature
■ Food from sealed packages	■ Food from street vendors
■ Hard-cooked eggs	■ Raw or soft-cooked (runny) eggs
■ Fruits and vegetables you have washed in safe water or peeled yourself	■ Raw or undercooked (rare) meat or fish
■ Pasteurized dairy products	■ Unwashed or unpeeled raw fruits and vegetables
	■ Condiments (such as salsa) made with fresh ingredients
	■ Salads
	■ Flavored ice or popsicles
	■ Unpasteurized dairy products
	■ Bushmeat (monkeys, bats, or other wild game)
Drink	**Do Not Drink**
■ Water, sodas, or sports drinks that are bottled and sealed (carbonated is safer)	■ Tap or well water
■ Water that has been disinfected (boiled, filtered, treated)	■ Fountain drinks
■ Ice made with bottled or disinfected water	■ Ice made with tap or well water
■ Hot coffee or tea	■ Drinks made with tap or well water (such as reconstituted juice)
■ Pasteurized milk	■ Unpasteurized milk

These recommendations are particularly important during travel to developing countries.

Source: Centers for Disease Control and Prevention. Travelers' health. Available from: https://wwwnc.cdc.gov/travel/page/food-water-safety

instead of deep fat fried–battered fish may not be possible, but the athlete would never know without asking.

Restaurants in transportation centers (airports, train stations, seaports, etc.) may be less likely to make a requested substitution to satisfy the request because they know they will probably never see the patron (or their business) again. Despite the possibility that the request may not be fulfilled, the athlete should request exactly what he or she would like. Even when ordering a baked potato, asking that all the toppings be provided on the side rather than on the potato is important. (See Table 12.5 from the Centers for Disease Control and Prevention for Safe and Risky foods and beverages while traveling.)

HIGH-ALTITUDE AND COLD ENVIRONMENTS

Performing physical work at **high altitude** presents enormous challenges that result from lower oxygen availability, lower air pressure, and lower temperature. Air temperature decreases by ~1°C for every 150 m above sea level, and this lower temperature is typically also associated with lower humidity (50). The lower oxygen availability results in automatic physiologic responses, including higher heart rate, vasodilation, and hyperventilation, that are intended to sustain tissue oxygen availability (51). Although the human system can adapt to doing work in higher elevations, this adaptation takes time to achieve. While there is individual variation, hypoxic conditions impact oxygen delivery to tissues in all individuals, requiring adaptation to the hypoxic (*i.e.*, high altitude) environment to achieve satisfactory performance. Athletes sometimes move quickly from lower to higher altitudes to enhance oxygen-carrying capacity. However, doing this without appropriate adaptation may result in **high-altitude illness** such as headache, nausea, and premature fatigue, all of which can negatively influence food and fluid consumption that may result in tissue loss that lowers cold tolerance (52). See Table 12.6 for the major nutritional issues associated with ascent to higher altitudes.

Table 12.6	Major Nutritional Issues Associated With Ascent to Moderately Higher Altitudes (1,500–3,000 m)	
Issue	**Problem**	**Recommendation**
Appetite	Rapid ascent to altitudes exceeding 2,000 m is associated with symptoms of acute mountain sickness, which is associated with nausea-induced loss of appetite.	Acute mountain sickness typically self-resolves in 2–4 days. Athletes should make every attempt to stay active and eat foods and fluids up to the maximal tolerance limit.
Fluids	Diuresis (increased urine production) occurs at high altitude, resulting in higher dehydration risk.	Take weight before and after exercise to determine water loss (16 oz = 1 lb), and drink sufficient fluids to minimize loss. Do not drink excess fluids.
Carbohydrates	Carbohydrates are utilized at a faster rate at high altitude, potentially increasing the risk of glycogen depletion and faster fatigue.	Try to consume high-carbohydrate foods/beverages as often as possible, including before, during, and after workouts.
Iron	High altitude increases red blood cell manufacture (erythropoiesis) as the body attempts to improve the capture of environmental oxygen. This process increases the iron requirement, with an initial decrease in stored iron (ferritin) as red blood cells are increased. Note: Producing sufficient additional red blood cells to enhance oxygen-carrying capacity is a slow process that may take weeks to months to achieve.	Regular consumption of foods high in iron helps to satisfy iron needs. For athletes who are unable or unwilling to consume high-iron foods (red meats, etc.), consumption of an iron supplement with vitamin C may be useful prior to and during exposure to high altitude. Cooking in an iron skillet also adds iron to the consumed foods. However, also need to be sure that if Fe supplementation is done and the athlete is monitored closely in the process to avoid Fe toxicity!

Source: Cheuvront SN, Ely BR, Wilber RL. Chapter 35: environment and exercise. In: Maughan RJ, editor. The encyclopaedia of sports medicine: an IOC Medical Commission Publication, sports nutrition. Chichester: Wiley Blackwell; 2014. p. 425–38.

High Altitude

Refers to any altitude significantly higher than that the athlete is accustomed to. Typically, high altitude is up to 2,500 m (8,200 ft), very high altitude is up to 5,500 m (18,045 ft), and extreme altitude is above 5,500 m. The lower oxygen air concentration at high altitudes results in adaptive physiologic events, including erythropoiesis to improve oxygen-carrying capacity.

High-Altitude Illness

Refers to a group of syndromes, including acute mountain sickness, high-altitude cerebral edema, and high-altitude pulmonary edema that may occur when training at an altitude to which a person has not well adapted.

Maintaining body fluid balance in extreme cold is just as difficult as maintaining fluid balance in hot and humid environments, with both increased urinary flow and voluntary dehydration potential contributing factors to dehydration. The practical aspect of keeping drinking fluids from freezing is a challenge in higher (and colder) altitudes and makes proper hydration even more difficult.

As a result, cold-weather exposure creates significant dehydration risk. It is common for soldiers in cold environments to lose up to 8% of body weight from dehydration, for several reasons (53):

- Difficulty obtaining adequate amounts of potable water
- High levels of water loss (particularly if excess clothing is worn or heavy equipment is being carried)
- Increased respiratory water loss
- Cold-induced diuresis

High-Altitude Training

There is less oxygen at higher altitudes, requiring that athletes adapt to the altitude prior to undergoing serious training activities. The higher the altitude, the lower the level of available oxygen. By definition, different degrees of high altitude are defined as follows:

- *High altitude*: 1,500–2,500 m (4,921–8,202 ft) (*e.g.*, Mount Washington, NH, USA, is 1,917 m)

- *Very high altitude*: 2,500–5,500 m (8,292–18,045 ft) (*e.g.*, Mont Blanc, France/Italy, is 4,810 m)
- *Extreme altitude*: Anything above 5,500 m (18,045 ft) (*e.g.*, K6, Pakistan, is 7,282 m)

Anaerobic events with lower reliance on oxidative metabolism may actually see some performance enhancement at higher elevations because of lower air resistance/atmospheric pressure. In addition, muscle strength and maximal muscle power are not negatively affected at high altitudes provided that muscle mass is maintained (54). It has been estimated that at an altitude of Mexico City (2,250 m), the lower air resistance imparts a 0.07 s advantage over a 100 m sprint (55,56). Despite the potential performance advantage of competing in an environment with lower air resistance, the reduced oxygen availability at high altitudes may negatively impact performance outcomes (57,58).

Important Factors to Consider

- High altitude is less likely to negatively impact high-intensity (anaerobic) activity than lower-intensity (aerobic) activity.
- The higher the altitude, the lower the oxygen availability, and the greater the negative impact on aerobic activity.

Lower oxygen concentrations at progressively higher altitudes require that athletes take a graduated approach to training at high altitudes for an efficient and illness-free adaptation. Those involved in higher altitude training can expect both faster respiration and faster heart rate because of the lower level of oxygen being pulled into the lungs with each breath. Only achieving a greater red blood cell (RBC) concentration, associated with higher oxygen-carrying capacity, will mediate the faster breathing and heart rate, but it often takes weeks for the higher RBC concentration to result in normal breathing and heart rate. Several nutrition factors are associated with production of new RBCs, including maintenance of energy balance coupled with sufficient intake of iron, folic acid, and vitamin B12. Most athletes find that consumption of an iron-rich healthy diet satisfies these requirements, but athletes who consume little or no meat may be at risk of compromising their ability to make sufficient new RBCs. These athletes may require supplementation and/or a major change in dietary intake to help ensure an appropriate adaptive response to high altitude. The maintenance of energy balance and adequate nutrient intake is also compromised by the loss of appetite that is common at high altitudes (Figure 12.4).

Heat loss in cold environments occurs through convection and conduction, but body temperature can be maintained through several means (59). The degree to which body heat is lost is lessened through vasoconstriction of the peripheral veins. Although this results in lower heat loss, it may also predispose individuals to frostbite of the fingers and toes. To lessen this risk of frostbite, *cold-induced vasodilation* is initiated about 10 minutes following initial exposure to the cold. The result is alternating vasoconstriction and vasodilation that not only helps to sustain core temperature but also fluctuates temperatures of feet and hands to lower frostbite risk (60).

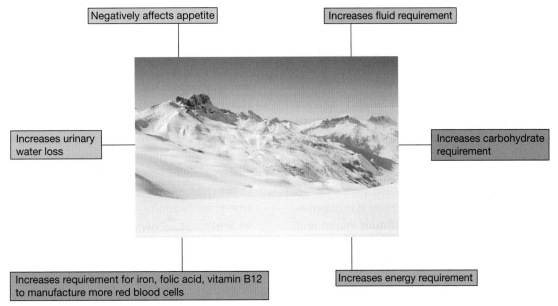

Negatively affects appetite

Increases fluid requirement

Increases urinary water loss

Increases carbohydrate requirement

Increases requirement for iron, folic acid, vitamin B12 to manufacture more red blood cells

Increases energy requirement

FIGURE 12.4: Nutritional requirements for high altitudes and cold environments. Monica Mayayo V/Shutterstock.com with added labels.

Another system for sustaining core body temperature is shivering, an involuntary central nervous system–induced mechanism that occurs when core body temperature drops by 3°C to 4°C (61,62). Shivering involves quick muscle contractions that result in a large increase (2.5 times higher than normal) in total energy expenditure, mainly from higher muscle glycogen (stored carbohydrate) utilization (63). Cold stress also increases muscle glycogen utilization as a result of increased plasma catecholamines, epinephrine, and norepinephrine (64). These systems for sustaining core body temperature are largely carbohydrate (glycogen) dependent, mandating that carbohydrate replacement be considered a highly important nutrition strategy when exercising at high altitudes and in the cold (65).

It should be noted that the reduced muscle mass associated with aging makes it more difficult for older individuals to adapt as quickly to high altitude and colder environments than for younger individuals. This is due to the lower heat production associated with lower musculature, both from exercise and from shivering (66).

Studies assessing gender differences in adaptation to high altitudes (4,300 m; 14,107 ft) suggest that, after 12 days of acclimatization, sympathetic nerve activity is similar in both men and women (67). It has also been found that high-altitude hypophagia (reduction in food intake), which is a common initial response of travel to high altitude (in the case of this study, Pikes Peak at 4,300 m; 14,107 ft), is similar in both men and women (68).

Many experienced athletes, including skiers and mountain climbers, who spend significant time at high altitudes are aware of the potential for nausea, confusion, and easy fatigue when working at high altitudes. It takes time to adapt to this relatively hypoxic environment, mainly by improving the capacity to deliver oxygen to working tissues through development of more RBCs. High-altitude exposure increases oxidative stress, and it is estimated that most humans are 80% acclimatized after 10 days at altitude and ~95% acclimatized by 45 days at altitude (69,70).

Common occurrences when at a higher altitude include faster breathing, shortness of breath, higher urination frequency, and more trouble sleeping than the person is accustomed to. The lower barometric pressure of high altitude lowers the oxygen concentration of every breath, forcing a more frequent breathing pattern in an attempt to pull in the same level of oxygen. It is impossible to obtain the same oxygen at high altitude when compared with sea level, no matter how rapid the breathing pattern. As a result, physical work will be more difficult and fatigue will occur more quickly at high altitude. Poor adaptation to high altitude from an excessively fast rate of ascent, inadequate carbohydrate consumption, or excess exertion will result in *altitude sickness,* which includes headaches, vomiting, anorexia, malaise, and nausea (71).

The common high-altitude illness syndromes include the following (72,73) (note: there are also drug-related treatments, including dexamethasone, not mentioned in the treatment recommendations below):

- *Acute mountain sickness:* A related disorder, acute mountain sickness commonly occurs at altitudes exceeding 2,000 m (6,600 ft), produces symptoms of nausea, dyspnea on exertion and at rest, poor sleep, ataxia, headache, altered mental state, lassitude, fluid retention from greater antidiuretic hormone production, and cough (74,75). It is thought to be the least serious and most common of the syndromes.
  - *Treatment:* Involves cessation of ascent, rest, and acclimatization to the current altitude/cold.
  - *Prevention:* Ascent slowly, with a maximum of 600 m/day (2,000 ft/day); avoid excess exertion; and avoid direct transport (*e.g.,* helicopter, ski lifts) to elevations greater than 2,750 m (9,000 ft).
- *High-altitude cerebral edema:* Symptoms of high-altitude cerebral edema, which can progress rapidly and result in death within a matter of a few hours, include gait ataxia (walking like someone intoxicated), confusion, psychiatric changes, and changes of consciousness that may progress to deep coma (76).
  - *Treatment:* Immediate descent to ~1,000 m (3,300 ft) and provide oxygen if available. If available and if the descent is delayed, should use portable hyperbaric chamber.
  - *Prevention:* Ascent slowly, with a maximum of 600 m/day (2,000 ft/day); avoid excess exertion; avoid direct transport (*e.g.,* helicopter, ski lifts) to elevations greater than 2,750 m (9,000 ft).
- *High-altitude pulmonary edema:* The cause(s) of high-altitude pulmonary edema (fluid in the lungs) are not well understood, but it is known that it rarely occurs at altitudes below 2,400 m (8,000 ft). Failure to treat this disorder immediately, typically by immediate descent, may result in death. Symptoms result from a lower oxygen–carbon dioxide exchange and include extreme fatigue, gurgling breaths, breathlessness at rest, tightness of the chest, cough with possible bloody sputum, and blue/gray lips and/or fingernails (77).
  - *Treatment:* Provide oxygen immediately and descend 500–1,000 m (1,600–3,300 ft) or more. If delayed descent, use portable hyperbaric chamber.
  - *Prevention:* Slow ascent with a maximum of 600 m/day (2,000 ft/day); sleep at lower altitude; avoid overexertion.

Studies assessing athletes in a high-altitude adventure race have found that 4.5% had altitude illness at the race onset; 14.1% had altitude illness during the race that required medical treatment; and 14.3% withdrew from the race because of altitude-related illness (78). It appears that the most significant nutrition-related changes are typically found at altitudes greater than 6,000 m. These include changes in eating patterns (typically hypophagia) with an associated loss of body weight and a negative nitrogen balance that is associated with loss of lean mass (79). As indicated earlier, illness occurring at high altitude should be treated by descent to a lower altitude and by administering oxygen, if available. Worsening symptoms should be taken seriously, with no delay in descent, as these symptoms may rapidly progress to high-altitude cerebral edema or high-altitude pulmonary edema, both of which are life threatening (80).

Body composition makes a difference in high-altitude sickness risk, with obese individuals more likely to suffer from acute mountain sickness (81). However, those with periodic high-altitude exposures appear to adapt and reduce the symptoms of acute mountain sickness, regardless of body composition (82). Other strategies, including magnesium supplementation and ginkgo biloba supplementation, have been tried for reducing acute mountain sickness, but without success (83,84). The combined impact of acute mountain sickness symptoms is a severe appetite depression with a concomitant reduction in foods and fluids. The high caloric requirements and fluid consumption difficulties of cold weather, combined with the anorexia of high altitude, create the two most serious problems of work at high altitude: maintenance of weight and fluid balance. Even those who are part of well-organized mountain-climbing expeditions and regularly exposed to high altitude typically fail to consume sufficient calories, resulting in body weight reduction. An assessment of participants in a Himalayan trek found that body weight was significantly reduced by the end of the trek, and energy intake was significantly lower at high altitude than at low altitude (85). Despite a greater need for energy, it has been found that food intakes are typically 10%–50% lower at high altitude, depending on the speed of the ascent (See Chapter 8 for strategies on predicting energy requirements.). This also appears to be true when people are in a hypobaric (lower air pressure) chamber and not exposed to severe cold (86). Individuals at high altitude must make a conscious effort to consume more food, often with forced eating, to obtain enough energy to satisfy physiologic needs (Box 12.2) (87).

Box 12.2   Sample Foods and Considerations for High-Altitude Eating

Sample Foods for High-Altitude Treks

- *Breakfasts:* Granola or energy bars, Pop-Tarts, oatmeal, bagels, hot sweet rice, couscous, grapenuts, hot cocoa, tea, and cider
- *Lunches:* Crackers (wheat thins, Ritz, Cheez-Its), cookies, bagels or rolls, jerky, sausages, cheese sticks, nuts, candy bars, dried fruits, flavored juice drink mixes, fruit leather, fig bars, hard candy, trail mix
- *Dinners:* Cocoa, cider, soups, hot Jello, and teas as the first course; freeze-dried meals with rice, noodles, vegetables; instant rice, stuffing, or mashed potatoes; pudding or mousse for desserts

How High Altitude Affects Cooking

At altitudes above 3,000 ft, preparation of food may require changes in time, temperature, or recipe. The reason is the lower atmospheric pressure due to a thinner blanket of air above. At sea level, the air presses on a square inch of surface with 14.7 lb (6.7 kg) pressure; at 5,000 ft (1,524 m) with 12.3 lb pressure; and at 10,000 ft (3,048 m) with only 10.2 lb (4.6 kg) pressure—a decrease of about 0.5 lb (0.23 m) per 1,000 ft (305 m). This decreased pressure affects food preparation in two ways:

- Water and other liquids evaporate faster and boil at lower temperatures.
- Leavening gases in breads and cakes expand more quickly.

As atmospheric pressure decreases, water boils at lower temperatures. At sea level, water boils at 212°F (100°C). With each 500-ft (152.4 m) increase in elevation, the boiling point of water is lowered by just under 1°F. At 7,500 ft (2,286 m), for example, water boils at about 198°F (92°C). Because water boils at a lower temperature at higher elevations, foods that are prepared by boiling or simmering will cook at a lower temperature, and it will take longer to cook.

(continued)

Box 12.2   Sample Foods and Considerations for High-Altitude Eating (*Continued*)

High-altitude areas are also prone to low humidity, which can cause the moisture in foods to evaporate more quickly during cooking. Covering foods during cooking will help retain moisture.

Why Cooking Time Must Be Increased

As altitude increases and atmospheric pressure decreases, the boiling point of water decreases. To compensate for the lower boiling point of water, the cooking time must be increased. Turning up the heat will not help cook food faster. No matter how high the cooking temperature, water cannot exceed its own boiling point—unless if using a pressure cooker. Even if the heat is turned up, the water will simply boil away faster and whatever is being cooked will dry out faster.

High Altitudes Affect How Meat and Poultry Are Cooked

Meat and poultry products are composed of muscle, connective tissue, fat, and bone. The muscle is ~75% water (although different cuts of meat may have more or less water) and 20% protein, with the remaining 5% representing a combination of fat, carbohydrates, and minerals. The leaner the meat, the higher the water content (less fat means more protein, thus more water).

With such high water content, meat and poultry are susceptible to drying out while being cooked if special precautions are not taken. Cooking meat and poultry at high altitudes may require adjustments in both time and moisture. This is especially true for meat cooked by simmering or braising. Depending on the density and size of the pieces, meats and poultry cooked by moist heat may take up to *one-fourth more cooking time* when cooked at 5,000 ft. Use the sea-level time and temperature guidelines when oven-roasting meat and poultry, as oven temperatures are not affected by altitude changes.

Use a Food Thermometer

A food thermometer is the only way to measure whether food has reached a safe internal temperature. In a high-altitude environment, it is easy to overcook meat and poultry or scorch casseroles. To prevent overcooking meat and poultry (which will result in dry, unappetizing food) or to prevent undercooking (which can result in food poisoning), check food with a food thermometer.

Where to Place the Food Thermometer

Meat: When taking the temperature of beef, pork, lamb, and veal roasts, steaks, or chops, the food thermometer should be placed in the thickest part of the meat, avoiding bone and fat. When the food being cooked is irregularly shaped, such as with a beef roast, check the temperature in several places.

Cook all raw beef, pork, lamb, and veal steaks, chops, and roasts to a minimum internal temperature of 145°F (63°C) as measured with a food thermometer before removing meat from the heat source. For safety and quality, allow meat to rest for at least 3 minutes before carving or consuming. For reasons of personal preference, consumers may choose to cook meat to higher temperatures.

Cook all raw ground beef, pork, lamb, and veal to an internal temperature of 160°F as measured with a food thermometer.

Poultry: A whole turkey, chicken, or other poultry is cooked to a safe minimum internal temperature of 165°F (74°C) as measured with a food thermometer. Check the internal temperature in the innermost part of the thigh and wing and the thickest part of the breast. For reasons of personal preference, consumers may choose to cook poultry to higher temperatures.

For optimum safety, do not stuff whole poultry. If stuffing whole poultry, the center of the stuffing must reach a safe minimum internal temperature of 165°F.

If cooking poultry parts, insert the food thermometer into the thickest area, avoiding the bone. The food thermometer may be inserted sideways if necessary. When the food is irregularly shaped, the temperature should be checked in several places.

Source: United States Department of Agriculture, Food Safety and Inspection Service. High altitude cooking and food safety. Available from: https://www.fsis.usda.gov/food-safety/safefood-handling-and-preparation/food-safety-basics/high-altitude-cooking

---

There is a reduction in fat-free mass at altitudes above 5,000 m, likely due to the combined results of hypophagia (typically 30% to 50% decrease in energy consumption) and an increase in energy expenditure (up to 1.85–3.0 times greater than at sea level in Mount Everest climbers) (88). Skeletal muscle represents a large proportion of normal total body protein turnover and typically there is homeostasis, with approximately the same amount of muscle protein gained as that lost. At high altitude, it appears that hypoxia is largely responsible for greater skeletal muscle loss than recovery, both because of the effects it has on reducing appetite and increasing energy metabolism (89). It should be noted that a reduction in total energy intake also results in the reduction in protein intake, the combination of which can have an impact on muscle protein status. It is well established that relatively higher protein intake (1.8 vs. 0.9 g/kg) is useful in sustaining skeletal muscle status when coupled with a total energy intake restriction (90). Given the difficulty of maintaining a sufficient calorie and protein intake when at high altitude and the fact that higher total protein intakes are thermogenic, requiring an additional 20%–30% of total calories for absorption and metabolism, providing a protein supplement relatively high in branched-chain amino acids (particularly leucine) may be a useful strategy for sustaining skeletal muscle mass (88).

Sweat loss in extremely cold environments can equal that of hot and humid environments, primarily because of the insulated clothing being worn. Moderate to heavy exercise in typically insulated winter clothing results in sweat loss estimated to be nearly 2 L of sweat per hour (53). The primary strategy to ensure adequate hydration is to have enough fluids readily available to allow for frequent consumption of appropriate quantities. This strategy is not easy to achieve, however, because in cold, high-altitude environments drinks can freeze unless there is a well-planned strategy for keeping the drinks fluid. Another problem is that fluids have a high density and are heavy to transport in sufficient quantities to satisfy needs. A potential option is to obtain fluids locally by melting and purifying ice and snow, but this process takes a great deal of time and a high level of heating fuel. This strategy is estimated to require more than 6 hours and 2 L of gas to melt enough ice/snow to satisfy fluid requirements for one person (53).

Meeting Energy and Nutrient Needs in the Cold at High Altitude

The main goal of exercising in a cold environment is to sustain normal core body temperature, which requires greater energy requirement. Energy expenditures at high altitude and cold are significantly higher (commonly 2.5–3.0 times greater) than at sea level. The energy requirement is sufficiently high that it is difficult to satisfy energy needs in this environment, resulting in loss of muscle and weight (91,92). Frequent eating at timed intervals, with a focus on high-carbohydrate foods, is important because carbohydrates take less oxygen to metabolize for energy than either fat or protein (Table 12.7). Insufficient carbohydrate may also result in low blood sugar, which negatively affects the central nervous system, resulting in mental confusion and disorientation. It has been found that some mountaineers prefer carbohydrates and may develop a dislike of fat (93). It has also been found, however, that many individuals at high altitudes maintain existing food preferences and do not shy away from higher-fat foods, despite a reduction in total food intake

Table 12.7	Nutrition Considerations for Exercise in Cold Environments	
Factor	**Issue**	**Recommended Action**
Fluid	High levels of body water loss occur even in cold weather because of the heat-preserving properties of insulated clothing. If insufficient clothing is worn, the lowering of core temperature results in diuresis.	Athletes should weigh themselves before and after exercise to determine the volume of water lost that was not adequately replaced. For every pound lost, 16 oz of fluids should be consumed during the activity to sustain pre-exercise weight (1 kg weight = 1,000 mL fluid).
Carbohydrates	Hypothermia (body temperature below 35°C) occurs when heat dissipation exceeds heat production, with shivering and other symptoms. Energy metabolism relies heavily on carbohydrate as a fuel, and shivering is mainly fueled by glycogen (stored carbohydrate).	Athletes should focus on consuming high-carbohydrate foods prior to exercise to ensure optimizing glycogen stores. Carbohydrates should be consumed during exercise to sustain blood sugar and mental function and to provide fuel to working muscles so as to diminish muscle glycogen utilization.

Source: Cheuvront SN, Ely BR, Wilber RL. Chapter 35: environment and exercise. In: Maughan RJ, editor. The encyclopaedia of sports medicine: an IOC Medical Commission Publication, sports nutrition. Chichester: Wiley Blackwell; 2014. p. 425–38.

as a result of a lowering of the sense of taste (94). The negative energy balance common at high altitude results in muscle and weight loss that reduces both strength and endurance and also the capability to produce sufficient heat to sustain core body temperature. Athletes at high altitudes should have as a primary goal the consumption of sufficient energy, regardless of the energy substrate distribution. A secondary goal would be the consumption of as much carbohydrate as is tolerated. None of this is easy to achieve, as even the time it takes to prepare/cook meals doubles for each 1,500 m (5,000 ft), as water boils at a lower temperature. Prepackaged, high-carbohydrate, moderate-protein foods are appropriate choices for most meals, with cooked meals reserved for times when there is adequate water and preparation time.

Vitamins and Minerals

Vitamin and mineral consumption should be considered well in advance of attempting to go to a high-altitude/cold environment. Iron status should be evaluated and determined to be excellent, with normal levels of iron stores (ferritin) prior to going to high altitude. It does little good to take supplemental iron while actively on a climb, as erythropoiesis (the process of making new RBCs) takes weeks and months to improve iron status (95). Oxidative stress may be higher in hot and cold environments, so consumption of foods that are good sources of antioxidants should be considered (96). A study of oxidative stress in humans at high altitudes found that those receiving an antioxidant mixture had lower markers of oxidative stress than those receiving single antioxidant supplements. If taking supplements, it appears that periodic consumption of a variety of antioxidants that include ascorbic acid, β-carotene, selenium, and vitamin E results in a better outcome than consuming a daily dose of a single antioxidant (97). (See Chapters 5 and 6 for specific information on vitamins and minerals, and Chapter 13 for information on supplements and ergogenic aids.)

Fluids

Having sufficient fluids available to consume in cold high-altitude environments is difficult but an absolute necessity to ensure that the individual can survive the environment. To ensure adequate fluid availability, each person should have easy access to a *minimum* of 2 L of fluids per day, with double that amount (4 L) the preferred volume (98). Consider that physical work in this environment may cause the loss of 2 L of sweat per hour. Climbers have developed a basecamp strategy, where large amounts of food, water, fuel, and other materials are moved to the highest possible altitude using helicopters or animal packs. Climbers then go from the basecamp to a higher altitude carrying just enough food and fluid to satisfy needs for the climb from the basecamp. Ideally, fresh potable water should be available at the basecamp as using snow and ice as a water source increases necessary resources in fuel, pots, stoves, etc. There are also reports that a diarrhea-causing intestinal parasite, *Giardia lamblia*, is present in high-altitude regions (93). Therefore, local fluid sources should be used only in emergencies, and preferably only if high-quality purification devices are available.

To avoid having fluids freeze, athletes should carry drinking fluids inside insulated clothing they wear, and also keep fluids inside sleeping bags when sleeping. It has been suggested that adding a small amount of glycerol has the double benefit of improving fluid retention while also reducing the risk that the water will freeze. As glycerol is a 3-carbon molecule metabolized like carbohydrate, it also adds a source of needed carbohydrate energy to the consumed fluid (53). (Note: Glycerol added to water was used for many years by endurance athletes competing in hot and humid environments. The effect of glycerol is to enhance water retention, resulting in a superhydrated state prior to the activity, which enables longer sustained sweat rates to dissipate the environmental and metabolic heat. Glycerol, however, has now been placed on the banned substance list by the World Anti-Doping Agency, so *it should not be used* by any athlete performing in sanctioned events.)

Athletes often consume less fluid while physically active than needed to sustain a state of normal hydration. This voluntary dehydration is likely to be a more serious problem when at high altitude, as appetite and the sensation of thirst are both blunted (53). To avoid this problem, athletes at high altitude should practice consuming fluids on a fixed time schedule, whether they feel thirsty or not (99). Consumption of smaller volumes at higher frequency may also reduce the need to urinate, which is more likely to occur following consumption of a large volume at one time (Please see Chapter 7 for additional information on hydration.).

HIGH HEAT AND HUMIDITY ENVIRONMENTS

It is difficult to dissipate the heat created from the metabolism of energy (humans are only ~30% efficient in converting burned fuel to muscular movement, with the remaining 70% heat creation) in addition to the heat of the environment imposed on the body on a hot day (100). This is even more difficult on a humid day, as sweat rates must increase because of the difficulty in evaporating sweat (the primary heat-removing system) into air that has a high water content (Figure 12.5). Humans cannot continually acquire the heat of exercise and the environment, as that would result in dangerously high core body temperature. Ultimately, there must be a balance between the production of heat plus the environmental heat, and the removal of excess heat to maintain core body temperature (Table 12.8).

The greater the amount of energy burned per unit of time, the greater the heat production and the greater the amount of excess heat that must be removed (101). Therefore, athletes who are unable to adequately remove the excess heat through the evaporation of sweat have only one option: lower the production of heat by lowering the energy burned per unit of time (*i.e.*, to slow down). It is now well established that heat stress results in earlier

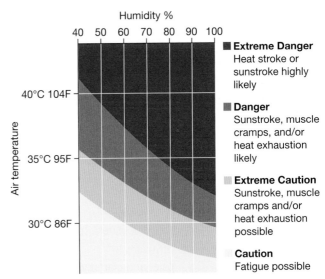

FIGURE 12.5: Risks of exercise in high temperatures and environments with high humidity. Heat danger increases with humidity. (Data from United States Department of Commerce, U.S. National Weather Service [Internet]. Accessed 2018 May 16. Available from: https://www.weather.gov/)

Table 12.8	Nutrition Considerations for Exercise in Hot/Humid Environments	
Factor	**Issue**	**Recommended Action**
Fluid	High environmental temperatures, particularly when coupled with high humidity, increase the sweat rate. Failure to match fluid consumption with sweat loss lowers total body water and blood volume, with a resultant lowering of the sweat rate. As the environmental and metabolic heat cannot be retained (it must be dissipated), a lowering of the sweat rate is inevitably associated with a slowing or cessation of physical activity.	Anyone exercising in a hot/humid environment should weigh themselves before and after exercise to determine the amount of fluid that was not adequately replaced during the exercise. The goal is to help the athlete understand the additional amount of fluid that should be consumed during physical activity to minimize the weight (*i.e.*, fluid) loss. Anything in excess of a 2% body weight loss is associated with a reduction in performance and may place the athlete at risk of heat illness.
Carbohydrates	Maintenance of blood sugar during physical activity is important to sustain central nervous system function and as a source of needed fuel to working muscles. During intense physical activity, blood sugar may drop to below-normal levels in less than 1 hr. In a stressful high-heat/humidity environment, blood sugar may drop more quickly.	Athletes should train with a sports beverage that contains ~6%–7% carbohydrate solution. Frequent consumption of this fluid will help to sustain blood sugar levels and has been established to be well-tolerated by the gastrointestinal tract.
Electrolytes	High sweat rates are associated with faster losses of sodium chloride and potassium. Poor blood sodium status is associated with low blood volume, lower stroke volume, and lower sweat rates.	Consumption of a sports drink that contains appropriate concentrations of electrolytes (typically ranging from 100 to 200 mg sodium/240 mL) can help to counteract the loss of electrolytes in sweat. It is also important for athletes to consume salt with meals to help ensure normal blood sodium levels.

Source: Cheuvront SN, Ely BR, Wilber RL. Chapter 35: environment and exercise. In: Maughan RJ, editor. The encyclopaedia of sports medicine: an IOC Medical Commission Publication, sports nutrition. Chichester: Wiley Blackwell; 2014. p. 425–38.

Table 12.9	Warning Signs and Symptoms of Heat-Related Illness	
Heat-Related Illness	**What to Look For**	**What to Do**
Heat stroke	▪ High body temperature (103°F or higher) ▪ Hot, red, dry, or damp skin ▪ Fast, strong pulse ▪ Headache ▪ Feeling dizzy ▪ Nausea ▪ Feeling confused ▪ Losing consciousness (passing out)	▪ Call 911 right away—heat stroke is a medical emergency ▪ Move the person to a cooler place ▪ Help lower the person's temperature with cool clothes or a cool bath ▪ Do *not* give the person anything to drink
Heat exhaustion	▪ Heavy sweating ▪ Cold, pale, and clammy skin ▪ Fast, weak pulse ▪ Nausea or vomiting ▪ Muscle cramps ▪ Feeling tired or weak ▪ Feeling dizzy ▪ Headache ▪ Fainting (passing out)	▪ Move to a cool place ▪ Loosen your clothes ▪ Put cool, wet clothes on your body or take a cool bath ▪ Sip water *Get medical help right away if:* ▪ You are throwing up ▪ Your symptoms get worse ▪ Your symptoms last longer than 1 hr
Heat cramps	▪ Heavy sweating during intense exercise ▪ Muscle pain or spasms	▪ Stop physical activity and move to a cool place ▪ Drink water or a sports drink ▪ Wait for cramps to go away before you do any more physical activity *Get medical help right away if:* ▪ Cramps last longer than 1 hr ▪ You're on a low-sodium diet ▪ You have heart problems

Source: United States Department of Health and Human Services, Centers for Disease Control and Prevention. Warning Signs and Symptoms of Heat-Related Illness [Internet]. Accessed 2017 July. Available from: https://www.cdc.gov/disasters/extremeheat/warning.html

fatigue (*i.e.*, shorter amount of time to exhaustion) and a reduction in exercise intensity (*i.e.*, to burn less energy and create less heat per unit of time), and acclimatization to the heat improves performance (102). However, even with acclimatization, there are risks of exercising in hot and humid environments, including **heat illness** such as heat stroke, heat exhaustion, and heat cramps (Table 12.9).

📖 Heat Illness

Refers to a group of syndromes, including heat exhaustion, heat cramps, and heat stroke, that most likely result from prolonged exposure to hot and humid environments that athletes have not been well adapted to. Nutritional factors, including failure to adequately replace fluid, electrolytes, and carbohydrate, will exacerbate the likelihood that heat illness, in one of its forms, may occur. It has become

increasingly clear that consumption of plain water during exercise increases the risk of hyponatremia, which increases the risk of serious problems that include encephalopathy, coma, or death (103). Symptoms of exercise-associated hyponatremia include confusion, headache, lethargy, seizures, and anorexia (104). (See Chapter 7 on hydration.)

Regardless of the sport, environmental heat stress has a negative impact on performance, with studies demonstrating this impact on cyclists, marathon runners, and soccer (105–107). However, athletes who have well acclimatized to the heat, typically over the course of 2 weeks, experience improved performance (101,108). It should also be noted that athletes who acclimatize to the heat are not likely to experience improved performance in a cool climate (109). To some extent, the well-conditioned athlete who has experience exercising in the heat may adapt the exercise intensity early to produce less metabolic heat, knowing that the environmental temperature will have an impact on performance. This was found in experienced runners competing in warm weather endurance events, who selected a slower pace at the onset of the race, whereas less-acclimatized/experienced runners begin the race at a faster pace only to find that they must quickly slow down because of the difficulty to adequately dissipate the acquired heat (110). This suggests that at least a portion of the benefit derived from acclimatizing to exercise in the heat is to have an improved understanding of its impact, allowing the athlete to appropriately modify exercise/racing strategy.

SUMMARY

- Advance planning is important for athletes who travel, with no assumptions about food/beverage availability necessary to satisfy the needs of athletes. As a safety measure, critical items (key foods, sports beverage powders, etc.) should be brought along to ensure availability.
- Athletes should be discouraged from trying new foods at the travel location until after the event to reduce the potential for an unwanted food reaction. Ample time should be built into the trip to ensure acclimatization to the new environment. As a general rule, the athlete should arrive 1 day early for each time zone crossed, up to a maximum of 7 days. Ample time should be made available for sufficient rest, and every effort should be made to get on the schedule of the new location as quickly as possible.
- Athletes should allow 1–2 weeks to become acclimated to a high-altitude environment. Training during the acclimatization period should be lower in volume and intensity so as to reduce the risk of altitude sickness.
- Especially for long-duration predominantly aerobic events, athletes should learn to make necessary adjustments in speed because of the lower oxygen availability. Athletes sometimes live at high altitude and train at lower altitude to enhance RBC formation. This provides a competitive advantage when competing at lower elevations because of the greater oxygen-carrying capacity.
- When training in a cold environment, the athlete should dress to stay warm. A failure to do so increases the risk of developing low body temperature with associated shivering, which is glycogen dependent, and may increase the risk of frostbite and other health problems.
- Athletes in high-heat environments should allow ample time, typically 1–2 weeks, to adapt to the heat. Training duration and intensity should be adjusted until the athlete has become acclimatized. If training for competition, athletes should do the more serious activity (*i.e.*, higher duration and/or intensity) during the coolest portion of the day (typically early morning), and try to become acclimated to the heat with more moderate activity during the middle of the day when it is the warmest.
- Goals, expectations, and strategies for competing in high heat should be adjusted to avoid heat stress disorders.

Practical Application Activity

Using online maps and the internet, and the online food analysis system used in previous chapters, do the following to see if you can make a food/beverage plan if you were a competing athlete:

For High-Altitude/Cold-Weather Competition
1. Select a high-altitude (minimum 1,500 meters elevation) competition site (*e.g.*, Val d'Isére. France; Aspen, Colorado, etc.) for a cold-weather winter sport such as cross-country or downhill skiing.
2. Find a hotel near the competition site where you could stay, keeping in mind that you should get there a minimum of 1 day early for each time zone you crossed (*i.e.*, if you crossed three time zones, you should be there 3 days before the competition begins, or even more days if you have not previously acclimated to the high altitude.)
3. Locate restaurants and, if available, grocery stores near the hotel where you can eat/buy food and beverages.
4. Analyze the foods available in the nearby restaurants (go through the online menu) and grocery stores with an eye toward cost (do you think you could afford it?), nutrient content (is it too high in fat?, is the carbohydrate content appropriate?, etc.), and familiarity (better to eat foods you are familiar with).
   a. Make a list of food items in the restaurant(s) and highlight those that satisfy your nutritional and cost criteria.
   b. Indicate which foods are available for breakfast, lunch, and dinner.

c. Where will you get snacks and beverages to consume? Are there nearby grocery stores that have what you need/like? Can you take foods with you from the restaurants? If so, make a list of what you can purchase.

5. Using known nutritional stresses associated with cold-weather/high-altitude environments and based on the lists created above, make a list of foods/beverages/beverage powders, etc. that you will need to bring with you. The amounts you will need to bring should be based on the number of days you have to be there to acclimate to the local time zone.

For Sea-Level/Hot and Humid Competition

1. Select a hot-humid competition site close to sea level (*e.g.*, Athens, Greece; Rio de Janeiro, Brazil, etc.) for a sport such as soccer or marathon.
2. Use the same procedure as described above, but consider the nutritional stresses associated with hot and humid weather environments to create your food and beverage lists, where you will obtain what you need, and what you will need to bring with you.

CHAPTER QUESTIONS

1. Which of the following travel diets are associated with improving cellular tryptophan levels, which help to enhance serotonin and improve a sense of relaxation and improved sleep?
   a. Higher protein and lower carbohydrate
   b. Higher fat and higher protein
   c. Lower protein and higher carbohydrate
   d. Lower fat, higher protein, and higher carbohydrate

2. To enhance epinephrine (adrenalin) production and alertness through an enhanced uptake of tyrosine, the athlete could consume a diet that is:
   a. Higher protein and lower carbohydrate
   b. Higher fat and higher protein
   c. Lower protein and higher carbohydrate
   d. Lower fat, higher protein, and higher carbohydrate

3. Diets that increase the amount of time it takes for athletes to adapt to a new environment are:
   a. Higher protein and lower carbohydrate
   b. Higher fat, with excess energy
   c. Lower protein and higher carbohydrate
   d. Lower fat, higher protein, and higher carbohydrate

4. Because air travel is dehydrating, athletes should keep sipping on fluids, particularly wine and beer, during the flight to maintain a moist mouth and throat.
   a. True
   b. False

5. It is important for athletes who have changed multiple time zones to:
   a. Try to maintain the schedule from the original time zone until at least 48 hours have passed to help the body adjust.
   b. Quickly get on the local schedule as soon as possible, as this helps the body adjust to the new time zone.
   c. Sleep upon arrival for a minimum of 10 hours to help the body adjust from the travel.
   d. Eat and drink foods and beverages that are familiar as soon as possible after arriving in the new time zone to help the GI tract adjust.

6. It takes ~_____ day(s) for each time zone change to fully adjust to the new time zone.
   a. 4
   b. 3
   c. 2
   d. 1

7. The change in circadian rhythm associated with travel may negatively affect the following:
   a. Leg strength
   b. Jumping
   c. Anaerobic activity
   d. Aerobic activity
   e. All the above

8. Although pasteurization is necessary for dairy foods produced in the United States, because bacterial infections in cows are far less common in Western Europe, it is not necessary to consume pasteurized dairy products when traveling to Western Europe.
   a. True
   b. False

9. Banned steroids are sometimes used in animal feed which can result in a positive blood/urine test if the athlete consumed meat that was fed this feed.
   a. True
   b. False

10. High-altitude environments may impact all of the following, except:
    a. Increased appetite
    b. Diuresis
    c. Faster glycogen depletion
    d. Erythropoiesis

ANSWERS TO CHAPTER QUESTIONS

1. c
2. a
3. b
4. b
5. b

6. d
7. e
8. b
9. a
10. a

Case Study Considerations

1. **Case Study Answer 1:** Perform a computer search to see what grocery stores are near your location that can be easily accessed to obtain familiar and well-tolerated foods. If uncertain, plan to bring snacks that are known to be well tolerated. If certain foods are known to affect you negatively, create some cards in the local language that contain information on the foods and food ingredients you must avoid. Have these cards available to give to the waiter/waitress when you're eating out just to be sure there is nothing lost in the translation.

2. **Case Study Answer 2:** Only bring foods that are known to be well tolerated and are shelf stable (*i.e.*, require no refrigeration), and focus on high-carbohydrate, high-protein, low-fat foods. Examples include instant oats, instant mashed potatoes, dry breakfast cereal, crackers, biscuits, dried fruit, chicken pouch, tuna pouch, and salmon pouch.

3. **Case Study Answer 3:** Make certain you stay well hydrated during the flight by frequently sipping on well-tolerated fluids (*e.g.*, water, fruit juices, and sports beverages). Avoid all alcohol and try to avoid excess consumption of caffeinated beverages, as these may result in a state of underhydration.

4. **Case Study Answer 4:** Try to get on the local eating and sleeping schedule as soon as you arrive. This will help you adjust to the local time zone and diminish the adaptation time adjustment to the impacted circadian rhythms.

5. **Case Study Answer 5:** Avoid consuming undercooked animal foods of any kind (*i.e.*, beef, chicken, fish, shellfish, etc.) and unpasteurized dairy products (*i.e.*, cheese made with unpasteurized milk, unpasteurized fresh milk, unpasteurized kefir, etc.). It is also important to avoid raw fruits and vegetables, as these may not have been adequately washed or the water they were washed in may not be free of bacteria. It is also important to avoid consuming food that is sold by street vendors, as the sanitation conditions may not be adequate.

REFERENCES

1. Maughan RJ, Shirreffs SM. Preparing athletes for competition in the heat: developing an effective acclimatization strategy. Sports Sci Exch. 1997;2(10):65.
2. Lei T-H, Wang F. Looking ahead of 2021 Tokyo summer Olympic Games: how does humid head affect endurance

performance? Insight into physiological mechanism and heat-related illness prevention strategies. J Therm Bio. 2021; 99:102975.

3. Lei T-H, Stannard SR, Perry BG, Schlader ZJ, Cotter JD, Mündel T. Influence of menstrual phase and arid vs. humid heat stress on autonomic and behavioural thermoregulation during exercise in trained but unacclimated women. J Physiol. 2017;595(9):2823–37.

4. Abbott SM, Reid K, Zee PC. Circadian rhythm sleep-wake disorders. Psychiatr Clin North Am. 2015;39:805–23.

5. Konturek PC, Brzozowski T, Konturek SJ. Gut clock: implication of circadian rhythms in the gastrointestinal tract. J Physiol Pharmacol. 2011;62(2):139–50.

6. Reilly T, Atkinson G, Edwards B, Waterhouse J, Farrelly K, Fairhurst E. Diurnal variation in temperature, mental and physical performance, and tasks specifically related to football (soccer). Chronobiol Int. 2007;24:507–19.

7. Reilly T, Waterhouse J, Burke LM, Alonso JM; International Association of Athletics Federations. Nutrition for travel. J Sports Sci. 2007;25(Suppl 1):S125–34.

8. Sanders SW, Moore JG. Gastrointestinal chronopharmacology: physiology, pharmacology and therapeutic implications. Pharmacol Ther. 1992;54:1–15.

9. Zisapel N. Circadian rhythm sleep disorders: pathophysiology and potential approaches to management. CNS Drugs. 2001;15(4):311–28.

10. Armstrong LE. Nutritional strategies for football: counteracting heat, cold, high altitude, and jet lag. J Sports Sci. 2006; 24(7):723–40.

11. Asher G, Sassone-Corsi P. Time for food: the intimate interplay between nutrition, metabolism, and the circadian clock. Cell. 2015;161(1):84–92.

12. Reilly T, Waterhouse J, Edwards B. Jet lag and air travel: implications for performance. Clin Sports Med. 2005;24(2):367–80.

13. Clayton GW, Librik L, Gardner RL, Guillemin R. Studies on the circadian rhythm of pituitary adrenocorticotropic release in man. J Clin Endocrinol Metab.1963;23:975–80.

14. David-Nelson MA, Brodish A. Evidence for a diurnal rhythm of corticotropin-releasing factor (CRF) in the hypothalamus. Endocrinology. 1969;85:861–6.

15. Hardeland R, Pandi-Perumal SR, Cardinali DP. Melatonin. Int J Biochem Cell Biol. 2006;38(3):313–6.

16. Lambert AE, Hoet JJ. Diurnal pattern of plasma insulin concentration in the human. Diabetologia. 1966;2:69–72.

17. Landgraf R, Häcker R, Buhl H. Plasma vasopressin and oxytocin in response to exercise and during a day-night cycle in man. Endokrinologie. 1982;79:281–91.

18. Liddle GW. An analysis of circadian rhythms in human adrenocortical secretory activity. Trans Am Clin Climatol Assoc. 1965;77:151–60.

19. Quay WB. Circadian and estrous rhythms in pineal melatonin and 5-hydroxy indole-3-acetic acid. Proc Soc Exp Biol Med. 1964;115:710–3.

20. Vosko AM, Schroeder A, Loh DH, Colwell CS. Vasoactive intestinal peptide and the mammalian circadian system. Gen Comp Endocrinol. 2007;152(2–3):165–75.

21. Leatherwood WE, Dragoo JL. Effect of airline travel on performance: a review of the literature. Br J Sports Med. 2013; 47:561–7.

22. Manfredini R, Manfredini F, Fersini C, Conconi F. Circadian rhythms, athletic performance, and jet lag. Br J Sports Med. 1998;32:101–6.

23. Angeles-Castellanos M, Amaya JM, Salgado-Delgado R, Buijs RM, Escobar C. Scheduled food hastens re-entrainment more than melatonin does after a 6-h phase advance of the light-dark cycle in rats. J Biol Rhythms. 2011;26(4):324–34.

24. Pivavarova O, Jürchott K, Rudovich N, et al. Changes of dietary fat and carbohydrate content alter central and peripheral clock in humans. J Clin Endocrinol Metab. 2015;100(6): 2291–302.

25. Parker-Simmons S, Andrew K. The traveling athlete. In: Maughan RJ, editor. Sports nutrition. John Wiley & Sons, Ltd.; 2014. p. 415–24.

26. Sports Nutrition Advisory Board-Gatorade. Eating on the road. Gatorade Sports Science Institute; 1996.

27. United States Department of Agriculture, Food Safety and Inspection Service. High Altitude Cooking and Food Safety [Internet]. Accessed 2024 June. Available from: https://www.fsis.usda.gov/food-safety/safe-food-handling-andpreparation/food-safety-basics/high-altitude-cooking

28. Mielcarek J, Kleiner S. Time zone changes. In: Benardot D, editor. Sports nutrition: a guide for the professional working with active people. American Dietetic Association; 1993.

29. Winget CM, DeRoshia CW, Markley CL, Holley DC. A review of human physiology and performance changes associated with desynchronosis of biological rhythms. Aviat Space Environ Med. 1984;55:1085–96.

30. McHill AW, Chinoy ED. Utilizing the National Basketball Association's COVID-19 restart "bubble" to uncover the impact of travel and circadian disruption on athletic performance. Scientific Reports. 2020;10(1):21827.

31. Rossiter A, Warrington GD, Comyns TM. Effects of long-haul travel on recovery and performance in elite athletes: a systematic Review. J Strength Cond Res. 2022;36(11):3234–45.

32. Yamanaka Y, Waterhouse J. Phase-adjustment of human circadian rhythms by light and physical exercise. J Phys Fitness Sports Med. 2016;5(4):287–99.

33. Chennaoui M, Arnal PJ, Sauvet F, Léger D. Sleep and exercise: a reciprocal issue? Sleep Med Rev. 2015;20:59–72.

34. Thun E, Bjorvatn B, Flo E, Harris A, Pallesen S. Sleep, circadian rhythms, and athletic performance. Sleep Med Rev. 2015;23:1–9.

35. Engle-Friedman M. The effects of sleep loss on capacity and effort. Sleep Sci. 2014;7(4):213–24.

36. Martin L, Thompson K. Reproducibility of diurnal variation in sub-maximal swimming. Int J Sports Med. 2000;21:387–92.

37. Souissi N, Gauthier A, Sesboüé B, Larue J, Davenne D. Circadian rhythms in two types of anaerobic cycle leg exercise: force-velocity and 30-s Wingate tests. Int J Sports Med. 2004; 25:114–49.

38. Nicolas A, Gauthier A, Bessot N, Moussay S, Davenne D. Time-of-day effects on myoelectric and mechanical properties of muscle during maximal and prolonged isokinetic exercise. Chronobiol Int. 2005;22:997–1011.

39. Coldwells A, Atkinson G, Reilly T. Sources of variation in back and leg dynamometry. Ergonomics. 1994;37:79–86.

40. Taylor KL, Cronin J, Gill N, Chapman D, Sheppard J. Sources of variability in iso-inertial jump assessments. Int J Sports Physiol Perform. 2010;5:546–58.

41. Lericollais R, Gauthier A, Bessot N, Sesboüé B, Davenne D. Time-of-day effects on fatigue during a sustained anaerobic test in well-trained cyclists. Chronobiol Int. 2009;26(8):1622–35.
42. Souissi N, Bessot N, Chamari K, Gauthier A, Sesboüé B, Davenne D. Effect of time of day on aerobic contribution to the 30-s Wingate test performance. Chronobiol Int. 2007;24:739–48.
43. Sack RL. Clinical practice. Jet lag. N Engl J Med. 2010;362(5):440–7.
44. Loat ER, Rhodes EC. Jet-lag and human performance. Sports Med. 1989;8:226–38.
45. Simmons E, McGrane O, Wedmore I. Jet lag modification. Curr Sports Med Rep. 2015;14(2):123–8.
46. Daly P, Gustafson R. Public health recommendations for athletes attending sporting events. Clin J Sport Med. 2011;21(1):67–70.
47. Stokes S. Italian rider Colo given a reduced ban for Clanbuterol Positive [Internet]. 2010. Accessed 2018 May 16. Available from: http://www.velonation.com/News/ID/5957/Italian-rider-Colo-given-a-reduced-ban-for-Clenbuterol-positive.aspx
48. Schiavone A, Tarantola M, Perona G, Pagliasso S, Badino P, Odore R, Cuniberti B, Lussiana C. Effects of dietary clenbuterol and cimaterol on muscle composition, β-adrenergic and androgen receptor concentrations in broiler chickens. J Anim Physiol Anim Nutr. 2004;88:94–100.
49. ESPN, Inc. Players warned too much meat abroad may lead to positive test [Internet]. 2016. Accessed 2016 December 13. Available from: http://www.espn.com/nfl/story/_/id/15454487/nfl-warns-eating-too-much-meat-mexico-china-result-positive-test
50. Ward MP, Milledge JS, West JB. High altitude medicine. 3rd ed. Arnold; 2000.
51. Hoyt RW, Arnold H. Environmental influences on body fluid balance during exercise: altitude. In: Buskirk ER, Susan MP, editors. Body fluid balance. CRC Press Inc.; 1996:183–96.
52. West JB. High-altitude medicine. Am J Respir Crit Care Med. 2012;186:1229–37.
53. Freund BJ, Sawka MN. Influence of cold stress on human fluid balance. In: Marriott BM, Carlson SJ, editors. Nutritional needs in cold and high altitude environments. National Academy Press; 1996. p. 161–71.
54. Fulco CS, Rock PB, Muza SR, Lammi E, Braun B, Cymerman A, Moore LG, Lewis SF. Gender alters impact of hypobaric hypoxia on adductor pollicis muscle performance. J Appl Physiol. 2001;91(1):100–8.
55. Linthorne NP. The effect of wind on 100-m sprint times. J Appl Biomech. 1994;10(2):110–31.
56. Linthorne NP. Improvement in 100-m sprint performance at an altitude of 2250 m. Sports. 2016;4(2):29.
57. Fulco CS, Rock PB, Cymerman A. Maximal and submaximal exercise performance at altitude. Aviat Space Environ Med. 1998;69:793–801.
58. Pugh LGCE. Oxygen intake in track and treadmill running with observations on the effect of air resistance. J Physiol. 1970;207(3):823–35.
59. Carlson SJ, Marriott BM, editors. Nutritional needs in cold and high-altitude environments: applications for military personnel in field operations. National Academy Press; 1996. 9 p.
60. Viscor G, Corominas J, Carceller A. Nutrition and hydration for high-altitude alpinism: A narrative review. International Journal of Environmental Research and Public Health. 2023;20(4):3186: https://doi.org/10.3390/ijerph20043186
61. Horvath SM. Exercise in a cold environment. Exerc Sport Sci Rev. 1981;9:221–63.
62. Webb P. Temperature of skin, subcutaneous tissue, muscle and core in resting men in cold, comfortable and hot conditions. Eur J Appl Physiol Occup Physiol. 1992;64:471–6.
63. Vallerand AL, Jacobs I. Rates of energy substrates utilization during human cold exposure. Eur J Appl Physiol Occup Physiol. 1989;58:873–8.
64. Young AJ, Muza SR, Sawka MN, Gonzalez RR, Pandolf KB. Human thermoregulatory responses to cold air are altered by repeated cold water immersion. J Appl Physiol. 1986;60:1542–8.
65. Febbraio MA. Exercise in climatic extremes. In: Maughan RJ, editor. Nutrition in sport. Blackwell Science; 2000. 498 p.
66. Young AJ. Effects of aging on human cold tolerance. Exp Aging Res. 1991;17(3):205–13.
67. Mazzeo RS, Reeves JT. Adrenergic contribution during acclimatization to high altitude: perspectives from Pikes Peak. Exerc Sport Sci Rev. 2003;31(1):13–8.
68. Hannon JP, Klain GJ, Sudman DM, Sullivan FJ. Nutritional aspects of high-altitude exposure in women. Am J Clin Nutr. 1976;29(6):604–13.
69. Jefferson JA, Simoni J, Escudero E, Swenson ER, Wesson DE, Schreiner GF, Schoene RB, Johnson RJ, Hurtado A. Increased oxidative stress following acute and chronic high altitude exposure. High Alt Med Biol. 2004;5(1):61–9.
70. Pena E, El Alam S, Siques P, Brito J. Oxitative stress and diseases associated with high-altitude exposure. Antioxidants. 2022;11(267): https://doi.org/10. 3390/antiox11020267
71. Askew EW. Work at high altitude and oxidative stress: antioxidant nutrients. Toxicology. 2002;180(2):107–19. Accessed 2018 June 29. Available from: https://doi.org/10.1016/S0300-483X(02)00385-2
72. Derby R, deWeber K. The athlete and high altitude. Curr Sports Med Rep. 2010;9(2):79–85.
73. Kale RM, Byrd RR. Altitude-related disorders. Medscape (Internet). Updated 2015. Accessed 2018 June 29. Available from: https://emedicine.medscape.com/article/303571-overview
74. Leppk JA, Icenogle MV, Maes D, Riboni K, Hinghofer-Szalkay H, Roach C. Early fluid retention and severe acute mountain sickness. J Appl Physiol. 2005;98(2):591–7.
75. Rodway GW, Hoffman LA, Sanders MH. High-altitude-related disorders–part I: pathophysiology, differential diagnosis, and treatment. Heart Lung. 2003;32(6):353–9.
76. Hackett PH, Roach RC. High altitude cerebral edema. High Alt Med Biol. 2004;5(2):136–46.
77. Savioli G, Ceresa IF, Gori G, Fumoso F, Gri N, Floris V, Varesi A, Martuscelli E, Marchisio S, Longhitano Y, Ricevuti G, Esposito C, Caironi G, Giadini G, Zanza C. Pathophysiology and therapy of high-altitude sickness: practical approach in emergency and critical care. J Clin Med. 2022;11:3937. https://doi.org/10.3390/jcm11143937
78. Talbot TS, Townes DA, Wedmore IS. To air is human: altitude illness during an expedition length adventure race. Wilderness Environ Med. 2004;15(2):90–4.

79. Guilland JC, Klepping J. Nutritional alterations at high altitude in man. Eur J Appl Physiol Occup Physiol. 1985;54(5):517–23.

80. Gallagher SA, Hackett PH. High-altitude illness. Emerg Med Clin North Am. 2004;22(2):329–55.

81. Ri-Li G, Chase PJ, Witkowski S, Wyrick BL, Stone JA, Levine BD, Babb TG. Obesity: associations with acute mountain sickness. Ann Intern Med. 2003;139(4):253–7.

82. Beidleman BA, Muza SR, Fulco CS, Cymerman A, Ditzler D, Stulz D, Staab JE, Skrinar GS, Lewis SF, Sawka MN. Intermittent altitude exposures reduce acute mountain sickness at 4300 m. Clin Sci. 2004;106(3):321–8.

83. Bartsch P, Bailey DM, Berger MM, Knauth M, Baumgartner RW. Acute mountain sickness: controversies and advances. High Alt Med Biol. 2004;5(2):110–24.

84. Dumont L, Lysakowski C, Tramer MR, Junod J-D, Mardirosoff C, Tassonyi E, Kayser B. Magnesium for the prevention and treatment of acute mountain sickness. Clin Sci. 2004; 106(3):269–77.

85. Major C, Doucet E. Energy intake during a typical Himalayan trek. High Alt Med Biol. 2004;5(3):355–63.

86. Rose MS, Houston CS, Fulco CS, Coates G, Sutton JR, Cymerman A. Operation Everest II: nutrition and body composition. J Appl Physiol. 1988;65:2545–51.

87. Butterfield GE. Maintenance of body weight at altitude: in search of 500 kcal/day. In: Marriott BM, Carlson SJ, editors. Nutritional needs in cold and high altitude environments: applications for military personnel in field operations. National Academy Press; 1996. 357 p.

88. Wing-Gaia SL. Nutritional strategies for the preservation of fat free mass at high altitude. Nutrients. 2014;6(2):665–81.

89. Brugarolas J, Lei K, Hurley RL, Manning BD, Reiling JH, Hafen E, Witters LA, Ellisen LW, Kaelin WG Jr. Regulation of mTOR function in response to hypoxia by REDD1 and the TSC1/TSC2 tumor suppressor complex. Genes Dev. 2004; 18:2893–904.

90. Pikosky MA, Smith TJ, Grediagin A, Castaneda-Sceppa C, Byerley L, Glickman EL, Young AJ. Increased protein maintains nitrogen balance during exercise-induced energy deficit. Med Sci Sports Exerc. 2008;40(3):505–12.

91. Reynolds RD, Lickteig JA, Deuster PA, Howard MP, Conway JM, Pietersma A, deStoppelaar J, Deurenberg P. Energy metabolism increases and regional body fat decreases while regional muscle mass is spared in humans climbing Mt. Everest. J Nutr. 1999;129(7):1307–14.

92. Westerterp-Plantenga MS. Effects of extreme environments on food intake in human subjects. Proc Nutr Soc. 1999;58(4): 791–8.

93. Ericsson CD, Steffen R, Basnyat B, Cumbo TA, Edelman R. Infections at high altitude. Clin Infect Dis. 2001;33(11): 1887–91.

94. Reynolds RD, Lickteig JA, Howard MP, Deuster PA. Intakes of high fat and high carbohydrate foods by humans increased with exposure to increasing altitude during an expedition to Mt. Everest. J Nutr. 1998;128(1):50–5.

95. Bateman AP, McArdle F, Walsh TS. Time course of anemia during six months follow up following intensive care discharge and factors associated with impaired recovery of erythropoiesis. Crit Care Med. 2009;37(6):1906–12.

96. Askew EW. Environmental and physical stress and nutrient requirements. Am J Clin Nutr. 1995;61(3):S631–7.

97. Chao WH, Askew EW, Roberts DE, Wood SM, Perkins JB. Oxidative stress in humans during work at moderate altitude. J Nutr. 1999;129(11):2009–12.

98. Gonzalez RR, Kenefick RW, Muza SR, Hamilton SW, Sawka MN. Sweat rate and prediction validation during high-altitude treks on Mount Kilimanjaro. J Appl Physiol. 2013; 114(4):436–43.

99. Murray R. Fluid needs in hot and cold environments. Int J Sport Nutr. 1995;5:S62–73.

100. Cheuvront SN, Kenefick RW, Montain SJ, Sawka MN. Mechanism of aerobic performance impairment with heat stress and dehydration. J Appl Physiol. 2010;109(6):1989–95.

101. Sawka MN, Wenger CB, Pandolf KB. Thermoregulatory responses to acute exercise-heat stress and heat acclimation. In: Blatties CM, Fregly MJ, editors. Handbook of physiology: section 4: environmental physiology. Vol 2. American Physiological Society; 1996. p. 157–185.

102. Cheuvront SN, Ely BR, Wilber RL. Environment and exercise. In: Maughan RJ, editor. Sports nutrition. Wiley Blackwell; 2014. p. 425–38.

103. Buck E, Miles R, Schroeder JD. Exercise-associated hyponatremia. [Updated 2022 Nov 25]. In: StatPearls [Internet]. StatPearls Publishing; 2022. Available from: https://www.ncbi.nlm.nih.gov/books/NBK572128/

104. Klingert M, Nikolaidis PT, Weiss K, Thuany M, Chlibková D, Knechtle B. Exercise-associated hyponatremia in marathon runners. J Clin Med. 2022;11:6755.

105. Ely MR, Cheuvront SN, Roberts WO, Montain SJ. Impact of weather on marathon-running performance. Med Sci Sports Exerc. 2007;39(3):489–93.

106. Galloway SD, Maughan RJ. Effects of ambient temperature on the capacity to perform prolonged cycle exercise in man. Med Sci Sports Exerc. 1997;29(9):1240–9.

107. Özgünen KT, Kurdak SS, Maughan RJ, Zeren C, Korkmaz S, Yazici Z, Ersöz G, Shirreffs SM, Binnet MS, Dvorak J. Effect of hot environmental conditions on physical activity patterns and temperature response of football players. Scand J Med Sci Sports. 2010;20(Suppl 3):140–7.

108. Racinais S, Périard JD, Karlsen A, Nybo L. Effect of heat and heat acclimatization on cycling time trial performance and pacing. Med Sci Sports Exerc. 2015;47(3):601–6.

109. Karlsen A, Racinais S, Jensen MV, Nørgaard SJ, Bonne T, Nybo L. Heat acclimatization does not improve VO$_{2max}$ or cycling performance in a cool climate in trained cyclists. Scand J Med Sci Sports. 2015;25(S1):269–76.

110. Ely MR, Martin DE, Cheuvront SN, Montain SJ. Effect of ambient temperature on marathon pacing is dependent on runner ability. Med Sci Sports Exerc. 2008;40(9):1679–80.

Dietary Supplements, Foods, and Ergogenic Aids Intended to Improve Performance: Myths and Realities

CHAPTER OBJECTIVES

- Explain the general problems associated with excess consumption of nutrients related to competitive absorption, cellular utilization, and excretion.
- Know the potential ergogenic benefits of caffeine and the optimal consumption strategies to achieve these benefits.
- List the potential dangers associated with consumption of ergogenic aids that target athletes.
- Understand how to find listings of banned substances for athletes competing in sanctioned events.
- Know the difference between nutritional and non-nutritional ergogenic aids.
- Describe the interaction effects between taking a nutrient supplement and the activity (mechanical loading) required to achieve a benefit that incorporates the consumed nutrient.
- Discuss the reasons why achieving a normal vitamin D status is important for optimizing performance.
- Understand how gut health is an integral and important component of maintaining health and athletic performance, and how prebiotics, probiotics, and synbiotics may help to achieve a healthy microbiome.
- List the possible ways that a misappropriation of perceived benefit may result from taking common protein-related supplements, including whey protein, branched-chain amino acids (BCAAs), β-alanine, and creatine.

Case Study

John was always at the cutting edge of everything having to do with the athletic endeavor. He had the latest shoes, wore water-releasing shirts to enhance sweat evaporation and cooling, and scoured athlete magazines for anything new that could improve his cycling performance. One day he read that a half-liter of beet juice consumed about an hour or two prior to exercise could significantly improve exercise time to fatigue. Perfect—he had been worried about taking supplements because there are problems that are periodically written about in the press, but this was FOOD. Beet juice! What could be better than that? He immediately went to his local grocery store and purchased his first case of organic beet juice in quart bottles.

The next day, about 2 hours before his exercise bout, he chugged down a half-liter of beet juice, and he could not wait to see the improvement. Nothing changed. He reached his fatigue point within 30 seconds of his usual time—but no matter, he had a whole case of beet juice and he was not about to give up. So, for the next 4 days, he followed the same procedure, but also with no improvement. He thought perhaps it was because he was already an elite cyclist that it would take more beet juice to make a discernible difference in performance, so he increased the volume by 100% and drank an entire liter before practice. He was convinced that this was his "magic bullet" to help differentiate him from his fellow cyclists. This continued for a month, with several cases of beet juice being consumed in ever-increasing quantity and frequency, but to no avail. There was simply no improvement in performance. He was not only not doing better, but also his muscles

(continued)

were getting more sore and he definitely felt weaker than before.

Finally, he decided to do what he should have done at the start and sat down for a conversation with his cycling club's sports dietitian. It took about 30 seconds for the dietitian to figure out the problems by just asking a few questions. The dietitian asked, "Do you use antibiotic mouthwash?" "Why yes, every day!" said John. The dietitian responded, "Well, that's why the beet juice is not working. The bacteria in your mouth that convert dietary nitrate to nitrite are not there because you have wiped out the bacteria with the mouthwash, so the conversion does not occur and there is *no benefit*." The dietitian pointed out that, to make matters worse, the high volume of beet juice that was being consumed was taking away from all the other foods that John should have been eating, so the right mix of nutrients was no longer present to enhance muscle recovery and reduce muscle soreness. John was stunned at his compounded mistakes, but he decided not to persevere. He gave up the antibacterial mouthwash for 1 month, started drinking half a quart of beet juice before practice, and his performance started to improve. Getting things right, he thought afterward, may be more complicated than just drinking some beet juice.

CASE STUDY DISCUSSION QUESTIONS

1. What would be the best strategy for consuming beet juice to improve exercise performance?
2. If a half-liter of beet juice is being consumed prior to exercise, are there any nutritional concerns that might arise by substituting beet juice for something else that may also be good to consume prior to exercise?
3. In this case study, overconsumption of beet juice may have created a nutritional imbalance by substituting beet juice for other important foods. Humans require a balance of needed nutrients and foods to help sustain the immune system, ensure normal metabolism, and maintain optimal production of hormones and enzymes. What kind of foods and beverages should this athlete be consuming throughout the day to help ensure good health?

INTRODUCTION

Competitive athletes are often interested in finding ways to be quicker and stronger with improved endurance. Since the time of the ancient Olympic Games, athletes have tried new training regimens and focused on consuming different foods and beverages with different intake patterns to improve performance (Table 13.1). The food patterns have evolved from focusing on cheese and vegetables to focusing on meat and fat, all with an eye toward improving performance more quickly. In more recent times, with our enhanced understanding of the human metabolic system and the chemicals we refer to as vitamins and minerals, athletes are increasingly turning to the use of these nutrients in a purified form rather than relying on obtaining them from foods. In addition, the improved understanding of metabolic pathways has enabled the creation of substances that can stimulate specific desired pathways to obtain the desired outcome.

Interestingly, the more that is known about what truly works to improve performance, the more scientists and practitioners are learning that there is no good substitute for regular consumption of a good distribution of health-promoting foods and beverages at the right time and in the right amounts to optimize performance. What also has been found is that many of the products advertised as *performance enhancing* (*i.e.*, ergogenic aids) have problems, either because they contain banned substances that are not on the label or because they expose tissues to excess nutrients in a single dose. We are increasingly learning that, for optimal nutrition, *more than enough is not better than enough*. As an example, a recent study found that long-term multivitamin use fails to prevent major cardiovascular disease events in men, regardless of baseline nutritional status (1), and a study assessing dietary supplement use in older women found a higher mortality rate in those taking multivitamin, vitamin B_6, folic acid, iron, zinc, or copper supplements (2). This is an important consideration before recommending high-dose vitamin supplements or ergogenic aids to athletes. It is also important to consider that a "food-first" approach is recommended by professional organizations that focus on athlete health, including the Academy of Nutrition and Dietetics, Dietitians of Canada, The National Athletic Trainers Association, and the American College of Sports Medicine (3,4).

Table 13.1	Historical Evolution of Sports Nutrition
Diogenes Laertius (died AD 222)	Wrote that Greek athletes trained originally on dried figs, moist fresh cheese, and wheat. The pattern then changed to focus on meat.
Epictetus (2nd century AD)	Wrote that Olympic champions avoided desserts and cold water and consumed wine sparingly.
Philostratus (born 170 AD)	Spoke badly about the athletic diet during his era, which was based on white bread sprinkled with poppy seeds and fish and pork.
Greek and Roman Gladiators (105 BCE to 404 CE)	Used certain wines, herbal teas, and mushrooms to enhance performance.
Americans at Berlin Olympic Games (1936)	Consumed beefsteak with an average daily intake of 125 g of butter (1,125 kcal!), three eggs, custard for dessert, and 1.5 L of milk, with ad libitum intake of breads, fresh vegetables, and salads.
Atlanta Olympic Games (1996)	Highly varied menu served at the athlete cafeteria that included fresh vegetables and dips, fruits, cheeses, breads, salads, pasta, rice, fruits, soups, meats and seafoods, cooked vegetables, desserts, and beverages.

Sources: Grivetti LE, Applegate EA. From Olympia to Atlanta: a cultural–historical perspective on diet and athletic training. J Nutr. 1997; 127(5S):860S–8S; Momaya A, Fawal M, Estes R. Performance-enhancing substances in sports: a review of the literature. Sports Med. 2015; 45(4):517–31.

NUTRITIONAL SUPPLEMENTS

The **Dietary Supplement Health and Education Act (DSHEA)** of 1994 of the United States defines a **dietary supplement** as a food product that is in addition to the total diet (5). The DSHEA clarifies that a dietary supplement cannot be represented as a conventional food or as the sole item of a meal or diet and should not be viewed as a partial or complete meal replacement. According to the DSHEA, a dietary supplement must contain at least one of the following:

- Vitamin
- Mineral
- Herb or other botanical substance
- Amino acid
- A substance that supplements the diet by serving to increase the total dietary intake
- Metabolite
- Concentrate
- Constituent
- Extract
- Combinations of any of the above ingredients

The DSHEA definition was not found to be satisfactory when applied to athletes as it does not clarify whether it is in addition to a "healthy" diet and has resulted in the following definition (6):

A food, food component, nutrient, or nonfood compound that is purposefully ingested in addition to the habitually consumed diet with the aim of achieving a specific health and/or performance benefit.

Dietary supplements may come in a number of forms, including nutrient-enriched foods (*e.g.,* in the United States, grains are enriched with folic acid); formulated foods that are intended to make it easy for athletes to consume before, during, or after exercise (*e.g.,* gels, sports bars, electrolyte/carbohydrate drinks); single nutrients consumed as a pill/capsule that are consumed in addition to foods; and combinations of these (6).

Dietary Supplement

Also referred to as a nutrient supplement, this is a high concentration of nutrients provided as a pill, capsule, or powder that is consumed orally (not put on skin, etc.) that provides high doses of vitamins, minerals, or related ingredients (*i.e.,* phytonutrients, metabolites, extracts). The Food and Drug Administration (FDA) defines dietary supplements as "products which are not pharmaceutical drugs, food additives like spices or preservatives, or conventional food."

Dietary Supplement Health and Education Act

This U.S. federal legislation of 1994 defines and regulates dietary supplements. Under this legislation, supplements are regulated by the FDA for "good manufacturing practices."

Under the DSHEA legislation, each manufacturer of a dietary supplement is responsible for the safety of the product (*i.e.*, no governmental oversight), but the dietary supplement manufacturer is not responsible for performing product safety testing, and it is not responsible for confirming/proving that the dietary supplement actually performs in a way that is consistent with claims made about the product. Therefore, although dietary supplements targeting athletes are often marketed as improving both health and performance, there is often little proof that this is the case. Although they may, and often do, contain essential vitamins, minerals, and amino acids, they may also contain other substances that are not essential nutrients such as *yohimbe*, *ma huang*, *ginkgo*, and other herb-based substances.

The purpose of drugs is to cure, treat, or prevent disease, and they must undergo intensive testing to determine optimal dosing, effectiveness, drug–drug and drug–nutrient/food interactions, and safety for FDA approval before a drug can be made available to the public. Dietary supplements, however, are not required to undergo any of these testing protocols before entering the marketplace. The general procedure, if a new ingredient is proposed to be added to a dietary supplement, is for the product manufacturer to gather relevant information on the ingredient to make a determination on safety and effectiveness and submit that determination to the FDA 75 days before the dietary supplement is made available to the public. Following this 75-day period, the new ingredient in the dietary supplement can be made available for public consumption if there is no FDA intervention to do so.

Ergogenic aids are those substances and/or activities that are performance enhancing (*i.e.*, create an **ergogenic effect**) and may take many forms, including physiologic aids, psychological aids, biomechanical aids, pharmacologic aids, and nutritional aids. Ergogenic aids are substances that have ergogenic effects (*i.e.*, are performance enhancing) and are, therefore, **ergolytic**:

- *Physiologic ergogenic aid:* An activity, typically provided by an athletic trainer or strength and conditioning coach, that improves the body's physiology (*i.e.*, more muscle for a bodybuilder) that has the effect of improving athletic performance.
- *Psychological ergogenic aid:* A strategy, typically provided by a sports psychologist, that improves the athlete's mental state (*i.e.*, relaxation technique) and has the effect of improving athletic performance.
- *Biomechanical ergogenic aid:* Any equipment or worn device (*i.e.*, muscle wraps, streamlined swimsuits) that has the effect of improving athletic performance.

- *Pharmacologic ergogenic aid:* A substance that has a drug or hormonal effect (*i.e.*, caffeine, anabolic steroids) and has the effect of improving athletic performance through enhanced musculature, blood flow, oxygen delivery, or other effect.
- *Nutritional ergogenic aid:* A supplement, food, or beverage that, when consumed at specific times and amounts (*i.e.*, vitamin D, beet juice, sports drinks, creatine), has the effect of enhancing athletic performance through improved endurance and/or power or muscle recovery.

Ergogenic Aid

A substance/strategy/technique that is used for the purpose of improving/enhancing athletic performance. The nutritional ergogenic aids are substances and nutrients that are food-derived (*e.g.*, beet juice), which can positively influence metabolism and muscle function, to improve performance. Other ergogenic aids are in the realm of pharmacologic aids (*i.e.*, drugs), physiologic aids (*i.e.*, exercise equipment), or psychological aids (*i.e.*, strategies to improve focus, attention span).

Ergogenic Effect

A performance-enhancing effect is observed through the consumption of an ergogenic aid or through a positive performance enhancement observed as a result of an exercise and/or nutritional protocol. (It is possible to achieve an ergogenic effect without consumption of a specific ergogenic substance.)

Ergolytic

Any substance or activity that can impair/reduce athletic performance. For instance, consumption of a substance that interferes with energy metabolism would be considered ergolytic, as would overtraining, which may also have a negative impact on performance.

The focus of this chapter is *nutritional ergogenic aids consumed in the form of dietary supplements* that are taken in addition to the normal and usual dietary intake of foods and fluids. As explained earlier, an ergogenic aid refers to a nutrient or related substance that is *performance enhancing*, but this term is often loosely used, as claims of performance enhancement are frequently made without evidence. The term *nutritional ergogenic aid* describes a substance that enters a known nutritional metabolic pathway, or consists of one or more nutrient. As an example, consumption of carbohydrates at the right time is known to improve performance, logically making carbohydrate a nutritional ergogenic aid. Creatine is a known component of food that enters a known metabolic

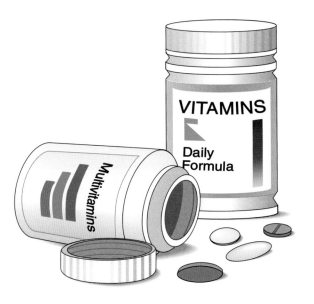
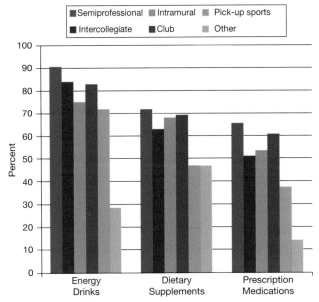

FIGURE 13.1: Prevalence of supplement use in the United States. (Part **A** from LifeART image copyright 2018. Lippincott Williams & Wilkins. All rights reserved. Part **B** reprinted by permission from Hoyte CO, Albert D, Heard KJ. The use of energy drinks, dietary supplements, and prescription medications by United States college students to enhance athletic performance. J Community Health. 2013;38:575–80.)

pathway and may improve sprint performance, so it could also be considered a nutritional ergogenic aid. Nonnutritional ergogenic aids, such as anabolic steroids, refer to products that have no food origin, are not nutrients, and have no known nutritional properties.

Although claims that supplements have ergogenic properties can be made in the United States without evidence or verification by the FDA (7), the relatively new Office of Dietary Supplements of the National Institutes of Health (NIH) has excellent fact sheets on supplement effectiveness and usage recommendations (Figure 13.1). This NIH office can be accessed at https://ods.od.nih.gov/. Table 13.2 contains a sample of a fact sheet provided by the Office of Dietary Supplements on supplements advertised as enabling weight loss.

Why Do Athletes Take Supplements?

There are multiple factors that differentiate athlete supplement use both by frequency and by magnitude of intake. There are differences in intake by sport, level of training, age (greater with higher age), sex (higher in men), and perceptions of what is "normal" for the sport (6,8). There are also a number of reasons why athletes take nutrient-based and other supplements, including (6):

■ To influence potential or current nutritional deficiency that could have an impact on athletic performance and/or health.

■ For the convenient consumption of nutrients and energy before, during, and after an exercise bout when the consumption of regular foods and beverages is not possible or less convenient.

■ To attain a performance enhancement, through improved training, improvement in body composition, lower muscle soreness and improved recovery, and/or lower injury/illness risk.

■ To derive financial benefit from sponsoring a product or because the consumed products are freely available.

■ To follow the supplement usage behavior of other athletes whom they admire.

■ To take steps that they believe will result in developing a lower risk of a nutrient deficiency.

Athletes are competitors who want to win. It is logical, therefore, that athletes will do what they believe will legally give them a winning edge. They train to improve physiologic adaptation to the sport, and they want to do the right things nutritionally to maximize the training benefit and diminish the potential negative side effects of training, such as muscle soreness. The marketing efforts that target supplement use in athletes emphasize that these supplements can provide precisely the things that the athlete desires: better health, more speed, more power, better endurance, bigger muscles, and a greater chance to win (9,10). However, there is a potential cost to taking some supplements, as they may contain prohibited substances that are not included on the label and may

Table 13.2	Common Ingredients in Weight-Loss Dietary Supplements		
Ingredient	**Proposed Mechanism of Action**	**Evidence of Efficacy**	**Evidence of Safety+**
Bitter orange (synephrine)	Increases energy expenditure and lipolysis, acts as a mild appetite suppressant	Small clinical trials of poor methodologic quality *Research findings:* Possible effect on resting metabolic rate and energy expenditure; inconclusive effects on weight loss	Some safety concerns reported *Reported adverse effects*: Chest pain, anxiety, and increased blood pressure and heart rate
Caffeine (as added caffeine or from guarana, kola nut, yerba mate, or other herbs)	Stimulates central nervous system, increases thermogenesis and fat oxidation	Short-term clinical trials of combination products *Research findings:* Possible modest effect on body weight or decreased weight gain over time	Safety concerns not usually reported at doses less than 400 mg/day for adults, significant safety concerns at higher doses *Reported adverse effects:* Nervousness, jitteriness, vomiting, and tachycardia
Calcium	Increases lipolysis and fat accumulation, decreases fat absorption	Several large clinical trials *Research findings:* No effect on body weight, weight loss, or prevention of weight gain based on clinical trials	No safety concerns reported at recommended intakes (1,000–1,200 mg/day for adults) *Reported adverse effects:* Constipation, kidney stones, and interference with zinc and iron absorption at intakes above 2,000–2,500 mg for adults
Chitosan	Binds dietary fat in the digestive tract	Small clinical trials, mostly of poor methodologic quality *Research findings:* Minimal effect on body weight	Few safety concerns reported, could cause allergic reactions *Reported adverse effects:* Flatulence, bloating, constipation, indigestion, nausea, and heartburn
Chromium	Increases lean muscle mass; promotes fat loss; and reduces food intake, hunger levels, and fat cravings	Several clinical trials of varying methodologic quality *Research findings:* Minimal effect on body weight and body fat	No safety concerns reported at recommended intakes (25–45 mcg/day for adults) *Reported adverse effects:* Headache, watery stools, constipation, weakness, vertigo, nausea, vomiting, and urticaria (hives)
Coleus forskohlii (forskolin)	Enhances lipolysis and reduces appetite	Few short-term clinical trials *Research findings:* No effect on body weight	No safety concerns reported *Reported adverse effects*: None known
Conjugated linoleic acid	Promotes apoptosis in adipose tissue	Several clinical trials *Research findings:* Minimal effect on body weight and body fat	Few safety concerns reported *Reported adverse effects*: Abdominal discomfort and pain, constipation, diarrhea, loose stools, dyspepsia, and (possibly) adverse effects on blood lipid profiles

Table 13.2	Common Ingredients in Weight-Loss Dietary Supplements (Continued)		
Ingredient	**Proposed Mechanism of Action**	**Evidence of Efficacy**	**Evidence of Safety+**
Ephedra (ma huang, ephedrine)	Stimulates central nervous system, increases thermogenesis, reduces appetite	Several short-term clinical trials of good methodologic quality, many of ephedra combined with caffeine *Research findings*: Modest effect on short-term weight loss	Significant safety concerns reported; banned as a dietary supplement ingredient *Reported adverse effects:* Anxiety, mood changes, nausea, vomiting, hypertension, palpitation, stroke, seizures, heart attack, and death
Fucoxanthin	Increases energy expenditure and fatty acid oxidation, suppresses adipocyte differentiation and lipid accumulation	Studied only in combination with pomegranate-seed oil in one trial in humans *Research findings*: Insufficient research to draw firm conclusions	No safety concerns reported but not rigorously studied *Reported adverse effects*: None known
Garcinia cambogia (hydroxycitric acid)	Inhibits lipogenesis, suppresses food intake	Several short-term clinical trials of varying methodologic quality *Research findings*: Little to no effect on body weight	Few safety concerns reported *Reported adverse effects*: Headache, nausea, upper respiratory tract symptoms, and gastrointestinal symptoms
Glucomannan	Increases feelings of satiety and fullness, prolongs gastric emptying time	Several clinical trials of varying methodologic quality, mostly focused on effects on lipid and blood glucose levels *Research findings:* Little to no effect on body weight	Significant safety concerns reported with tablet forms, which might cause esophageal obstructions, but few safety concerns with other forms *Reported adverse effects:* Loose stools, flatulence, diarrhea, constipation, and abdominal discomfort
Green coffee bean extract (*Coffea arabica, Coffea canephora, Coffea robusta*)	Inhibits fat accumulation, modulates glucose metabolism	Few clinical trials, all of poor methodologic quality *Research findings:* Possible modest effect on body weight	Few safety concerns reported but not rigorously studied; contains caffeine *Reported adverse effects:* Headache and urinary tract infections
Green tea (*Camellia sinensis*) and green tea extract	Increases energy expenditure and fat oxidation, reduces lipogenesis and fat absorption	Several clinical trials of good methodologic quality on green tea catechins with and without caffeine *Research findings:* Possible modest effect on body weight	No safety concerns reported when used as a beverage, contains caffeine; some safety concerns reported for green tea extract *Reported adverse effects (for green tea extract):* Constipation, abdominal discomfort, nausea, increased blood pressure, liver damage
Guar gum	Acts as bulking agent in gut, delays gastric emptying, increases feelings of satiety	Several clinical trials of good methodologic quality *Research findings:* No effect on body weight	Few safety concerns reported with currently available formulations *Reported adverse effects*: Abdominal pain, flatulence, diarrhea, nausea, and cramps

(continued)

Table 13.2	Common Ingredients in Weight-Loss Dietary Supplements (Continued)		
Ingredient	Proposed Mechanism of Action	Evidence of Efficacy	Evidence of Safety+
Hoodia (*Hoodia gordonii*)	Suppresses appetite, reduces food intake	Very little published research on humans *Research findings*: No effect on energy intake or body weight based on results from one study	Some safety concerns reported; increases heart rate and blood pressure *Reported adverse effects*: Headache, dizziness, nausea, and vomiting
Pyruvate	Increases lipolysis and energy expenditure	Few clinical trials of weak methodologic quality *Research findings*: Possible minimal effect on body weight and body fat	Few safety concerns reported *Reported adverse effects*: Diarrhea, gas, bloating, and (possibly) decreased high-density lipoprotein levels
Raspberry ketone	Alters lipid metabolism	Studied only in combination with other ingredients *Research findings*: Insufficient research to draw firm conclusions	No safety concerns reported but not rigorously studied *Reported adverse effects*: None known
White kidney bean (*Phaseolus vulgaris*)	Interferes with breakdown and absorption of carbohydrates by acting as a "starch blocker"	Several clinical trials of varying methodologic quality *Research findings*: Possible modest effect on body weight and body fat	Few safety concerns reported *Reported adverse effects*: Headache, soft stools, flatulence, and constipation
Yohimbe (*Pausinystalia yohimbe*)	Has hyperadrenergic effects	Very little research on yohimbe for weight loss *Research findings*: No effect on body weight; insufficient research to draw firm conclusions	Significant safety concerns reported *Reported adverse effects*: Headache, anxiety, agitation, hypertension, and tachycardia

Source: United States Department of Health and Human Services, National Institutes of Health, Office of Dietary Supplements. 2017. Accessed 2018 May 17. Available from: https://ods.od.nih.gov/factsheets/WeightLoss-HealthProfessional

result in a positive doping result (8,11). There should be a decision-making procedure for determining whether an athlete should take a supplement (11):

- Athlete Evaluation
  - The athlete wishes to take a supplement.
  - What is the expected effect of taking the supplement?
  - What are the motivational reasons for taking the supplement?
- Professional Evaluation
  - The athlete should be screened to determine if nutrient deficiencies or other medical issues are present.

- Would a supplement be appropriate given the athlete's condition?
- Are there other nutritional issues that would not be addressed with the supplement being evaluated?
- Product Evaluation
  - Is there a science-based rationale for using the supplement?
  - Were the protocols used for assessing the supplement science and evidence-based?
  - Are there any potential acute or long-term side effects from taking the supplement?

- Risk Evaluation
  - Has the supplement been tested by an independent laboratory to determine if there are any substances present that are on the World Antidoping Agency (WADA) banned substance list? There are now multiple reports of supplement contamination with substances that are prohibited (12).
- Practical and General Evaluation
  - Is there an established protocol for taking the supplement (*i.e.*, daily, morning, prior to exercise, etc.) to optimize the performance effect
  - Are there any unwanted effects, such as interfering with the absorption of other nutrients, or delaying gastric emptying?

A review of multiple studies assessing dietary supplement intake in athletes found that elite athletes were far more likely than nonelite athletes to take dietary supplements (10) (Figure 13.1). It was found that the prevalence of use in men and women was similar, but that a greater proportion of women took iron, whereas a greater proportion of men took protein, creatine, and vitamin E (10). There is also evidence that greater than 25% of preadolescent runners regularly use supplements, with athletes who restrict food intake and those with bone injuries more likely to take supplements (13). It was found in this preadolescent group that female runners had higher intakes of supplements (particularly multivitamins/minerals, calcium, vitamin D, iron, and probiotics), while male runners took creatine and consumed sports foods more often. It was recommended that this group of athletes should satisfy their energy needs from nutrient-rich foods and should only take supplements after a consultation with a registered dietitian/nutritionist. A study of adults seeking to improve fitness, including those who compete and those who do not, found that over 85% took supplements with no difference between those involved in competitions and those who were not (14). The common reasons that athletes take dietary supplements include (10,15):

- The supplement has a direct beneficial effect on exercise performance.
- The supplement will help the athlete recover from exercise.
- To help maintain health, as compensation for a diet that is believed to be inadequate in fulfilling the needs of an athlete.
- To satisfy what is believed to be heavy nutrient demands that are created by regular training.
- Because an admired and successful athlete is taking them, and at least a portion of the athlete's success is *believed to be* based on the consumption of the dietary supplement(s)

There is also evidence that supplement use in athletes (11):

- Varies across different sports and activities
- Increases with the level of training/performance
- Increases with age
- Is higher in men than in women
- Is strongly influenced by perceived cultural norms (both sporting and nonsporting)

Do Dietary Supplements Help?

Several reviews have suggested that performance is not improved with the intake of vitamin supplements/ergogenic aids in athletes who consume a balanced diet providing sufficient energy, but there may be some circumstances that warrant dietary supplement intake if consumption of a balanced diet is not possible (16–20):

- Pregnant and lactating women have higher requirements for many nutrients, including iron and folic acid (see recommended dietary allowance [RDA] table), so are at higher risk for deficiency. The need for folic acid in women of childbearing age is now well established to lower the risk of having a baby with a neural tube defect (*e.g.*, spina bifida or anencephaly). To minimize this risk, the United States has instituted a program for fortifying cereal grains with folic acid (21).
- Athletes appear to be at higher risk of iron deficiency than nonathletes as a result of foot-strike hemolysis, iron sweat loss, and increased iron losses in urine and feces (see Chapter 6). Therefore, athletes may require iron intakes greater than the RDA. For athletes with iron deficiency or iron deficiency anemia, as measured by serum ferritin, hemoglobin, and hematocrit, supplemental intake of iron may be required. However, oral supplements of iron should not be taken without the presence of deficiency, and supplements should only be taken with the direct supervision of a health professional (6).
- Approximately 10%–30% of older adults experience lower gastric production of intrinsic factor, which is necessary for the absorption of B_{12}. The Institute of Medicine recommends consumption of sublingual vitamin B_{12} supplements for anyone over the age of 50 to lower the risk of B_{12} deficiency and associated megaloblastic anemia (22).
- Vegans (*i.e.*, those who consume no meat, fish, or dairy products) are at greater risk than omnivores and lacto-ovo vegetarians for developing vitamin B_{12} deficiency because animal foods are the natural source of

vitamin B_{12}. While a limited number of foods, such as fermented beans (*e.g.*, tempe, natto, douche, tofu, etc.) contain vitamin B_{12}, vitamin supplementation with vitamin B_{12} and/or consumption of breakfast cereals fortified with vitamin B_{12} can lower the risk of developing a deficiency in vegans (22,23).

■ Consumption of antibiotics may diminish intestinal bacteria and lower the bacterial production of vitamin K, which is necessary for normal blood clotting and bone health. Supplemental intake of vitamin K and the consumption of probiotics to help return the gut microbiome to a normal state may diminish the risk of deficiency (24,25).

■ People who are lactose intolerant and avoid dairy products as a result of this condition may be at risk for vitamin B_2 (riboflavin), vitamin D, and calcium deficiency. As a result, they may benefit from the consumption of supplements containing these nutrients (26,27).

■ Because of a high variability in calcium absorption and calcium loss via urine and feces, assessment of bone mineral density may be the only effective means of determining the adequacy of long-term calcium consumption. Athletes should have daily intakes of calcium that are ~1,500 mg/day from a combination of foods and supplements (if necessary to achieve this level of intake), with good vitamin D status to ensure normal calcium absorption (see Chapter 6). Poor bone density that predisposes an athlete to fracture is a complex nutritional issue, involving maintenance of good energy balance, adequate calcium intake, and adequate vitamin D status (6).

Dietary Supplement Intake in Athletes

There are clearly multiple nutrients that are related to exercise performance, both directly and indirectly (Table 13.3). Ideally, these nutrients would be best provided through the consumption of a balanced diet, but it is clear that many athletes now consume supplements with the hope of positively influencing athletic performance. There are clear benefits of supplement use if dietary modification to correct a nutrient deficiency is not possible, and if there is a specific supplement effect that may improve training and/or competition (12). It has been found that a high proportion of elite adolescent athletes consume dietary supplements daily, with some of these athletes *required* to consume dietary supplements by their sporting organizations. Supplements commonly consumed in this elite adolescent athlete population include creatine, protein, and magnesium, with the *belief* that these supplements are needed to improve performance, that failure to take them may be harmful to health or that failure to take supplements will result in illness (28). A study of Canadian athletes found that 87% of assessed athletes (N = 440, including 63% women and 37% men) took at least three dietary supplements over the previous 6 months, including sports drinks, multivitamin and mineral supplements, high-carbohydrate sports bars, protein powder, and meal replacement products (29).

The general reasons athletes take supplements and recommendations for taking them include the following (4,17,26,30):

■ There is little evidence to suggest that it is common for physically active individuals to suffer from inadequate dietary intakes of vitamins and minerals. Athletes at highest risk are those with restricted intakes (*i.e.*, vegetarian athletes and athletes on calorie-restricted diets).

■ Some physically active people/athletes, including ballet dancers, gymnasts, long-distance runners, and wrestlers, may have inadequate exposure to vitamins and minerals because they limit energy consumption in an attempt to meet sport-specific weight requirements or to satisfy aesthetic requirements of the sport/activity.

■ Physically active people should consume a wide variety of foods to optimize exposure to vitamins, minerals, and phytonutrients to eliminate the requirement for dietary supplements.

■ Only people with a biologically confirmed nutrient deficiency are likely to benefit from the consumption of the deficient nutrient through dietary supplements.

■ Athletes with questions about the adequacy of their diet should meet with an appropriately credentialed licensed/registered dietitian to help determine how well nutrient needs are satisfied, rather than self-prescribe dietary supplements.

■ To reduce fat mass and boost muscle building, with many supplements sold promising to help athletes achieve these goals.

■ To increase energy stores, particularly glycogen, for which we have limited stores and which is needed for high-intensity activity.

■ To support the immune system. Many supplements (particularly vitamins, polyphenols, echinacea) are sold with this promise.

■ To improve bone health, which is far more complex than simply taking calcium and/or vitamin D supplements.

Table 13.3	Vitamins and Minerals: Exercise Relationships	
Nutrient	**Major Function**	**Deficiency**
Thiamin (vitamin B_1)	Metabolism of carbohydrates and amino acids	Weakness, poor endurance, muscle loss, weight loss
Riboflavin (vitamin B_2)	Oxidative energy metabolism, electron transport in adenosine triphosphate (ATP) production	Weakness, photophobia, altered nervous system function, altered skin and mucous membranes (cheilosis, angular stomatitis, inflamed nasolabial folds, swollen tongue)
Niacin (vitamin B_3)	Oxidative energy metabolism, electron transport in ATP production	Irritability, diarrhea, dermatitis
Pyridoxine/pyridoxal/pyridoxamine (vitamin B_6)	Gluconeogenesis, protein metabolism (deamination and transamination reactions)	Dermatitis, swollen tongue, convulsions
Cyanocobalamin (vitamin B_{12})	Formation of red blood cells/hemoglobin	Macrocytic anemia, neurologic symptoms
Folic acid	Formation of red blood cells/hemoglobin, formation of nucleic acids	Macrocytic anemia, early fatigue
Ascorbic acid (vitamin C)	Antioxidant, protein (connective tissue collagen) synthesis, improve iron absorption	Poor appetite (potentially resulting in other micronutrient deficiencies), early fatigue, poor wound healing
Retinol (vitamin A)	Antioxidant, maintains disease resistance, vision	Loss of appetite, poor immunity, eye problems
α-Tocopherol (vitamin E)	Antioxidant	Nerve and muscle damage
Chromium	Glucose metabolism (insulin sensitivity)	Glucose intolerance, poor blood glucose control, early fatigue
Iron	Hemoglobin synthesis, oxygen delivery to tissues	Anemia, poor concentration, poor immune system, early fatigue
Magnesium	Energy metabolism, nerve conduction, muscle contraction	Muscle weakness and cramping, nausea, irritability
Zinc	Immune system health, glycolysis, nucleic acid synthesis, carbohydrate metabolism, sense of smell and taste	Poor immunity, poor appetite (potentially resulting in other micronutrient deficiencies), skin rashes, diarrhea

More information on these vitamins and minerals can be found in Chapters 5 and 6.
Source: Lukaski H. Vitamin and mineral status: effects on physical performance. Nutrition. 2004;20:632–44.

POTENTIAL RISKS OF DIETARY SUPPLEMENTS AND ERGOGENIC AIDS

Some products sold as ergogenic aids often have an unknown origin (the substances in the package are not clearly indicated), contain no known nutrient, and have no substance that is known to enter a nutritional pathway. To make matters even more confusing, several studies evaluating the composition of ergogenic aids that have marketing programs targeting athletes have found that a large proportion of the products have significantly less of the active ingredient than advertised (31). Potentially dangerous and career damaging is the finding in several studies that a number of ergogenic aids targeting athletes contain banned substances not listed on the label (32). This may also be the cause of a certain amount of misattribution related to the product. The athlete believes he or she is simply taking a certain proprietary mix of vitamins and finds that, incredibly, his or her muscle mass starts to enlarge. The athlete attributes this change to the vitamin mix, when it may actually be due to the *anabolic steroid* that the athlete unknowingly has been taking with the vitamin mix. Current doping rules are clear: The athlete is responsible for what he or she consumes, and should the athlete compete in a sanctioned event and have a positive urine test for a banned substance, that athlete cannot claim ignorance that what he or she was consuming contained a banned substance (33). Given that between 40% and 70% of athletes use supplements, with 10%–15% of supplements containing banned substances, this should be a real concern for athletes (34). This concern is made worse by the relative absence of regulation and enforcement of issues that would help to ensure athletes and the public that dietary supplements are safe to consume (35).

Athletes should be concerned with excessive supplement use and the potentially adverse reactions from high doses of different supplements. Although consistent adverse reactions to taking dietary supplements have not been documented (36), the widespread use of dietary supplements by elite athletes, with no apparent health or performance benefits, suggests a need for educational programs focused on dietary supplement use in athletes (37). The amount, quantity, and combinations of dietary supplements used by athletes have raised a concern about the potential risk of side effects (37).

It is difficult to discern whether certain consumed substances have a performance-enhancing effect. Where improvements are seen, it is possibly due to a **placebo** effect: The athletes taking the supplement *believe* it will help, so it actually helps even though there is no biochemical basis for the improvement. In other cases, improvements may occur because the product is filling a need that is missing from the foods that an athlete commonly consumes. For instance, bodybuilders often consume insufficient energy, forcing a larger than desired proportion of the consumed protein to be used to satisfy energy needs rather than tissue-building needs. The protein supplements that are consumed by bodybuilders help to satisfy the energy requirement and enable a greater proportion of protein to be available for muscle protein synthesis. The benefit of the protein may be due to the larger energy (*i.e.*, kcal) intake rather than protein per se, suggesting that simply eating more energy would help to better satisfy the protein requirement and would be a less expensive and equally effective means of sustaining and/or enlarging the muscle mass (38). Of course, there must also be physical stress in conjunction with sufficient energy/nutrients to encourage the muscular adaptation that bodybuilders seek (Figure 13.2). It simply is not feasible for performance enhancement to occur without the combination of mechanical loading (*i.e.*, exercise) and

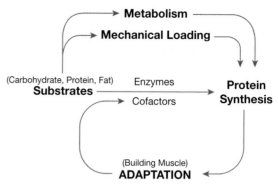

FIGURE 13.2: Physical activity (loading) plus adequate nutrient consumption is necessary to achieve the desired body/performance adaptation. Simply taking a supplement achieves nothing. (Adapted from Coyle EF. Workshop on the role of dietary supplements for physically active people. Bethesda (MD): National Institute of Health, Office of Education; 1996. 22 p.)

sufficient nutrients. The following is a practical guide to minimize the risk of taking a supplement (Maughn & Sherriffs, 2018):

- "Do not rely on advice from friends, fellow athletes, or coaches but undergo a proper evaluation by a qualified physician and/ or sports nutrition professional familiar with sport and antidoping rules. It is quite likely that dietary supplements are not necessary and nutrient deficiencies may be corrected from food sources.
- Avoid any product making claims of performance enhancement or any exaggerated claims or uses of the words: stimulant, energy or muscle booster, enhancer, legal or alternate steroid, extreme, blast, or weight loss. Even if no prohibited substance is listed on the label, the product may be spiked with one.
- Herbal stimulants and prohormones are especially high risk. Use of the terms herbal or natural does not in any way mean that the product does not contain a prohibited substance.
- Some companies offer guarantees of purity or are certified by other companies that do quality control. Verify the third-party testing system's reputation and remember there are no absolute guarantees.
- Avoid any company that states their products are WADA-approved. WADA or its accredited laboratories never test supplements or any products when not part of a doping control process. WADA cannot recommend any company or quality control system. In order to guarantee purity, each product batch would have to be tested for all prohibited substances.
- Avoid products containing multiple ingredients as there is a higher risk of contamination. Vitamins and

minerals (often classified as supplements) should be from reputable pharmaceutical companies and should not be mixed with other products.

- Seek guidance from your antidoping organization about recent information on contaminated or dangerous products in your part of the world (*e.g.*, U.S. Anti-Doping Agency High-Risk List)."

📖 Placebo

In research, a placebo contains no active ingredient but is typically indistinguishable from a pill/capsule/drink that contains the active ingredient. The placebo allows the researcher to make a clear statistical differentiation between the observed effects of the consumed active ingredient and the placebo. The *placebo effect* refers to a phenomenon in which a placebo can have an effect, despite the fact that it has no active ingredient because the person taking it believes or has the expectation that the placebo will be useful.

Although athletes may feel that consumption of dietary supplements/ergogenic aids permits them to eat less carefully, the literature is increasingly clear that these products do not take the place of a good diet. At best, if a supplement or ergogenic aid were to provide any benefit, the athlete must have a special need that a well-balanced diet that is consumed in a way that sustains a good energy balance fails to meet. There are few such substances, so the athlete must be cautious as the costs of these products are high, the benefits are limited, and the potential adverse effects are real. Ideally, rather than focusing on a "magic bullet" to enhance performance, athletes should take a realistic approach. Nothing is better than the consumption of a balanced intake of foods and beverages that provides sufficient energy and nutrients to support growth, activity, and tissue maintenance.

What follows is a review of nutritional supplements/ergogenic aids commonly consumed by athletes. Not included are a number of supplements that are available to athletes, but that do not yet have the popular acceptance of those reviewed. These include *epicatechins* from dark chocolate, *niacin* (vitamin B_3) found in meats, the antioxidant and muscle protectant *resveratrol* found in red-colored fruits and red wine, the cellular metabolism regulator *phosphatidic acid*, and the muscle protein simulator *ursolic acid*. As of the writing of this book, there are insufficient studies to clearly discern if these substances do or do not have a performance-enhancing effect.

NUTRITIONAL SUPPLEMENTS AND ERGOGENIC AIDS COMMONLY CONSUMED BY ATHLETES

Caffeine

Caffeine is a trimethylxanthine and one of several methylxanthines found in coffee, tea, cola, chocolate, and a variety of other foods and beverages (Table 13.4). It is important to consider that not all coffee provides the same level of caffeine, so understanding how a specific brand of coffee impacts an individual athlete is important (39). There is no apparent influence of caffeine consumption on energy intake, gastric emptying, and appetite (40). In addition, there does not appear to be a differential impact on anaerobic performance in individual athletes with different gene profiles (41). As a supplement, caffeine is a stimulant with established benefits for endurance, supramaximal, and sprint athletic endeavors (6). A review of studies found that when compared to a placebo, endurance athletes are likely to experience a clear performance enhancement of approximately 3%, regardless of sex, age, athlete VO_2 max, or timing of caffeine ingestion prior to competition (42). It is one of the most popularly consumed food and beverage ingredients, with a large proportion

Table 13.4	Caffeine Content of Commonly Consumed Foods and Beverages	
Food/Beverage	Serving	Caffeine Content (mg)
Ground coffee	12 oz	50–100
Black tea	8 oz	30–80
Green tea	8 oz	35–60
Herbal tea	8 oz	0
Cola	20 oz	50–65
Root beer, most brands	12 oz	0
Ginger ale	12 oz	0
Common energy drinks	Varies	30–134+
Caffeinated snack foods	Varies	20–150
Over-the-counter caffeine	1 capsule	200
Caffeine powder	1/16 tsp	200
Caffeine citrate solution	½ tsp	415

Source: Center for Science in the Public Interest. Accessed 2018 May 17. Available from: https://cspinet.org/

of the adult population consuming caffeine-containing products (43). For athletes, these products include caffeine-containing beverages, gels, and gums, many of which have been tested for efficacy as ergogenic substances (44). Although most studied with endurance athletes, caffeinated products are also commonly used by athletes in high-intensity and team sports (45). Caffeine has two primary effects: (i) as an adenosine antagonist it is a central nervous system stimulant and (ii) it is a muscle relaxant, resulting in a lower level of perceived effort and lowering the feeling of pain and fatigue associated with exercise (44,46). Although caffeine is generally considered safe to use when consumed within the range of 3–13 mg/kg, athletes should be cautious to avoid taking other stimulants and/or alcohol when consuming high levels of caffeine (45). For endurance athletes consuming relatively moderate quantities of 3–6 mg/kg of anhydrous caffeine in pill or powder form, typically consumed about 60 minutes prior to exercise, it has been found to be an effective ergogenic aid by increasing time to fatigue (47). Caffeine doses of <3 mg/kg provided before and during exercise as part of a carbohydrate-containing beverage have also been found to be effective in increasing time to fatigue (44). Low doses of caffeine (100–300 mg) when consumed after the first 15–80 minutes of physical activity have been found to improve cycling time trial performance by 3%–7% (48). Doses of caffeine greater than 9 mg/kg do not appear to have a performance-enhancing effect and may result in negative side effects, including anxiety, restlessness, and nausea (45). It is important to consider that there are insufficient studies differentiating ergogenesis between male and female athletes (49). However, the current recommendations for caffeine (3–6 mg/kg) prior to exercise to enhance endurance are likely to also be appropriate for women (50). A summary of the influence caffeine has on performance includes (51):

- Central nervous system stimulant because of its ability to block adenosine receptors.
- Enhances lipid oxidation.
- Promotes the metabolism of glucose and lipids.
- Enhances the accumulation of muscle glycogen postexercise.
- Enhances the contractile power of muscle by improving cell calcium content.
- Enhances vasodilation by promoting production of endothelial nitric oxide synthase, which increases nitric oxide.
- Increases β-endorphins, which positively impacts time to fatigue.

Some studies indicate that, as with all drugs, caffeine has a reduced-dose effect (i.e., it is less effective when consuming caffeine in the same amounts chronically, as the athlete adapts to this level of intake), so abstaining from heavy caffeine intake for at least 7 days prior to consuming it for a competition will enhance the potential ergogenic benefit (52). However, more recent findings indicate that habitual caffeine intake may not influence the ergogenic benefits of acute caffeine supplementation on anaerobic power and endurance, resistance exercise, and jumping (53,54). Not all athletes respond to caffeine, as it has been found that some athletes have a genetic inability to respond to its potential ergogenic properties, regardless of the caffeine ingestion strategy (55).

Concern has been raised that excess consumption of caffeine may result in unwanted side effects, including tremor, anxiety, and a higher heart rate (46). It should be noted that the National Collegiate Athletic Association (NCAA) prohibits the consumption of large quantities of caffeine that result in urinary caffeine levels exceeding 15 mcg/mL. This would require in excess of 700–900 mg caffeine (~5–7 cups of coffee) consumed in a relatively short period of time to reach this level (44). Athletes competing in NCAA-sanctioned events should know that caffeine-containing products may not have the caffeine or other stimulant content disclosed on the product label (4).

There is little reason to consume arbitrarily high levels of caffeine, as the maximal benefit appears to be reached at a level of 6 mg/kg body mass (Figure 13.3) (56). Even lower doses (<3 mg/kg) appear capable of imparting an ergogenic benefit for specific performance benefits (57,58). It is thought that low-dose caffeine intake may have certain other benefits, including potentially fewer side effects and a better mood state (44). Current recommendations for caffeine consumption include (51):

- Consume caffeine 60 minutes prior to exercise to ensure sufficient time for absorption.
- Performance enhancement for a variety of exercise types has been observed when consumed in moderate doses of 3–6 mg/kg.
- No additional benefit has been observed when the consumption dose exceeds 9 mg/kg.
- Following a period of no caffeine consumption, resuming intake is likely to have a similar ergogenic benefit, and perhaps even better.
- Caffeine may improve mental acuity during performance, which may be important when an athlete does not have sufficient sleep as may happen because of long travel.

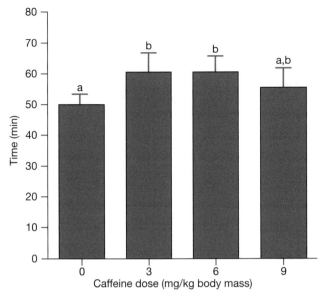

FIGURE 13.3: Effects of ingesting no caffeine (0) or 3, 6, or 9 mg/kg body mass of caffeine (dose) on running time to exhaustion at 85% of maximum oxygen uptake. Data are means ± standard error ($n = 8$). Bars with different letters are significantly different, and bars with the same letters are not significantly different. (From Graham TE, Spriet LL. Metabolic, catecholamine and exercise performance responses to varying doses of caffeine. J Appl Physiol. 1995; 78:867–74.)

- Caffeine should not be used prior to a major competition if its effect has not been tested in practice.
- The optimal dose within the recommended level of 3–6 mg/kg should be tested during practice to determine the individual athlete's optimal consumption level.

Although caffeine use is typically associated with improved endurance time to exhaustion, there is some limited information on the impact of caffeine on power/anaerobic work. Athletes who ingested caffeine at a level of 5 mg/kg lifted significantly more weight and performed a significantly higher number of bench press repetitions when compared with consumption of a placebo (59). This same study also found that consumption of caffeine resulted in greater vigor and less fatigue on a mood state score questionnaire than for those consuming the placebo. There is also contradictory evidence finding that caffeine intake does not improve total work capacity, best sprint, or time of last sprint performance in team sport athletes when compared to a placebo (60). These findings imply that athletes should independently determine whether caffeine imparts the desired ergogenic effect.

Carbohydrates (Gels, Drinks, Foods)

Carbohydrate has a critically important role in physical activity and is the macronutrient that provides the greatest amount of dietary energy in most people. In high-intensity, primarily anaerobic, exercise, carbohydrate is the primary fuel used by the muscles, as it has the capacity to be metabolized for energy anaerobically. Ideally, athletes should periodize carbohydrate intake to match the carbohydrate demand of training and/or competition (61). Athletes who periodize dietary intake to more closely match requirements are also likely to have a more stable gut microbiome, which is associated with improved endurance performance (62). The glycemic index of the carbohydrates consumed also makes a difference in endurance performance, which lower glycemic index foods having an advantage over higher glycemic index foods (63). In low-intensity but long-duration exercise, fat may be the primary fuel, but fat requires carbohydrates to burn completely (64). However, because carbohydrate storage is limited (~100 g glycogen in liver; ~400–500 g glycogen in muscles), it is typically the limiting energy substrate in physical activity. That is, carbohydrate is likely to "run out" more quickly than either fat or protein, and when carbohydrate runs out it is difficult to continue exercising (65). In a recent review of 50 of 61 (82%) studies assessing carbohydrate supplementation on exercise performance of varying durations, it was found to have statistically significant performance benefits (66). Care should be taken to avoid carbohydrate-loading strategies that the individual athlete has not adequately adapted to. As indicated in a recent study on bodybuilders, carbohydrate loading may result in GI symptoms that include constipation and diarrhea (67,68).

One strategy to help ensure that carbohydrate stores do not run out during exercise is to begin exercise with glycogen stores at their maximal level. This strategy, commonly referred to as *glycogen loading*, has as its goal the storage of as much carbohydrate in the tissues as they can hold. The traditional or classical regimen for **carbohydrate loading** (referred to as the Astrand regimen for the person who first described it) achieves maximal muscle glycogen stores by first completely depleting the muscles of glycogen (69). This is followed by a phase in which muscle glycogen is restored to maximal levels through the consumption of a high-carbohydrate diet while avoiding activity that may be glycogen-depleting (*i.e.*, high-intensity activity). Although successful in optimizing glycogen tissue stores, this regimen is no longer recommended because of the potential dangers associated with glycogen depletion, which include irregular heartbeats and a sudden loss of blood pressure (BP) (70).

📖 Carbohydrate Loading

A strategy for maximizing muscle glycogen stores in advance of an athletic event. Typically, this involves consumption of relatively high carbohydrate while reducing activities (*i.e.*, higher intensity) that may use muscle glycogen for several days.

Sherman/Costill method is the commonly recommended strategy for carbohydrate loading. This method was developed after the Astrand regimen and was found to be safer than the Astrand method but equally effective in optimizing glycogen storage. This approach is based on maintaining carbohydrate stores at all times and avoiding carbohydrate depletion. Using the recommended Sherman/Costill method, the athlete should do the following (71):

- Regularly consume a diet that is 55%–65% of carbohydrate daily, which is slightly increased to 60%–70% of carbohydrate in preparation for competition. This represents a carbohydrate intake of ~7–12 g/kg of body mass/day.
- For 4–7 days prior to competition, exercise (particularly intense exercise) should be gradually reduced to avoid using up a significant amount of muscle glycogen. During this tapering phase, a high-carbohydrate intake is maintained.

It has been found that this method is equally effective in maximizing glycogen stores as the Astrand regimen, but it avoids the difficulties associated with glycogen depletion. A recent study on basketball players found that 4 weeks on a low-carbohydrate diet decreased total work capacity but returned to predepletion levels after a carbohydrate loading procedure. In addition, this strategy of low-carbohydrate intake followed by carbohydrate loading did not ultimately impact peak power (72). This strongly implies that glycogen depletion is not a valid strategy for optimizing muscle glycogen stores. It should be noted that glycogen storage increases water storage in a 1:3 ratio (*i.e.*, for every gram of stored glycogen, the body stores ~3 g of water). Athletes should consider carefully if their sport would benefit from glycogen loading, as this strategy may improve endurance, but may also add some degree of weight and initial muscle stiffness (73). Where flexibility and high strength: weight ratio are important (*e.g.*, gymnastics, figure

skating, diving), maximizing glycogen stores may not be desirable (69).

The type of carbohydrate consumed does appear to make a difference. Glucose polymer products, including *polycose* (an easily digestible carbohydrate polymer with rapid absorption) and *maltodextrins* (a polysaccharide manufactured from starch via partial hydrolysis that is easy to digest and absorb), are found in several sports beverages and sports gels and are easily digested into glucose and appear to be effective in glycogen production, as are starches from pasta, bread, rice, and other cereal grains (64,74).

To summarize, the following strategies should be followed to optimize carbohydrate availability (4,75,76):

- To optimize muscle glycogen storage in preparation for an event/exercise or to recover muscle glycogen following exercise.
  - 7–12 g of carbohydrate/kg body mass/day.
- Rapid recovery of muscle glycogen following exercise when there are fewer than 8 hours available to recover prior to the next exercise bout.
  - 1–1.2 g/kg carbohydrate immediately following exercise, repeated every hour until a regular meal schedule is resumed.
  - There is evidence that consumption of carbohydrate as small snacks every 15–60 minutes may be advantageous early in the recovery period following exercise.
- Pre-event meal before a prolonged exercise session.
  - 1–4 g/kg carbohydrate consumed 1–4 hours prior to exercise.
- Carbohydrate consumption during moderate-intensity or intermittent exercise 1 hour or longer in duration.
- Insufficient total energy consumption, even with a relatively high consumption of carbohydrate, will result in diminished glycogen stores.
  - Exercise duration ~1 hour: small amounts of carbohydrate from a sports beverage providing 6%–7% carbohydrate solution. There is also evidence that mouth rinsing with a carbohydrate drink may provide some benefit.
  - Exercise duration greater than 90 minutes: 0.5–1.0 g/kg/hr (30–60 g/hr).
  - Exercise duration greater than 4 hours: ~1.5–1.8 g/min of multiple transportable carbohydrates (*i.e.*, the consumed carbohydrate contains more than a single source of carbohydrate. For instance, it is better to have a combination of sucrose and glucose than the caloric equivalent of glucose alone to optimize intestinal carbohydrate receptors).

- Typical daily intake. (Assumes carbohydrate is spread out over the day, with consumption that optimizes carbohydrate availability before, during, and immediately after exercise.)
  - Athletes performing a light training program.
    - 3–5 g/kg/day
  - Athletes with moderate exercise program.
    - 5–7 g/kg/day
  - Endurance athletes with 1–3 hours of moderate to higher intensity training.
    - 7–12 g/kg/day
  - Athletes with extreme exercise of long duration (greater than 4–5 hours), such as Tour de France.
    - A minimum of 10–12 g/kg/day

β-Alanine

Exercise results in reduced muscle energy substrates, including adenosine triphosphate (ATP), phosphocreatine (PCr), and glycogen, and an accumulation of metabolites, including adenosine diphosphate, H^+, and magnesium (Mg^{2+}), with a greater potential for cell-damaging free radicals (77). It appears that the dipeptide carnosine helps to limit muscular fatigue by buffering the accumulating H^+. Carnosine consists of the two amino acids β-alanine and histidine and increases with the consumption of β-alanine (78,79). A study assessing the muscle carnosine response to β-alanine supplementation found that nearly all studied subjects experienced elevated carnosine, regardless of sex (80). The effect of the increased buffering capacity is to enable an improvement in high-intensity exercise performance (6). There are dietary sources of β-alanine, primarily from the meat of predominantly anaerobic animals, such as poultry, or from animals in low-oxygen environments, such as fish and whales. Providing a standard supplemental dose of >800 mg β-alanine may result in unpleasant side effects that include skin rashes and/or transient paresthesia (tingling of the skin). However, this can be managed through consumption of slow-release tablets of β-alanine that may also be effective in elevating carnosine (79,81). Some studies suggest that intake of 3–6 g/day (0.8–1.6 g every 3–4 hours) for 10–12 weeks increases cellular buffering capacity by 50%–85% (79,82). Importantly, consumption of β-alanine within the recommended dose does not appear to have an adverse reaction to those consuming it (83). Interestingly, the muscle carnosine loading effect of supplemented β-alanine appears to be more pronounced in trained versus untrained muscles, but the effectiveness of supplemental β-alanine in producing a performance enhancement appears harder to realize in athletes who are already well-trained (84,85). Although there is a large between-athlete variation in performance benefit, athletes consuming β-alanine as per the usual protocol generally realize performance benefits ranging from 0.2%–3.0% during continuous and/or intermittent exercise lasting 30 seconds to 10 minutes (6). Different sports appear to have different outcomes when athletes consume β-alanine. A meta-analysis found that athletes involved in 4-km cycling, 2,000-m rowing, swimming sprints of 100 and 200 m, combat sports, and water polo may find a benefit from β-alanine supplementation (86). There is, however, contradictory evidence. For instance, it has been found that an 8-week training program resulted in significant strength improvements, but the addition of β-alanine did not enhance the improvement in strength (87). In addition, a study of β-alanine–supplemented rugby players had findings that could not support the use of β-alanine in these players (88). There is also some evidence that β-alanine may have a body fat-lowering effect, but a careful review of studies assessing the body composition impact of β-alanine found that it was unlikely to improve body composition, regardless of dosage, when combined with exercise training (89). Another study found that, when taken by itself or with sodium bicarbonate, β-alanine supplementation increases glycolysis but does not improve short-duration cycling time-trial performance (90).

Nitrate and Other Nitric Oxide Stimulators

Supplementation of dietary nitrate and other products, including citrus flavonoids, that increase plasma nitrite concentration or directly increase the production of nitric oxide. **Nitric oxide** (NO) has multiple functions, all of which are important for competitive athletes. These functions include (91–93):

- Regulation of blood flow and BP (vasodilation)
- Muscle contractility
- Glucose homeostasis
- Calcium homeostasis
- Mitochondrial respiration and biogenesis

A review of studies has found a clear ergogenic benefit of NO in recreationally active, young, healthy men in a variety of exercise formats, but the beneficial effects are not as clear in women or well-trained athletes (94).

Nitric Oxide

Commonly abbreviated as NO, nitric oxide is a powerful vasodilator that improves oxygen delivery to cells. The improved oxygen delivery has the effect of lowering heart rate and BP, as the heart does not have to work as hard to deliver the required oxygen. In children and adolescents, there is a robust L-arginine pathway for producing NO. With aging, this pathway is not as active and BP rises. However, consumption of high-nitrate foods (*i.e.*, beet juice, spinach, lettuce rocket, celery, cress, chervil) results in higher nitric acid, improved oxygen delivery, and lower BP.

It was originally thought that NO was only generated through oxidation of the amino acid L-arginine in a reaction catalyzed by nitric oxide synthase (NOS) (95). However, it has since been found that NO may also be produced from consumed foods through reduction of nitrate to nitrite, and then nitrite to NO (96). This pathway is particularly important in conditions of low oxygen availability, including high oxygen demand in skeletal muscle during exercise. It has also been found that supplementation with citrus flavonoid, an antioxidant and also a stimulator of NO production, has a positive impact on exercise performance. Using a double-blind, randomized study of healthy trained males, 4 weeks of supplementation with 500-mg citrus flavonoid resulted in a significant improvement in power production (time trial on cycle ergometer) when compared with a placebo (92).

Nitrate sources come in either organic or inorganic forms. The organic form is typically consumed as sodium nitrate or sodium nitrite, which are common pharmaceutical agents used in individuals with a heart condition, such as angina. Sodium nitrate and nitrite are also commonly used as food preservatives in some processed meats, such as bacon. Organic nitrate/nitrite has potent vasodilatory effects, but its chronic use may result in endothelial dysfunction that eventually results in elevated oxidative stress (97). The inorganic form is typically consumed from dietary sources such as beetroot juice or green leafy vegetables. Chronic consumption of inorganic naturally occurring food-based nitrate, however, does not result in negative effects with chronic intake because of its participation in the enterosalivary circulation, which naturally inhibits excess oxidative stress by controlling and preventing excess production of NO (98). Inorganic food-borne nitrate appears to also have a cytoprotective effect against ischemia-reperfusion injury, while continuous use of organic nitrate may increase the potential for the injury (98).

Recent studies have found that both inorganic and organic nitrate supplements can significantly increase plasma nitrate and nitrite concentration with a resultant reduction in systolic BP resulting from enhanced NO production. However, chronic use of the organic form, typically as sodium nitrate, has a reduced benefit. In healthy individuals, a single administration of beetroot juice or other vegetable juices that contain inorganic nitrate ranging from 400 mg to 800 mg, has been found to decrease BP in both males and females (99). Similarly, a single administration of either sodium nitrate or nitrite was also found to decrease BP in healthy individuals (100,101). Although both organic and inorganic nitrate have potent vasodilatory effects, it has been determined that food-based inorganic nitrate had a greater effect in lowering the BP than organic nitrate (sodium nitrate) when individuals were provided with the same amount of nitrate (100). In healthy young men and postmenopausal women, food-based inorganic nitrate supplementation provided in a single dose or over 14 consecutive days also significantly decreased BP (102,103). In addition, in patients with health comorbidities and Raynaud syndrome, the BP-lowering effect of food-based inorganic nitrate persistently lowered both systolic and diastolic BP (104). It is important to note that an abundance of nitrate-reducing bacteria in the oral cavity was found to be associated with lower systolic BP in healthy individuals, likely the result of an enhanced nitrate—nitrite–NO conversion (105,106).

There is increasing evidence that improving NO production through consumption of food-based inorganic nitrate is also beneficial in time to exhaustion and oxygen cost during exercise, which may improve exercise performance (107). Nitrate reduction by oral bacteria regulates postexercise hypotension and skeletal muscle oxygenation by lowering BP and increasing muscle oxygenation, which results in a proportionately higher fat metabolism, in healthy individuals (108). The higher fat metabolism diminishes reliance on carbohydrate, for which humans have limited storage, and is likely the primary reason associated with greater fatigue resistance. Dietary inorganic nitrate supplementation using beetroot juice (the juice form enhances surface contact with oral bacteria) may also increase time to fatigue by reducing exercise-associated leg muscle pain (107). Similar treatment with beetroot juice may also reduce oxygen cost of exercise, which improves exercise economy and enhances tolerance to high-intensity exercise (109).

Nitrate in foods, particularly beets and green leafy vegetables, can be reduced to nitrite by oral bacteria, resulting in higher plasma nitrite concentrations. The higher plasma nitrite concentration serves as reservoir for NO production (110). Beet juice and vegetable juices are preferred because they have better surface area contact than solid foods between the food-derived nitrate and the oral bacteria (111). The importance of the healthy oral microbiome is clearly an important factor in deriving a benefit from high-nitrate foods, as the oral bacteria converts nitrate to nitrite, which is the precursor to the vasodilator nitric oxide (112).

There have been multiple other studies that have investigated whether dietary nitrate supplementation impacts the physiologic response to exercise. In one such study, it was found that 3 days of sodium nitrate supplementation (0.1 mmol/kg/day) reduced resting BP and oxygen cost of submaximal cycle exercise (113). Other studies found that enhancing NO bioavailability through the dietary intake of beetroot juice reduced resting BP, reduced the oxygen cost of submaximal exercise by 5%, and extended the time to exhaustion during high-intensity exercise by 16% (114). Interestingly, food nitrate supplementation also reduces the oxygen cost of submaximal exercise and may also enhance exercise tolerance and performance (91,115). Other recent studies have found that acute dietary intake of 0.5 L of beetroot juice before 4-km and 16.1-km cycle time trial performance in competitive cyclists resulted in greater power output for same oxygen uptake, and a 2.7% reduction in time to complete both time trial distances (109,116–117). It was determined that this effect can be maintained for at least 15 days if supplementation at the same dose (~0.5 L beetroot juice) is continued. Importantly, nitrate-depleted beetroot (placebo) was found to have no effect, suggesting that nitrate is a key bioactive component of beetroot juice. As a word of caution, because nitrate is converted to nitrite by oral bacteria, use of antiseptic mouthwash may inhibit NO production. A recent study assessed BP in 19 healthy volunteers during an initial 7-day control period, followed by a 7-day treatment period with a chlorhexidine-based antiseptic mouthwash (111). The antiseptic mouthwash treatment significantly reduced oral nitrite production by 90% and plasma nitrite levels by 25% compared with the control period. This resulted in a significant increase in systolic and diastolic BP. Results of this study suggest that oral bacteria play an important role in plasma nitrite levels and in the physiologic control of BP.

Creatine

Creatine supplementation, typically as creatine monohydrate, has been found to improve performance of repeated bouts of high-intensity exercise with short recovery periods (4,118). The potential benefits of creatine supplementation represent a good reason to have the following dietary strategy: "Food first but not always food only" (119). A recent review has also found that, when taken in recommended doses, there are no apparent negative side effects found in adolescent athletes who take creatine supplements (120). In addition, studies have found that creatine supplementation may enhance the adaptive response to exercise, including an increase in lean mass, strength, and muscular endurance (6,121,122). PCr serves as a storage depot for maintaining ATP levels during high-intensity activities, such as sprinting, which can quickly deplete ATP. Creatine is made from three amino acids, and it joins with phosphorus to make PCr (123). It is believed that saturating muscles with creatine will enhance the ability to maintain, through effective resynthesis, the high-energy compound ATP, thereby delaying fatigue in high-intensity activities (64). There is also some evidence that creatine supplementation may lower oxidative stress and markers of tissue inflammation (124). Humans mainly synthesize creatine in the liver and other metabolically active tissues from the amino acids arginine, glycine, and methionine, and we can also obtain preformed creatine from meats (125). However, normal cooking reduces the availability of preformed creatine in the diet, and given the ever-increasing importance of fully cooking meat products to reduce the chance of bacterial infection, the amount of creatine delivered by the diet is likely to be small. Because of a net lower intake of preformed creatine from meat and typically lower protein intakes that provide the amino acids necessary for creatine synthesis, pure vegans may be at risk for low intakes of creatine (4,126). However, a recent review has found that the benefits derived from creatine supplementation did not differentially help vegetarians more than omnivores (122). While there are limited studies on the impact of creatine supplementation on paralympic athletes, it has been found that paralympic powerlifters taking a placebo experienced earlier muscle fatigue when compared to those taking creatine (127).

Creatine is now one of the most popular performance-enhancing supplements taken by athletes (128). A typical creatine loading regimen involves an initial loading phase of 20 g/day, divided into four equal daily doses of 5 g/dose, for 5–7 days, followed by a maintenance phase of 3–5 g/day for differing periods of time (1 week to 6 months) (125). Recent studies suggest that creatine monohydrate supplementation at doses of 0.1 g/kg body weight that is combined with resistance training improves the potential for a performance benefit (128). Earlier studies have suggested that taking daily creatine supplements results in muscle tissue saturation of creatine after 5 days (129). This finding suggests that creatine should not be taken for longer than 5 days, with some studies suggesting that taking creatine supplements 5 days per month is adequate to saturate muscle tissue (130). There is also evidence that consuming the creatine monohydrate supplement with additional protein and carbohydrate (~100 calories protein + ~100 calories carbohydrate) may improve the uptake of creatine by cells because of the higher insulin response from the additional energy substrates (131). There are multiple potential benefits from creatine supplementation, which include (132,133):

- Enhanced sprint performance
- Lower fatigue during multiple maximal effort muscle contractions
- Elevated muscle mass and strength resulting from training
- Improved glycogen synthesis
- Elevated anaerobic threshold
- Better training tolerance
- Potential for improving cognitive function and alleviating mental fatigue.

Although no negative health effects have been documented with creatine supplementation (using the recommended intake protocol) for up to 4 years, athletes should be aware that the long-term safety of creatine monohydrate supplementation has never been tested on children, adolescents, or adults (134). Creatine supplementation is associated with acute weight gain from water retention (0.6–2 kg following creatine loading), which may cause difficulties for athletes in weight-sensitive sports, and there are also reports that creatine may cause GI discomfort (4,135,136). In a study comparing creatine monohydrate supplementation with a supplement of 250-kcal carbohydrate for 5 days using a repeated jump height test, it was found that the carbohydrate group performed as effectively as the creatine monohydrate group, but without the added weight gain associated with creatine consumption (135). Creatine supplementation has also been linked to transient renal (kidney) dysfunction (137). It was found that the athlete with renal dysfunction had been taking oral creatine supplements to prepare for the soccer season. He had not been exceeding the recommended doses, and once he stopped the supplements renal function recovered. It has been advised that high-dose (>3–5 g/day) creatine supplementation should not be used by those with preexisting renal disease or those with a potential risk for renal dysfunction (*i.e.*, diabetics, hypertensives) (138). A test of kidney function would,

therefore, be logical in advance of creatine supplementation. A meta-analysis of major creatine issues has found the following (139):

- Creatine supplementation may increase intracellular water volume, but studies are inconsistent in determining that water retention is a by-product of creatine supplementation.
- When taken in recommended doses, creatine supplementation is not associated with kidney damage or dysfunction in healthy individuals.
- There is no evidence that creatine supplementation increases testosterone or results in hair loss.
- There is no evidence that creatine supplementation is associated with dehydration and associated muscle cramping.
- Fat mass is not increased because of creatine supplementation.
- Low daily doses of creatine supplements (3–5 g/day) are associated with elevated intramuscular creatine stores and enhanced muscle performance/recovery.
- Older adults who exercise may achieve enhanced benefits from creatine supplementation.
- While resistance/power activities have been shown to experience benefits from creatine supplementation, other combination and endurance activities may also experience benefits.
- Creatine monohydrate appears to be the optimal formulation for creatine supplements.

Sodium Bicarbonate/Sodium Citrate

Supplementation with sodium bicarbonate or sodium citrate enhances extracellular buffering capacity, with performance improvements observed in athletic events that would otherwise be affected by acid-based disturbances, typically associated with anaerobic glycolysis and including repeated high-intensity sprints and high-intensity events lasting 1–7 minutes (140,141). Researchers have found that both sodium bicarbonate and sodium citrate have a buffering effect on the acidity (lactic acid) that is primarily created not only in anaerobic sports but also in team sports that involve repeated sprinting, allowing for prolonged maintenance of force or power (142,143). Because many activities involve mainly anaerobic metabolic processes, it would appear that some athletes could derive a benefit from consumption of these buffers.

The typical consumption protocol for sodium bicarbonate and sodium citrate is to consume 200–400 mg/kg ~1–2 hours prior to exercise (144). However, there are reported GI problems related to consumption of sodium bicarbonate that may include vomiting and diarrhea, but these may be somewhat mediated through coingestion of small high-carbohydrate snacks (4,142,145). These negative side effects from taking sodium bicarbonate should give athletes reason to be cautious before taking this potential ergogenic aid. It has been found that sodium bicarbonate may induce minor symptoms earlier than sodium citrate, but that GI symptoms were mostly minor regardless of whether sodium citrate or sodium bicarbonate was consumed (146). Enteric-coated sodium bicarbonate supplementation consumed prior to exercise has been found to eliminate GI symptoms and improves 4-km cycling time-trial performance (147). The enteric coating resists gastric acidity, thereby reducing the buffering of gastric pH and helping to eliminate GI symptoms. As an alternative, sodium citrate appears to result in less GI distress, but the tolerance of this supplement should also be tested prior to use at a competition (6,148). In addition, it has been determined that sodium citrate should be consumed over a period of less than 60 minutes and completed 2.5–4.5 hours prior to exercise (149).

While some studies have found a significant benefit from sodium bicarbonate ingestion on intermittent exercise time to exhaustion, other studies have conflicting results (150–153). A meta-analysis of team sports has found that, when compared to a placebo, sodium bicarbonate failed to improve total work capacity, best sprint time, and last sprint time, suggesting that individual athletes should determine if sodium bicarbonate intake results in the desired outcomes (60). An analysis of female athletes using sodium bicarbonate supplements has also found that there is no sex-specific dosing recommendation and that athletes wishing to supplement with sodium bicarbonate should consume approximately 0.2–0.3 g/kg 1–3 hours prior to high-intensity exercise (154). Because of the wide variety of individual responses observed with either sodium bicarbonate or sodium citrate, individual athletes should carefully determine when either supplement should be taken, the amount that appears beneficial, and whether there is a clear ergogenesis (155).

Branched-Chain Amino Acids

BCAAs include valine, leucine, and isoleucine, and all are amino acids that cannot be produced by the body so must be consumed. The BCAAs can bypass the liver to be oxidized directly by muscle tissue to derive energy (156). One of the BCAAs, leucine, is a muscle protein synthesis stimulator that enables size and strength muscle adaptations that relate to the activities being performed (157).

Dairy proteins appear to have benefits relative to other protein sources, perhaps largely due to the relatively high leucine content and the high digestibility and absorption qualities of the BCAAs in dairy products (158). BCAA metabolism appears to be elevated in endurance activities, and there appears to be an energy balance component to BCAA availability because plasma concentrations are affected by changes in total energy availability as well as the intake of protein, fat, and carbohydrate (159). It is theorized that intense physical activity may break down muscle tissue at a fast rate, but that supplementation with BCAA minimizes this muscle degradation and results in improved fat-free mass (160). It has also been theorized that supplemental intake of BCAA may result in central fatigue by releasing more tryptophan to cross the blood–brain barrier, which stimulates the production of serotonin (161). Serotonin induces sleep, suppresses appetite, and induces physiologic fatigue. However, a recent study assessing the effects of BCAA supplementation on fatigue found no significant effects on central fatigue (162), and it was previously found that the coingestion of carbohydrate with BCAA appears to minimize central fatigue (163).

A number of studies assessing the supplemental intake of BCAA on athletic performance have mixed results. The studies combining BCAA with carbohydrate appear to have more improvement than the BCAA alone, whereas some studies found that carbohydrate alone provided the ergogenic benefit while combining BCAA with carbohydrate resulted in performance improvements (156). Supplementation of BCAA is typically in the range of 20–25 g (equivalent to 80–100 kcal). The findings suggest that athletes consuming good-quality protein with sufficient carbohydrate are likely to achieve the same or more benefit than might be derived from the consumption of BCAA supplements alone. The current upper-level recommendation of approximately 1.6 g/kg/day of well-distributed protein appears to be sufficient to optimize muscle mass, putting into question the potential benefits of additional BCAAs on muscle strength and hypertrophy (164).

Gut and Oral Microbiome: Prebiotics/Probiotics[1]

The health-enhancing impact of exercise occurs through several mechanisms, including the positive impact it has

---

[1]Special thanks to Megan Rossi, PhD, RD for providing information for this section on prebiotics and probiotics. Dr. Rossi is a research associate in Diabetes and Nutritional Sciences at King's College, London and is a specialist in the area of the gut microbiome.

Table 13.5   Prebiotics, Probiotics, and Synbiotics

Prebiotics	Nondigestible food components that help the growth and activity of beneficial bacteria (*i.e.*, food for beneficial bacteria)	Prebiotics are a type of dietary fiber that passes through the upper GI tract indigested providing substrate for colonic bacteria. Prebiotics are naturally found in many foods including: artichokes, onion, garlic, asparagus, and leeks
Probiotics	Live bacteria that provide a health benefit when consumed in adequate amounts (*i.e.*, good bacteria)	Common probiotics include *Lactobacillus* and *Bifidobacterium*, which naturally occur in a range of foods including: yogurts (with active live cultures), kefir, kombucha, kimchi, and natto
Synbiotics	Combination of prebiotics and probiotics	Synbiotics provide both the beneficial bacteria to the GI tract and the substrate (*i.e.*, food) to help the bacteria thrive in the colon. Examples of synbiotic foods include live culture yogurt with sliced nectarine; beans and fresh sour dill pickles; kefir and cashew nuts; greens sautéed with garlic and sour cream added

on the immune system, its anti-inflammatory impact, and its metabolism-improving effects (165). Recent studies on the gut and oral **microbiome** suggest a major role in immunity and metabolism, and disruption of the gut microbiome can result in chronic inflammatory disease that can negatively affect athletic performance (166). In addition, the oral microbiome plays an important role in converting dietary inorganic nitrate to nitrite, which is a precursor to the vasodilator nitric oxide (167). As a result, gut and oral-microbial modulating therapies, including prebiotics and probiotics, are gaining popularity among athletes (Table 13.5).

📖 Microbiome

Also referred to as the microbiota, microbiome refers to the microbial organisms that inhabit the GI system and have many functions related to human health, including the immune system, hormone production, and metabolism. The gut microbiome is influenced by dietary intake, exercise habits, age, sex, genetics, ethnicity, antibiotics, health state, and disease state (168). The microbiome has a critically important role in the metabolism of nutrients, the inflammatory response to exercise, and immune system function. As a result of long-duration high-intensity exercise, the gut microbiota is dysregulated. However, long-term exposure to the same exercise enhances the immune response with associated positive changes to the gut microbiota (168), The microbiome may be degraded through antibiotics and/or consumption of foods that fail to support the bacteria (*i.e.*, prebiotics), and/or fail to provide bacteria such as *Lactobacillus* and *Bifidobacterium* found in live culture yogurts and other fermented foods (*i.e.*, probiotics).

Prebiotics and probiotics work by modifying the community of bacteria that resides in the large intestine, termed the gut *microbiota*, which has been shown to play a pivotal role in health and disease. There is a growing body of evidence suggesting this therapeutic target may benefit athletes by influencing immune function, reducing gut mucosal permeability, and decreasing the systemic inflammatory response associated with intense exercise (169). Beyond exercise-specific targets, prebiotics and probiotics may also have other benefits in athletes including reducing stress-related symptoms such as insomnia, poor concentration, anxiousness, depression, and fatigue (170). There is also evidence, using a randomized double-blind placebo protocol, that *Lactobacillus casei* Shirota, a common bacterium in probiotic capsules, may help to reduce upper respiratory tract infection incidence in athletes (171). The brain-gut connection is now well established, and it has been found that there are alterations in the gut microbiome following a sport-related head injury, and monitoring these microbiome changes may enable a better concussion diagnosis (172).

Common probiotic foods include yogurt, kefir, sauerkraut, pickles, tempeh, kimchi, and kombucha tea. Where regular consumption of these foods is not possible, athletes can find a wide array of probiotic capsules that are available for sale. Summary points for the athlete gut microbiome (173):

- Studies suggest a different gut microbiome makeup between athletes and nonathletes, with health-associated bacteria commonly being associated with athletes.

- While probiotics and prebiotics have been shown to positively influence several outcomes, the mechanism(s) for this positive relationship are not well understood.
- Intense exercise is associated with GI and respiratory infections, and the makeup of the oral and gut microbiome may influence the infections commonly seen in athletes.

Vitamin D

Vitamin D affects multiple body systems and may impact muscle soreness, muscle recovery, calcium homeostasis, immunity, bone mineral density, and other skeletal and extraskeletal cellular processes that include cardiopulmonary function (174,175). It is this increasing understanding of vitamin D that has resulted in an enhanced interest in vitamin D and the multiple roles it plays in athletic performance (see Table 13.6).

Recent studies have found that vitamin D–deficient athletes are at higher risk for all types of skeletal fracture, but also increases in total body inflammation, infectious illness, and muscle function (176). A study assessing vitamin D supplementation found that vitamin D_2 and D_3 supplementation was safe and protected against acute respiratory tract infection (177). A study of 98 young athletes and dancers found that 73% of the assessed athletes were vitamin D deficient and that athletes involved in indoor sports had nearly double the prevalence of vitamin D deficiency when compared with athletes in outdoor sports (178). Athletes associated with specific sports, experience different vitamin D deficiency risks. It was found that 32% of basketball players were deficient and 47% had insufficient levels; 26% of American football players were deficient, and 42%–80%

had insufficient levels (175). Interestingly, it was found in the 1950s that athletes exposed to ultraviolet light that produces vitamin D improved athletic performance, primarily through lower muscle soreness and improved muscle recovery (145). Both the faster recovery in muscle soreness and improved muscle recovery are likely a function of increased muscle protein synthesis, which is enhanced with good vitamin D status (179,180). It should be noted that darker-skinned athletes are likely to require more sunlight (ultraviolet B [UVB]) exposure than light-skinned athletes to derive the same vitamin D–forming benefit. It has been estimated that light-skinned individuals require up to 40% less UVB exposure to achieve the same vitamin D status than darker-skinned individuals, placing darker-skinned athletes at higher risk of deficiency, assuming equivalence in food intake (181).

The problem is clear: Vitamin D production is nearly absent during the winter, in athletes living in areas with changing seasons, and in athletes living at high latitudes (182), and forces athletes to rely on vitamin D stores that were acquired during the summer. Dietary vitamin D is relatively low, and in athletes who train and compete indoors all year, the acquisition of vitamin D even during the summer is inadequate, placing them at high risk for fractures (176,183,184) (Figure 13.4).

The Institute of Medicine classifies adequate vitamin D as a serum value of >50 nmol/L, inadequate vitamin D as 30–50 nmol/L, and vitamin D deficiency as <30 nmol/L (174). However, there is no clear consensus for the level of serum vitamin D (25-hydroxyvitamin D) that is associated with an optimal level, deficiency, or insufficiency in athletes (185). Typically, UVB exposure contributes to 80%–90% of serum vitamin D, whereas dietary sources contribute 10%–20% (186). There is now good evidence

Table 13.6		**Forms of Vitamin D Supplements**
Vitamin D_2	Ergocalciferol (from plants)	Vitamin D_2 is produced by plants with exposure to ultraviolet radiation. The vitamin D_2 content of foods may be increased through postharvest ultraviolet light irradiation. This also occurs in soy milk, almond milk, and coconut milk, which is exposed to ultraviolet light to increase the vitamin D_2 content.
Vitamin D_3	Cholecalciferol (from animals)	This is the most biologically active form of vitamin D for humans and appears to be the superior supplemental form as it has better absorption and utilization than vitamin D_2. In humans, sunlight exposure to the fat layer under the skin converts cholesterol to vitamin D_3.

Sources: Data from Lehmann U, Hirche F, Stangl GI, Hinz K, Westphal S, Dierkes J. Bioavailability of vitamin D(2) and D(3) in healthy volunteers, a randomized placebo-controlled trial. J Clin Endocrinol Metab. 2013;98(11):4339–45; Logan VF, Gray AR, Peddie MC, Harper MJ, Houghton LA. Long-term vitamin D3 supplementation is more effective than vitamin D2 in maintaining serum 25-hydroxyvitamin D status over the winter months. Br J Nutr. 2013;109(6):1082–8.

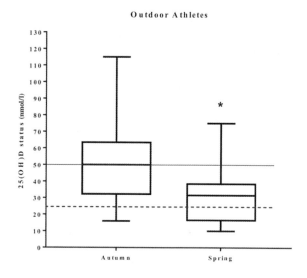

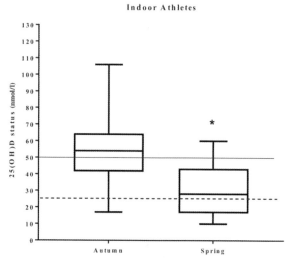

FIGURE 13.4: Different vitamin D status of indoor and outdoor athletes in the autumn and spring. (Reprinted from Wilson-Barnes SL, Hunt JEA, Williams EL, Allison SJ, Wild JJ, Wainwright J, Lanham-New SA, Manders RJF. Seasonal variation in vitamin D status, bone health and athletic performance in competitive university student-athletes: a longitudinal study. J Nutr Sci. 2020;9(e8):1–10.)

that supplemental consumption of vitamin D in athletes with serum vitamin D below 40 nmol/L is a performance-improving strategy. It appears that >40 ng/mL serum vitamin D is needed for fracture prevention in athletes, with no additional benefits observed with serum vitamin D >50 nmol/L (187). Vitamin D supplemental doses vary widely, ranging from 1,000–50,000 IU, with typical supplemental doses in the range of 1,000–2,000 IU. The European Food Safety Authority recently stated that 4,000 IU is the maximum reasonable dose for vitamin D supplementation (188). Daily supplementation above this level should involve careful monitoring of serum vitamin D to avoid toxicity (189). Even among older adults

experiencing muscular and strength declines, providing 1,000 IU of ergocalciferol per day for 2 years was found to significantly increase muscle strength and size (190). Studies of supplemented and nonsupplemented athletes demonstrate performance improvement in the vitamin D–supplemented group, particularly in athletes living in northern climates (191,192). It is generally recognized now that athletes with low serum vitamin D should be placed on vitamin D supplementation (193). However, given the potential for toxicity, vitamin D supplementation should be undertaken under the guidance of a health professional.

Green Tea and Other Polyphenol Containing Foods

Past studies suggest that consumption of antioxidants, either through antioxidant foods or through supplementation, may be protective against exercise-associated oxidative stress from reactive oxygen species (ROS-Free Radicals) and muscle damage (194,195). There have also been studies suggesting that antioxidant-supplemented athletes may not adapt well to training, predisposing them to a greater degree of oxidative damage (196–198). Green tea consumption may be useful in lowering the potential damage caused by ROS because it contains catechins and polyphenols, which have antioxidant and anti-inflammatory properties (199). A double-blind, randomized, placebo-controlled crossover study assessing two 4-week periods with either a green tea extract (980-mg polyphenols daily) or a placebo on sprinters found that the green tea extract prevented oxidative stress following repeated cycle sprint tests (200). This is a finding consistent with previous studies assessing green tea extract (201,202). It was also found that green tea supplement consumption ~90 minutes prior to aerobic exercise lowered inflammation and oxidative stress and enhanced VO_2 max in athletes training in a hot environment (203).

As indicated in Table 13.7, there are different types and sources of polyphenols, requiring a balanced and varied diet to obtain them. It has been found that consumption of different polyphenol-containing foods may be associated with different beneficial effect, with some associated with enhanced recovery, while others associated with enhanced fatigue resistance (204). It is recommended, therefore, that nutritional habits should incorporate polyphenol-risk foods (*i.e.*, fresh fruits, tea, etc.) rather than becoming excessively reliant on a supplement, which is likely to focus on a single polyphenol.

Supplements to Enhance the Immune System

A number of nutritional supplements are consumed for the purpose of enhancing immune function in athletes. These include vitamins C and E, zinc, and other substances not previously covered in this chapter, including bovine colostrum, glutamine, echinacea, and omega-3 fatty acids. It is important to consider that it is the position of the American College of Sports Medicine that micronutrient supplements are not needed for athletes consuming a balanced energy-adequate diet. However, the literature commonly reports that total food/energy intake in many athletes is inadequate, resulting in a high risk of micronutrient deficiency and raising the possible necessity for nutrient supplements in these athletes (205). A summary of their potential action and effectiveness is provided in the following sections (6).

Vitamin C

Vitamin C (ascorbic acid) is involved in removing ROS and is involved in immune function. There is limited evidence that supplemental vitamin C may help to prevent upper respiratory symptoms and no supporting evidence that supplementation with >200 mg/day vitamin C is useful in treating or resolving upper respiratory symptoms. Based on current findings, it appears that the higher antioxidant need resulting from regular exercise can easily be satisfied through a diet that provides a regular consumption of fresh fruits and vegetables (206). It has been hypothesized that the combination of beetroot juice (a good source of nitrate) plus 200 mg of vitamin C would result in higher nitric oxide formation that could enhance performance. However, current findings do not support this hypothesis (207).

Vitamin E

Vitamin E is involved in removing ROS and is involved in immune function. There is no evidence that vitamin E supplementation aids immune function, with some evidence that high doses may increase oxidative damage and increase upper respiratory symptoms. Importantly, regular supplementation of vitamin E may inhibit normal tissue adaptation to physical activity, with a failure to attenuate delayed onset muscle soreness (208).

Current findings suggest that vitamin E supplementation is not effective in reducing exercise-induced inflammation (209). There are two possible areas that show a potential for benefiting athletes who supplement with Vitamin E (210). One is that vitamin E supplementation shows promise in athletes involved in high-altitude training.

Initial data suggest that these athletes are less likely to experience deformation of newly formed red blood cells. Another possible area is that acute supplementation of vitamin E may benefit athletes involved in high-intensity exercise with short recovery intervals. More research is needed to further explore these areas, as the majority of studies have found that chronic vitamin supplementation does not improve performance and may inhibit performance (211). It is important to consider that beneficial effects of vitamin E are likely to occur when low doses are consumed (typically from foods), and negative effects are likely to occur when high doses (5–17 times higher than the RDA) are consumed (typically from supplements) (212). It is also important to consider that high levels of vitamin E may result in the reduced absorption of other fat-soluble vitamins, creating unwanted deficiencies (213).

Zinc

Zinc is an essential mineral found in many proteins and appears to be in especially high demand in exercising skeletal muscle (214). This mineral is required as an enzyme cofactor for immune cells, with a deficiency associated with impaired immunity. There is evidence that zinc deficiency with associated exercise impairment occurs in athletes, particularly following exhaustive exercise (215,216). However, study limitations have resulted in limited evidence that zinc supplementation (20–30 mg/day) results in the desired ergogenic benefits (217). Studies assessing the differences in zinc status between male and female athletes have found only minor differences that are likely due to differences in muscle mass, and muscle damage (218). There are claims that zinc supplementation may reduce the incidence of upper respiratory symptoms, but only moderate research supports that it is useful for treating upper respiratory symptoms. For a zinc supplement to be useful, it should be consumed within 24 hours of the onset of upper respiratory symptoms for the duration of the illness. Potential side effects include hypogeusia (low taste sensation), dysgeusia (altered taste sensation), and nausea. Ideally, athletes should consume foods that are rich in zinc to counteract potential exercise-associated deficiencies. These include meats, shellfish, legumes (chickpeas, lentils, beans), seeds (hemp, pumpkin, squash), nuts and peanuts, cheese and milk, eggs, and dark chocolate.

Bovine Colostrum

This is the first milk produced by a cow following delivery of a calf and includes antibodies, growth factors, and

Table 13.7   Polyphenol Compounds in Foods

Polyphenol Type	Subclass	Common Food Sources
Flavonoids	Flavanols	Lentils, green tea, black tea, grapes, chocolate, cranberry juice, apples, yellow onions, deep green vegetables, broccoli, spinach, tomatoes
	Flavones	Celery, pepper, grapes, parsley
	Flavanones	Oranges, grapefruit, lemons, rosemary, peppermint
	Anthocyanins	Blackberries, blueberries, black grapes, cherries, plums, strawberries
Phenolic Acids	Hydroxybenzoic acids; hydroxycinnamic acids	Strawberries, grapes, bananas, tea, coffee, chicory, peas, oats, wheat, rice, artichokes
Stilbenes	Resveratrol	Legumes, grapes, soy, peanuts
Lignans	Enterolignans, enterodiol, enterolactone	Flax seeds, sesame seeds, legumes, whole grain cereals (rye, wheat, oat, barley)

Source: Adapted from D'Angelo S. Polyphenols: potential beneficial effects of these phytochemical in athletes. Curr Sports Med Rep. 2020;19(7): 260–5.

other chemicals involved in immunity. There is limited support for use of bovine colostrum, with some information suggesting that it can help to sustain salivary antimicrobial proteins following heavy exercise. (These salivary antimicrobial proteins typically decrease following heavy exercise.) While there is some beginning evidence that bovine colostrum may benefit gut health in athletes, more research support is required to better understand the usefulness of bovine colostrum supplementation (219,220).

Glutamine

Glutamine is the most prevalent nonessential amino acid in human muscle and plasma and is used as a source of energy for immune cells, is involved in acid-base regulation, is available for gluconeogenesis, and is a precursor of the antioxidant glutathione (221,222). Following prolonged exercise and heavy training, glutamine availability is reduced, providing the rationale for using glutamine supplements as an ergogenic aid. The typical supplemental dose of L-glutamine ranges from 250 to 100 mg/capsule (221). However, there is no evidence that consumption of glutamine supplements before and after exercise benefits immune function. There is limited evidence that there may be a reduction in upper respiratory symptoms following endurance events in athletes who supplement with glutamine. While glutamine supplementation may improve some fatigue parameters, there does not appear to be a clear benefit on performance outcomes related to aerobic performance, the athlete's immune system, or body composition (223,224).

Echinacea

This is a herbal extract that claims to enhance immune function, but there is limited support for this claim. Recent studies suggest that there is no effect of echinacea on infection incidence or severity. In nontrained females, 8 weeks of echinacea extract supplementation coupled with resistance training had no significant impact on inflammatory factors (225).

Omega-3 Fatty Acids

Omega-3 fatty acids are found in cold water fish oils, flax seeds, walnuts, and chia seeds, and may positively influence immune function, anxiety, BP, and inflammation. There are also claims that omega-3 fatty acids, typically supplemented as eicosapentaenoic acid (EPA) and docosahexaenoic acid (DHA), also have anti-inflammatory and recovery benefits following exercise (226). There is no evidence that omega-3 fatty acids reduce upper respiratory symptoms in athletes and limited support suggests that it lowers inflammation following muscle-damaging eccentric exercise. There is some evidence that supplementation improves cognitive function in healthy older adults, but it is unclear if this effect benefits younger, healthy athletes with either health or athletic performance. The general claims that omega-3 fatty acid supplementation helps to promote muscle recovery or promotes muscle growth are not well supported in studies that followed athletes for less than 6 weeks (226). However, longer studies that followed athletes for 8 weeks or longer were more likely to observe positive changes in athletes

(227). It is possible that these longer-term benefits relate to a dietary change that focuses more on omega-3 fatty acids, which may result in a lower consumption of saturated fatty acids, which are known to be more inflammatory (228).

Energy Drinks

The popularity of energy drinks (not to be confused with sports beverages) has grown dramatically since their introduction over 30 years ago. It has been reported that a large proportion of college students consume energy drinks for a variety of reasons, including insufficient sleep, more energy, greater alertness to study, driving for a long time, mixing with alcohol while partying, and treating a hangover (229). There is increasing awareness that high and/or regular consumption of energy drinks have dangers associated with them (230). Collegiate athletes also commonly consume energy drinks, which are high in caffeine, sugars, and other substances including vitamins, herbal extracts, and amino acids, because of the belief that they are performance enhancing (231). Children and adolescents, a marketing target for energy drinks, are also heavy consumers of this product (232,233). Although popular, serious concerns have been raised regarding the potential negative effects of consuming energy drinks because they have an extremely high concentration of caffeine, typically in the range of 30–134 mg/100 mL. (The maximum FDA recommended limit for caffeine is 20 mg/100 mL.) Some low-volume energy "shots" provided in small containers have a concentration of caffeine that is up to 12 times the FDA recommended limit (234). Despite this all-too-common use, there are clear concerns about the use of energy drinks because they place athletes in clear peril. These concerns include (231,234–238):

- Many energy drinks contain ingredients (B vitamins, glucuronolactone, ginseng extract, guarana, ephedra, yohimbe, ginkgo, kola nut, theophylline, herbs, and/or L-carnitine) for which the health consequences, when consumed alone or in combination, are not well understood.
- There is evidence for an ergogenic benefit for caffeine, but the optimal functional dose demonstrating a performance enhancement is typically in the range of 3–6 mg/kg. Most energy drinks have caffeine concentrations that far exceed this range.
- There have been documented reports of adverse effects from consumption of energy drinks while engaged in physical activity, including palpitations,

agitation, tremor, and GI upset. The acute effects of energy drink consumption include the following:
- Abnormal endothelial function, suggestive of an inflammatory effect that could negatively impact cardiovascular function.
- Elevated norepinephrine levels, resulting in high BP and a fast increase in blood sugar from rapid liver glycogen breakdown. This dramatic lowering of liver glycogen may make it difficult for an athlete to sustain normal blood sugar during an event, with associated lowering of mental acuity and reduced muscle function.
- Sudden death has been documented in individuals who have consumed energy drinks in conjunction with exercise.
- Abnormal neurologic symptoms that include epileptic seizures, reversible cerebral vasoconstriction, and intracerebral hemorrhage.
- GI effects that include diarrhea, nausea, and vomiting.
- Acute renal failure and metabolic acidosis.
- Higher obesity risk, which is likely the result of an acute excess glucose uptake by tissues, resulting in higher tissue fat manufacture.
- Acute psychosis, including mind-racing, restlessness, jitteriness, trouble sleeping, and greater likelihood of risk-taking behavior.
- Fatalities have been reported in individuals who combine energy drinks with alcohol.

Because children are typically smaller than adults, children consuming a standard container of an energy drink will receive a higher relative dose of the contents, resulting in an even greater frequency of the adverse effects described above. As a result, the American College of Sports Medicine's position on energy drinks is that *they should not be consumed by children or adolescents for any reason or purpose* (231). This recommendation has become increasingly difficult to apply, as there are persistent beliefs in adolescent athletes that, while they have different beliefs about sports beverages and energy drinks, many maintain beliefs that energy drinks cause no harm and are effective (239,240). In addition, it is important to note that the American College of Sports Medicine also recommends that *health care providers, athletic trainers, sports medicine physicians, personal trainers, should educate their patients or clients about energy drink use and potential adverse events* (231). The goal is to provide sufficient science-based information about the potential adverse effects of energy drinks so that athletes and clients can make an informed choice about whether to consume them.

FIGURE 13.5: Common supplements with strong evidence of performance effect (green); moderate evidence of performance effect (amber); or lack of evidence of performance effect or prohibited substance. (From Close GL, Hamilton DL, Philp A, Burke LM, Morton JP. New strategies in sport nutrition to increase exercise performance. Free Radic Biol Med. 2016;98:144–58.) *ZMA refers to a supplement containing zinc, magnesium, and vitamin B-6.

	Green	Amber	Red
Endurance	Caffeine Carbohydrate gels/drinks Beta-alanine Beetroot juice Sodium bicarb/citrate Antioxidants	Taurine Cherry active L-Carnitine	Ephedrine Methylhexanamine Herbal supplements Citrulline malate L-Arginine Synephrine
Strength/Size	Creatine Protein	Leucine BCAAs	ZMA* Anything "Anabolic" Testosterone Boosters Herbal supplements Colostrum
Health	Probiotics Electrolytes Vitamin D	Vitamin C Multivitamin Glucosamine Quercetin Glutamine Fish oil Collagen	Magnesium Herbal supplements

SUMMARY

There is an expanding, wide array of products that manufacturers imply will result in athletic performance enhancement:

- On balance, it appears that the most effective performance enhancement that athletes can achieve will result from exposure to a wide array of nutrients from a varied and well-balanced diet, maintenance of good energy balance throughout the day and, in particular, during the athletic endeavor, and sustaining a well-hydrated state.

- Certain supplements, such as vitamin D and/or carbohydrate, help to fulfill what may be difficult for some athletes to obtain because of the nature of the sport (*e.g.*, indoors away from sunlight), or a tradition that encourages low body weight through restrictive eating.

- There may well be a benefit for some supplements for certain athletes, such as creatine monohydrate for power athletes. However, athletes should consider carefully if the money spent on creatine would be better spent on good-quality foods that can help maintain a satisfactory energy balance (Figure 13.5).

- Importantly, anyone purchasing a consumable item should expect that the label contains an accurate list of the ingredients and the amounts of each contained within each serving.

- There is evidence, however, that this is not the case with all supplement products, that a significant proportion of them contain WADA banned substances not listed on the label, and that protein powders were found to be contaminated with lead at a level considered unhealthy (33,241).

- Other reports found excessive levels of heavy metals (arsenic, lead, and mercury) in protein powders and drinks (33).

- Male bodybuilders from Iran who were taking combinations of dietary supplements were found to develop hepatitis as a result of product contamination (242).

- Athletes who decide to consume an ergogenic aid/supplement should proceed cautiously. Although the risks may be small, the risk exists.

- Athletes should not rely on the person or company selling the supplement to provide an unbiased view of what it may do. They should have a conversation with an appropriately credentialed health professional to determine if there are any negative aspects to the supplement to be taken.

- Athletes should take objective measures on whether the consumed supplement is actually benefiting them in the expected way, and whether there are any negative side effects (*i.e.*, GI discomfort) that may be attributed to the consumed product.

- Of the ergogenic aids reviewed in this chapter, the ones with the greatest promise are food or sunshine-based: vitamin D, carbohydrate, food-based probiotics, and naturally occurring nitrate (*i.e.*, beet juice). Athletes should consider these first before experimenting with other products.

- The benefits achieved from consumption of a well-balanced diet coupled with regular doses of sunlight may well eliminate the desire to look elsewhere to improve performance.

Practical Application Activity

Using the procedure described in earlier chapters, create a spreadsheet with calcium, iron, and folic acid (folate) consumed from foods and beverages in a typical day by accessing the online USDA Food Composition Database (https://ods.od.nih.gov/factsheets/list-all/).

1. If your intake is low in any of these nutrients, modify your diet to see what foods you would require to help ensure an adequate intake of these nutrients.

2. Now take a typical multivitamin supplement that you find on the internet that targets athletes and add the nutrients/amounts listed on the label into the spreadsheet for each of the three nutrients.
3. Add the recommended intake to your daily intake and analyze these nutrients again.
4. Find what the possible problems and benefits are with daily consumption of this level of nutrient intake by looking up the nutrients on the Office of Dietary Supplements of the NIH website (https://ods.od.nih.gov/).

CHAPTER QUESTIONS

1. Athletes commonly take dietary supplements because they believe the supplement
   a. Will improve athletic performance
   b. Will help to satisfy the nutritional needs associated with heavy training
   c. Will help them become successful like the athlete who is taking the same supplement
   d. All the above
   e. a and b only

2. The term *ergogenic aid* refers to a substance that
   a. Improves flexibility
   b. Is performance enhancing
   c. Helps to satisfy the need for energy during physical activity
   d. Helps an athlete achieve a good night's sleep

3. A nutritional ergogenic aid
   a. Must be a known vitamin
   b. Must be a substance naturally and normally consumed in foods
   c. Must be a protein that improves energy metabolism
   d. Must be a mineral that enhances blood volume and aids the sweat rate

4. A significant proportion of ergogenic aids and vitamin supplements that target athletes in advertisements contain banned substances that are not listed on the label.
   a. True
   b. False

5. The *placebo effect* refers to
   a. The benefit derived from a consumed substance that unexpectedly resulted in a cellular improvement in energy metabolism.

   b. The performance benefit derived from a consumed substance that had no biologic benefit, but resulted in an improvement because the athlete believed it would help.
   c. The improvement in exercise performance resulting from regular consumption of an ergogenic aid rather than periodic/irregular consumption.
   d. The synergistic performance benefit derived from the intake of two different substances when the intake of either substance by itself results in no benefit.

6. The performance benefit derived from an increase in protein consumption may be the result of an improved energy balance resulting from the protein rather than any other protein-specific anabolic function.
   a. True
   b. False

7. Of the following, which is *not* a known primary effect of caffeine in athletes?
   a. It stimulates the central nervous system
   b. It increases muscle mass
   c. It lowers perceived effort during exercise
   d. It lowers the feeling of pain and fatigue associated with exercise

8. The maximal performance benefit from caffeine is reached at an intake level of
   a. 3 mg/kg
   b. 3 g/kg
   c. 6 mg/kg
   d. 15 mg/kg

9. Regular consumption of carbohydrate at a level of _____ is useful for optimizing muscle glycogen storage in preparation for a sporting event.
   a. 7–12 g/kg/day
   b. 3–4 g/kg/day
   c. 15–20 mg/kg/day
   d. 15–20 g/kg/day

10. Beetroot juice has been shown to improve _____ availability.
    a. NOS
    b. Nitric oxide
    c. L-Arginine
    d. Red blood cell concentration

ANSWERS TO CHAPTER QUESTIONS

1. d
2. b
3. b
4. a
5. b

6. a
7. b
8. c
9. a
10. b

Case Study Considerations

1. **Case Study Answer 1:** The best strategy for consuming beet juice is to make certain that (1) it does not negatively impact your digestive system, and (2) assure that the conversion of the nitrate in beet juice can be converted to nitrite via oral bacteria. Nitrite is the precursor to nitric oxide, which is a vasodilator. This can only occur if the bacteria are present, so it is necessary to avoid use of antibiotic mouthwash. Ideally, the beet juice should be consumed slowly with no other foods or beverages to enhance time of contact with oral bacteria. Studies show that half a liter consumed 1–2 hours prior to exercise is effective.

2. **Case Study Answer 2:** Consumption of beet juice is not a substitute for the pregame meal that should be relatively high in low-fiber carbohydrate with low fat and moderate protein…all consumed with plenty of water. The purpose of the beet juice is to enhance the production of nitric oxide, which is a vasodilator. The nitric oxide lowers blood pressure while enhancing oxygen and nutrient delivery to cells. The improved oxygen delivery enhances fat metabolism while lowering carbohydrate utilization. The lower carbohydrate utilization enhances time to fatigue.

3. **Case Study Answer 3:** An important lesson from this case study is that "More than enough is not better than enough." Typically, having too much of one food or beverage limits the consumption of other foods/beverages that are also needed to ensure optimal tissue exposure to required nutrients (vitamins, minerals, carbohydrate, protein, fat). It is far too common for athletes to believe that a certain substance is "good" for them, so they tend to overconsume that substance at the expense of other foods/beverages. Ideally, athletes should strive to have a dynamic relationship between their eating patterns and nutrient needs. This requires planning for what to consume, and when it is best to consume it to stay in a good energy/nutrient balanced state. High-fiber foods, for instance, should not be consumed prior to exercise because they cause bloating and delayed gastric emptying. However, several hours prior to exercise and after exercise high-fiber foods are important to consume because they provide "food" for the gut microbiome, and also help to mediate the delivery of nutrients to cells. So, it's not just what to eat, but when to eat it that are important considerations. In general, a variety of high-carbohydrate, moderate protein, low-fat meals should be consumed with plenty of water. Protein should be distributed well throughout the day (~30 g/meal) with meals that enable a good energy-balanced state.

REFERENCES

1. Rautiainen S, Gaziano JM, Christen WG, Bubes V, Kotler G, Glynn RJ, Mansn JE, Buring JE, Sesso HD. Effect of baseline nutritional status on long-term multivitamin use and cardiovascular disease risk: a secondary analysis of the Physicians' Health Study II Randomized Clinical Trial. JAMA Cardiol. 2017:2(6):617–25.

2. Mursu J, Robien K, Harnack LJ, Park K, Jacobs DR Jr. Dietary supplements and mortality rate in older women: the Iowa Women's Health Study. Arch Intern Med. 2011;171(18): 1625–33.

3. Buell JL, Franks R, Ransone J, Powers ME, Laquale KM, Carlson-Phillips A; National Athletic Trainers' Association. National Athletic Trainers' Association position statement: evaluation of dietary supplements for performance nutrition. J Athl Train. 2013;48(1):124–36.

4. Thomas DT, Erdman KA, Burke LM. American College of Sports Medicine joint position statement. Nutrition and athletic performance. Med Sci Sports Exerc. 2016;48(3):543–68.

5. United States Department of Health and Human Services, National Institutes of Health. Public Law 103–417. 103rd Congress. Dietary supplement Health and Education Act of 1994.

6. Maughan RJ, Burke LM, Dvorak J, Larson-Meyer DE, Peeling P, Phillips SM, Rawson ES, Walsh NP, Garthe I, Geyer H, Meeusen R, van Loon LJC, Shirreffs SM, Spriet LL, Stuart M, Vernec A, Currell K, Ali VM, Budgett RG, Ljungqvist A, Mountjoy M, Pitsiladis YP, Soligard T, Erdener U, Engebretsen L. IOC consensus statement: dietary supplements and the high-performance athlete. Br J Sports Med. 2018;52(7): 439–55.

7. Juhn M. Popular sports supplements and ergogenic aids. Sports Med. 2003;33(12):921–39.

8. Maughan RJ, Depiesse F, Geyer H; International Association of Athletics Federations. The use of dietary supplements by athletes. J Sports Sci. 2007;25(Suppl 1):S103–13.

9. Froiland K, Koszewski W, Hingst J, Kopecky L. Nutritional supplement use among college athletes and their sources of information. Int J Sport Nut Exerc Metab. 2004;14(1):104–20.

10. Knapik JJ, Steelman RA, Hoedebecke SS, Austin KG, Farina EK, Lieberman HR. Prevalence of dietary supplement use by athletes: systematic review and meta-analysis. Sports Med. 2016;46:103–23.

11. Garthe I, Ramsbottom R. Elite athletes, a rationale for the use of dietary supplements: a practical approach. PharmaNutrition. 2020;14:100234.

12. Maughan RJ, Shirreffs SM. Making decisions about supplement use. Int J Sport Nutr Exerc Metab. 2018;28 212–9.

13. Barrack MT, Sassone J, Dizon F, Wu AC, DeLuca S, Ackerman KE, Tenforde AS. Dietary supplement intake and factors associated with increased use in preadolescent endurance runners. J Acad Nutr Diet. 2022;122(3):573–82.

14. Mazzilli M, Macaluso F, Zambelli S, Picerno P, Luciano E. The use of dietary supplements in fitness practitioners: a cross-sectional observation study. Int J Environ Res Public Health. 2021;18:5005.

15. Slesinski MJ, Subar AF, Kahle LL. Trends in the use of vitamin and mineral supplements in the United States: the 1987 and 1992 National Health Interview Surveys. J Am Diet Assoc. 1995;95(8):921–3.

16. Fairfield KM, Fletcher RH. Vitamins for chronic disease prevention in adults: scientific review. JAMA. 2002;287(23): 3116–26.

17. Lukaski HC. Vitamin and mineral status: effects on physical performance. Nutrition. 2004;20:632–44.

18. Manore MM. Dietary supplements for improving body composition and reducing body weight: where is the evidence? Int J Sport Nutr Exerc Metab. 2012;22(2):139–54.

19. Manore MM. Vitamins and minerals: part I. How much do I need? ACSM's Health Fit J. 2001;5(3):33–5.

20. Manore MM. Vitamins and minerals: part II. Who needs to supplement? ACSM's Health Fitness J. 2001;5(4):30–4.

21. Williams J, Mai CT, Mulinare J, Isenburg J, Flood TJ, Ethen M, Frohnert B, Kirby RS; Centers for Disease Control and Prevention. Updated estimates of neural tube defects prevented by mandatory folic acid fortification — United States, 1995–2011. MMWR Morb Mortal Wkly Rep. 2015;64(01):1–5.

22. Institute of Medicine, Food and Nutrition Board. Dietary reference intakes: thiamin, riboflavin, niacin, vitamin B_6, folate, vitamin B_{12}, pantothenic acid, biotin, and choline. Washington (DC): National Academy Press; 1998.

23. Watanabe F, Yabuta Y, Bito T, Teng F. Vitamin B_{12}-containing plant food sources for vegetarians. Nutrients. 2014;6: 1861–73.

24. LeBlanc JG, Milani C, de Giori GS, Sesma F, van Sinderen D, Ventura M. Bacteria as vitamin suppliers to their host: a gut microbiota perspective. Curr Opin Biotechnol. 2013;24(2): 160–8.

25. Nowak JK, Grzybowczyka-Chlebowczyk U, Landowski P, Szaflarska-Poplawska A, Klincewicz B, Adamczak D, Banasiewicz T, Plawski A, Walkowiak J. Prevalence and correlates of vitamin K deficiency in children with inflammatory bowel disease. Sci Rep. 2014;4:4768.

26. Manore MM. Effect of physical activity on thiamine, riboflavin, and vitamin B-6 requirements. Am J Clin Nutr. 2000;72: 598S–606S.

27. United States Department of Health and Human Services, National Institutes of Health, NIDDK. Lactose intolerance. Accessed 2017 November. Available from: https://www.niddk.nih.gov/health-information/digestive-diseases/lactose-intolerance

28. Diehl K, Thiel A, Zipfel S, Mayer J, Schnell A, Schneider S. Elite adolescent athletes' use of dietary supplements: characteristics, opinions, and sources of supply and information. Int J Sport Nutr Exerc Metab. 2012;22:165–74.

29. Lun V, Erdman KA, Fung TS, Reimer RA. Dietary supplementation practices in Canadian high-performance athletes. Int J Sport Nutr Exerc Metab. 2012;22:31–7.

30. Freschi M, Pollastri L. Injury and health risk management sports . In: Krutsch W, editor. ESKKA; 2020. Chapter 60, Nutritional supplements; p. 399–403.

31. Catlin DH, Leder BZ, Ahrens B, Starcevic B, Hatton CK, Green GA, Finkelstein JS. Trace contamination of over-the-counter androstenedione and positive urine test results for a nandrolone metabolite. JAMA. 2000;284(20):2618–21.

32. Geyer M, Parr MK, Mareck U, Reinhart U, Schrader Y, Schänzer W. Analysis of non-hormonal nutritional supplements for

anabolic-androgenic steroids—results of an international study. Int J Sports Med. 2004;25(2):124–9.

33. Maughan RJ. Sports nutrition. International Olympic Committee. In: Maughan RJ, editor. 1st ed. London: John Wiley & Sons, Ltd.; 2014. Chapter 23, Risks and rewards of dietary supplement use by athletes.

34. Outram S, Stewart B. Doping through supplement use: a review of available empirical data. Int J Sport Nutr Exerc Metab. 2015;25(1):54–9.

35. Petroczi A, Taylor G, Naughton DP. Mission impossible? Regulatory and enforcement issues to ensure safety of dietary supplements. Food Chem Toxicol. 2011;49(2):393–402.

36. Huang H-Y, Caballero B, Chang S, Alberg AJ, Semba RD, Schneyer CR, Wilson RF, Cheng TY, Vassy J, Prokopowicz G, Barnes GJ II, Bass EB. The efficacy and safety of multivitamin and mineral supplement use to prevent cancer and chronic disease in adults: a systematic review for a National Institute of Health State-of-the-Science Conference. Ann Intern Med. 2006;145(5):372–85.

37. Lazic JS, Dikic N, Radivojevic N, Mazic S, Radovanovic D, Mitrovic N, Lazic M, Zivanic S, Suzic S. Dietary supplements and medications in elite sport—polypharmacy or real need? Scand J Med Sci Sports. 2011;21(2):260–7.

38. Butterfield G, Cady C, Moynihan S. Effect of increasing protein intake on nitrogen balance in recreational weight lifters. Med Sci Sports Exerc. 1992;24:S71.

39. Desbrow B, Hall S, Irwin C. Caffeine content of Nespresso® pod coffee. Nutr Health. 2019;25(1):3–7.

40. Schubert MM, Irwin C, Seay RF, Clarke HE, Allegro D, Desbrow B. Caffeine, coffee, and appetite control: a review. Int J Food Sci Nutr. 2017;68(8):901–12.

41. Sicova M, Guest NS, Terrell PN, El-Sohemy A. Caffeine, genetic variation and anaerobic performance in male athletes: a randomized controlled trial. Eur J Appl Physiol. 2021; 121(12):3499–513.

42. Shen JG, Brooks MB, Cincotta J, Manjourides JD. Establishing a relationship between the effect of caffeine and duration of endurance athletic time trial events: a systematic review and meta-analysis. J Sci Med Sport. 2019;22(2):232–8.

43. Burke L, Desbrow B, Spriet L. Caffeine for sports performance. Champaign (IL): Human Kinetics; 2013.

44. Spriet LL. Exercise and sport performance with low doses of caffeine. Sports Med. 2014;44(Suppl 2):S175–84.

45. Burke LM. Caffeine and sports performance. Appl Physiol Nutr Metab. 2008;33(6):1319–34.

46. Tarnopolsky MA. Caffeine and creatine use in sport. Ann Nutr Metab. 2010;57(2):1–8.

47. Ganio MS, Klau JF, Casa DJ, Armstrong LE, Maresh CM. Effect of caffeine on sport-specific endurance performance: a systematic review. J Strength Cond Res. 2009;23(1):315–24.

48. Talanian JL, Spriet LL. Low and moderate doses of caffeine late in exercise improve performance in trained cyclists. Appl Physiol Nutr Metab. 2016;41(8):850–5.

49. Murphy MJ, Rushing BR, Summer SJ, Hackney AC. Dietary supplements for athletic performance in women: beta-alanine, caffeine, and nitrate. Int J Sport Nutr Exerc Metab. 2022; 32(4):311–23.

50. Skinner TL, Desbrow B, Arapova J, Schaumberg MA, Osborne J, Grant GD, Anoopkumar-Dukie S, Leveritt MD. Women experience the same ergogenic response to caffeine as men. Med Sci Sports Exerc. 2019;51(6):1195–202.

51. Tambalis KD, Arnaoutis G. The role of caffeine consumption on individuals' health and athletic performance: an overview. Int J Physiol Nutr Phys Educ. 2022;7(1):215–24.

52. Ganio MS, Klau JF, Casa DJ, Armstrong LE, Maresh CM. Effect of caffeine on sport-specific endurance performance: a systematic review. J Strength Cond Res. 2009;23(1):315–24.

53. Grgic J, Mikulic P. Acute effects of caffeine supplementation on resistance exercise, jumping, and Wingate performance: no influence of habitual caffeine intake. Eur J Sport Sci. 2021; 21(8):1165–75.

54. Clarke ND, Richardson DL. Habitual caffeine consumption does not affect the ergogenicity of coffee ingestion during a 5 km cycling time trial. Int J Sport Nutr Exerc Metab. 2021; 31(1):13–20.

55. Womack CJ, Saunders MJ, Bechtel MK, Bolton DJ, Martin M, Luden ND, Dunham W, Hancock M. The influence of a CYP1A2 polymorphism on the ergogenic effects of caffeine. J Int Soc Sports Nutr. 2012;9(1):7.

56. Graham TE, Spriet LL. Metabolic, catecholamine, and exercise performance responses to varying doses of caffeine. J Appl Physiol (1985). 1995;78(3):867–74.

57. Lane SC, Areta JL, Bird SR, Coffey VG, Burke LM, Desbrow B, Karagounis LG, Hawley JA. Caffeine ingestion and cycling power output in a low or normal muscle glycogen state. Med Sci Sports Exerc. 2013;45(8):1577–84.

58. Jiménez SL, Diaz-Lara J, Pareja-Galeano H, Del Coso J. Caffeinated drinks and physical performance in sport: a systematic review. Nutrients. 2021;13(9):2944.

59. Duncan MJ, Oxford SW. The effect of caffeine ingestion on mood state and bench press performance to failure. J Strength Cond Res. 2011;25(1):178–85.

60. Lopes-Silva JP, Choo HC, Franchini E, Abbiss CR. Isolated ingestion of caffeine and sodium bicarbonate on repeated sprint performance: a systematic review and meta-analysis. J Sci Med Sport. 2019;22(8):962–72.

61. Podlogar T, Wallis GA. New horizons in carbohydrate research and application for endurance athletes. Sports Med. 2022;52(Suppl 1):S5–23.

62. Furber MJW, Young GR, Holt GS, Pyle S, Davison G, Roberts MG, Roberts JD, Howatson G, Smith DL. Gut microbial stability is associated with greater endurance performance in athletes undertaking dietary periodization. mSystems. 2022;7(3):e0012922.

63. Zdzieblik D, Friesenborg H, Gollhofer A, König D. Effect of a high fat diet vs. high carbohydrate diets with different glycemic indices on metabolic parameters in male endurance athletes: a pilot trial. Front Nutr. 2022;9:802374.

64. Nagle FJ, Bassett DR. Nutrition in exercise and sport. In: Hickson JF, Wolinsky I, editors. Boca Raton (FL): CRC Press; 1989. Energy metabolism; p. 87–106.

65. Valeriani A. The need for carbohydrate intake during endurance exercise. Sports Med. 1991;12(6):349–58.

66. Stellingwerff T, Cox GR. Systematic review: carbohydrate supplementation on exercise performance or capacity of varying durations. Appl Physiol Nutr Metab. 2014;39(9):998–1011.

67. De Moraes WMAM, de Almeida FN, dos Santos LEA, Cavalcante KDG, Santos HO, Navata JW, Prestes J. Carbohydrate

loading practice in bodybuilders: effects on muscle thickness, photo silhouette scores, mood states and gastrointestinal symptoms. J Sports Sci Med. 2019;18(4):772–9.

68. King AJ, Etxebarria N, Ross ML, Garvican-Lewis L, Heikura IA, McKay AKA, Tee N, Forbes SF, Beard NA, Saunders PU, Sharma AP, Gaskell SK, Costa RJS, Burke LM. Short-term very high carbohydrate diet and gut-training have minor effects on gastrointestinal status and performance in highly trained endurance athletes. Nutrients. 2022;14(9):1929.

69. Hawley JA, Schabort EJ, Noakes TD, Dennis SC. Carbohydrate-loading and exercise performance. An Update. Sports Med. 1997;24(2):73–81.

70. Bergstrom J, Hermansen L, Hultman E, Saltin B. Diet, muscle glycogen, and physical performance. Acta Physiol Scand. 1967;71(2):140–50.

71. Costill DL, Hargreaves M. Carbohydrate nutrition and fatigue. Sports Med. 1992;13(2):86–92.

72. Michalczyk MM, Chycki J, Zajac A, Maszczyk A, Zydek G, Langford J. Anaerobic performance after a low-carbohydrate diet (LCD) followed by 7 days of carbohydrate loading in male basketball players. Nutrients. 2019;11(4):778.

73. Shiose K, Takahashi H, Yamada Y. Muscle glycogen assessment and relationship with body hydration status: a narrative review. Nutrients. 2023;15(1):155.

74. Coyle EF. Ross symposium on nutrient utilization during exercise. In: Fox EL, editor. Columbus (OH): Ross Laboratories; 1983. Effects of glucose polymer feedings on fatigability and the metabolic response to prolonged strenuous exercise; p. 4–11.

75. Castell LM, Burke LM, Stear SJ, Maughan RJ. BJSM reviews: A-Z of nutritional supplements: dietary supplements, sports nutrition foods and ergogenic aids for health and performance part 8. Br J Sports Med. 2010;44(6):468–70.

76. Mountjoy M, Sundgot-Borgen J, Burke L, Carter S, Constantini N, Lebrun C, Meyer N, Sherman R, Steffen K, Budgett R, Ljungqvist A. The IOC consensus statement: beyond the female athlete triad–Relative Energy Deficiency in Sport (RED-S). Br J Sports Med. 2014;48(7):491–7.

77. Begum G, Cunliffe A, Leveritt M. Physiological role of carnosine in contracting muscle. Int J Sport Nutr Exerc Metab. 2005;15:493–514.

78. Blancquaert L, Everaert I, Derave W. Beta-alanine supplementation, muscle carnosine and exercise performance. Curr Opin Clin Nutr Metab Care. 2015;18(1):63–70.

79. Stellingwerff T, Decombaz J, Harris RC, Boesch C. Optimizing human in vivo dosing and delivery of beta-alanine supplements for muscle carnosine synthesis. Amino Acids. 2012; 43(1):57–65.

80. Rezende NS, Swinton P, de Oliveira LF, da Silva RP, da Eira Silva V, Nemezio K, Yamaguchi G, Artioli GG, Gualano B, Saunders B, Dolan E. The muscle carnosine response to beta-alanine supplementation: a systematic review with Bayesian individual and aggregate data E-max model and meta-analysis. Front Physiol. 2020;11:913.

81. Stegen S, Bex T, Vervaet C, Vanhee L, Achten E, Derave W. Beta-alanine dose for maintaining moderately elevated muscle carnosine levels. Med Sci Sports Exerc. 2014;46(7):1426–32.

82. Saunders B, Elliott-Sale K, Artioli GG, Swinton PA, Dolan E, Roschel H, Sale C, Gualano B. β-alanine supplementation to improve exercise capacity and performance: a systematic review and meta-analysis. Br J Sports Med. 2017;51(8): 658–69.

83. Dolan E, Swinton PA, Painelli VS, Hemingway BS, Mazzolani B, Smaira FI, Saunders B, Artioli GG, Gualano B. A systematic risk assessment and meta-analysis on the use of oral β-alanine supplementation. Adv Nutr. 2019;10(3):452–63.

84. Bellinger PM. β-Alanine supplementation for athletic performance: an update. J Strength Cond Res. 2014;28(6):1751–70.

85. Bex T, Chung W, Baguet A, Stegen S, Stautemas J, Achten E, Derave W. Muscle carnosine loading by beta-alanine supplementation is more pronounced in trained vs. untrained muscles. J Appl Physiol(1985). 2014;116(2):204–9.

86. Brisola GMP, Zagatto AM. Ergogenic effects of β-alanine supplementation on different sports modalities: strong evidence or only incipient findings? J Strength Cond Res. 2019; 33(1):253–82.

87. De Camargo JBB, Brigitte FA, Zaroni RS, Germano D, Souza D, Bacurau RF, Marchetti PH, Braz TV, Aoki MS, Lopes CR. Does beta-alanine supplementation enhance adaptations to resistance training? A randomized, placebo-controlled, double-blind study. Biol Sport. 2023;40(1):217–24.

88. Smith CF, Harty PS, Stecker RA, Kerksick CM. A pilot study to examine the impact of beta-alanine supplementation on anaerobic exercise performance in collegiate rugby athletes. Sports. 2019;7(11):231.

89. Ashtary-Larky D, Bagheri R, Ghanavati M, Asbagh O, Wong A, Stout JR, Suzuki K. Effects of beta-alanine supplementation on body composition: a GRADE-assessed systematic review and meta-analysis. J Int Soc Sports Nutr. 2022;19(1):196–218.

90. da Silva RP, de Oliveira LF, Saunders B, Kratz CA, Painelli VS, Silva VE, Marins JCB, Franchini E, Gualano B, Artioli GG. Effects of β-Alanine and sodium bicarbonate supplementation on the estimated energy system contribution during high-intensity intermittent exercise. Amino Acids. 2019; 51(1):83–96.

91. Jones AM. Dietary nitrate supplementation and exercise performance. Sports Med. 2014;44(Suppl 1):S35–45.

92. Overdevest E, Wouters JA, Wolfs KHM, van Leeuwen JJM, Possemiers S. Citrus flavonoid supplementation improves exercise performance in trained athletes. J Sports Sci Med. 2018;17(1):24–30.

93. Stamler JS, Meissner G. Physiology of nitric oxide in skeletal muscle. Physiol Rev. 2001;81(1):209–37.

94. Senefeld JW, Wiggins CC, Regimbal RJ, Dominelli PB, Baker SE, Joyner MJ. Ergogenic effect of nitrate supplementation: a systematic review and meta-analysis. Med Sci Sports Exerc. 2020;52(10):2250–61.

95. Moncada S, Higgs A. The L-arginine-nitric oxide pathway. N Engl J Med. 1993;329(27):2002–12.

96. Duncan C, Dougall H, Johnston P, Green S, Brogan R, Leifert C, Smith L, Golden M, Benjamin N. Chemical generation of nitric oxide in the mouth from the enterosalivary circulation of dietary nitrate. Nat Med. 1995;1(6):546–51.

97. Münzel T, Daiber A. Inorganic nitrite and nitrate in cardiovascular therapy: a better alternative to organic nitrates as nitric oxide donors? Vasc Pharmacol. 2018;102:1–10.

98. Omar SA, Artime E, Webb AJ. A comparison of organic and inorganic nitrates/nitrites. Nitric Oxide, 2012;26(4):229–40.

99. O'Gallagher K, Cardona SB, Hill C, Al-Saedi A, Shahed F, Floyd CN, McNeill K, Mills CE, Webb AJ. Grapefruit juice enhances the systolic blood pressure-lowering effects of dietary nitrate-containing beetroot juice. Br J Clin Pharmacol. 2021;87(2):577–87.

100. Jonvik KL, Nyakayiru J, Pinckaers PJ, Senden JM, van Loon LJ, Verdijk LB. Nitrate-rich vegetables increase plasma nitrate and nitrite concentrations and lower blood pressure in healthy adults. J Nutr. 2016;146(5):986–93.

101. Hughan KS, Wendell SG, Delmastro-Greenwood M, Helbling N, Corey C, Bellavia L, Potti G, Grimes G, Goodpaster B, Kim-Shapiro DB, Shiva S, Freeman BA, Gladwin M. Conjugated linoleic acid modulates clinical responses to oral nitrite and nitrate. Hypertension. 2017;70(3):634–44.

102. Sweazea KL, Johnston CS, Miller B, Gumpricht E. Nitrate-rich fruit and vegetable supplement reduces blood pressure in normotensive healthy young males without significantly altering flow-mediated vasodilation: a randomized, double-blinded, controlled trial. J Nutr Metab. 2018;2018:1729653.

103. Kim DJ-K, Roe CA, Somani YB, Moore DJ, Barrett MA, Flanagan M, Kim-Shapiro DB, Basu S, Muller MD, Proctor DN. Effects of acute dietary nitrate supplementation on aortic blood pressures and pulse wave characteristics in post-menopausal women. Nitric Oxide. 2019;85:10–16.

104. Shepherd AI, Costello JT, Bailey SJ, Bishop N, Wadley AJ, Young-Min S, Gilchrist M, Mayes H, White D, Gorczynski P, Saynor ZL, Massey H, Eglin CM. "Beet" the cold: beetroot juice supplementation improves peripheral blood flow, endothelial function, and anti-inflammatory status in individuals with Raynaud's phenomenon. J Appl Physiol. 2019;127(5):1478–90.

105. Goh CE, Trinh P, Colombo PC, Genkinger JM, Mathema B, Uhlemann A-C, LeDuc C, Leibel R, Rosenbaum M, Paster BJ, Desvarieux M, Papapanou PN, Jacobs DR Jr, Demmer RT. Association between nitrate-reducing oral bacteria and cardiometabolic outcomes: results from origins. J Am Heart Assoc. 2019;8(23):e013324.

106. Tribble GD, Angelov N, Weltman R, Wang B-Y, Eswaran SV, Gay IC, Parthasarathy K, Dao D-HV, Richardson KN, Ismail NM, Sharina IG, Hyde ER, Ajami NJ, Petrosino JF, Bryan NS. Frequency of tongue cleaning impacts the human tongue microbiome composition and enterosalivary circulation of nitrate. Front Cell Infect Microbiol. 2019;9:39.

107. Husmann F, Bruhn S, Mittlmeier T, Zschorlich V, Behrens M. Dietary nitrate supplementation improves exercise tolerance by reducing muscle fatigue and perceptual responses. Front Physiol. 2019;10:404.

108. Cutler C, Kiernan M, Willis JR, Gallardo-Alfaro L, Casas-Agustench P, White D, Hickson M, Gabaldon T, Bescos R. Post-exercise hypotension and skeletal muscle oxygenation is regulated by nitrate-reducing activity of oral bacteria. Free Radical Biol Med. 2019;143:252–9.

109. Lansley KE, Winyard PG, Bailey SJ, Vanhatalo A, Wilkerson DP, Blackwell JR, Gilchrist M, Benjamin N, Jones AM. Acute dietary nitrate supplementation improves cycling time trial performance. Med Sci Sports Exerc. 2011;43(6):1125–31.

110. Lundberg JO, Govoni M. Inorganic nitrate is a possible source for systemic generation of nitric oxide. Free Radic Biol Med. 2004;37:395–400.

111. Kapil V, Haydara SMA, Pearl V, Lundbergh JO, Weitzbergh E, Ahluwaliaa A. Physiological role for nitrate-reducing oral bacteria in blood pressure control. Free Radic Biol Med. 2013;55:93–100.

112. Liddle L, Burleigh MC, Monaghan C, Muggeridge DJ, Sculthorpe N, Pedlar CR, Butcher J, Henriquez FL, Easton C. Variability in nitrate-reducing oral bacteria and nitric oxide metabolites in biological fluids following dietary nitrate administration: an assessment of the critical difference. Nitric Oxide. 2019;83:1–10.

113. Larsen FJ, Weitzberg E, Lundberg JO, Ekblom B. Effects of dietary nitrate on oxygen cost during exercise. Acta Physiol (Oxf). 2007;191:59–66.

114. Bailey SJ, Winyard P, Vanhatalo A, Blackwell JR, Dimenna FJ, Wilkerson DP, Tarr J, Benjamin N, Jones AM. Dietary nitrate supplementation reduces the O_2 cost of low-intensity exercise and enhances tolerance to high-intensity exercise in humans. J Appl Physiol(1985). 2009;107(4):1144–55.

115. Larsen FJ, Weitzberg E, Lundberg JO, Ekblom B. Dietary nitrate reduces maximal oxygen consumption while maintaining work performance in maximal exercise. Free Radic Biol Med. 2010;48:342–7.

116. Lansley KE, Winyard PG, Fulford J, Vanhatalo A, Bailey SJ, Blackwell JR, DiMenna FJ, Gilchrist M, Benjamin N, Jones AM. Dietary nitrate supplementation reduces the O_2 cost of walking and running: a placebo-controlled study. J Appl Physiol(1985). 2011;110(3):591–600.

117. Vanhatalo A, Bailey S, Blackwell JR, DiMenna FJ, Pavey TG, Wilkerson DP, Benjamin N, Winyard PG, Jones AM. Acute and chronic effects of dietary nitrate supplementation on blood pressure and the physiological responses to moderate-intensity and incremental exercise. Am J Physiol Regul Integr Comp Physiol. 2010;299(4):R1121–31.

118. Volek JS, Rawson ES. Scientific basis and practical aspects of creatine supplementation for athletes. Nutrition. 2004;20(7–8):609–14.

119. Close GL, Kasper AM, Walsh NP, Maughan RJ. Food first but not always food only: recommendations for using dietary supplements in sport. Int J Sport Nutr Exerc Metab. 2022;32(5):371–86.

120. Machado M. A narrative review on athletic performance and safety of creatine supplementation for adolescents. J Biomed Sci. 2022;4(2):OAJBS.ID.000419.

121. Rawson ES, Volek JS. Effects of creatine supplementation and resistance training on muscle strength and weightlifting performance. J Strength Cond Res. 2003;17(4):822–31.

122. Kaviani M, Shaw K, Chilibeck PD. Benefits of creatine supplementation for vegetarians compared to omnivorous athletes: a systematic review. Int J Environ Res Public Health. 2020;17(9):3041.

123. Poortmans JR, Rawson ES, Burke LM, Stear SJ, Castell LM. A-Z of nutritional supplements: dietary supplements, sports nutrition foods and ergogenic aids for health and performance Part 11. Br J Sports Med. 2010;44:765–6.

124. Deminice R, Rosa FT, Franco GS, Jordao AA. Effects of creatine supplementation on oxidative stress and inflammatory markers after repeated-sprint exercise in humans. Nutrition. 2013;29:1127–32.

125. Bemben MG, Lamont HS. Creatine supplementation and exercise performance: recent findings. Sports Med. 2005;35(2):107–25.

126. Burke DG, Chilibeck PD, Parise G, Candow DG, Mahoney D, Tarnopolsky M. Effect of creatine and weight training on muscle creatine and performance in vegetarians. Med Sci Sports Exerc. 2003;35(11):1946–55.

127. Sampaio CRSF, Aidar FJ, Ferreira ARP, dos Santos JL, Marçal AC, de Matos DG, de Souza RF, Moreira OC, Guerra I, Filho JF, Marcucci-Barbosa LS, Nunes-Silva A, de Almeida-Neto PF, Cabral BGAT, Reis VM. Can creatine supplementation interfere with muscle strength and fatigue in Brazilian national level Paralympic powerlifting? Nutrients. 2020;12(9):2492.

128. Cooper R, Naclerio F, Allgrove J, Jimenez A. Creating supplementation with specific view to exercise/sports performance: an update. J Int Soc Sports Nutr. 2012;9(1):33.

129. Harris RC, Soderlund K, Hultman E. Elevation of creatine in resting and exercised muscle of normal subjects by creatine supplementation. Clin Sci (Lond). 1992;83:367–74.

130. Maughan RJ. Creatine supplementation and exercise performance. Int J Sport Nutr. 1995;5(2):94–101.

131. Steenge GR, Simpson EJ, Greenhaff PL. Protein- and carbohydrate-induced augmentation of whole body creatine retention in humans. J Appl Physiol (1985). 2000;89(3):1165–71.

132. Wax B, Kerksick CM, Jagim AR, Mayo JJ, Lyons BC, Kreider RB. Creatine for exercise and sports performance, with recovery considerations for healthy populations. Nutrients. 2021;13(6):1915.

133. Hall M, Manetta E, Tupper K. Creatine supplementation: an update. Curr Sports Med Rep. 2021;20(7): 338–44.

134. Schilling BK, Stone MH, Utter A, Kearney JT, Johnson M, Coglianese R, Smith L, O'Bryant HS, Fry AC, Starks M, Keith R, Stone ME. Creatine supplementation and health variables: a retrospective study. Med Sci Sports Exerc. 2001;33(2):183–8.

135. Koenig CA, Benardot D, Cody M, Thompson WR. Comparison of creatine monohydrate and carbohydrate supplementation on repeated jump height performance. J Strength Cond Res. 2008;22(4):1081–6.

136. Powers ME, Arnold BL, Weltman AL, Perrin DH, Mistry D, Kahler DM, Kraemer W, Volek J. Creatine supplementation increases total body water without altering fluid distribution. J Athl Train. 2003;38(1):44–50.

137. Pritchard NR, Kalra PA. Creatine supplements linked to renal damage. Lancet. 1998;351(19111):1252–3.

138. Kim HJ, Kim CK, Carpentier A, Poortmans JR. Studies on the safety of creatine supplementation. Amino Acids. 2011;40(5):1409–18.

139. Antonio J, Candow DG, Forbes SC, Gualano B, Jagim AR, Kreider RB, Rawson ES, Smith-Ryan AE, VanDusseldorp TA, Willoughby DS, Ziegenfuss TN. Common questions and misconceptions about creatine supplementation: what does the scientific evidence really show? J Int Soc Sports Nutr. 2021;18(13): https://doi.org/10.1186/s12970-021-00412-w

140. Carr AJ, Slater GJ, Gore CJ, Dawson B, Burke LM. Effect of sodium bicarbonate on [HCO_3^-], pH, and gastrointestinal symptoms. Int J Sport Nutr Exerc Metab. 2011;21(3):189–94.

141. Lancha AH Jr, Painelli VS, Saunders B, Artioli GG. Nutritional strategies to modulate intracellular and extracellular buffering capacity during high-intensity exercise. Sports Med. 2015;45(Suppl 1):S71–81.

142. Close GL, Hamilton DL, Philp A, Burke LM, Morton JP. New strategies in sport nutrition to increase exercise performance. Free Radic Biol Med. 2016;98:144–58.

143. Montgomery DL, Beaudin PA. Blood lactate and heart rate response of young females during gymnastic routines. J Sports Med. 1982;22(3):358–65.

144. Siegler JC, Marshall PWM, Bray J, Towlson C. Sodium bicarbonate supplementation and ingestion timing: does it matter? J Strength Cond Res. 2012;26(7):1953–8.

145. Cannell JJ, Hollis BW, Sorenson MB, Taft TN, Anderson JJB. Athletic performance and vitamin D. Med Sci Sports Exerc. 2009;41(5):1102–10.

146. Urwin CS, Snow RJ, Condo D, Snipe RMJ, Wadley GD, Convit L, Carr AJ. A comparison of sodium citrate and sodium bicarbonate ingestion: blood alkalosis and gastrointestinal symptoms. Int J Sport Nutr Exerc Metab. 2023;33:1–10.

147. Hilton NP, Leach NK, Hilton MM, Sparks SA, McNaughton LR. Enteric-coated sodium bicarbonate supplementation improves high-intensity cycling performance in trained cyclists. Eur J Appl Physiol. 2020;120(7):1563–73.

148. Requena B, Zabala M, Padial P, Belén F. Sodium bicarbonate and sodium citrate: ergogenic aids? J Strength Cond Res. 2005;19(1):213–24.

149. Urwin CS, Snow RJ, Orellana L, Condo D, Wadley GD, Carr AJ. Does varying the ingestion period of sodium citrate influence blood alkalosis and gastrointestinal symptoms? PLoS One. 2021;16(5):e0251808.

150. Grgic J, Garofolini A, Pickering C, Duncan MJ, Tinsley GM, Del Coso J. Isolated effects of caffeine and sodium bicarbonate ingestion on performance in the Yo-Yo test: a systematic review and meta-analysis. J Sci Med Sport. 2020;23:41–47.

151. Lino RS, Lagares LS, Oliveira CVC, Queiroz CO, Pinto LLT, Almeida LAB, Bonfim ES, dos Santos CPC. Effect of sodium bicarbonate supplementation on two different performance indicators in sports: a systematic review with meta-analysis. Phys Act Nutr. 2021;25(1):7–15.

152. Hadzic M, Eckstein ML, Schugardt M. The impact of sodium bicarbonate on performance in response to exercise duration in athletes: a systematic review. J Sports Sci Med. 2019;18(2):271–81.

153. Cunha VCR, Aoki MS, Zourdos MC, Gomes RV, Barbosa WP, Massa M, Moreira A, Capitani CD. Sodium citrate supplementation enhances tennis skill performance: a crossover, placebo-controlled, double blind study. J Int Soc Sports Nutr. 2019;16(1):32.

154. Saunders B, de Oliveira LF, Dolan E, Durkalec-Michalsi K, McNaughton L, Artioli GG, Swinton PA. Sodium bicarbonate supplementation and the female athlete: a brief commentary with small scale systematic review and meta-analysis. Eur J Sport Sci. 2022;22(5):745–54.

155. Cerullo G, Parimbelli M, Perna S, Pecoraro M, Liguori G, Negro M, D'Antona G. Sodium citrate supplementation: an updated revision and practical recommendations on exercise performance, hydration status, and potential risks. Transl Sports Med. 2020;1–8.

156. Beduschi G. Current popular ergogenic aids used in sports: a critical review. Nutr Diet. 2003;60(2):104–18.

157. Martinho DV, Nobari H, Faria A, Field A, Duarte D, Sarmento H. Oral branched-chain amino acids supplementation in athletes: a systematic review. Nutrients. 2022;14(19):4002.

158. Pennings B, Boirie Y, Senden JMG, Gijsen AP, Kuipers H, van Loon LJC. Whey protein stimulates postprandial muscle protein accretion more effectively than do casein and casein hydrolysate in older men. Am J Clin Nutr. 2011;93(5): 997–1005.

159. Adibi SA. Metabolism of branched-chain amino acids in altered nutrition. Metabolism. 1976;25(11):1287–302.

160. Kreider RB, Miriel V, Bertun E. Amino acid supplementation and exercise performance: proposed ergogenic value. Sports Med. 1993;16(3):190–209.

161. Gastmann UA, Lehman MJ. Overtraining and the BCAA hypothesis. Med Sci Sports Exerc. 1998;30:1173–8.

162. Quiroga N, Dinunzio C, Van Scoy J, Woolley B, McKenzie J. Effects of branched chain amino acid supplementation in delaying central fatigue. Int J Exerc Sci. 2017;8(5). Accessed 2018 May 17. Available from: https://digitalcommons.wku. edu/ijesab/vol8/iss5/77

163. Davis JM, Bailey SP, Woods JA, Galiano FJ, Hamilton M, Bartizi WP. Effects of carbohydrate feeding on plasma free tryptophan and branched-chain amino acids during prolonged cycling. Eur J Appl Physiol. 1992;65:513–19.

164. Plotkin DL, Delcastillo K, Van Every DW, Tipton KD, Aragon AA, Schoenfeld BJ. Isolated leucine and branched-chain amino acid supplementation for enhancing muscular strength and hypertrophy: a narrative review. Int J Sport Nutr Exerc Metab. 2021:31:292–301.

165. Karstoft K, Pedersen BK. Exercise and type 2 diabetes: focus on metabolism and inflammation. Immunol Cell Biol. 2016; 94(2):146–50.

166. Lancaster GI, Febbraio MA. Exercise and the immune system: implications for elite athletes and the general population. Immunol Cell Biol. 2016;94:115–6.

167. Bryan NS, Burleigh MC, Easton C. The oral microbiome, nitric oxide, and exercise performance. Nitric Oxide. 2022; 125;23–30.

168. Miranda-Comas G, Petering RC, Zaman N, Chang R. Implications of the gut microbiome in sports. Sports Health. 2022;14(6):894–98.

169. Mach N, Fuster-Botella D. Endurance exercise and gut microbiota: a review. J Sport Health Sci. 2017;6(2):179–97.

170. Clark A, Mach N. Exercise-induced stress behavior, gut-microbiota-brain axis and diet: a systematic review for athletes. J Int Soc Sports Nutr. 2016;13:43.

171. Gleeson M, Bishop NC, Oliveira M, Tauler P. Daily probiotic's (*Lactobacillus* casei Shirota) reduction of infection incidence in athletes. Int J Sport Nut Exerc Metab. 2011;21(1): 55–64.

172. Soriano S, Curry K, Sadrameli SS, Wang Q, Nute M, Reeves E, Kabir R, Wiese J, Criswell A, Schodrof S, Britz GW, Gadhia R, Podell K, Treangen T, Villapol S. Alterations to the gut microbiome after sport-related concussion in a collegiate football players cohort: a pilot study. Brain Behav Immun Health. 2022;21:100483.

173. O'Brien MT, O'Sullivan O, Claesson MJ, Cotter PD. The athlete gut microbiome and its relevance to health and performance: a review. Sports Med. 2022;52(Suppl 1):S119–28.

174. Todd JJ, Pourshahidi KL, McSorley EM, Madigan SM, Magee PJ. Vitamin D: recent advances and implications for athletes. Sports Med. 2015;45(2):213–29.

175. de la Puente Yagüe M, Yurrita LC, Cabañas MJC, Cenzual MAC. Role of vitamin D in athletes and their performance: current concepts and new trends. Nutrients. 2020;12(2):579.

176. Larson-Meyer DE, Willis KS. Vitamin D and athletes. Curr Sports Med Rep. 2010;9:220–6.

177. Martineau AR, Jolliffe DA, Hooper RL, Greenberg L, Aloia JF, Bergman P, Dubnov-Raz G, Esposito S, Ganmaa D, Ginde AA, Goodall EC, Grant CC, Griffiths CJ, Janssens W, Laaksi I, Manaseki-Holland S, Mauger D, Murdoch DR, Neale R, Rees JR, Simpson S Jr, Stelmach I, Kumar GT, Urashima M, Camargo CA Jr. Vitamin D supplementation to prevent acute respiratory tract infections: systematic review and meta-analysis of individual participant data. BMJ. 2017;356:i6583.

178. Constantini NW, Arieli R, Chodick G, Dubnov-Ras G. High prevalence of vitamin D insufficiency in athletes and dancers. Clin J Sport Med. 2010;20(5):368–71.

179. Birge SJ, Haddad JG. 25-hydroxycholecalciferol stimulation of muscle metabolism. J Clin Invest. 1975;56(5):1100–7.

180. Wassner SJ, Li JB, Sperduto A, Norman ME. Vitamin D deficiency, hypocalcemia, and increased skeletal muscle degradation in rats. J Clin Invest. 1983;72(1):102–12.

181. Hall LM, Kimlin MG, Aronov PA, Hammock BD, Slusser JR, Woodhouse LR, Stephensen CB. Vitamin D intake needed to maintain target serum 25-hydroxyvitamin D concentrations in participants with low sun exposure and dark skin pigmentation is substantially higher than current recommendations. J Nutr. 2010;140(3):542–50.

182. Krzywanski J, Mikulski T, Krysztofiak H, Mlynczak M, Gaczynska E, Ziemba A. Seasonal vitamin D status in Polish elite athletes in relation to sun exposure and oral supplementation. PLoS One. 2016;11(10):e0164395.

183. Holick MF. Vitamin D deficiency. N Engl J Med. 2007; 357:266–81.

184. Wilson-Barnes SL, Hunt JEA, Williams EL, Allison SJ, Wild JJ, Wainwright J, Lanham-New SA, Manders RJF. Seasonal variation in vitamin D status, bone health and athletic performance in competitive university student athletes: a longitudinal study. J Nutr Sci. 2020;9:e8.

185. Larson-Meyer DE, Woolf K, Burke LM. Assessment of nutrient status in athletes and the need for supplementation. Int J Sport Nutr Exerc Metab. 2018;28(2):139–58.

186. Owens DJ, Allison R, Close GL. Vitamin D and the athlete: current perspectives and new challenges. Sports Med. 2018; 48(Suppl 1):3–16.

187. Shuler FD, Wingate MK, Moore GH, Giangarra C. Sports health benefits of vitamin D. Sports Health. 2012;4(6): 496–501.

188. European Food Safety Authority. Vitamin D: EFSA sets dietary reference values. 2016. Accessed 2016 December 1. Available from: https://www.efsa.europa.eu/en/press/news/161028

189. Heaney RP. Vitamin D: criteria for safety and efficacy. Nutr Rev. 2008;66:S178–81.

190. Sato Y, Iwamoto J, Kanoko T, Satoh K. Low-dose vitamin D prevents muscular atrophy and reduces falls and hip fractures in women after stroke: a randomized controlled trial. Cerebrovasc Dis. 2005;20(3):187–92.

191. Close GL, Russell J, Cobley JN, Owens DJ, Wilson G, Gregson W, Fraser WD, Morton JP. Assessment of vitamin D concentration in non-supplemented professional athletes and healthy

adults during the winter months in the UK: implications for skeletal muscle function. J Sports Sci. 2013;31(4):344–53.

192. Ksiażek A, Zagrodna A, Słowińska-Lisowska M. Vitamin D, skeletal muscle function and athletic performance in athletes-a narrative review. Nutrients. 2019;11(8):1800.

193. Abushamma AA. The effects of vitamin D supplementation on athletic performance and junior prevention. J Allied Health Sci. 2022;8(2):1–15.

194. Bloomer RJ, Goldfarb AH. Anaerobic exercise and oxidative stress: a review. Can J Appl Physiol. 2004;29(3):245–63.

195. Powers SK, Ji LL, Leeuwenburgh C. Exercise training-induced alterations in skeletal muscle antioxidant capacity: a brief review. Med Sci Sports Exerc. 1999;31(7):987–97.

196. Close GL, Ashton T, Cable T, Doran D, Holloway C, McArdle F, MacLaren DPM. Ascorbic acid supplementation does not attenuate post-exercise muscle soreness following muscle-damaging exercise but may delay the recovery process. Br J Nutr. 2006;95(5):976–81.

197. Gomez-Cabrera MC, Domenech E, Romagnoli M, Arduini A, Borras C, Pallardo FV, Sastre J, Viña J. Oral administration of vitamin C decreases muscle mitochondrial biogenesis and hampers training-induced adaptations in endurance performance. Am J Clin Nutr. 2008;87(1):142–9.

198. Teixeira VH, Valente HF, Casal SI, Marques AF, Moreira PA. Antioxidants do not prevent postexercise peroxidation and may delay muscle recovery. Med Sci Sports Exerc. 2009; 41(9):1752–60.

199. Nobari H, Saedmocheshi S, Chung LH, Suzuki K, Maynar-Mariño M, Pérez-Gómez J. An overview on how exercise with green tea consumption can prevent the production of reactive oxygen species and improve sports performance. Int J Environ Res Public Health. 2021;19:218.

200. Jówko E, Długołęcka B, Makaruk, Cieśliński I. The effect of green tea extract supplementation on exercise induced oxidative stress parameters in male sprinters. Eur J Nutr. 2015; 54:783–91.

201. Jówko E, Sacharuk J, Balasińska B, Ostaszewski P, Charmas M, Charmas R. Green tea extract supplementation gives protection against exercise-induced oxidative damage in healthy men. Nutr Res. 2011;31(11):813–21.

202. Panza VSP, Wazlawik E, Schütz GR, Comin L, Hecht KC, da Silva EL. Consumption of green tea favorably affects oxidative stress markers in weight-trained men. Nutrition. 2008;24(5):433–42.

203. Sobhani V, Mehrtash M, Shirvani H, Fasihi-Ramandi M. Effects of short-term green tea extract supplementation on VO2 Max and inflammatory and antioxidant responses of healthy young men in a hot environment. Int J Prev Med. 2020;11:170.

204. D'Angelo S. Polyphenols: potential beneficial effects of these phytochemical in athletes. Curr Sports Med Rep. 2020; 19(7):260–65.

205. Jordan SL, Albracht-Schulte K, Robert-McComb JJ. Micronutrient deficiency in athletes and inefficiency of supplementation: is low energy availability a culprit? PharmaNutrition. 2020;14:100229.

206. Sukri NM. Does vitamin C minimize exercise-induced oxidative stress? Sport Sci Health. 2021;17(2):505–33.

207. Miller GD, Nesbit BA, Kim-Shapiro DB, Basu S, Berry MJ. Effect of vitamin C and protein supplementation on plasma nitrate and nitrite response following consumption of beetroot juice. Nutrients. 2022;14(9):1880.

208. De Oliveira DCX, Rosa FT, Simões-Ambrósio L, Jordan AA, Deminice R. Antioxidant vitamin supplementation prevents oxidative stress but does not enhance performance in young football athletes. Nutrition. 2019;63-64:29–35.

209. Kim M, Eo H, Lim JG, Lim H, Lim Y. Can low-dose of dietary vitamin E supplementation reduce exercise-induced muscle damage and oxidative stress? A meta-analysis of randomized controlled trials. Nutrients. 2022;14(8):1599.

210. Higgins MR, Izadi A, Kaviani M. Antioxidants and exercise performance: with a focus on vitamin E and C supplementation. Int J Environ Res Public Health. 2020;17(22):8452.

211. Beck KL, von Hurst PR, O'Brien WJ, Badenhorst CE. Micronutrients and athletic performance: a review. Food Chem Toxicol. 2021;158:112618.

212. Li S, Fasipe B, Laher I. Potential harms of supplementation with high doses of antioxidants in athletes. J Exerc Sci Fit. 2022;20(4):269–75.

213. Brancaccio M, Mennitti C, Cesaro A, Fimiani F, Vano M, Gargiulo B, Caiazza M, Amodio F, Coto I, D'Alicandro G, Mazzaccara C, Lombardo B, Pero R, Terracciano D, Limongelli G, Calabro P, D'Argenio V, Frisso G, Scudiero O. The biological role of vitamins in athletes' muscle heart and microbiota. Int J Environ Res Public Health. 2022;19(3):1249.

214. Hernández-Camacho JD, Vicente-García C, Parsons DS, Navas-Enamorado I. Zinc at the crossroads of exercise and proteostasis. Redox Biol. 2020;35:101529.

215. Tarmast D. Effect of an incremental exercise to exhaustion on plasma concentrations of iron and zinc in athletes and non-athletes. Acta Health Medica. 2019;4(3):284–94.

216. Toro-Román V, Siquier-Coll J, Bartolomé I, Grijota FJ, Muñoz D, Maynar-Mariño M. Influence of physical training on intracellular and extracellular zinc concentrations. J Int Soc Sports Nutr. 2022;19(1):110–25.

217. Heffernan SM, Horner K, De Vito G, Conway GE. The role of mineral and trace element supplementation in exercise and athletic performance: a systematic review. Nutrients. 2019;11:696.

218. Toro-Román V, Robles-Gil M, Muñoz D, Bartolomé I, Sequier-Coll J, Maynar-Mariño M. Extracellular and intracellular concentrations of molybdenum and zinc in soccer players: sex differences. Biology. 2022;11:1710.

219. Dziewiecka H, Buttar HS, Kasperska A, Ostapiuk-Kaolczuk J, Domagalska M, Chichoń J, Skarpańska-Stejnborn A. A systematic review of the influence of bovine colostrum supplementation on leaky gut syndrome in athletes: diagnostic biomarkers and future directions. Nutrients. 2022;14: 2512.

220. Davison G. The use of bovine colostrum in sport and exercise. Nutrients. 2021;13(6):1789.

221. Trivedi K, Hussain MS, Mohapatra C. Role of glutamine as an ergogenic amino acid during fatigue. J Clin Med Rev Reports. 2022;4(2).

222. Grucza K, Cholbinski P, Kwiatkowska D, Szutowski M. Effects of supplementation with glutathione and its precursors on athlete performance. Biomed J Sci Tech Res. 2019;12(4):9434–41.

223. Coqueiro AY, Rogero MM, Tirapegui J. Glutamine as an anti-fatigue amino acid in sports nutrition. Nutrients. 2019; 11:863.

224. Ahmadi L, Ghaedi H, Lamerd I. The effect of echinacea extract supplementation with resistance training on selected inflammatory markers in non-athlete females. J Exerc Physiol Health. 2019;2(2):24–9.

225. Ahmadi AR, Rayant E, Bahraini M, Mansoori A. The effect of glutamine supplementation on athletic performance, body composition, and immune function: a systematic review and a meta-analysis of clinical trials. Clin Nutr. 2019;38(3):1076–91.

226. Philpott JD, Witard OC, Galloway SDR. Applications of omega-3 polyunsaturated fatty acid supplementation for sport performance. Res Sports Med. 2019;27(2):219–37.

227. Thielecke F, Blannin A. Omega-3 fatty acids for sport performance-are they equally beneficial for athletes and amateurs? A narrative review. Nutrients. 2020;12:3712.

228. Fritsche KL. The science of fatty acids and inflammation. Adv Nutr. 2015;6(3):293S–301S.

229. Malinauskas BM, Aeby VG, Overton RF, Carpenter-Aeby T, Barber-Heidal K. A survey of energy drink consumption patterns among college students. Nutr J. 2007;6:35.

230. Erdmann J, Wiciński M, Wódkiewicz E, Nowaczewska M, Słupski M, Otto SW, Kubiak K, Huk-Wieliczuk E, Malinowski B. Effects of energy drink consumption on physical performance and potential danger of inordinate usage. Nutrients. 2021;13:2506.

231. Higgins JP, Babu K, Deuster PA, Shearer J. Energy drinks: a contemporary issues paper. Curr Sports Med Rep. 2018; 17(2):65–72.

232. Schneider MB, Benjamin HJ; Committee on Nutrition and the Council on Sports Medicine and Fitness. Sports drinks and energy drinks for children and adolescents: are they appropriate? Pediatrics. 2011;127(6):1182–9.

233. Terry-McElrath YM, O'Malley PM, Johnston LD. Energy drinks, soft drinks, and substance use among United States secondary school students. J Addict Med. 2014;8(1):6–13.

234. Higgins JP, Yarlagadda S, Yang B. Cardiovascular complications of energy drinks. Beverages. 2015;1(2):104–26.

235. Goldfarb M, Tellier C, Thanassoulis G. Review of published cases of adverse cardiovascular events after ingestion of energy drinks. Am J Cardiol. 2014;113(1):168–72.

236. Gunja N, Brown JA. Energy drinks: health risks and toxicity. Med J Aust. 2012;196(1):46–9.

237. Higgins JP, Tuttle TD, Higgins CL. Energy beverages: content and safety. Mayo Clin Proc. 2010;85(11):1033–41.

238. MacKnight JM. Energy drink use in sport: all risk, no gain. Curr Sports Med Rep. 2020;19(3):102–3.

239. Pfender E, Bleakley A, Ellithorpe M, Hennessy M, Maloney E, Jordan A, Stevens R. Perceptions of sports and energy drinks: factors associated with adolescent beliefs. Am J Health Promot. 2023;37(1):84–8.

240. Hennessy M, Bleakley A, Ellithorpe ME, Maloney E, Jordan AB, Stevens R. Reducing unhealthy normative behavior: the case of sports and energy drinks. Health Educ Behav. 2023;50(3):394–405.

241. Maughan RJ. Contamination of dietary supplements and positive drug tests in sport. J Sports Sci. 2005;23(9):883–9.

242. Timcheh-Hariri A, Balali-Mood M, Aryan E, Sadeghi M, Riahi-Zanjani B. Toxic hepatitis in a group of 20 male body-builders taking dietary supplements. Food Chem Toxicol. 2012;50(10):3826–32.

Nutritional Issues Related to Athlete Health, Disease, and Injury

CHAPTER OBJECTIVES

- Recognize the relationships between nutrition, physical activity, and disease risks.
- List the general ways that physical activity influences nutritional requirements.
- Demonstrate an understanding for the reasons why physical activity and nutrient/energy consumption should be dynamically linked.
- Identify the exercise recommendations of the Centers for Disease Control and Prevention (CDC), World Health Organization (WHO), and American College of Sports Medicine (ACSM) for children and adults.
- Recognize the specific disease-reducing impact of good nutrition and regular physical activity.

- Appraise the impact of inactivity and poor nutrition on risk for common chronic health disorders, including heart disease, diabetes, cancer, and poor bone health.
- Identify major points of current dietary guidelines for Americans.
- Discuss consequences of low-calorie weight loss diets specific to the prevalence of obesity and associated health problems.
- Explain the basis for different types of dietary fat and respective risk for heart disease.
- Differentiate behaviors of disordered eating frequently observed in athletes.

Case Study

John was an amazing football player in high school and in college. People would watch him play and would comment about how he could suddenly change direction and go just as fast sideways and backward as he could go forward. This quickness made him an ideal defensive back, being able to suddenly move to the ball carrier for a clean tackle. Everyone who knew anything about football noticed, and even those who were just casual onlookers would comment, "Who is that guy?" His college team made the playoffs, in no small part because of his amazing capacity to shut down running plays. He was so observant and intuitive that he even managed a few quarterback sacks during his final season. The professional ranks were looking at him as a great rookie prospect. He was not just an athlete; he was a scholar-athlete with superb grades. Some people thought it came easy to him, but they did not know the hours he spent studying and the time he spent in the weight room

making sure he was always in top academic and physical condition.

After his last collegiate football season successfully ended, he was recruited to join his favorite professional team with an amazing offer, which he accepted. He was now a professional player, working to make the playing squad of a historically successful team. One of his first interactions with the defensive coach was interesting. The coach was concerned that John was 10 lb lighter than everyone else in the same position, and told him that to be successful he needed to put on some "weight" and that 10 lb would make all the difference in his survivability as a defensive back. John thought that was curious, because his weight had not changed in 4 years, a stable 180 lb. He was recruited and offered a contract at his current weight, but now they wanted him to be 190 lb. OK, he thought, the defensive coach must know best, so he looked at some strategies for how he could increase his weight.

(continued)

Easy—he would eat more than usual (mainly protein) at breakfast and dinner to put on some muscle weight and spend a bit more time in the gym to work out. This strategy resulted in him getting bigger, but it was mainly in his belly and not his muscles. For the first time in his life he started hearing coaches yell at him, "Can't you move faster?" One of his fellow players suggested that he take some vitamin E, as it was suggested that vitamin E would help to reduce the muscle soreness he was feeling, and that within 1 week he would likely feel great. It did not work and he continued getting sore and prematurely fatigued. This was not the way he wanted to start his professional career. There was only one thing to do—ask to speak with the defensive coach. John started the discussion by saying that he would prefer to stay at his accustomed weight and, if that did not work during the season, then he would be happy to work to add weight. The defensive coach was speechless, but managed an "OK." He was sure that his 180-lb player would perform poorly over the course of the season, but felt that maybe that would be an important lesson for John to learn. John made the starting lineup, and then started piling up enough positive stats that there was talk that he might be rookie of the year. Weight change was no longer discussed.

CASE STUDY
DISCUSSION QUESTIONS

1. What are the potential difficulties associated with increasing weight in an already fit athlete?
2. Is there any evidence that supplemental vitamin E intake is useful for reducing muscle soreness?
3. Is greater consumption of protein the only nutritional consideration when trying to increase muscle mass?

With few exceptions, as has been observed in ultra-endurance running and other sports that induce overuse injuries, athletes involved in most sports achieve good health and lower risk of all-cause mortality (1,2). However, the traditions in many sports sometimes interfere with athletes achieving both good health and good performance. Some traditions may be more obviously bad than others. For instance, telling a small female gymnast that she has to lose even more weight before a major competition is obviously bad, but being small in gymnastics has been a long-time tradition in the sport. The common tradition of many athletes exercising prior to the consumption of breakfast may also diminish the benefit derived from the exercise as a result of low energy availability (LEA) and/or exercising in a low blood sugar state. Think about some of these traditions in the different sports listed below, and see if you can identify some that may interfere with good nutrition practices and have a negative impact on performance. Where both genders participate in the sport, indicate if you think there is a nutrition tradition that is different in male and female sports, and whether these nutritional differences have an impact on performance.

- Volleyball (men and women)
- American football (men only)
- Basketball (men and women)
- Soccer (men and women)
- Long-distance running (men and women)
- Sprinting (men and women)
- Weight lifting (men and women)
- Bodybuilding (men and women)
- Rhythmic gymnastics (women only)
- Artistic gymnastics (men and women)

INTRODUCTION

Physical activity, when performed correctly and with appropriate nutritional support, has many potential health benefits, including (3):

- Increased longevity
- Improved muscle strength
- Lower risk of cardiovascular disease
- Lower risk of type II diabetes
- Stronger bones
- Lower risk of certain cancers
- Improved immune system
- Improved mental health
- Healthier weight

While these health benefits are an important reason for individuals to exercise on a regular basis, a failure to satisfy nutritional needs in real time can have a profoundly negative impact on health and may also increase injury risk. It has been found that 1 in 12 athletes incur an injury during international competitions, which impacts future training and competition (4). A particular problem that is likely to exacerbate the health problems observed in athletes is that nutrition knowledge in athletes has been found to be inadequate, making it far too easy for them to follow a training/nutrition path that is not supportive of good health (5).

A screening of Olympic and Paralympic athletes who completed health screenings found health-related issues in 37% of athletes training for the Olympic Games, and 48% of athletes training for the Paralympic games (6). Health issues in male and female, Olympic and Paralympic, athletes found issues related to allergies, anxiety, depression, sleep apnea, and sleep quality. Sleep disturbance commonly occurs in athletes prior to competition and/or following long travel, and this is likely to negatively impact performance (7). While the issues associated with anxiety/mental health in elite athletes are only now being carefully assessed, there is a known association between mental health issues and performance, injury, reinjury, and illness (8). This study documented multiple mental health symptoms and disorders observed in elite athletes, including:

- Sleep disorders and sleep concerns
- Major depressive disorder and depression symptoms
- Suicide
- Anxiety and related disorders
- Posttraumatic stress disorder and other trauma-related disorders
- Eating disorders
- Attention-deficit/hyperactivity disorder
- Bipolar and psychotic disorders
- Sport-related concussion
- Substance use and substance use disorders
- Gambling disorder and other behavioral addictions.

University scholarship male and female athletes were assessed for mental health disorders and mental health problems were found in 51.7% in this population (9). It appears that depression and anxiety disorders may occur in athletes at least as often as in the general population (10). Some of the mental health disorders have nutritional relationships and are discussed in this chapter.

For everyone involved in physical activity there is a requirement for increased energy and nutrient needs to satisfy exercise-associated requirements. Although a seemingly simple task, ensuring that cellular needs are met may be more complex than it originally appears. Energy requirements must be satisfied in "real time" rather than randomly, and the intake of the **energy substrates**, carbohydrate, protein, and fat, should be considered as well. An athlete who requires between 1.2 and 2.0 g/kg of protein should consider how to best satisfy this need by planning how to consume both the total requirement and the optimal distribution of protein during the day. Consumption

of carbohydrate, protein, and fluids available immediately postexercise is a well-established strategy for optimizing **muscle protein synthesis (MPS)** and improving muscle recovery, but this requires planning and ensuring that the appropriate foods and beverages are available when the athlete needs them the most.

Energy Substrate

A nutrient that can be metabolized to provide cellular energy. In human nutrition, the energy substrates are carbohydrate (4 calories/g), protein (4 calories/g), and fat (9 calories/g). Alcohol is also capable of providing energy (7 calories/g), but because it also interferes with B-vitamin metabolism and, thus, interferes with normal energy metabolism, it is not usually considered an energy substrate.

Muscle Protein Synthesis

This represents the desired adaptive response to exercise, which is to synthesize muscle in a way that allows adaptation to the exercise being performed, with the ultimate aim of improving exercise performance. Providing nutrients in the right amounts, of the right kind, and at the right times enables enhanced muscle protein synthesis. Athletes should understand that if sufficient dietary protein is consumed in a way that the body can use it, consuming additional protein intake will not lower muscle injury risk or reduce postexercise muscle soreness (4). However, a small increase in dietary protein may be desirable as a muscle injury repair strategy by helping to limit muscle atrophy and helping to promote muscle repair (4,11).

Physically active people who understand the basic nutrition and exercise principles will help to ensure that the activity they do will contribute to rather than detract from a state of good health.

Physical activity affects:

- *Energy requirement:* Physical activity increases energy expenditure, which must be satisfied through consumption of more foods, or the resulting energy balance deficit may result in loss of muscle, loss of bone density, and a relative increase in fat mass. The downregulation of lean mass (a logical survival adaptation to adjust to the insufficient provision of energy) and upregulation of fat mass may cause athletes in weight or appearance sports (*i.e.,* wrestling, gymnastics, figure skating) to further reduce energy intake, leading to eating disorders and multiple health risks (12–15).
- *Energy substrate requirements:* Physical activity increases the utilization of carbohydrate and places greater demands on protein to sustain, repair, and increase musculature. Consumption of carbohydrate and

protein foods in the right amounts and at the right times helps to satisfy these needs.

- *Vitamin requirements:* Physical activity alters the requirement for certain vitamins, particularly for B-vitamins, which are involved in energy metabolism. The foods containing the energy substrates typically also contain these B-vitamins, provided the foods consumed are of reasonably good quality. For instance, the simple carbohydrate sucrose (table sugar) provides a source of energy but is devoid of any B-vitamins that are needed for its metabolism. On the other hand, starchy carbohydrates derived from rice, potatoes, breads, and so forth contain the vitamins needed for the energy they provide.
- *Mineral requirements:* Physical activity is associated with greater loss of some minerals via sweat and urine, and intense physical activity may interfere with the retention of some minerals. Established strategies for athletes work nicely in helping to ensure mineral adequacy. For instance, consumption of electrolyte-containing sports beverages during physical activity helps to offset the loss of minerals in sweat. Both male and female athletes are known to be at higher risk of iron deficiency and iron deficiency anemia, suggesting a greater need for iron. Ideally, anyone involved in regular physical activity should have iron status assessed at regular yearly intervals to determine if the foods consumed are satisfying iron needs.
- *Fluid requirements:* Because more energy is being metabolized as a result of the physical activity, more metabolic heat is being created that must be dissipated. The primary mechanism for this heat dissipation is the production of sweat, which can volumetrically exceed a human's capacity to easily replace it. As a result, athletes should make their state of hydration a high priority by initiating exercise in a well-hydrated state, learning to drink frequently and early (before the sensation of thirst occurs), and drinking enough fluids after exercise to offset the weight loss (*i.e.,* body water loss) resulting from the exercise. **Dehydration**, **underhydration**, and **euhydration** describe different states of hydration.

Dehydration

Represents a condition of inadequate body water, commonly caused by insufficient fluid consumption that fails to match fluid and electrolyte loss through sweat and urine, or conditions that result in high body water and electrolyte loss, including diarrhea and vomiting.

Underhydration

Often used synonymously with dehydration, referring to a state of inadequate body water.

Euhydration

Refers to a state of normal body water content, with normal body water in both the intercellular and extracellular spaces.

NUTRITION CONSIDERATIONS FOR REDUCING INJURY AND HEALTH RISKS

Not all athletes are the same, and differences in age, sex, dietary preferences (*i.e.,* vegan, omnivore, food intolerances, food allergies, etc.) training time, training intensity, and competition venues all have an influence on the nutrition strategies that should be followed to minimize injury and health risks. Importantly, the information in this chapter should be considered a guide rather than a prescription, as athlete differences may require significantly different nutrition strategies. Ideally, athletes facing health and/or injury issues should have a credentialed sports medicine team provide an appropriate risk-reduction strategy.

Consuming sufficient good-quality foods with well-timed intake is a key strategy for athletes to benefit from training and reduce injury and health risks. It has become increasingly clear that supplementation of vitamins and minerals is not needed for athletes consuming sufficient energy from a variety of foods (16,17). In addition, consumption of sufficient and appropriately constituted fluid intake before, during, and after exercise training/competition is extremely important, and critically important for athletes exercising/competing in hot and humid climates (18).

HEALTH ISSUES RELATED TO SUPPLEMENT INTAKE

The current literature strongly suggests that well-nourished athletes do not require supplements to enhance physical performance, and supplements may actually negatively influence the athlete's adaptation to training stress (19). However, it is common for athletes to treat the recommended nutrient intakes as minimum requirements, despite the fact that there is an ever-increasing body of evidence suggesting that excessive consumption of nutrients through high-dose supplements may create more problems than it resolves (20). Evidence of **vitamin toxicity**, even for water-soluble vitamins that were once thought to be benign at any level of intake (after all, you just "urinate away the excess"), is now well documented. As an example, too much vitamin B_6 may result in the same peripheral neuropathy, with loss of sensation in the fingers and toes, that is associated with vitamin B_6 deficiency; and too much vitamin C (>2,000 mg/day) may result in diarrhea or, worse, may increase the risk of kidney stones (21–24). (Note: The adult recommended dietary allowance [RDA] for vitamin B_6 is 1.3 mg/day with the tolerable upper intake level set at 100 mg/day, and supplements commonly provide 100 mg or more. Combined with the vitamin B_6 consumed from foods, the tolerable upper intake level for vitamin B_6 is likely to be exceeded in those consuming supplements. The adult RDA for vitamin C is between 75 and 90 mg/day, and supplements commonly provide 1,000 mg or more. Combined with the vitamin C consumed from foods, it is possible for the tolerable upper intake level of 2,000 mg to be exceeded in those consuming supplements.) Excess iron intake may result in higher cancer risk, as much of the iron consumed goes unabsorbed and is inflammatory to the intestines, resulting in an increased colon cancer risk (25,26). This represents a clear nutritional balancing act, as both poor iron status and iron excess are associated with elevated colon cancer risk (27,28). Importantly, the source of iron does not appear to influence colorectal cancer risk. Low intake of iron from plants and white meat, and higher intake of iron from red meat and supplements are all associated with higher colorectal cancer risk (29). It is clear that the goal is to have enough without getting too much. In addition, the competitive absorption of iron and zinc may result in reduced zinc absorption with increased risk of zinc deficiency in people who chronically consume iron supplements (30). Ideally, athletes should consider regular blood screening to determine iron status, as follows (31):

- Annually
  - No history of iron deficiency
  - No history of irregular menses
  - No reports of fatigue after extended rest
  - Strength-Power athletes with minimal endurance component
  - No restriction of iron-containing foods
  - No evidence of low energy availability (LEA)
  - No pathology that may negatively impact iron absorption (*i.e.*, Crohn disease; celiac disease; etc.)

- Biannually
  - Female
  - Previous history of poor iron status
  - Previous history of irregular menses
  - Undertaking high endurance and/or team-based sports training
  - No evidence of prolonged fatigue after extended rest
  - No diet that may limit iron intake or absorption
  - No evidence of LEA
- Quarterly
  - Recent history of iron deficiency/depletion (regardless of sex)
  - Evidence of irregular menses
  - High training loads in team and endurance-based sports
  - Reporting prolonged fatigue, even after extended rest
  - Early fatigue during training
  - Poor athletic performance without obvious cause
  - Restrictive diet that limits food variety and calories
  - Evidence of LEA

Put simply, the nutrition paradigm that "more than enough is not better than enough" is important to remember, but it is also important to consider that the daily requirement for a nutrient is not meant to be consumed at a single time with a single dose, but should be consumed through multiple meals throughout the day. As an example, studies on the water-soluble vitamin *folic acid* have found that consuming a high level in a single dose through supplementation rather than distributing the daily requirement throughout the day may accelerate the progression of preneoplastic lesions, increasing colorectal, prostate, and other cancer risks (Figure 14.1) (32–36). Perhaps more than for any other reason, this is precisely why meals and snacks with good-quality foods and beverages should be considered a better strategy for exposing tissues to needed nutrients than supplements (37). In addition, these are some of the reasons why major sports organizations, including the International Association of Athletics Federations, recommends a "food first" approach to satisfying nutritional needs, with supplements only used to treat deficiencies when satisfying nutrient needs via food is not possible (38).

Vitamin Toxicity

Refers to a level of vitamin intake that exceeds cellular capacity and may lead to toxicity symptoms, which vary by vitamin. The dietary reference intakes provide a tolerable upper intake level, which is the upper limit for human consumption to avoid risk of vitamin toxicity.

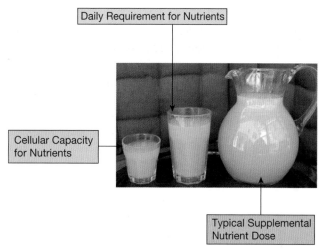

Daily Requirement for Nutrients

Cellular Capacity
for Nutrients

Typical Supplemental
Nutrient Dose

FIGURE 14.1: The daily requirement for nutrients is not intended to be provided in a single dose, as this is likely to exceed cellular capacity to deal with it optimally.

Although increasing physical activity may add a greater challenge for how to best satisfy nutritional requirements, every major health organization has concluded that staying active through regular involvement in physical activity or sport is a critically important component of lifelong health. It is also important to start exercising early. The WHO, the CDC, and the Exercise is Medicine, a global health initiative of the ACSM, all recommend exercise strategies for children, adolescents, and adults to enhance cardiorespiratory and muscular fitness, bone health, and cardiovascular and metabolic health biomarkers. These recommendations include the following (39–42):

- Children and youth should accumulate at least 60 minutes of moderate- to vigorous-intensity physical activity daily.
- Amounts of physical activity greater than 60 minutes provide additional health benefits.
- Most of the daily physical activity should be aerobic. Vigorous-intensity activities should be incorporated, including those that strengthen muscle and bone, at least three times per week.

Regarding the vigorous-intensity activities, bone-loading activities can be performed as part of playing games, running, turning, or jumping. It is generally recommended that 60 minutes of exercise be accumulated (does not need to be continuous) per day (*e.g.*, two exercise bouts of 30 minutes each per day). It is also encouraged that those with disabilities should work with health care providers to find strategies that will also encourage daily physical activity. For those who are not currently

active, the recommendation is gradually to increase activity to achieve the goal of 60 minutes per day. The benefits of doing so are clear:

- develop healthy **musculoskeletal** tissues (*i.e.*, bones, muscles, and joints);
- develop a healthy cardiovascular system (*i.e.*, heart and lungs);
- develop neuromuscular awareness (*i.e.*, coordination and movement control) to help avoid a **neuromuscular disorder**;
- maintain a healthy body weight;
- reduce psychological symptoms of anxiety and depression; and
- reduce unhealthy behaviors, such as smoking and drug and alcohol abuse, and improve academic performance.

Musculoskeletal

Refers to skeletal muscles, the skeleton, and related tendons, ligaments, joints, and connective tissues that enable body movement.

Neuromuscular Disorder

Refers to disorders affecting nerve control of muscles under a person's direct control (*i.e.*, arms and legs). Often of genetic origin, neuromuscular disorders may also be the result of poor nutritional status affecting the immune system.

Important Factors to Consider

- The importance of physical activity in reducing chronic disease is clear. Worldwide, it is estimated that attributable contribution to chronic disease as a result of physical inactivity is an increase in:
  - the global burden of disease from coronary heart disease;
  - type II diabetes; and
  - breast and colon cancer cases.
- Inactivity is the 4th leading cause of premature mortality worldwide, or about 3.3 million deaths per year. On the other hand, regular physical activity:
  - reduces mortality and the risk of recurrent breast cancer by ~50%;
  - reduces the risk of developing Alzheimer disease;

- lowers the risk of all-cause, cardiovascular, and cancer-specific mortality in adults with higher levels of muscle strength; and
- leads to higher academic performance in children and adults.
- Despite these health concerns of being physically inactive:
  - More than half of adults in the United States (56%) do not meet the recommendations for sufficient physical activity set forth by the 2008 Physical Activity Guidelines for Americans.
  - US adolescents and adults spend almost 8 hours a day in sedentary behaviors, and as much as 36% of adults engage in no leisure-time physical activity at all.

Source: American College of Sports Medicine. Exercise is medicine: Fact sheet. Available from: https://www.exerciseismedicine.org/assets/page_documents/EIM%20Fact%20Sheet%20 2014_update%20March%202018.pdf

DIETARY GUIDELINES FOR AMERICANS, 2020–2025

Exercise alone cannot resolve chronic disease prevalence, as there is also a strong nutritional and genetic relationship to disease risk. Ideally, physical activity and nutrition should be considered as integrated and dynamically related factors that should be considered together. Although the prevalence of infectious diseases has dropped, that of noncommunicable diseases related to lifestyle, including exercise and nutrition, has increased sharply (Box 14.1).

The dietary guidelines for Americans (43) make the following four basic recommendations:

- *Follow a healthy dietary pattern at every life state.* All food and beverage choices matter. Choose a healthy eating pattern at an appropriate calorie level to help achieve and maintain a healthy body weight, support nutrient adequacy, and reduce the risk of chronic disease. The goal is to "Make Every Bite Count."
- *Customize and enjoy nutrient-dense food and beverage choices to reflect personal preferences, cultural traditions, and budgetary considerations.* Everyone has a role in helping to create and support healthy eating patterns in multiple settings nationwide, from home to school to work to communities.
- *Focus on meeting food group needs with nutrient-dense foods and beverages, and stay within calorie limits.* To

meet nutrient needs within calorie limits, choose a variety of nutrient-dense foods across and within all food groups in recommended amounts.
- *Limit foods and beverages higher in added sugars, saturated fat, and sodium, and limit alcoholic beverages.* Consume an eating pattern low in added sugars, saturated fats, and sodium. Cut back on foods and beverages higher in these components to amounts that are within healthy eating patterns.

An important addition to the 2020–2025 Dietary Guidelines is that the pattern of eating is critically important for sustaining health and reducing disease risks. This update to the dietary guidelines is because there is an ever-increasing body of evidence showing that the individual's *pattern* of eating has the greatest impact on their health. A comprehensive document on the Dietary Guidelines for Americans is available at the following website: https://www.dietaryguidelines.gov/sites/default/files/2021-03/Dietary_Guidelines_for_Americans-2020-2025.pdf

OBESITY AND RELATED CONDITIONS

Obesity affects 78 million adults and 12.5 million children, with the prediction that, if obesity rates continue at their current pace, 44% of all Americans will be obese by the year 2030. In 2013, there were 112,000 obesity-related deaths in the United States, and obese children were twice as likely as their nonobese peers to die before reaching the age of 55. Chronic disease risks associated with obesity include increased risk of heart disease, respiratory disease, liver disease, hypertension, osteoarthritis, cancer, and type II diabetes (44). Reducing obesity has a risk reduction effect for all of these conditions (Figure 14.2, Table 14.1).

Metabolic Syndrome

Refers to a cluster of metabolic disorders that increase risk of cardiovascular disease. An individual with a combination of two or three of the following conditions is thought to have metabolic syndrome: high abdominal obesity, high triglyceride level, low high-density lipoprotein cholesterol, high BP, and high fasting blood glucose. Lowering fat mass through appropriate dietary strategies and exercise is the standard strategy for lowering metabolic syndrome risk.

Box 14.1   Facts About Nutrition and Physical Activity–Related Health Conditions in the United States

Overweight and Obesity

- For more than 25 years, more than half of the adult population has been overweight or obese.
- Obesity is most prevalent in those aged 40 years and older and in African-American adults and is least prevalent in adults with highest incomes.
- Since the early 2000s, abdominal obesity has been present in about half of US adults of all ages. Prevalence is higher with increasing age and varies by sex and race/ethnicity.
- In 2009–2012, 65% of adult females and 73% of adult males were overweight or obese.
- In 2009–2012, nearly one in three youth aged 2–19 years were overweight or obese.

Cardiovascular Disease and Risk Factors

- Coronary heart disease
- Stroke
- Hypertension
- High total blood cholesterol
- In 2010, cardiovascular disease affected about 84 million men and women aged 20 years and older (35% of the population).
- In 2007–2010, about 50% of adults who were of normal weight and nearly three-fourths of those who were overweight or obese had at least one cardiometabolic risk factor (*i.e.*, high blood pressure [BP], abnormal blood lipids, smoking, or diabetes).
- Rates of hypertension, abnormal blood lipid profiles, and diabetes are higher in adults with abdominal obesity.
- In 2009–2012, almost 56% of adults aged 18 years and older had either prehypertension (27%) or hypertension (29%).
- In 2009–2012, rates of hypertension among adults were highest in African-Americans (41%) and in adults aged 65 years and older (69%).

- In 2009–2012, 10% of children aged 8–17 years had either borderline hypertension (8%) or hypertension (2%).
- In 2009–2012, 100 million adults aged 20 years or older (53%) had total cholesterol levels >200 mg/dL; almost 31 million had levels >240 mg/dL.
- In 2011–2012, 8% of children aged 8–17 years had total cholesterol levels >200 mg/dL.

Diabetes

- In 2012, the prevalence of diabetes (type I plus type II) was 14% for men and 11% for women aged 20 years and older (more than 90% of total diabetes in adults is type II).
- Among children with type II diabetes, about 80% were obese.

Cancer

- Breast cancer
  - Breast cancer is the third leading cause of cancer death in the United States.
  - In 2012, an estimated 3 million women had a history of breast cancer.
- Colorectal cancer
  - Colorectal cancer is the second leading cause of cancer death in the United States.
  - In 2012, an estimated 1.2 million adult men and women had a history of colorectal cancer.

Bone Health

- A higher percent of women are affected by osteoporosis (15%) and low bone mass (51%) than men (about 4% and 35%, respectively).
- In 2005–2010, ~10 million (10%) adults aged 50 years and older had osteoporosis and 43 million (44%) had low bone mass.

Source: United States Department of Health and Human Services and United States Department of Agriculture. 2015–2020 Dietary Guidelines for Americans. 8th ed. December 2015. Accessed 2018 May 21. Available from: http://health.gov/dietaryguidelines/2015/guidelines/

Factors That Contribute to Obesity

Obesity is the result of several factors, including (59,60):

- *Excess energy consumption relative to energy expenditure.* Excess energy is stored as fat, resulting in obesity.

- *Inactivity.* The human system has a "use it or lose it" protocol related to survival, particularly for tissue that is energy expensive. Inactivity lowers the need for muscle, so the body lowers this energy-expensive tissue. As a result, there is less tissue with which to

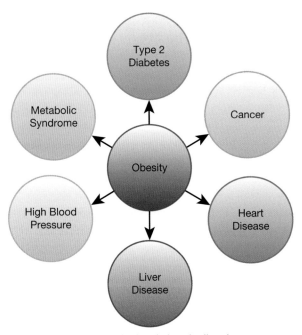

FIGURE 14.2: Obesity and related chronic disorders.

metabolize consumed energy, resulting in greater fat storage.

- *Environment.* Many environments make it difficult to sustain activity as a normal part of daily living, thereby lowering activity and the opportunity to metabolize energy. The environment we live in often overemphasizes unhealthy foods with low nutrient densities, such as high-sweetened beverages and desserts, and underemphasizes healthy foods with high nutrient densities, such as fresh fruits and vegetables.
- *Genetic background.* Obesity may be familial, with a greater chance of becoming obese if one or both parents are obese. To a certain extent, having an obese parent may also increase obesity risk because the food environment created by the obese parent is adapted by the children in the household.
- *Preexisting disease state.* Certain diseases are associated with obesity, including hypothyroidism, Cushing syndrome, and polycystic ovarian syndrome. Resolving the disease state may help to resolve the associated obesity.
- *Medications.* Some medications that are taken to control or resolve a health condition may predispose an individual to obesity. For instance, corticosteroids that are often taken for allergies may lower lean mass and, therefore, lower the tissues that metabolize energy. The difference in a person's capacity to metabolize energy is small, but over time may predispose the person to obesity.

- *Smoking.* The addictive substance in cigarette smoke, nicotine, elevates the rate of energy expenditure. Stopping smoking without finding a means of increasing energy expenditure (*i.e.*, physical activity) may predispose the person to obesity. However, the mortality risk from obesity is far lower than the mortality risk from smoking, suggesting that smokers should most definitely stop smoking and also find a way to become regularly physically active.
- *Age.* Aging is associated with a loss of lean mass and an increase in fat mass, greatly increasing obesity risk. Menopause in women is also associated with an increase in fat mass. These age-related changes in body composition, referred to as *sarcopenia*, are best addressed through regular physical activity that is matched with a diet that sustains energy balance. There are also data to show that evenly distributing relatively small amounts of protein intake during meals throughout the day may improve the older person's ability to sustain muscle mass.
- *Pregnancy.* Weight gain is a necessary part of a normal pregnancy, as the extra tissue helps to satisfy the energy needs of the growing fetus and, after delivery, the energy needs associated with lactation. However, many women find it difficult to return to the prepregnancy weight after pregnancy. This is likely due to multiple reasons, not the least of which is increased difficulty to find time to be physically active because of the increased responsibilities associated with child rearing.
- *Poor sleep.* Insufficient sleep is associated with higher obesity risk across all age groups. This may be due to better maintenance of the hormones leptin (lowers hunger) and ghrelin (increases hunger), but may also be associated with altered food preferences. Insufficient sleep is associated with greater consumption of high-calorie, high-sweet foods that are associated with obesity.

Of the factors related to activity, the ones over which most people have direct control over, energy balance and activity, may appear relatively simple. However, there are complexities that must be considered when addressing these issues to prevent or resolve an obese state.

Weight and Body Mass Index

Weight and body mass index (BMI) are often used as measures of whether an individual is obese or whether the obesity is getting better or worse. Obesity is defined

Table 14.1	Conditions Closely and Commonly Linked to Obesity
Condition	**Links to Obesity**
Heart disease	Also referred to as cardiovascular disease, this disease is associated with elevated blood lipids (including cholesterol), high blood pressure (BP), obesity, smoking, diabetes, and insufficient physical activity (45). There is also evidence that regular consumption of nuts lowers heart attack risk (45). It has been estimated that most heart disease can be prevented through obesity reduction, cessation of smoking, and moderating alcohol consumption (41,42).
Type II diabetes	Type II diabetes is the most common form of diabetes, resulting from high blood sugar (hyperglycemia), insulin resistance, and eventually insufficient functional insulin. Complications include heart disease, strokes, and poor blood flow to the extremities and eyes. Type II diabetes is commonly associated with obesity and insufficient physical activity. The prevalence of type II diabetes has increased in parallel with the prevalence of obesity. Consumption of refined carbohydrates results in hyperglycemia, exacerbating the diabetes, and diets with more protein/less refined carbohydrate appear to ameliorate the symptoms (46–48).
Metabolic syndrome	**Metabolic syndrome** has four major components, including visceral obesity (*i.e.*, large levels of stored fat in the trunk), dyslipidemia (*i.e.*, high blood lipids with low high-density lipoprotein cholesterol and elevated very low-density lipoprotein cholesterol and triglycerides), hyperglycemia (*i.e.*, high blood glucose), and hypertension (*i.e.*, high BP), and a proinflammatory state. There is increased risk of type II diabetes with metabolic syndrome, and all of these components are associated with obesity and insufficient physical activity (49,50).
Liver disease	Obesity is associated with elevated risk of developing nonalcoholic fatty liver disease (NAFLD), with up to 85% of obese individuals having NAFLD (51,52). Overfeeding in laboratory animals has been linked to development of NAFLD, whereas energy intakes that sustain energy balance, which results in lower obesity, appear to be an effective strategy for lowering NAFLD risk (53).
Hypertension	Obesity and hypertension are closely linked and are associated with heart muscle enlargement (left ventricular) and kidney damage, which are associated with high cardiac output, high plasma volume, and peripheral tissue resistance. Sodium (salt) retention is a common feature of the obese hypertensive (54). Recent evidence suggests that elevated leptin production seen in obesity may also contribute to hypertension (55).
Cancer	It has been estimated that obesity-related cancer risk is high, with 20% of cancers attributable directly to obesity. Obesity-related cancer risk is particularly high of endometrial, esophageal, colorectal, breast, prostate, and renal cancers. These cancers are associated with excess production of insulin, insulin-like growth factor I, sex hormones (primarily testosterone, estrogen, and progesterone), and adipokines (the cell signaling proteins produced by fat cells) (56).
Osteoarthritis	Osteoarthritis is a joint disease that is associated with the deterioration of joints, with symptoms associated with pain and stiffness. It has been found that obesity and osteoarthritis are clearly linked, affecting both weight- and non–weight-bearing joints (57). It has been found that lowering weight/obesity by 10%, particularly when coupled with a regular exercise program, can result in significant improvement in pain relief and physical function (58).

as having excess body *fat*, not excess weight (61). BMI is an appropriate population indicator of obesity prevalence, but as it does not differentiate between fat mass and lean mass, it is not a good individual indicator of obesity. Weight, therefore, is a poor measure because it fails to consider what component of weight (muscle mass? fat mass?) is changing. Low-calorie weight loss diets may cause a lowering of weight, but studies now show that these diets often result in a greater loss of lean mass than fat mass. The resultant greater proportion of fat mass (*i.e.*, higher body fat percent) is suggestive of greater obesity, despite a lowering of weight.

Higher Lean Mass and Lower Fat Mass

Athletes typically have a greater proportion of lean mass and a lower proportion of fat mass than nonathletes, and this greater presence of lean mass often makes them appear to be obese on a BMI index (*i.e.*, BMI >30), when they are not (62). Because BMI has a low sensitivity to detect excess body fat, it fails to identify over a quarter of children and adolescents as obese who have normal BMI but excess body fat (63).

Energy Balance

The concept of *energy-in, energy-out* (*i.e.*, energy balance) is often assessed in 24-hour units, but data suggest that such an assessment fails to address the expected endocrine response to real-time deviations in energy balance that could affect obesity (13,64,65). For instance, an athlete who has no energy intake prior to the morning workout will achieve a severe negative energy balance and low blood sugar (*i.e.*, the body used significantly more energy than was provided), resulting in elevated cortisol production that breaks down both muscle and bone tissue (*i.e.*, lean mass goes down), and a hyperinsulinemic response at the next eating opportunity that results in greater fat acquisition, even if the total calories consumed later in the day suggest that the daily energy balance appears to satisfy energy needs (65–67). It is likely for this reason that low-calorie fad diets have a poor record of lowering obesity and also increasing health risks (12).

Infrequent Meals

Studies have found that decreasing meal frequency may create problems in controlling obesity, likely because such a strategy is likely to result in larger energy balance deviations than more frequent eating patterns. It has been found, for instance, that people with infrequent eating patterns are likely to have greater total energy intakes than those with more frequent eating patterns, likely because of an upregulation of the appetite-stimulating hormone *ghrelin* (68). Insulin release following a meal typically suppresses ghrelin, but if a long period of time between meals leads to low blood sugar, there is a hyperinsulinemic response at the next eating opportunity and ghrelin is not suppressed, resulting in sustained high appetite (69,70).

Physical Activity and Controlled Energy Consumption

Programs that increase physical activity but fail to simultaneously address the additional energy/nutrient requirements associated with this physical activity with strategies that ensure good relative energy availability may not be as beneficial as they could be in lowering obesity risk. There is evidence that the combination of an exercise program coupled with controlled energy consumption to sustain energy balance rather than place the subject on a severe calorie restriction is a more successful strategy for losing body fat and reducing obesity than either diet alone or exercise alone (71,72).

Basic Strategies for Reducing Obesity

Limit Foods High in Saturated Fats and Trans-Fats

A basic strategy for reducing obesity is to limit the chronic consumption of foods that are high in saturated and trans-fats, including processed meats, fatty cuts of red meats, and fried foods, and that result in higher per-meal energy intakes. Although the reduction of the total consumption of fat has been seen as a desirable strategy for lowering obesity risk, the evidence suggests that the type and the amount of fat consumed per meal may be more important predictors of obesity (73,74). To some extent, this is because lower fat intake is often associated with higher intake of refined carbohydrates, such as white bread and white rice, which tend to produce hyperinsulinemia and higher fat storage. An assessment of a large cohort of women found that greater consumption of unhealthy fats (*i.e.*, saturated and trans-fats) was associated with greater obesity risk, but that consumption of more healthy fats (*i.e.*, mono- and polyunsaturated fats) was not (75). The type of meat consumed also has a direct impact on cancer risk separate from obesity. Regular consumption of red meats and processed meats (*e.g.*, bacon, sausage) is associated with higher risk of diabetes, heart disease, and colon cancer (48,76,77).

Limit High-Sugar Beverages

Limit the consumption of drinks that are high in sugar, including sodas and fruit juices. Sugary beverages are clearly associated with greater obesity risk, as they tend to result in both hyperinsulinemia and greater fat manufacture, and also greater total energy consumption (78–81). It has also been found that there is a significant association between artificially sweetened soda consumption and obesity (79). When possible, consumption of fresh whole fruit is a better option than juices made from fruit (82). However, sports beverages when consumed correctly (*i.e.*, small amounts consumed at regular intervals during physical activity), and which typically contain sugar as the primary source of energy, are appropriate and unlikely to contribute to obesity risk when consumed in this fashion. Appropriate use of sugar-containing sports beverages may help the athlete achieve better within-day energy balance, which would *lower* obesity risk (13,66,67,83).

Increase Daily Physical Activity

Increase regular, daily physical activity. According to the CDC, people should accrue a minimum of 150 minutes of weekly physical activity (3). The CDC notes that more time spent in physical activity (even beyond 300 minutes/week) results in greater health benefits. The CDC recommends one of the following three guidelines for physical activity:

- 2 hours and 30 minutes (150 minutes) of moderate-intensity aerobic activity (*i.e.*, brisk walking) every week; and muscle-strengthening activities on 2 or more days per week that work all major muscle groups (legs, hips, back, abdomen, chest, shoulders, and arms). A total of 1 hour and 15 minutes (75 minutes) of vigorous-intensity aerobic activity (*i.e.*, jogging or running) every week; and muscle-strengthening activities on 2 or more days a week that work all major muscle groups (legs, hips, back, abdomen, chest, shoulders, and arms).
- An equivalent mix of moderate- and vigorous-intensity aerobic activity; and muscle-strengthening activities on 2 or more days a week that work all major muscle groups (legs, hips, back, abdomen, chest, shoulders, and arms).

Improve Sleep Duration and Quality

Insufficient sleep is associated with greater inflammation and higher risk of obesity and cardiovascular disease (84). It has been found that improving sleep duration and/or sleep quality significantly improves body composition (*i.e.*, lowers body fat) and also positively affects other energy balance–associated factors (85). An analysis of the first National Health and Nutrition Examination Survey found that individuals who averaged less than 7 hours of sleep per night were more likely to be obese that those who averaged at least 7 hours of sleep. Insufficient sleep was associated with sweet cravings and additional energy intakes, but with no compensatory increase in energy expenditure (86). Short sleep duration appears to particularly affect younger age groups, which appear to be even more likely to experience weight gain with sleep deprivation than older groups (Figure 14.3) (87).

Participate in Activities That Lower Stress

Stress influences eating behavior, resulting in over- or undereating, and also increases the preference for energy-dense foods that are high in sugar and fat (88). Studies have found that *mindfulness-based stress reduction* strategies, including nonreligious meditation, significantly reduce stress and, therefore, provide a coping strategy for lowering obesity risk (89).

Regularly Assess Body Fat Level/Weight

Find a way to regularly assess body fat level in conjunction with weight, to determine if weight loss is the

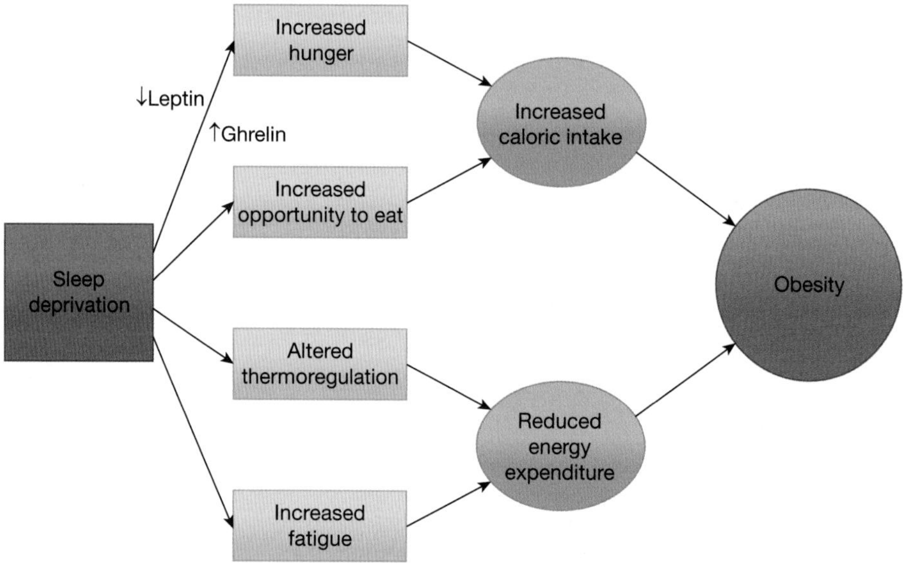

FIGURE 14.3: Proposed mechanisms causing predisposition to obesity with sleep deprivation. (From Patel SR, Hu FB. Short sleep duration and weight gain: a systematic review. Obesity. 2008; 16:643–53.)

result of primarily fat mass or lean mass. (See Chapter 8 for information on assessment of body composition.) It is important for people to understand that lowering fat mass while retaining lean mass is not something that can occur quickly and involves creating an eating pattern that dynamically matches energy expenditure to sustain a reasonable energy balance throughout the day (13,17,56).

Improve Meal Frequency and Eating Patterns

Avoid meal skipping and eat in a pattern that dynamically matches energy expenditure to sustain a reasonable energy balance throughout the day. Skipping breakfast, for instance, is associated with greater obesity risk. Subjects who skipped breakfast as adults had significantly higher waist circumference and BMI, and those who skipped breakfast as children and as adults had even higher waist circumference and BMI, along with more cardiometabolic risk factors (68,90). Findings of studies assessing eating frequency are inconsistent, likely because randomly increasing eating frequency will not necessarily help to sustain a desirable energy balance. Rather, eating frequency should be patterned in a way that will reduce large energy balance deficits and surpluses, to limit cortisol production and avoid losses in lean mass and increases in fat mass (64,66,67,83).

Follow the Mediterranean Diet

The traditional Mediterranean diet is rich in olive oil, fruits, vegetables, nuts, and fish. Studies of individuals consuming this type of diet have generally found lower risk of obesity, heart disease, and type II diabetes (91).

Improve the Microbiome

The gut **microbiome** (*i.e.*, the collection of bacterial colonies that reside in the colon) is involved in multiple metabolic functions, including energy balance. The gut microbiome is influenced by several factors, including diet, genetics, antibiotic intake, exercise, and the environment (92). The diet plays a major role in microbiome composition, and it appears that dietary composition and caloric intake quickly regulate the composition of microbes in the intestines and their functions (93). Obesity risk may be increased through microbiome-enhanced energy extraction from foods and by contributing to the regulation of fat storage (94,95). The increased obesity risk is the result of higher body fat, higher liver triglycerides, higher fasting plasma glucose, and greater

tissue insulin resistance. It was observed in a study on mice that switching from a low-fat, plant-based diet high in polysaccharides to a typical Western diet high in fat and sugar altered the **microbiota** in a single day and altered the metabolic pathways toward increased fat storage (96). It has become increasingly clear that certain strains of bacteria that are part of the gut microbiome can have a positive impact on metabolic health and obesity risk (97). These and other studies suggest that consumption of a Mediterranean-type diet high in fresh fruits and vegetables and lower in meat-based fats facilitates lower obesity risk, at least in part through beneficial alterations in the gut microbiome (98).

There is increasing evidence that higher consumption of polyphenols, which can be obtained from fruits (principally berries), vegetables, and supplements provide health and performance benefits in athletes by enhancing the microbiome (99). There is also developing evidence that other nutrients/food compounds/foods, including caffeine, vitamin D, omega-3 fatty acids, and carbohydrate/electrolyte sports beverages may also enhance microbiome health in athletes (100). Importantly, commonly taken protein supplements that result in protein overconsumption appear to have a harmful effect on the human gut, especially when consumed with otherwise restrictive and/or unbalanced diets (101).

An assessment of track and field athletes found that an increasing number of them implement special diets, without the clinical necessity to do so, in an attempt to enhance performance. The commonly implemented diets include:

- Gluten-Free
- FODMAP diet (low fermentable oligo-, di-, and monosaccharides and polyols)
- Vegetarian
- Fasting

It was found that there were no direct beneficial outcomes from these diets, and there may actually be an adverse impact because of the food restrictions associated with these diets. However, vegetarian diets have been found to enhance the gut microbiome, but must be carefully applied to assure an adequate and balanced energy/nutrient intake (102). Athletes often experience GI problems, and the removal of foods from the diet is an attempt to lower these problems, but doing so should be guided by an appropriately credentials sports nutritionist to help assure that the restricted foods do not result in nutrient or energy deficiency, and also likely to improve gut health (103).

> ### 📖 Microbiome
>
> Microorganisms in any defined area of the body. The gut microbiome refers to the microorganisms in the intestines. These gut microorganisms are involved in metabolism and immune function and are highly influenced by the foods consumed. A poor gut microbiome (referred to as a dysbiotic state) is associated with irritable bowel syndrome (IBS), inflammatory bowel disease, obesity, and type II diabetes.
>
> ### 📖 Microbiota
>
> Synonymous with microbiome.

OXIDATIVE STRESS

Oxidative stress is created through an accumulation of reactive oxygen species (ROS) and is a common component of intense physical activity, particularly when coupled with fatigue (104). Tissue damage may occur when ROS has created damage to the cellular structures, cellular DNA, and cellular proteins and lipids (see Chapter 9) (105). Although it is seemingly logical to consume more of the antioxidant vitamins, including vitamins C and E, through supplementation, studies have not found this strategy to be useful in reducing markers of oxidative stress (106,107). Some studies have found that taking commonly available supplemental doses of these vitamins has precisely the opposite of the desired effect by increasing oxidative stress with a resultant decrease in performance (108). It appears that exercise-induced oxidative stress will cause an adaptive response by promoting production of more antioxidant defenses. However, supplementation with antioxidant vitamins appears to blunt this natural adaptive response, thus lowering potential adaptive benefits that the exerciser should obtain, including promotion of endogenous antioxidant defense capacity (109). A study assessing 1–2 months of vitamin E supplementation (800 IU) compared with a placebo in triathletes found that vitamin E supplementation resulted in more oxidative stress and inflammation following a competitive triathlon (107). These data strongly suggest that athletes wishing to achieve a normal adaptive response to the potentially damaging effects of exercise-associated oxidative stress should rely on a good-quality healthy diet that satisfies energy needs (37). Consumption of antioxidant vitamin supplements appears to be counterproductive unless there is a known biologic deficiency to a vitamin as a result of food allergies, intolerances, or sensitivities (37).

PHYTONUTRIENTS AND HEALTH

Phytonutrients are chemicals found naturally in plants and generally refer to nonnutrient (*i.e.*, nonvitamin or mineral) substances. The phytonutrients are not necessary for human survival, so there are no recommended dietary intakes of these chemicals. Plants produce phytonutrients as self-protection, and there is evidence that these same phytonutrients may also be cell protective/health enhancing, through reduction of cellular inflammation and oxidative stress, for humans (110). The flavonoids are receiving a great deal of attention because of their health and performance potential (Table 14.2).

Table 14.2	Food Sources of Dietary Flavonoids
Flavonoid	**Food Sources**
Anthocyanidins and anthocyanins	Berries that are red, blue, and purple in color; red and purple grapes; red wine
Flavan-3-ols	*Monomers:* Teas, including white, green, and oolong; cocoa-based products, grapes, berries, and apples *Dimers and polymers:* Apples, berries, cocoa-based products, red grapes, red wine *Theaflavins:* Black tea
Flavonols (including quercetin)	Onions, scallions, kale, broccoli, apples, berries, teas
Flavones	Parsley, thyme, celery, hot peppers
Flavanones	Citrus fruit and juices
Isoflavones	Soybeans, soy-based foods, legumes

Data from Linus Pauling Institute. Resveratrol. Accessed January 2, 2017. http://lpi.oregonstate.edu/mic/dietary-factors/phytochemicals/resveratrol

Several companies are now including phytochemicals in sports drinks and energy bars, but these have not yet been investigated to determine if they benefit the athlete through enhanced performance, improved mental acuity, reduced injury risk, or enhanced injury recovery. Several phytochemicals have been undergoing testing to determine their potential usefulness with athletes, including possible performance and health benefits, and these include anthocyanin; curcumin; green tea extract and a chemical within this extract, epigallocatechin gallate; flavonol; and polyphenol.

Anthocyanin

Anthocyanin flavonoids are responsible for the blue color of blueberries and other deep blue/deep red berries. A study of wild blueberries that are high in anthocyanins found that consumption for 6 weeks resulted in a significant reduction in oxidatively induced DNA damage (111). A similar finding was observed with consumption of strawberry-based anthocyanin, which was found to lower cardiovascular risk by improving the plasma lipid profile and oxidative stress in humans (112). In a study of athletes, anthocyanin supplementation was found to significantly improve VO_{2max} compared with a placebo, despite no body composition difference following the 6-week intervention (113). Other studies have found improvements in strength or lower strength reductions following exercise in athletes consuming fruits high in anthocyanins (*i.e.*, pomegranate juice or tart cherry juice) (114,115). A study of endurance athletes consuming anthocyanin through blackcurrant powder found that it increased stroke volume and cardiac output significantly and improved lactate clearance, both of which have implications for exercise performance (116).

Curcumin

Curcumin is a polyphenol derived from the spice turmeric and has historically been used medicinally in different parts of the world. Studies have suggested that curcumin lowers the risk of oral, gastrointestinal (GI), liver, and colon cancers and may also lower oxidative stress and inflammation associated with the onset of type II diabetes (117–122). In athletes, it has been found that curcumin lowered the pain associated with delayed-onset muscle soreness following exercise, and there is also evidence suggesting improved muscle recovery following exercise (123).

Green Tea Extract and Epigallocatechin Gallate

Green tea is made from the plant *Camellia sinensis L.*, which is rich in polyphenol catechins and caffeine that may have anticarcinogenic, anti-inflammatory, oxidative, and cardiac protective effects. A study of the effect of green tea extract on healthy humans during rest and exercise found that it may increase fat metabolism through improved oxidative stress biomarkers (124). A similar result was found in a study of trained and untrained males, who consumed either a cellulose placebo or green tea prior to two exercise sessions. It was observed that the green tea significantly improved resting and postexercise fat oxidation (125). In a study assessing green tea on oxidative stress and muscle damage in soccer players, it was found that it was beneficial in reducing oxidative stress but not muscle damage in these athletes (126).

Quercetin

Quercetin, a polyphenol (flavonoid) antioxidant, appears to have anti-inflammatory and antioxidant properties (127). However, an analysis of multiple studies assessing the effect of quercetin on endurance performance found that the effect of supplementation is likely to be small with no ergogenic benefit for both trained and untrained people (128). A study assessing oxidative damage and inflammation following intense exercise using laboratory mice found that quercetin was effective in lowering both muscle and liver inflammatory markers (129). These and other data suggest that quercetin has the potential for lowering tissue inflammation and improving peripheral tissue circulation that may have a small benefit on endurance performance, suggesting that athletes should consume quercetin and other antioxidant polyphenols as a regular part of the diet. (See Table 14.2 for quercetin-containing foods.) There are limited data at this time to suggest that regular supplemental intake of quercetin would impart additional beneficial effects in athletes (128).

Resveratrol

The flavonoid resveratrol is found in red wine, grape skins and seeds, peanuts, blueberries, raspberries, mulberries, lingonberries, and senna. Because it is found in red wine, red wine consumption has for some been attributed to lowering cardiovascular disease risk. However, studies assessing nonalcoholic red grapes containing 8 mg/day of resveratrol found that it lowered inflammation, atherosclerosis, and risk of cardiovascular disease (130,131). There is no additional evidence suggesting that the resveratrol in red wine would have similar benefits (132). An early animal study assessing the potential benefits of resveratrol on endurance exercise found that it improved aerobic capacity and fat metabolism while increasing insulin sensitivity (133). However, a study assessing the effect on inflammation and delayed-onset muscle soreness in male marathoners found no benefits associated with the resveratrol consumption (134).

FOOD SAFETY, FOOD ALLERGIES, INTOLERANCES, AND SENSITIVITIES

Food safety, allergies, intolerances, and sensitivities are important to consider for an athlete's health and performance. The federal government has made headway in labeling foods for allergenic ingredients (the Food Allergen Labeling and Consumer Protection Act of 2004; effective January 1, 2006), but this law does not yet have an impact on food labeling requirements on restaurant menus. In addition, this law does not address common food intolerances and food sensitivities. Nutritional menu labeling legislation is currently an important area of interest as the obesity epidemic has initiated efforts that mandate restaurants to list calorie counts and nutritional information on every menu offering. The current food labeling requirements almost exclusively deal with the caloric values of menu items and ignore other equally important factors that could help people with food intolerances, food sensitivities, and food allergies. To exacerbate this issue, many states require food service employees to obtain some form of certification on food sanitation and safety practices, but these certifications fail to address the equally important areas of food allergies, food intolerances, and food sensitivities (135,136). This leaves affected customers at risk, because those who serve the food have little or no idea about the issues related to these other areas that can affect health.

Food Safety

The existing food safety and sanitation laws deal with the preparation, storage, and serving of food that is safe for customers to consume. Depending on the statistical strategy used to estimate the prevalence of disease and mortality, it has been estimated that there are between 9.4 and 76 million foodborne diseases in the United States every year, with between 55,961 and 325,000 hospitalizations and between 1,251 and 5,000 fatalities (137,138). The number of individuals who experience foodborne illnesses and recover amounts to over a million per year, and it is estimated that an equivalent number of cases is never reported. The cause of these illnesses goes well beyond commercial restaurants. Foodborne illnesses also include private homes and social meal functions where state food safety and sanitation regulations are not mandated by law. Given the close proximity with which athletes live and train with each other, the possible transfer of disease from one athlete to another, through shared foods and drinks, is an important consideration in avoiding the transfer of illness from one athlete to another. The generally recommended strategies for avoiding transfer of contaminated foods and preventing foodborne illness are:

- Athletes should avoid sharing bottled beverages (*i.e.*, water, sports beverages). Toward this end, athletes should have bottles with their name clearly imprinted on it.
- Pathogens (bacteria, viruses, etc.) can be transferred via food from infected individuals. Therefore, food sharing should be limited to avoid pathogen transfer. As an additional caution, athletes should be encouraged to frequently and thoroughly wash their hands to limit pathogenic transfer via food and other means (equipment, etc.).

Food Allergies

It has been estimated that 2.5% of the US population has a **food allergy**, with higher allergy risks found in African-Americans, males, and children (139). Food allergies are caused by the ingestion of a specific antigen with an ensuing immunoglobulin E (IgE)-mediated allergic response. The symptoms of food allergies are usually immediate, occurring within 2 minutes to 2 hours after ingestion, and can involve the GI tract, respiratory system, eyes, and skin (140). Symptom severity can be unpredictable and life threatening in the case of anaphylaxis (141). The most common food allergies are related to the consumption of peanuts, tree nuts, egg, milk, wheat, soybeans, fish, and crustacean shellfish, with a food-specific protein the usual offending substance (140). Athletes should be completely aware of any allergen-containing food and avoid the consumption of it. If the athlete is unsure about the contents of a food, they should err on the side of caution and avoid consuming the food. Athletes with known food allergies should also be extremely cautious about accepting foods and beverages from other athletes without firm assurance that the offered foods and beverages are free of a potential allergen. On a rare occasion, an athlete may have a food-dependent, exercise-induced anaphylactic reaction (142). In this condition, the allergic reaction only occurs when food and exercise are combined, but does not occur when the food is consumed without exercise. With such a condition, athletes should avoid the offending food for a minimum of 4 hours before exercise and should always have immediately available a self-injectable EpiPen (a self-injectable dose of adrenaline) should a reaction occur. Even with appropriate caution, however, allergic reactions are possible. Therefore, the following steps should be taken with any athlete who has a known allergy:

1. The team's health care professionals (athletic trainer, doctor) should make an inquiry on the initial contact with an athlete as to whether the athlete has an allergy and, if so, the nature and severity of the allergy.

2. If the allergy is to a commonly consumed food, food alternatives should be made available at team meetings, competitions, travel, etc., with the knowledge that even passive contact with that food may result in an allergic response.

3. There should be a plan in place should the athlete experience an allergic reaction, including knowledge of whether the athlete has available medications, often an EpiPen or antihistamine, and where the medications are kept.

4. Should an athlete experience an allergic reaction, which may include anaphylaxis (throat tightness, tongue swelling, and loss of consciousness), the medications should be immediately administered and the emergency action plan activated (call 911, etc.). On arrival, the ambulance personnel should be notified whether a medication was already provided.

Food Intolerance

Food intolerance typically involves insufficient or missing digestive substances, such as enzymes or bile salts, causing a usually rapid onset of distressing GI symptoms, such as gas, bloating, and diarrhea. For example, symptoms of lactose intolerance are present in about 10% of the population and occur when the enzyme lactase is not produced in sufficient amounts to adequately break down the lactose in dairy products. Some athletes may experience a food intolerance from consuming carbohydrates that are not well absorbed but are rapidly fermentable. These carbohydrates are known as "fermentable oligo-, di-, and monosaccharides and polyols" (FODMAP), and limiting their intake in individuals with food intolerances may help to manage the symptoms. Common FODMAP foods that are typically listed on food labels include: fructose, fructans, lactose, sorbitol, and xylitol. (See: https://www.aboutibs.org/low-fodmap-diet/effects-of-fodmaps-on-the-gut.html for more information on the FODMAP diet approach.)

Celiac Disease

Celiac disease is an autoimmune disease that results from exposure to gluten, which causes an inflammation in the small intestine and affects nutrient absorption (143). The resulting malabsorption is associated with iron deficiency resulting in anemia and poor calcium absorption resulting in low bone mineral density (144). Other nutrient deficiencies may also occur, including deficiencies of vitamins D and B_{12}, and folate and the mineral zinc (145). It takes an extremely small exposure to gluten to trigger a response. In most celiac patients, only 20 parts per million (equal to approximately two crumbs of bread on a large dinner plate) is sufficient to create the celiac-associated GI symptoms of abdominal pain, bloating, nausea, vomiting, and alternating constipation and diarrhea. Other signs, including myalgia, arthralgia, low bone density, menstrual irregularities, and dermatitis, are also associated with celiac disease (145). Athletes with celiac disease must totally avoid the consumption of gluten. Because gluten is found in many carbohydrate products commonly consumed by athletes (breads, energy bars, etc.), it is important for athletes to find gluten-free alternatives that can provide the necessary carbohydrate required to satisfy energy needs, including fruits, vegetables, legumes, quinoa, millet, potato, corn, rice, pumpkin, and squash. Many gluten-free products are now available, making this task easier, but the athlete with celiac disease should seek the guidance of a dietitian to ensure that both energy and nutrient needs are being met. It is important to note that consuming diets that are gluten-free has become popular, even in athletes without celiac disease or gluten sensitivity, but there is no evidence of a performance benefit derived from adopting a gluten-free diet in

FIGURE 14.4: Food sensitivity inflammatory reactions. GERD, gastroesophageal reflux disease. (Adapted from Oxford Biomedical Technologies, Inc. How food sensitivities cause inflammation. Available from: http://nowleap.com/how-food-sensitivities-cause-inflammation © 2016 All Rights Reserved.)

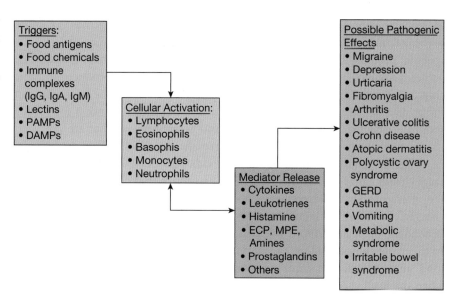

athletes without celiac disease or other nonceliac gluten intolerance (146).

Food Sensitivities

Food sensitivities are non–IgE-mediated inflammatory reactions involving the immune system (Figure 14.4). There has recently been an increase in the popularity of gluten-free diets, in large part due to an increase in nonceliac disease gluten sensitivity which, if not properly managed, can result in irritable bowel syndrome (IBS), chronic fatigue, and autoimmunity issues (147,148). There is a fad diet component to consumption of a gluten-free diet, which would unnecessarily limit the consumption of a wide spectrum of carbohydrate foods if celiac disease or nonceliac gluten sensitivity is not present (149). The prevalence of food sensitivities has not been estimated, but is now thought to be a major contributor to chronic GI disease in the population (150). Symptoms occur as a result of cytokine and mediator release from granulocytes and T-cells. These released mediators, including prostaglandins, histamines, cytokines, and serotonin, adversely affect gut function through tissue inflammation, smooth muscle contraction, mucus secretion, and pain receptor activation. The mechanisms underlying food sensitivities are complex, requiring time and the sleuthing skills of an astute diagnostician. There are many possible food sensitivities, and because the inflammatory response may occur more than 24 hours following consumption (unlike an allergy or intolerance that can have a response soon after consumption), it is difficult to find the offending food(s). As a result, the food source of symptoms may remain elusive without food sensitivity testing and

a personalized elimination diet under the supervision of a registered dietitian or other appropriately credentialed health professional.

📖 Food Allergy

A reaction that occurs when the body's immune system overreacts to a food or a food substance. Symptoms of food allergy may range from mild (*i.e.*, slight skin rash) to severe (*i.e.*, impaired breathing, altered heart rate, sudden drop in BP). There is a wide variation in the individual causes of food allergies, but they often result from exposure to one of these foods/food categories: eggs, milk, peanuts, tree nuts, fish, shellfish, wheat, and soy.

📖 Food Intolerance

The difficulty a person may have in consuming a particular food, often because of a missing or inadequate level of a specific digestive enzyme. For instance, lactose intolerance is the result of insufficient lactase (the enzyme that digests lactose). The undigested lactose results in bloating and diarrhea. Food intolerance is not a food allergy.

📖 Food Sensitivity

Refers to nonallergic (*i.e.*, non-IgE) and nonfood intolerance inflammatory reactions to specific foods or food components that, over time, may result in a number of clinical outcomes that affect the gut as well as the immune and neurologic systems.

A healthy gut microbiome is necessary to help migrate or metabolize potential inflammatory agents, such as gluten, out of the gut before it can become an inflammatory agent (151,152). Besides GI symptoms that include bloating and diarrhea, other common symptoms of nonceliac gluten sensitivity include problems with attention span, lowered immunity, skin rash, joint and muscle aches, and chronic fatigue.

DISORDERED EATING AND EATING DISORDERS

Important Factors to Consider

- Disordered eating and eating disorders are important conditions that affect many athletes, particularly if they are involved in aesthetic/appearance sports that have a large subjective component in the scoring (*i.e.*, how you appear doing a skill, not just if the skill is completed) (13,17,153,154). While more commonly affecting female athletes, eating disorders also occur in male athletes. Female athletes who have low energy availability (LEA) experience low estrogen and low bone mineral density, while male athletes experience low testosterone and low bone mineral density (155). It is important to consider that athletes with Relative Energy Deficiency in Sport (RED-S) or LEA limit nutrient intake as a result of the caloric restriction, placing them at health risk (156). LEA has been found to induce a variety of health problems, including undesirable changes to the endocrine system, mental disorders, and thyroid suppression (157). Female athletes with LEA face several nutrition-related issues that can predispose them to an eating disorder or are a result of an eating disorder. This includes (18,158–160):
- Female athletes have a higher requirement for iron and other nutrients associated with red blood cell replacement (*i.e.*, folate, vitamin B_{12}, etc.). This increased requirement is a result of monthly menstrual blood loss, which can also impact thermoregulation because of the body fluid imbalance.
- Females athletes often have a high expectation for a "thin" appearance in a number of sports that have a subjective component to scoring. These include gymnastics, synchronized swimming, diving, and figure skating. This expectation may result in inadequate energy and nutrient consumption that can result in loss of lean mass and a number of health associated with related to RED-S.
- LEA is also likely to negatively impact other athletes. In female track and field athletes, LEA was reported in 60% of the middle-and long-distance athletes

and 23% of elite sprinters, and was associated with amenorrhea (161). It has also been found that LEA has long-term health effects, including low bone mineral density with increased stress fracture risk, and other health effects, including (161):
- Reproductive dysfunction
- Impaired bone health
- Abnormal blood lipids
- Irregular heart rhythm and hypotension
- Hypoglycemia
- Low resting metabolic rate
- Immunologic suppression
- Higher injury risk
- Impaired performance
- GI problems
- Reduced appetite
- Eating disorders and depression
- Because eating disorders are psychometric disorders, it is important that you not try to resolve a disordered eating/eating disorder problem by yourself. These are complicated disorders that require a trained health professional (typically a psychiatrist or psychologist trained in eating disorder treatment) to work with anyone with this health problem.
- Be careful what you say to an athlete, as there is often an excess level of importance placed on appearance rather than performance, which may exacerbate an eating problem (162). For instance, imagine seeing an athlete and as a greeting, you say, "You look really good today!" Sounds innocent enough, but what if this athlete had just finished purging (vomiting) in the bathroom? Your statement could be viewed by the athlete as reinforcement for what was just done in the bathroom that helped to make the athlete look "really good." Rather than focusing on appearance, try sticking to more important things like: "Good to see you!" and "I hear you're doing really well in biology!"

Some athletes, particularly those involved in sports where appearance or making weight is a common aspect of the sport and are often subjectively scored (*i.e.*, wrestling, gymnastics, figure skating, diving), are at risk of developing disordered eating patterns that may develop into classical eating disorders, including anorexia nervosa (AN) and bulimia nervosa (BN) (163–165). It has been found that the prevalence of eating disorders in athletes is nearly four times higher than in nonathletes (18% vs. 5%) and is particularly high in athletes involved in sports where

FIGURE 14.5: Possible relationship between energy deficits and disordered eating. (From Benardot D, Thompson W. Energy from food for physical activity: enough and on time. ACSM Health Fit J. 1999;3(4):14–8.)

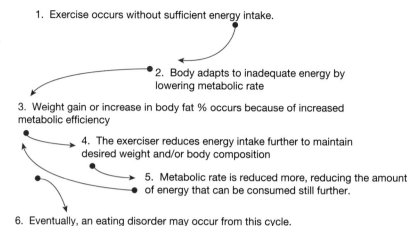

1. Exercise occurs without sufficient energy intake.

2. Body adapts to inadequate energy by lowering metabolic rate

3. Weight gain or increase in body fat % occurs because of increased metabolic efficiency

4. The exerciser reduces energy intake further to maintain desired weight and/or body composition

5. Metabolic rate is reduced more, reducing the amount of energy that can be consumed still further.

6. Eventually, an eating disorder may occur from this cycle.

appearance or weight is considered important (153,166). The route taken is often the following:

Normal Eating → Disordered Eating → Eating Disorders

A *normal eater* is someone who has a flexible eating pattern, tends to feel no guilt about eating a wide variety of foods, and eats with little restraint when hunger occurs (167). A **disordered eating** pattern is characterized by restrained eating behaviors that tend to ignore physiologic signals of hunger, often because of an excessive emphasis on body weight and the potential that eating will contribute to excess weight (168). Greater difficulty in regulating emotion and body dissatisfaction are important predictors of disordered eating in female athletes (169). An **eating disorder** is a psychological condition that is associated with distorted body image, low self-esteem, and an excessive emphasis on food (170). There is likely to be an energy-deficiency relationship in the progression of disordered eating patterns to diagnosable eating disorders, as insufficient energy intake is associated with a proportionately greater loss of lean mass than fat mass, resulting in a larger body size because of the higher relative fat mass. The lower density of fat mass makes the athlete look bigger at the same weight (12). As illustrated in Figure 14.5, the adaptation to a lower level of tissue capable of metabolizing energy (*i.e.*, *adaptive thermogenesis*) causes a progressive lowering of energy intake that further reduces lean tissue and, eventually, leads to an eating disorder.

📖 Disordered Eating

Characterized by restrained eating behaviors that tend to ignore physiologic signals of hunger, often because of an excessive emphasis on body weight and the potential that eating will contribute to excess weight.

📖 Eating Disorder

One of several psychological conditions, including anorexia nervosa, bulimia nervosa, and binge eating disorder (BED), that are associated with distorted body image, low self-esteem, and an excessive emphasis on food.

There are also changing cultural expectations for what a healthy person should look like, potentially encouraging athletes in appearance sports to resort to restrained eating behaviors in an attempt to achieve the unachievable (171,172). The *female athlete triad*, which is often seen in female athletes participating in appearance sports, consists of the following (Figure 14.6) (173,174):

1. LEA
2. Low bone mineral density
3. Abnormal menstrual status

It has become increasingly clear that the poor energy availability commonly seen in eating disorders may be directly responsible for lower bone mineral density and the low estrogen that is associated with abnormal menstrual status (175). However, LEA may also be the result of a failure to adequately consume sufficient energy to support the exercise, separate from an eating disorder (13). It has also become evident that male athletes also develop a series of problems associated with LEA, recently reported as *relative energy deficiency in sport (RED-S)*. (See Chapter 8 for additional information on RED-S.) To help determine if an athlete may have the female athlete triad, a series of questions have been developed as part of the preparticipation physical examination (*i.e.*, an examination that should occur *before* an athlete is allowed to participate in sport). The recommended screening questions for the preparticipation physical examination are (176):

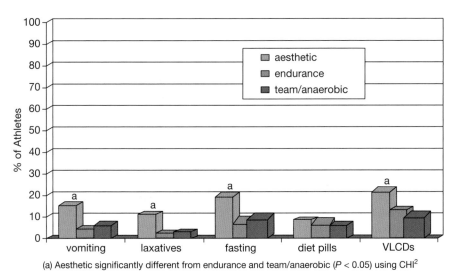

FIGURE 14.6: Athletes in "aesthetic" sports have higher rates of pathogenic weight control practices (VLCD: "Very Low Calorie Diets"). (From Beals KA, Manore MM. Disorders of the female athlete triad among collegiate athletes. Int J Sport Nutr Exerc Metab. 2002;12(3):281–93.)

(a) Aesthetic significantly different from endurance and team/anaerobic ($P < 0.05$) using CHI^2 analysis.

1. Have you ever had a menstrual period?
2. How old were you when you had your first menstrual period?
3. When was your most recent menstrual period?
4. How many periods have you had in the past 12 months?
5. Are you presently taking any female hormones (estrogen, progesterone, birth control pills)?
6. Do you worry about your weight?
7. Are you trying to or has anyone recommended that you gain or lose weight?
8. Are you on a special diet or do you avoid certain types of foods or food groups?
9. Have you ever had an eating disorder?
10. Have you ever had a stress fracture?
11. Have you ever been told you have lost bone mineral density (osteopenia or osteoporosis)?

The American Medical Society for Sports Medicine and the ACSM have developed guidelines for a preparticipation physical examination that include questions meant to determine the likelihood of disordered eating or an eating disorder. These questions relate to whether the athlete worries about weight, if anyone has recommended weight change, if the athlete is on a special diet that avoids certain foods, if the athlete was ever diagnosed with an eating disorder, of if he or she is taking supplements for the express purpose of altering weight (177).

Eating disorders have a psychological component, sometimes associated with a coping strategy used to deal with deeper problems that are too difficult to address directly. For instance, a young female may find it difficult to deal with the increased attention she is receiving as she begins developing into an adult woman. An eating disorder that dramatically lowers energy intake is also seen as a coping strategy in adolescent girls who have experienced sexual abuse (171,178,179). There may also be a genetic component to the development of eating disorders, with certain individuals having a genetic predisposition to its development (180).

Reasons for the development of eating disorders in athletes have also been assessed in athletes who were diagnosed as having an eating disorder (181):

- Prolonged dieting/weight fluctuations (37%)
- New coach (30%)
- Injury/illness (23%)
- Casual comments about weight (19%)
- Leaving home coupled with failure at school or work (10%)
- Problem in a relationship (10%)
- Illness or injury to family members (7%)
- Death of significant other(s) (4%)
- Sexual abuse (4%)

In the United States, it has been estimated that 10 million women and 1 million men will suffer from an eating disorder during their lifetime (182). According to the American College of Obstetricians and Gynecologists, the prevalence of eating disorders is between 16% and 47% of females trying to achieve a slender appearance, which places them at risk for hypothalamic amenorrhea (183). Using a questionnaire and clinical interview to determine the presence of eating disorders in 1,620 athletes and 1,696 nonathlete controls, it was found that 13.5% of the athletes had an eating disorder, whereas significantly fewer (4.6%) nonathletes had an eating disorder (184). Eating disorder prevalence was higher in female than in male athletes, and it was also found that the eating disorder prevalence in a subsample of female athletes participating in aesthetic sports was significantly higher than that of females in endurance sports (42% vs. 24%), technical sports (42% vs. 17%), and ball sports (42% vs. 16%). Involvement in early weight-control behaviors (*i.e.*, dieting at a young age) is a predictor of disordered eating later in life, for both men and women (185). It is critical, therefore, that young and adolescent athletes satisfy the nutritional needs for both physical activity and growth/development, as failure to do so is likely to result in multiple health issues, including delayed puberty, poor bone health, failure to achieve predicted stature, eating disorders, and elevated injury risk (16). In females, problems associated with poor energy availability appear to be even more pronounced (186). The health risks associated with eating disorders are high, with the risk of premature death 6–13 times higher in females diagnosed with AN (187). Strategies for encouraging good feeding practices in young athletes include the following (16,188):

- Involve children/adolescents in menu planning for family meals, with the goal of satisfying the type and amounts of foods to be consumed at appropriate times to satisfy exercise requirements.
- Encourage positive feedback for young athletes who are making positive steps to consume appropriate foods and beverages that satisfy the dual requirements for exercise and development.
- Enable and encourage participation of young athletes in the preparation of nutrient-rich meals and snacks as an integral part of the athletic endeavor.

Types and Dangers of Eating Disorders

Eating disorders are complex and potentially life-threatening psychological conditions that require a multidisciplinary care team of health professionals trained in working with eating disorders, typically a physician, psychiatrist or psychologist, and dietitian, to diagnose and/or treat the disorder (189) (Figure 14.7).

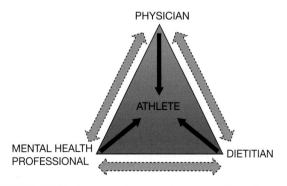

FIGURE 14.7: Dietitians, physicians, and mental health professionals should work as a team when working with eating disordered athletes.

Those without formal training should *not* be involved in attempting to resolve an eating disorder, as any well-intentioned action may be counterproductive. What follows is a summary of the basic criteria for each of the more commonly seen eating disorders in athletes, with common symptoms. The purpose of this information is to help you understand the complexity of the condition and, if you suspect that someone you know or work with may have an eating disorder, to bring them to the attention of an appropriately credentialed health professional.

The major eating disorders seen in athletes include: AN, BN, BED, and other specified feeding or eating disorder (OSFED). These are potentially life-threatening conditions, with diagnostic criteria published by the American Psychiatric Association in the 5th edition of *Diagnostic and Statistical Manual of Mental Disorders (DSM-5)* (190). When matched for age and gender, mortality ratios for those with AN are 5.35 times higher, with BN 1.50 times higher, and with OSFED 1.70 times higher than in those without eating disorders (191).

Anorexia Nervosa

AN is an extremely serious and potentially life-threatening eating disorder that is characterized by self-induced starvation that is coupled with extreme weight loss (Box 14.2) (192). The generally accepted criteria for AN include:

- Refusal to maintain weight within a normal range for height and age (more than 15% below ideal body weight)
- Fear of weight gain, with severe restriction of energy intake to reduce weight
- Severe body image disturbance in which body image is the predominant measure of self-worth with denial of the seriousness of the illness
- In postmenarchal females, absence of the menstrual cycle, or amenorrhea (greater than three cycles)

Bulimia Nervosa

This eating disorder, also referred to as *bulimia*, is associated with secretively binging on large amounts of food, followed with a purging strategy (vomiting, laxative abuse, diuretics, enemas, etc.) to eliminate the calories consumed during the binge (193). In extreme cases, the purging may occur after consumption of relatively small quantities of foods. It has been reported that, during a binge, 10,000–20,000 kcal may be consumed in a single day, typically in secret and often from forbidden foods such as cookies, candy, chips, and ice cream (194). The typical cause is preoccupation with body image and weight, coupled with low self-esteem. The current diagnostic criteria (DSM-5)

Box 14.2	Common Signs and Symptoms of Anorexia Nervosa

Following are common signs and symptoms of AN:

- Dry skin
- Cold intolerance and hypothermia
- Blue hands and feet
- Constipation
- Bloating
- Delayed puberty
- Primary amenorrhea (never experienced a menstrual period) or secondary amenorrhea (experienced a menstrual period, but without one for 3 months or longer)
- Nerve compression

- Fainting and orthostatic hypotension (sudden drop in BP on changing position, as from sitting to standing)
- Lanugo hair (increase in body hair in physiologic attempt to sustain body heat)
- Scalp hair loss
- Early satiety
- Weakness, fatigue
- Short stature for age
- Osteopenia (low bone mineral density)
- Sexual immaturity for age (breast atrophy, etc.)
- Pitting edema (typically from poor protein status and poor electrolyte status)
- Cardiac murmurs and arrhythmias

Source: Data from Harrington BC, Haxton C, Jimerson DC. Initial evaluation, diagnosis, and treatment of anorexia nervosa and bulimia nervosa. *Am Fam Physician.* 2015;91(1):46–52.

required for BN is now a binge once per week over a 3-month period. The previous diagnostic criterion was binge twice per week for 3 months, a change that has resulted in an increase in the diagnosis of BN (195). Eating disorders are often associated with anxiety disorders, with many also suffering from depression, which has been associated with suicidal attempts in this population (196,197). In those with BN, 23% of deaths occur as a result of suicide or cardiac arrhythmia (187,196). Common warning signs of BN include (193):

- Evidence of binge eating, including disappearance of large amounts of food in short periods of time or the discovery of wrappers and containers indicating the consumption of large amounts of food.
- Evidence of purging behaviors, including frequent trips to the bathroom after meals, signs and/or smells of vomiting, presence of wrappers or packages of laxatives or diuretics.
- Excessive, rigid exercise regimen—despite weather, fatigue, illness, or injury, the compulsive need to "burn off" calories taken in.
- Unusual swelling of the cheeks or jaw area.
- Calluses on the back of the hands and knuckles from self-induced vomiting (Figure 14.8). Discoloration or staining of the teeth (see Figure 14.7).
- Creation of lifestyle schedules or rituals to make time for binge-and-purge sessions.
- Withdrawal from usual friends and activities.
- In general, behaviors and attitudes indicating that weight loss, dieting, and control of food are becoming primary concerns.
- Continued exercise despite injury; overuse injuries.

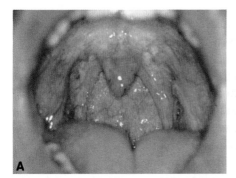 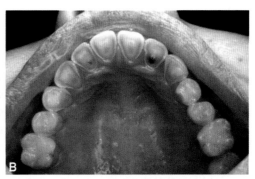

FIGURE 14.8: Oral manifestations of purging-type eating disorders. Signs of purging include (**A**) irritation and inflammation of the pharynx and esophagus from chronic vomiting and (**B**) erosion of the lingual surface of the teeth, loss of dental enamel, periodontal disease, and extensive dental caries. (From Wilkins EM. Clinical practice of the dental hygienist. 12th ed. Philadelphia (PA): LWW (PE); 2016.)

Binge Eating Disorder

BED is characterized by frequent episodes of consuming large quantities of foods, often to the point of discomfort. Unlike with BN, there is no purging following a binging episode with BED. As with other eating disorders, BED is life threatening, often from increased suicide risk. It is the most common of the diagnosable eating disorders, affecting 3.5% of women, 2% of men, and up to 1.6% of adolescents (182,198). The diagnostic criteria and symptoms associated with BED include (190):

A. Recurrent episodes of binge eating. An episode of binge eating is characterized by both of the following:
   ● Eating, in a discrete period of time (*e.g.*, within any 2-hour period), an amount of food that is definitely larger than what most people would eat in a similar period of time under similar circumstances.
   ● A sense of lack of control over eating during the episode (*e.g.*, a feeling that one cannot stop eating or control what or how much one is eating).
B. The binge eating episodes are associated with three (or more) of the following:
   ● Eating much more rapidly than normal.
   ● Eating until feeling uncomfortably full.
   ● Eating large amounts of food when not feeling physically hungry.
   ● Eating alone because of feeling embarrassed by how much one is eating.
   ● Feeling disgusted with oneself, depressed, or very guilty afterward.
C. Marked distress regarding binge eating is present.
D. The binge eating occurs, on average, at least once a week for 3 months.

The binge eating is not associated with the recurrent use of inappropriate compensatory behaviors (*e.g.*, purging) as in BN and does not occur exclusively during the course of BN or AN.

Other Specified Feeding or Eating Disorder

The criteria for OSFED are similar as for AN, except that regular menses are accepted in the diagnosis and weight is still within the normal range. It is the most prevalent of the eating disorders, with about 60% of those with an eating disorder diagnosed as having OSFED (199). A major criterion for OSFED is that the individual does not meet the criteria for AN or BN, but does engage in inappropriate compensatory behavior after just consuming a small quantity of food. Examples include: engaging in self-induced vomiting after consuming two cookies or, something commonly seen, chewing and spitting out large amounts of foods without swallowing. This disorder is typically observed in young females between the ages of 15 and 30 and is present in 3%–5% of women living in Western countries. Sample criteria for OSFED include (198):

■ Atypical AN (although there is restrictive eating, weight is not below normal)
■ BN (tends to have gorge–purge behavior, but less often than in BN)
■ BED (will exhibit binge eating, but does so less often than in BN)
■ Purging disorder (may purge, but without the binge eating typical of BN)

Night eating syndrome (exhibits excessive nighttime food consumption).

HIGH-ALTITUDE TRAINING

It has become increasingly common for athletes to train at a high altitude in advance of a major competition, with the goal of enhancing erythropoiesis to enable improved oxygen carrying capacity. It has also become clear that the greater the hypoxic environment the greater the risk of poor energy availability and inadequate iron provision. Current findings suggest that athletes in a hypoxic environment will enhance hemoglobin when consuming high doses of iron of between 100 and 200 mg (200). It has also become clear that the best strategy for dealing with the increased oxidative stress associated with high-altitude training is to try to resolve the elevated oxidative stress with consumption of more antioxidant-rich foods rather than rely on antioxidant supplements, which typically supply excessively high levels of antioxidants. There have also been investigations on consumption of foods that will enhance nitric oxide (typically beetroot juice), but the combination of low oxygen availability and slow hemoglobin production it is still not clear that higher nitrate consumption to enhance nitric oxide is useful (201,202). See Table 14.3 to illustrate the nutrition-related impact in athletes training at different altitudes.

It is clear that an important consideration of high-altitude training is to maintain food availability strategies that will help to avoid poor energy availability, as this can clearly negatively impact the athlete's health (200).

Table 14.3	**Potential Nutrition-Related Physiologic Changes or Nutrition Interventions for Various Altitudes (Relative Level of Importance/ Evidence for Consideration *Compared* to Sea Level)**					
Altitude	Energy Requirements (EI, EEE, EA, and BM)	Increased Glycogen Use/ CHO Needs	Increased Oxidative Stress	Increased Antioxidant Requirements	Increased Iron Requirements	Various Ergogenic Supplements
Extreme altitude (>5,500 m)	✓✓✓✓	✓✓✓✓	✓✓✓✓	?	✓✓✓✓	✓?
High altitude (3,000 m–5,500 m)	✓✓✓	✓✓✓✓	✓✓✓	?	✓✓✓	✓?
Moderate altitude (2,000 m–3,000 m)	✓?	?	✓✓	?	✓✓✓	✓?
Low altitude (500 m–2,000 m)	=?	?	✓	?	✓✓	✓?

Potential nutrition-related physiologic/metabolic changes or nutrition interventions for various altitudes. Altitude cut-offs are as established by Bartsch P, Saltin B. General introduction to altitude adaptation and mountain sickness. Scand J Med Sci Sports. 2008;18(Suppl 1):1–10.

All rankings are reflective of the relative level of importance and impact, and/or evidence, compared to sea level. An equal (=) sign represents equivalent evidence and importance as at sea level. ✓✓✓✓ is convincing evidence, ✓✓✓ is strong evidence, ✓✓ is moderate evidence, and ✓ is low or emerging evidence for a physiologic/metabolic change or for nutrition intervention consideration. ? indicates emerging evidence or potentially theoretical rationale, but no published studies at specific altitude or requires more scientific confirmation.

BM, body mass; CHO, carbohydrate; EA, energy availability; EEE, exercise energy expenditure; EI, energy intake.

Based on information from Stellingwerff T, Peeling P, Garvican-Lewis LA, Hall R, Koivisto AE, Heikura IA, and Burke LM. Nutrition and altitude: strategies to enhance adaptation, improve performance and maintain health: a narrative review. Sports Med. 2019;49(Suppl 2):S169–84.

BASIC HEALTH ENHANCING STRATEGIES FOR ATHLETES

- Eat sufficient energy to:
  - Support the desired level of lean body mass.
  - Avoid RED-S and/or LEA
- Eat enough carbohydrates to fuel training and maintain glycogen store. A greater proportion of carbohydrate: total energy is needed with activities that have a higher proportion of strength/power (*i.e.*, glycogen).
- Consume sufficient energy in a well-distributed manner to avoid RED-S. This generally requires more eating opportunities than the standard 3 meals/day, and should consider the pre-, during-, and postactivity energy intake.
- Choose a meal prior to training and competition that provides needed energy but that does not result in GI distress.
- Eat a high-quality protein source (20–25 g/meal) that is distributed throughout the day to satisfy total protein requirement. Example: A 100 kg power athlete who wishes to consume 2 g/kg of protein (200 g)

should have approximately eight opportunities during the day to consume 25 g of protein per opportunity.
- If competing in a weight class sport, select a weight class that can be safely achieved without a major dietary change, with minimal stress and without anxiety.
- Select low-fat, nonfried foods, as the fats in these foods may be inflammatory.
- Avoid extreme weight shifts, as this is likely to result in excess loss of lean tissue.
- Satisfy fluid needs by maintaining relatively clear urine. This requires ample water consumed with foods, a chronic sipping protocol of a well-formulated sport drink during training/competition, and sufficient fluid postexercise to return to a well-hydrated state.
- Seek the advice of a credential sports nutrition expert if you wish to make major changes to your diet or you wish to discuss the intake of nutrient supplements.
- Have a regular blood test (*e.g.*, annually) to understand your iron and vitamin D status.
- Maintain a healthy gut microbiome through regular consumption of fresh fruits, fresh vegetables, and whole grains.
- Carefully examine the use of sports foods and establish tolerance during training rather than competition.

- With any sign of ill health, seek the advice of a credential health professional.

SUMMARY

- Physical activity should and can be health promoting, and if the right activities are matched with an appropriate nutrient/energy intake, there is good evidence to suggest that the activity will result in better health, lower disease risks, and improve longevity. There is also good evidence to suggest that the well-nourished individual who has regular physical activity has lower risk of major chronic disorders, including cardiovascular disease, obesity, diabetes, and osteoporosis.

- The greater the energy expenditure, the greater the requirement for consumed energy to satisfy the need. However, the required energy cannot be provided randomly. Rather, there should be a dynamic relationship between energy expended and energy consumed so that a wide shift in energy balance during the day (*i.e.*, within-day energy balance) does not occur.

- The higher requirement for energy in physically active people also results in a higher requirement for many vitamins and minerals. However, consumption of insufficient energy with vitamin and mineral supplements fails to satisfy this need, whereas consumption of good-quality foods (*i.e.*, fresh fruits and vegetables, whole grains, fish, and meats) helps to satisfy both energy and vitamin/mineral needs. After all, what good are vitamins that are involved in energy metabolism if insufficient energy is consumed for the vitamins to metabolize? The best way for athletes to satisfy nutritional requirements is through consumption of foods, not supplements.

- Vitamin supplements typically contain high multiples of RDA for any given nutrient. For instance, although the RDA for vitamin C is ~60 mg, vitamin C supplements often contain 1,000–2,000 mg. There is scant evidence that chronic overconsumption of vitamins is useful in the athletic endeavor and an increasing body of evidence that many vitamin supplements are counterproductive. As a simple rule, remember: More than enough is not better than enough. (If a small amount is good for you, it does not hold that more is better.)

- There is an increasing body of evidence suggesting that athletes who are on "weight loss diets" and fail to consume sufficient energy to support the combined demands of age, sex, and physical activity are likely to develop higher body fat percent, have greater risk of eating disorders, and are at increased health risk.

- Staying well hydrated should be a high priority for physically active people. Poor hydration inhibits physical activity, inhibits benefiting from the desired physiologic changes the physical activity should result in, and may result in a life-threatening increase in heat stress risk.

- With the possible exception of swimming, physical activity place multiples of normal gravitational forces on bones, which causes a desired adaptation: an increase in bone mineral density and lower risk of later osteoporosis. However, physical activity also increases the requirement for energy, and a failure to satisfy energy needs in real time increases cortisol production, which results in a *decrease* in bone mineral density.

- Lowering obesity risk is an important goal, as the obesity rate is now of epidemic proportions in the United States and many other industrialized nations. Nutritional factors that can help to lower obesity risk include maintenance of a reasonably good energy balance, limiting the consumption of beverages that are high in sugar, increasing daily physical activity, ensuring good-quality sleep of at least 7 hours, regular assessment of body composition to be able to intervene early if there is a rise in body fat level or an lowering of lean mass, develop an eating plan with sufficient frequency to avoid hunger, eat foods typical of the Mediterranean diet (fresh fruits, nuts, vegetables, fish, and olive oil), and ensure a healthy gut microbiome through ample consumption of plant-based foods that are not heavily processed.

- Although exercise-induced oxidative stress is a normal component of physical activity, there is good evidence to suggest that consumption of a good-quality, healthy diet that satisfies energy needs and is coupled with regular physical activity results in a positive adaptive response to the oxidative stress. There is also evidence to suggest that consumption of antioxidant vitamins may inhibit the desired adaptive response to exercise, with a resultant increase in oxidative stress.

- It is increasingly being recognized that phytonutrients (*i.e.*, plant-based chemicals with nutrient qualities that are not vitamins or minerals) are an important component of a healthy diet. Phytonutrients are derived from plants (*i.e.*, fruits and vegetables) and include substances such as resveratrol, curcumin, anthocyanin, and quercetin, all of which impart health benefits when consumed as part of a well-balanced healthy diet.

- Food allergies are important factors to consider when planning what to eat. It is also important to consider food intolerances, food sensitivities, and food safety as all of these may negatively impact health and athletic performance if not properly planned for and dealt with.

- Athletes involved in weight control and appearance sports appear to be at particularly high risk of developing disordered eating and/or eating disorders, which are serious conditions that should be addressed by a medical professional trained to work with these conditions. There are different types of eating disorders, all of which are considered psychological disorders. These include AN, BN, and BED.

Practical Application Activity

Phytonutrients are increasingly being studied and it is being found that, although they are not directly essential for maintaining human life the way that vitamins are, they are important for protecting cells and enhancing health in humans. One way of categorizing phytonutrients is by color, because many phytonutrients are related to the color of foods (*e.g.*, the red/purple color of blueberries is due to the phytonutrient *anthocyanin*). To determine if you are exposing yourself to a wide array of phytonutrients, do the following:

1. Write down all the fruits and vegetables and their color that you consume over a 3-day period.
2. Find the phytonutrient(s) associated with each color.
3. Determine if there are colors missing in your diet and see what fruits and vegetables you could eat that have those colors.

CHAPTER QUESTIONS

1. If an athlete's daily requirement for protein is 1.5 g/kg, there is no difference in how this protein is consumed (*i.e.*, in a single meal, in three meals, in six meals)
   a. True
   b. False

2. For children, the combination of physical activity and good nutrition should help them develop:
   a. Healthy body weight
   b. Healthy cardiovascular system
   c. Healthy self-esteem with lower risk of anxiety and depression
   d. Better academic performance
   e. All of the above
   f. a, b, and c only

3. Worldwide, the prevalence of physical inactivity and type II diabetes is:
   a. 2%
   b. 7%
   c. 10%
   d. 90%

4. What proportion of the US adult population fails to meet the recommendations for physical activity?
   a. 10%
   b. 23%
   c. 56%
   d. 72%

5. A high proportion of women develop osteoporosis, and this is likely to lead to an inadequate acquisition of bone mineral density during adolescence.
   a. True
   b. False

6. Of the following, which is *not* a recommendation of the dietary guidelines for Americans?
   a. Consume more protein, but only from low-fat sources
   b. Limit the intake of sugar and salt
   c. Eat a wide variety of high nutrient-dense foods
   d. Limit the consumption of saturated fats

7. Of the following conditions, which are related to obesity?
   a. Nonalcoholic fatty liver disease
   b. Hypertension
   c. Colon cancer
   d. Type II diabetes
   e. All of the above
   f. b, c, and d only

8. Obesity refers to:
   a. High body weight
   b. High body fat
   c. High abdominal fat
   d. High lower body fat

9. Assessment of 24-hour energy balance is a good means of determining if body fat level will increase.
   a. True
   b. False

10. Examples of phytonutrients include all of the following, except:
    a. Flavonols
    b. Cobalamin
    c. Anthocyanins
    d. Isoflavones

ANSWERS TO CHAPTER QUESTIONS

1. b
2. e
3. b
4. c
5. a

6. a
7. f
8. b
9. b
10. b

Case Study Considerations

1. **Case Study Answer 1:** Fit athletes typically have a good strength:weight ratio (*i.e.*, muscle to fat differential), and focusing on "weight" fails to discriminate on *what* weight should change. Ideally, athletes would want to increase muscle weight while keeping fat weight the same, with a resultant improvement in the strength:weight ratio. The sudden increased caloric intake, above the usual intake, is likely to result in more of the excess energy being stored as fat, which is the opposite of the desired outcome. More fat weight means that now the muscle has to expend more energy to move more total weight and is likely to result in a slower acceleration and movement, with a negative impact on performance. Ideally, energy intake and energy expenditure should be dynamically linked, so that the athlete can support lean mass while limiting the potential for increasing fat mass.

2. **Case Study Answer 2:** Having sufficient vitamin E and other antioxidant vitamins/nutrients is important for reducing the potential negative impact of reactive oxygen species (ROS) on muscle soreness. However, there is limited data to suggest that having more than the requirement for vitamin E is useful in lowering the negative impact of ROS. In fact, there is evidence that having high daily doses of vitamin E, as typically supplied via supplements, may inhibit the muscle tissue adaptation to exercise, resulting in more muscle soreness and making matters worse. It is also important to consider that antioxidant vitamins work together. For instance, vitamin E is fat soluble and "lives" in the cell membrane. Vitamin C is water soluble and is carried in the blood. When vitamin E captures an ROS, it gives it off to vitamin C to carry it away, so that vitamin E is capable of capturing another ROS. This is a clear example of why nutrient balance is important.

3. **Case Study Answer 3:** Muscle increases slowly, so requires only a subtle increase in extra protein with appropriate amino acids (*e.g.*, leucine, which is a muscle protein synthesis stimulator). But the muscle must be physically worked harder than usual to make the muscle enlargement possible. This requires more energy, primarily from carbohydrate, to satisfy energy needs. Trying to satisfy energy needs from consuming extra protein is problematic, as the protein must be denitrogenated, and the elevated blood urea nitrogen must be excreted. This elevates urinary fluid loss and increases the risk of developing dehydration, which would be contraindicated for someone wishing to increase musculature.

REFERENCES

1. Scheer V, Tiller NB, Doutreleau S, Khodaee M, Knechtle B, Pasternak A, Rojas-Valverde D. Potential long-term health problems associated with ultra-endurance running: a narrative review. Sports Med. 2022;52:725–40.

2. Clarsen B, Bahr R, Myklebust G, Andersson SH, Docking SL, Drew M, Finch CF, Fortington LV, Harøy J, Khan KM, Moreau B, Moore IS, Møller M, Nabhan D, Nielsen RO, Pasanen K, Schwellnus M, Soligard T, Verhagen E. Improved reporting of overuse injuries and health problems in sport: an update of the Oslo Sport Trauma Research Center questionnaires. Br J Sports Med. 2020;54:390–6.

3. United States Department of Health and Human Services, Centers for Disease Control and Prevention. The benefits of physical activity. Accessed 2017 November 8. Available from: https://www.cdc.gov/physicalactivity/basics/pa-health/index.htm

4. Close GL, Sale C, Baar K, Berman S. Nutrition for the prevention and treatment of injuries in track and field athletes. Int J Sport Nutr Exercise Metab. 2019;19:189–97.

5. Condo D, Lohman R, Kelly M, Carr A. Nutritional intake, sports nutrition knowledge and energy availability female Australian rules football players. Nutrients. 2019;11:971.

6. Nabhan D, Lewis M, Taylor D, Bahr R. Expanding the screening toolbox to promote athlete health: how the US Olympic & Paralympic Committee screened for health problems in 940 athletes. Br J Sports Med. 2021;55:226–30.

7. Walsh NP, Hanson SL, Sargent C, Roach GD, Nédélec M, Gupta L, Leader J, Fullagar HH, Coutts AJ, Edwards BJ, Pullinger SA, Robertson CM, Burniston JG, Lastella M, Meur YL, Hausswirth C, Bender AM, Grandner MA, Samuels CH. Sleep and the athlete: narrative review and 2021 expert consensus recommendations. Br J Sports Med. 2020:bjsports-2020-102025.

8. Reardon CL, Hainline B, Aron CM, Baron D, Baum AL, Binder A, Budgett R, Campriani N, Mauricio J, Castaldelli-Maia JM, Currie A, Derevensky JL, Glick ID, Gorczynski P, Gouttebarge V, Grandner MA, Han DH, McDuff D, Mountjoy M, Polat A, Purcell R, Putukian M, Rice S, Sills A, Still T, Swartz L, Zhu LJ, Engebretsen L. Mental health in elite athletes: international Olympic Committee consensus statement (2019). Br J Sports Med. 2019;53:667–99.

9. Åkesdotter C, Kenttä G, Eloranta S, Franck J. The prevalence of mental health problems in elite athletes. J Sci Med Sport. 2020;23:329–35.

10. Reardon CL. Psychiatric comorbidities in sports. Neurol Clin. 2017;35:537–46.

11. Wall BT, Snijders T, Senden JM, Ottenbros CL, Gijsen AP, Verdijk LB, van Loon LJ. Disuse impairs the muscle protein synthetic response to protein ingestion in healthy men. J Clin Endocrinol Metab. 2013;98:4872–81.

12. Duloo AG, Montani JP. Pathways from dieting to weight regain, to obesity and to the metabolic syndrome: an overview. Obes Rev. 2015;16(Suppl 1):1–6.

13. Mountjoy M, Sundgot-Borgen J, Burke L, Carter S, Constantini N, Lebrun C, Meyer N, Sherman R, Steffen K, Budgett R, Ljungqvist A. The IOC consensus statement: beyond the Female Athlete Triad-Relative Energy Deficiency in Sport (RED-S). Br J Sports Med. 2014;48:491–7.

14. Ochner CN, Tsai AG, Kushner RF, Wadden TA. Treating obesity seriously: when recommendations for lifestyle change confront biological adaptations. Lancet Diabetes Endocrinol. 2015;3(4):232–4.

15. Helms ER, Prnjak K, Linardon J. Towards a sustainable nutrition paradigm in physique sport: a narrative review. Sports (Basel). 2019;7(7):172.

16. Tambalis KD. Special nutritional needs for athletes and exercisers. Eur J Physiother. 2022;3(1):1–22.

17. Thomas DT, Erdman KA, Burke LM. American College of Sports Medicine Joint Position Statement. Nutrition and athletic performance. Med Sci Sports Exerc. 2016;48(3):543–68.

18. Casa D, Cheuvront SN, Galloway SD, Shirreffs SM. Fluid needs for training, competition and recovery in track-and-field athletes. Int J Sport Nutr Exercise Metab. 2019;29(2):175–80.

19. Beck KL, von Hurst PR, O'Brien WJ, Badenhorst CE. Micronutrients and athletic performance: a review. Food Chem Toxicol. 2021;158:112618.

20. Mursu J, Robien K, Harnack LJ, Park K, Jacobs DR Jr. Dietary supplements and mortality rate in older women: the Iowa Women's Health Study. Arch Intern Med. 2011;171(18):1625–33.

21. Institute of Medicine, Food and Nutrition Board. Vitamin C. Dietary reference intakes for vitamin C, vitamin E, selenium, and carotenoids. Washington (DC): National Academy Press; 2000. p. 95–185.

22. Taylor EN, Stampfer MJ, Curhan GC. Dietary factors and the risk of incident kidney stones in men: new insights after 14 years of follow-up. J Am Soc Nephrol. 2004;15(12):3225–32.

23. Thomas LDK, Elinder C-G, Tiselius H-G, Wolk A, Akesson A. Ascorbic acid supplements and kidney stone incidence among men: a prospective study. JAMA Intern Med. 2013;173(5):386–8.

24. Vrolijk MF, Opperhuizen A, Jansen EHJM, Hageman GJ, Bast A, Haenen GRMM. The vitamin B6 paradox: supplementation with high concentrations of pyridoxine leads to decreased vitamin B6 function. Toxicol In Vitro. 2017;44:206–12.

25. Nelson RL. Iron and colorectal cancer risk: human studies. Nutr Rev. 2001;59(5):140–8.

26. Wen CP, Lee JH, Tai Y-P, Wen C, Wu SB, Tsai MK, Hsieh DPH, Chiang H-C, Hsiung CA, Hsu CY, Wu X. High serum iron is associated with increased cancer risk. Cancer Res. 2014;74(22):6589–97.

27. Aksan A, Farrag K, Aksan S, Schroeder O, Stein J. Flipside of the coin: iron deficiency and colorectal cancer. Front Immunol. 2021;12:635899.

28. Phipps O, Al-Hassi HO, Quraishi MN, Kuman A, Brookes MJ. Influence of iron on the gut microbiota in colorectal cancer. Nutrients. 2020;12:2512.

29. Luo H, Zhang N-Q, Huang J, Zhang X, Feng X-L, Pan Z-Z, Chen Y-M, Fang Y-J, Zhang C-X. Different forms and sources of iron in relation to colorectal cancer risk: a case-control study in China. Br J Nutr. 2019;121:735–47.

30. Schümann K, Borch-Iohnsen B, Hentze MW, Marx JJM. Tolerable upper intakes for dietary iron set by the US food and Nutrition Board. Am J Clin Nutr. 2002;76(3):499–500.

31. Sim M, Garvican-Lewis LA, Cox GR, Govus A, McKay AKA, Stellingwerff T, Peeling P. Iron considerations for the athlete: a narrative review. Eur J Appl Physiol. 2019;119(7):1463–78.

32. Figueiredo JC, Grau MV, Haile RW, Sandler RS, Summers RW, Bresalier RS, Burke CA, McKeown-Eyssen GE, Baron JA. Folic acid and risk of prostate cancer: results from a randomized clinical trial. J Natl Cancer Inst. 2009;101(6):432–5.

33. Kim Y-I. Folate: a magic bullet or a double edged sword for colorectal cancer prevention? Gut. 2006;55(10):1387–9.

34. Lee JE, Willett WC, Fuchs CS, Smith-Warner SA, Wu K, Ma J, Giovannucci E. Folate intake and risk of colorectal cancer and adenoma: modification by time. Am J Clin Nutr. 2011;93(4):817–25.

35. Mason JB. Unraveling the complex relationship between folate and cancer risk. Biofactors. 2011;37(4):253–60.

36. Ulrich CM, Potter JD. Folate supplementation: too much of a good thing? Cancer Epidemiol Biomarkers Prev. 2006;15(2):189–93.

37. Maughan RJ, Depiesse F, Geyer H; International Association of Athletics Federations. The use of dietary supplements by athletes. J Sports Sci. 2007;25(S1):S103–13.

38. Burke LM, Castell LM, Casa DJ, Close GL, Costa RJS, Desbrow B, Hanson SL, Lis DM, Melin AK, Peeling P, Saunders PU, Slater GJ, Sago J, Wizard OC, Bermon S, Stellingwerff T. International association of athletics federations consensus statement 2019: nutrition for athletics. Int J Sport Nutr Exerc Metab. 2019;29:73–84.

39. American College of Sports Medicine. Exercise is medicine: physical activity-far reaching! Accessed 2024 May 23. Available from: https://www.exerciseismedicine.org/wpcontent/uploads/2021/02/EIM-miracle-drug-handout.pdf

40. United States Department of Health and Human Services, Centers for Disease Control and Prevention. Division of nutrition, physical activity, and obesity, national center for chronic disease prevention and health promotion. How much physical activity do adults need? 2015. Accessed 2017 January 6. Available from: https://www.cdc.gov/physicalactivity/basics/adults/index.htm

41. World Health Organization. Global atlas on cardiovascular disease prevention and control. Geneva: World Health Organization; 2011.

42. World Health Organization. Global strategy on diet, physical activity and health: information sheet: global recommendations on physical activity for health 5–17 years old. Accessed 2024 May 23. Available from: https://www.who.int/publications/i/item/9241592222

43. Dietary Guidelines for Americans: 2020–2025. Accessed 2024 May 23. Available from: https://www.dietaryguidelines.gov/2020-2025-dietary-guidelinesonline-materials/top-10-things-you-need-know

44. Cawley J, Biener A, Meyerhoefer C, Ding Y, Zvenyach T, Smolarz BG, Ramasamy A. Direct medical costs of obesity in the United States and the most populous states. J Manag Care Spec Pharm. 2021;27(3):354–366. doi: 10.18553/jmcp.2021.20410. Epub 2021 Jan 20.

45. Mente A, de Koning L, Shannon HS, Anand SS. A systematic review of the evidence supporting a causal link between dietary factors and coronary heart disease. Arch Intern Med. 2009;169:659–69.

46. Barclay AW, Petocz P, McMillan-Price J, Flood VM, Prvan T, Mitchell P, Brand-Miller JC. Glycemic index, glycemic load, and chronic disease risk—a meta-analysis of observational studies. Am J Clin Nutr. 2008;87(3):627–37.

47. Malik VS, Popkin BM, Bray GA, Després JP, Willett WC, Hu FB. Sugar-sweetened beverages and risk of metabolic syndrome and type 2 diabetes: a meta-analysis. Diabetes Care. 2010;33:2477–83.

48. Pan A, Sun Q, Bernstein AM, Schulze MB, Manson JE, Willett WC, Hu FB. Red meat consumption and risk of type 2 diabetes: 3 cohorts of US adults and an updated meta-analysis. Am J Clin Nutr. 2011;94(4):1088–96.

49. Alberti KGMM, Zimmet P, Shaw J; IDF Epidemiology Task Force Consensus Group. The metabolic syndrome–a new worldwide definition. Lancet. 2005;366(9491):1059–62.

50. Grundy SM, Brewer HB, Cleeman JI, Smith SC, Lenfant C; American Heart Association; National Heart, Lung, and Blood Institute. Definition of metabolic syndrome: report of the National Heart, Lung, and Blood Institute/American Heart Association conference on scientific issues related to definition. Circulation. 2004;109:433–8.

51. Fabbrini E, Sullivan S, Klein S. Obesity and nonalcoholic fatty liver disease: biochemical, metabolic, and clinical implications. Hepatology. 2010;51(2):679–89.

52. Gholam PM, Kotler DP, Flancbaum LJ. Liver pathology in morbidly obese patients undergoing Roux-en-Y gastric bypass surgery. Obes Surg. 2002;12:49–51.

53. Dixon JB, Bhathal PS, Hughes NR, O'Brien PE. Nonalcoholic fatty liver disease: improvement in liver histological analysis with weight loss. Hepatology. 2004;39:1647–54.

54. Kurukulasuriya LR, Stas S, Lastra G, Manrique C, Sowers JR. Hypertension in obesity. Med Clin North Am. 2011;95(5):903–17.

55. Simonds SE, Cowley MA. Hypertension in obesity: is leptin the culprit? Trends Neurosci. 2013;36(2):121–32.

56. De Pergola G, Silvestris F. Obesity as a major risk factor for cancer. J Obes. 2013;2013: 291546.

57. van Saase JL, Vandenbroucke JP, van Romunde LK, Valkenburg HA. Osteoarthritis and obesity in the general population. A relationship calling for an explanation. J Rheumatol. 1988;15(7):1152–8.

58. Bliddal H, Leeds AR, Christensen R. Osteoarthritis, obesity and weight loss: evidence, hypotheses and horizons-a scoping review. Obes Rev. 2014;15(7):578–86.

59. United States Department of Health and Human Services, Centers for Disease Control and Prevention. Adult obesity causes & consequences. Accessed 2024 May 23. Available from: https://www.cdc.gov/obesity/basics/consequences.html

60. United States Department of Health and Human Services, National Institutes of Health, National Heart, Lunch, and Blood Institute. What causes overweight and obesity? Updated 2012. Accessed 2017 January 6. Available from: https://www.nhlbi.nih.gov/health/health-topics/topics/obe/causes

61. Harvard School of Public Health. Obesity definition. Accessed 2017 January 2. Available from: https://www.hsph.harvard.edu/obesity-prevention-source/obesity-definition/

62. Mridha S, Barman P. Comparison of height-weight matched young-adult female athletes and non-athletes in selected anthropometric measurements. Int J Sci Res. 2014;3(1):265–8.

63. Javed A, Jumean M, Murad MH, Okorodudu D, Kumar S, Somers VK, Sochor O, Lopez-Jimenez F. Diagnostic performance of body mass index to identify obesity as defined by body adiposity in children and adolescents: a systematic review and meta-analysis. Pediatr Obes. 2015;10(3):234–44.

64. Benardot D. Energy thermodynamics revisited: energy intake strategies for optimizing athlete body composition and performance. J Exerc Sci Health. 2013;11(2):1–13.

65. Benardot D. Timing of energy and fluid intake: new concepts for weight control and hydration. ACSM Health Fit J. 2007;11(4):13–9.

66. Deutz RC, Benardot D, Martin DE, Cody MM. Relationship between energy deficits and body composition in elite female gymnasts and runners. Med Sci Sports Exerc. 2000;32:659–68.

67. Fahrenholtz IL, Sjödin A, Benardot D, Tornberg ÅB, Skouby S, Faber J, Sundgot-Borgen JK, Melin AK. Within-day energy deficiency and reproductive function in female endurance athletes. Scand J Med Sci Sports. 2018:28(3):1139–46.

68. Smith KJ, Gall SL, McNaughton SA, Blizzard L, Dwyer T, Venn AJ. Skipping breakfast: longitudinal associations with cardiometabolic risk factors in the Childhood Determinants of Adult Health Study. Am J Clin Nutr. 2010;92(6):1316–25.

69. Anderwald C, Brabant G, Bernroider E, Horn R, Brehm A, Waldhäusl W, Roden M. Insulin-dependent modulation of plasma ghrelin and leptin concentrations is less pronounced in type 2 diabetic patients. Diabetes. 2003;52(7):1792–8.

70. Solomon TPJ, Chambers ES, Jeukendrup AE, Toogood AA, Blannin AK. The effect of feeding frequency on insulin and ghrelin responses in human subjects. Br J Nutr. 2008;100(4):810–9.

71. Miller WC, Koceja DM, Hamilton EJ. A meta-analysis of the past 25 years of weight loss research using diet, exercise or diet plus exercise intervention. Int J Obes Relat Metab Disord. 1997;21:941–7.

72. Ross R, Dagnone D, Jones PJH, Smith H, Paddags A, Hudson R. Reduction in obesity and related comorbid conditions after diet-induced weight loss or exercise-induced weight loss in men. A randomized, controlled trial. Ann Intern Med. 2000;133(2):92–103.

73. Sacks FM, Bray GA, Carey VJ, Smith SR, Ryan DH, Anton SD, McManus K, Champagne CM, Bishop LM, Laranjo N, Leboff MS, Rood JC, de Jonge L, Greenway FL, Loria CM, Obarzanek E, Williamson DA. Comparison of weight-loss diets with different compositions of fat, protein, and carbohydrates. N Engl J Med. 2009;360(9):859–73.

74. Willett WC, Leibel RL. Dietary fat is not a major determinant of body fat. Am J Med. 2002;113(Suppl 9B):47S–59S.

75. Field AE, Willett WC, Lissner L, Colditz GA. Dietary fat and weight gain among women in the Nurses' Health Study. Obes. 2007;15:967–76.

76. Aune D, Ursin G, Veierød MB. Meat consumption and the risk of type 2 diabetes: a systematic review and meta-analysis of cohort studies. Diabetologia. 2009;52:2277–87.

77. Bernstein AM, Sun Q, Hu FB, Stampfer MJ, Manson JE, Willett WC. Major dietary protein sources and risk of coronary heart disease in women. Circulation. 2010;122:876–83.

78. Hu FB, Malik VS. Sugar-sweetened beverages and risk of obesity and type 2 diabetes: epidemiologic evidence. Physiol Behav. 2010;100(1):47–54.

79. Ruanpeng D, Thongprayoon C, Cheungpasitporn W, Harindhanavidhi T. Sugar and artificially sweetened beverages linked to obesity: a systematic review and meta-analysis. QJM. 2017;110(8):513–20.

80. Te Morenga L, Mallard S, Mann J. Dietary sugars and body weight: systematic review and meta-analyses of randomized controlled trials and cohort studies. BMJ. 2012;346:e7492.

81. Vartanian LR, Schwartz MB, Brownell KD. Effects of soft drink consumption on nutrition and health: a systematic review and meta-analysis. Am J Public Health. 2007;97:667–75.

82. Mozaffarian D, Hao T, Rimm EB, Willett WC, Hu FB. Changes in diet and lifestyle and long-term weight gain in women and men. N Engl J Med. 2011;364:2392–404.

83. Torstveit MK, Fahrenholtz I, Stenqvist TB, Sylta Ø, Melin A. Within-day energy deficiency and metabolic perturbation in male endurance athletes. Int J Sport Nutr Exerc Metab. 2018:28(4):419–27.

84. Miller MA, Cappuccio FP. Inflammation, sleep, obesity, and cardiovascular disease. Curr Vasc Pharmacol. 2007;5(2): 93–102.

85. Capers PL, Fobian AD, Kaiser KA, Borah R, Allison DB. A systematic review and meta-analysis of randomized controlled trials of the impact of sleep duration on adiposity and components of energy balance. Obes Rev. 2015;16:771–82.

86. Gangwisch JE, Malaspina D, Boden-Albala B, Heymsfield SB. Inadequate sleep as a risk factor for obesity: analysis of the NHANES I. Sleep. 2005;28(10):1289–96.

87. Patel SR, Hu FB. Short sleep duration and weight gain: a systematic review. Obes. 2008;16:643–53.

88. Torres SJ, Nowson CA. Relationship between stress, eating behavior, and obesity. Nutrition. 2007;23(11–12):887–94.

89. Grossman P, Niemann L, Schmidt S, Walach H. Mindfulness-based stress reduction and health benefits: a meta-analysis. J Psychosom Res. 2004;57(1):35–43.

90. Isacco L, Lazaar N, Ratel S, Thivel D, Aucouturier J, Doré E, Meyer M, Duché P. The impact of eating habits on anthropometric characteristics in French primary school children. Child Care Health Dev. 2010;36(6):835–42.

91. Buckland G, Bach A, Serra-Majem L. Obesity and the Mediterranean diet: a systematic review of observational and intervention studies. Obes Rev. 2008;9:582–93.

92. Hughes RL. A review of the role of the gut microbiome in personalized sports nutrition. Front Nutr. 2020;6:191.

93. Tilg H, Kaser A. Gut microbiome, obesity, and metabolic dysfunction. J Clin Invest. 2011;121(6):2126–32.

94. Bäckhed F, Ding H, Wang T, Hooper LV, Koh GY, Nagy A, Semenkovich CF, Gordon JI. The gut microbiota as an environmental factor that regulates fat storage. Proc Natl Acad Sci U S A. 2004;101(44):15718–23.

95. Ley RE, Backhed F, Turnbaugh P, Lozupone CA, Knight RD, Gordon JI. Obesity alters gut microbial ecology. Proc Natl Acad Sci U S A. 2005;102(31):11070–5.

96. Turnbaugh PJ, Ridaura VK, Faith JJ, Rey FE, Knight R, Gordon JI. The effect of diet on the human gut microbiome: a metagenomic analysis in humanized gnotobiotic mice. Sci Transl Med. 2009;1(6):6ra14.

97. Patterson E, Ryan PM, Cryan JF, Dinan TG, Ross RP, Fitzgerald GF, Stanton C. Gut microbiota, obesity and diabetes. Postgrad Med J. 2016;92:286–300.

98. De Filippis F, Pellagrini N, Vannini L, Jeffery IB, La Storia A, Laghi L, Serrazanetti DI, Di Cagno R, Ferrocino I, Lazzi C, Turroni S, Cocolin L, Brigidi P, Neviani E, Gobbetti M, O'Toole PW, Ercolini D. High-level adherence to a Mediterranean diet beneficially impact the gut microbiota and associated metabolome. Gut. 2016;65:1812–21.

99. Zeppa SD, Agostini D, Gervasi M, Annibalini G, Amatori S, Ferrini F, Sisti D, Piccoli G, Barbieri E, Sestili P, Stocchi V.

Mutual interactions among exercise, sport supplements and microbiota. Nutrients. 2020;12:17.

100. Close GL, Hamilton DL, Philip A, Burke LM, Morton JP. New strategies in sport nutrition to increase exercise performance. Free Radic Biol Med. 2016;98:144–58.

101. Kårlund A, Gómez-Gallego C, Turpeinen AM, Palo-oja O-M, El-Nezami H, Kolehmainen M. Protein supplements and their relation with nutrition, microbiota composition and health: is more protein always better for sportspeople? Nutrients. 2019;11:829.

102. Lis DM, Kings D, Larson-Meyer DE. Dietary practices adopted by track-and-field athletes: gluten-free, low FOD-MAP, vegetarian, and fasting. Int J Sport Nutr Exerc Metab. 2019;29:236–45.

103. Lis DM. Exit gluten-free and enter low FODMAPs: a novel dietary strategy to reduce gastrointestinal symptoms in athletes. Sports Medicine. 2019;49(Suppl 1):S87–97.

104. Reid MB, Shoji T, Moody MR, Entman ML. Reactive oxygen in skeletal muscle. II. Extra cellular release of free radicals. J Appl Physiol. 1992;73(5):1805–9.

105. Halliwell B, Gutteridge J. Free radicals in biology and medicine. New York (NY): Oxford University Press; 2007.

106. Gleeson M, Nieman DC, Pedersen BK. Exercise, nutrition and immune function. J Sports Sci. 2004;22(1):115–25.

107. Nieman DC, Henson DA, McAnulty SR, McAnulty LS, Morrow JD, Ahmed A, Heward CB. Vitamin E and immunity after the Kona Triathlon World Championship. Med Sci Sports Exerc. 2004;36(8):1328–35.

108. Gomez-Cabrera MC, Domenich E, Romagnoli M, Arduini A, Borras C, Pallardo PV, Sastre J, Viña J. Oral administration of vitamin C decreases muscle mitochondrial biogenesis and hampers training-induced adaptations in endurance performance. Am J Clin Nutr. 2008;87(1):142–9.

109. Ristow M, Zarse K, Oberbach A, Klöting N, Birringer M, Kiehntopf M, Stumvoll M, Kahn CR, Blüher M. Antioxidants prevent health-promoting effects of physical exercise in humans. Proc Natl Acad Sci U S A. 2009;106:8665–870.

110. Riccioni G, Speranza L, Pesce M, Cusenza S, D'Orazio N, Glade MJ. Novel phytonutrient contributors to antioxidant protection against cardiovascular disease. Nutrition. 2012;28(6):605–10.

111. Riso P, Klimis-Zacas D, Del Bo' C, Martini D, Campolo J, Vendrame S, Møller P, Loft S, De Maria R, Porrini M. Effect of a wild blueberry (Vaccinium angustifolium) drink intervention on markers of oxidative stress, inflammation and endothelial function in humans with cardiovascular risk factors. Eur J Nutr. 2013;52(3):949–61.

112. Alvarez-Suarez JM, Giampieri F, Tulipani S, Casoli T, Di Stefano G, González-Paramás AM, Santos-Buelga C, Busco F, Quiles JL, Cordero MD, Bompadre S, Mezzetti B, Battino M. One-month strawberry-rich anthocyanin supplementation ameliorates cardiovascular risk, oxidative stress markers and platelet activation in humans. J Nutr Biochem. 2014;25(3):289–94.

113. Yarahmadi M, Askari G, Kargerfard M, Ghiasvand R, Hoseini M, Mohamadi H, Asadi A. The effect of anthocyanin supplementation on body composition, exercise performance and muscle damage indices in athletes. Int J Prev Med. 2104; 5(12):1594–1600.

114. Connolly DA, McHugh MP, Padilla-Zakour OI, Carlson L, Sayers SP. Efficacy of a tart cherry juice blend in preventing the symptoms of muscle damage. Br J Sports Med. 2006;40(8):679–83.

115. González-Gallego J, García-Mediavilla MV, Sánchez-Campos S, Tuñón MJ. Fruit polyphenols, immunity and inflammation. Br J Nutr. 2010;104(S3):S15–27.

116. Willems MET, Myers SD, Gault ML, Cook MD. Beneficial physiological effects with blackcurrant intake in endurance athletes. Int J Sport Nutr Exerc Metab. 2015;25;367–74.

117. Carroll RE, Benya RV, Turgeon DK, Vareed S, Neuman M, Rodriguez L, Kakarala M, Carpenter PM, McLaren C, Meyskens FL Jr, Brenner DE. Phase IIa clinical trial of curcumin for the prevention of colorectal neoplasia. Cancer Prev Res (Phila). 2011;4(3):354–64.

118. Epstein J, Sanderson IR, MacDonald TT. Curcumin as a therapeutic agent: the evidence from in vitro, animal and human studies. Br J Nutr. 2010;103(11):1545–57.

119. Huang MT, Lou YR, Ma W, Newmark HL, Reuhl KR, Conney AH. Inhibitory effects of dietary curcumin on forestomach, duodenal, and colon carcinogenesis in mice. Cancer Res. 1994; 54(22):5841–7.

120. Rivera-Mancía S, Lozada-García MC, Pedraza-Chaverri J. Experimental evidence for curcumin and its analogs for management of diabetes mellitus and its associated complications. Eur J Pharmacol. 2015;756:30–7.

121. Sahebkar A, Cicero AFG, Simental-Mendía LE, Aggarwal BB, Gupta SC. Curcumin downregulates human tumor necrosis factor-α levels: a systematic review and meta-analysis of randomized controlled trials. Pharmacol Res. 2016;107:234–42.

122. Taylor RA, Leonard MC. Curcumin for inflammatory bowel disease: a review of human studies. Altern Med Rev. 2011; 16(2):152–6.

123. Nicol LM, Rowlands DS, Fazakerly R, Kellett J. Curcumin supplementation likely attenuates delayed onset muscle soreness (DOMS). Eur J Appl Physiol. 2015;115(8):1769–77.

124. Sugita M, Kapoor MP, Nishimura A, Okubo T. Influence of green tea catechins on oxidative stress metabolites at rest and during exercise in healthy humans. Nutrition. 2016;32(3): 321–31.

125. Gahreman DE, Boutcher YN, Bustamante S, Boutcher SH. The combined effect of green tea and acute interval sprinting exercise on fat oxidation of trained and untrained males. J Exerc Nutrition Biochem. 2016;20(1):1–8.

126. Hadi A, Pourmansoumi M, Kafeshani M, Karimian J, Maracy MR, Entezari MH. The effect of green tea and sour tea (Hibiscus sabdariffa L.) supplementation on oxidative stress and muscle damage in athletes. J Diet Suppl. 2017;14(3):346–57.

127. Askari G, Hajishafiee M, Ghiasvand R, Hariri M, Darvishi L, Ghassemi S, Iraj B, Hovsepian V. Quercetin and vitamin C supplementation: effects on lipid profile and muscle damage in male athletes. Int J Prev Med. 2013;4(S1):S58–62.

128. Pelletier DM, Lacerte G, Goulet EDB. Effects of quercetin supplementation on endurance performance and maximal oxygen consumption: a meta-analysis. Int J Sport Nutr Exerc Metab. 2013;23:73–82.

129. Tang Y, Li J, Gao C, Xu Y, Li Y, Yu X, Wang J, Liu L, Yao P. Hepatoprotective effect of quercetin on endoplasmic reticulum stress and inflammation after intense exercise in mice

through phosphoinositide 3-kinase and nuclear factor-kappa B. Oxid Med Cell Longev. 2016;2016:8696587.

130. De Curtis A, Murzilli S, Di Castelnuovo A, Rotilio D, Donati MB, De Gaetano G, Iacoviello L. Alcohol-free red wine prevents arterial thrombosis in dietary-induced hypercholesterolemic rats: experimental support for the "French paradox." J Thromb Haemost. 2005;3(2):346–50.

131. Stocker R, O'Halloran RA. Dealcoholized red wine decreases atherosclerosis in apolipoprotein E gene-deficient mice independently of inhibition of lipid peroxidation in the artery wall. Am J Clin Nutr. 2004;79(1):123–30.

132. Linus Pauling Institute. Resveratrol. Accessed 2017 January 2. Available from: http://lpi.oregonstate.edu/mic/dietary-factors/phytochemicals/resveratrol

133. Lagouge M, Argmann C, Gerhart-Hines Z, Meziane H, Lerin C, Daussin F, Messadeq N, Milne J, Lambert P, Elliott P, Geny B, Laakso M, Puigserver P, Auwerx J. Resveratrol improves mitochondrial function and protects against metabolic disease by activating SIRT1 and PGC-1alpha. Cell. 2006;127:1109–22.

134. Laupheimer MW, Perry M, Benton S, Malliaras P, Maffulli N. Resveratrol exerts no effect on inflammatory response and delayed onset muscle soreness after a marathon in male athletes: a randomised, double-blind, placebo-controlled pilot feasibility study. Transl Med UniSa. 2014;10:38–42.

135. Algeo S. Opinion: Food allergy training needs to be mandated. Restaurant Hospitality Exclusive Insight. 2017. p. 1. Accessed 2024 May 23. Available from: https://www.restaurant-hospitality.com/food-trends/opinion-foodallergy-training-needs-be-mandated

136. Lipcsei L, Radke T. Food safety innovations in federal guidelines. J Environ Health. 2017;80(2):42–4.

137. Mead PS, Slutsker L, Dietz V, McCaig LF, Bresee JS, Shapiro C, Griffin PM, Tauxe RV. Food-related illness and death in the United States. Emerg Infect Dis. 1999;5(5):607–25.

138. Scallan E, Hoekstra RM, Angulo FJ, Tauxe RV, Widdowson M-A, Roy SL, Jones JL, Griffin PM. Foodborne illness acquired in the United States—major pathogens. Emerg Infect Dis. 2011;17(1):7–15.

139. Liu AH, Jaramillo R, Sicherer SH, Wood RA, Bock SA, Burks AW, Massing M, Cohn RD, Zeldin DC. National prevalence and risk factors for food allergy and relationship to asthma: results from the National Health and Nutrition Examination Survey 2005–2006. J Allergy Clin Immunol. 2010;126(4):798–806.

140. Sicherer SH, Sampson HA. Food allergy: epidemiology, pathogenesis, diagnosis, and treatment. J Allergy Clin Immunol. 2014;133(2):291–305.

141. Muraro A, Agache I, Clark A, Sheikh A, Roberts G, Akdis AC, Borrego LM, Higgs J, Hourihane JO'B, Jorgensen P, Mazon A, Parmigiani D, Said M, Schnadt S, van Os-Medendorp H, Vlieg-Boerstra BJ, Wickman M; European Academy of Allergy and Clinical Immunology. EAACI food allergy and anaphylaxis guidelines: managing patients with food allergy in the community. Allergy. 2014;69(8):1046–57.

142. Romano A, De Fonso M, Giuffreda F, Papa G, Artesani MC, Viola M, Venuti A, Palmieri V, Zeppilli P. Food-dependent exercise-induced anaphylaxis: clinical and laboratory findings in 54 subjects. Int Arch Allergy Immunol. 2001;125(3):264–72.

143. Dagmar R, Piper TJ. Celiac disease: a review for the athlete and interdisciplinary team. Strength Cond J. 2016;38(4):66–71.

144. Freeman HJ. Iron deficiency anemia in celiac disease. World J Gastroenterol. 2015;21(31):9233–8.

145. Mancini LA, Trojian T, Mancini AC. Celiac disease and the athlete. Curr Sports Med Rep. 2011;10(2):105–8.

146. Volpe SL. Gluten-free diets and exercise performance. ACSM's Health Fit J. 2018;22(1):35–6.

147. Fasano A, Sapone A, Zevallos V, Schuppan D. Nonceliac gluten sensitivity. Gastroenterology. 2015;148(6):1195–204.

148. Vazquez-Roque M, Oxentenko AS. Nonceliac gluten sensitivity. Mayo Clin Proc. 2015;90(9):1272–7.

149. Lis DM, Stellingwerff T, Shing CM, Ahuja KDK, Fell JW. Exploring the popularity, experiences, and beliefs surrounding gluten-free diets in nonceliac athletes. Int J Sport Nutr Exerc Metab. 2015;25(1):37–45.

150. Lee D, Albenberg L, Compher C, Baldassano R, Piccoli D, Lewis JD, Wu GD. Diet in the pathogenesis and treatment of inflammatory bowel diseases. Gastroenterology. 2015;148(6):1087–106.

151. Corley DA, Shuppan D. Introduction—food, the immune system, and the gastrointestinal tract. Gastroenterology. 2015;148(6):1083–6.

152. Khanna S, Tosh PK. A clinician's primer on the role of the microbiome in human health and disease. Mayo Clin Proc. 2014;89(1):107–14.

153. Bratland-Sanda S, Sundgot-Borgen J. Eating disorders in athletes: overview of prevalence, risk factors and recommendations for prevention and treatment. Eur J Sport Sci. 2013;13(5):499–508.

154. Melin A, Torstveit MK, Burke L, Marks S, Sundgot-Borgen J. Disordered eating and eating disorders in aquatic sport. Int J Sport Nutr Exerc Metab. 2014;24(4):450–9. https://doi.org/10.1123/ijsnem.2014-0029

155. De Souza MJ, Koltun KJ, Williams NI. The role of energy availability in reproductive function in the female athlete triad and extension of its effects to men: an initial working model of a similar syndrome in male athletes. Sports Med. 2019;49(Suppl2): S125–37.

156. Peklaj E, Rešćič N, Seljuk BK, Kozjek NR. Is RED-S in athletes just another face of malnutrition? Clin Nutr ESPEN. 2022;48:298–307.

157. Wasserfurth P, Palmowski J, Hahn A, Krüger K. Reasons for and consequences of low energy availability in female and male athletes: social environment, adaptations, and prevention. Sports Med Open. 2020;6:44.

158. Desbrow B, Burd NA, Tarnopolsky M, Moore DR, Elliott-Sale KJ. Nutrition for special populations: young, female, and masters athletes. Int J Sport Nutr Exerc Metab. 2019;29(2):220–7.

159. Pedlar CR, Brugnara C, Bruinvels G, Burden R. Iron balance and iron supplementation for the female athlete: a practical approach. Eur J Sport Sci. 2018;18(2):295–305.

160. Hashimoto H, Ishijima T, Suzuki K, Higuchi M. The effect of the menstrual cycle and water consumption on physiological responses during prolonged exercise at moderate intensity in hot conditions. J Sports Med Phys Fitness. 2016;56(9):951–60.

161. Melin AK, Heikura IA, Tenfold A, Mountjoy M. Energy availability in athletics: health, performance, and physique. Int J Sport Nutr Exercise Metab. 2019;29:152–64.

162. Stoeber J, Yang H. Physical appearance perfectionism explains variance in eating disorder symptoms above general perfectionism. Pers Individ Dif. 2015;86:303–7.

163. Holland LA, Brown TA, Keel PK. Defining features of unhealthy exercise associated with disordered eating and eating disorder diagnoses. Psychol Sport Exerc. 2014;15(1)116–23.

164. Sundgot-Borgen J, Meyer NL, Lohman TG, Ackland TR, Maughan RJ, Stewart AD, Müller W. How to minimize the health risks to athletes who compete in weight-sensitive sports review and position statement on behalf of the Ad Hoc Research Working Group on Body Composition, Health and Performance, under the auspices of the IOC Medical Commission. Br J Sports Med. 2013;47(16):1012–22.

165. Mancine RP, Gusta DW, Moshrefi A, Kennedy SF. Prevalence of disordered eating in athletes categorized by emphasis on leanness and activity type-a systematic review. J Eat Disord. 2020;8:47.

166. Sundgot-Borgen J. Prevalence of eating disorders in elite female athletes. Int J Sport Nutr. 1993;3(1):29–40.

167. Freeland-Graves JH, Nitzke S. Position of the Academy of Nutrition and Dietetics: total diet approach to healthy eating. J Acad Nutr Diet. 2013;113(2):307–17.

168. Polivy J, Heatherton T. Spiral model of dieting and disordered eating: encyclopedia of feeding and eating disorders. New York (NY): Springer; 2015. p. 1–3.

169. Shriver LH, Wollenberg G, Gates GE. Prevalence of disordered eating and its association with emotion regulation in female college athletes. Int J Sport Nutr Exerc Metab. 2016; 26(3):240–8.

170. Geil KE, Hermann-Werner A, Mayer J, Diehl K, Schneider S, Thiel A, Zipfel S; GOAL study group. Eating disorder pathology in elite adolescent athletes. Int J Eat Disord. 2016;49(6):553–62.

171. Polivy J, Herman CP. Causes of eating disorders. Annu Rev Psychol. 2002;53:187–213.

172. Rosen JC. Body-image disturbances in eating disorders. In: Cash TF, Pruzinsky T, editors. Body images: development, deviance, and change. New York (NY): Guilford Press; 1990. p. 190–214.

173. Nattiv A, Loucks AB, Manore MM, Sanborn CF, Sundgot-Borgen J, Warren MP; American College of Sports Medicine. American College of Sports Medicine position stand: the female athlete triad. Med Sci Sports Exerc. 2007;39(10): 1867–82.

174. Beals KA, Manore MM. Disorders of the female athlete triad among collegiate athletes. Int J Sport Nutr Exerc Metab. 2002;12(3):281–93.

175. Fredericson M, Kent K. Normalization of bone density in a previously amenorrheic runner with osteoporosis. Med Sci Sports Exerc. 2005;37:1481–6.

176. De Souza MJ, Nattiv A, Joy E, Misra M, Williams NI, Mallinson RJ, Gibbs JC, Olmsted M, Goolsby M, Matheson G; Expert Panel. 2014 Female Athlete Triad coalition consensus statement on treatment and return to play of the female athlete triad: 1st International Conference held in San Francisco, California, May 2012 and 2nd International Conference held in Indianapolis, Indiana, May 2013. Br J Sports Med. 2014;48:289.

177. Bernhardt DT, Roberts WO, editors. PPE: preparticipation physical evaluation. 4th ed. Elk Grove Village (IL): American Academy of Pediatrics; 2010.

178. Castellini G, Lelli L, Ricca V, Maggi M. Sexuality in eating disorders patients: etiological factors, sexual dysfunction and identity issues. A systematic review. Horm Mol Biol Clin Investig. 2015;25(2):71–90.

179. Killen JD, Hayward C, Litt I, Hammer LD, Wilson DM, Taylor CB, Varady A, Shisslak C. Is puberty a risk factor for eating disorders? Am J Dis Child. 1992;146(3):323–5.

180. Klump KL, Miller KB, Keel PK, McGue M. Genetic and environmental influences on anorexia nervosa syndromes in a population-based twin sample. Psychol Med. 2001;31(4): 737–40.

181. Sundgot-Borgen J. Eating disorders in female athletes. Sports Med. 1994;17(3):176–88.

182. Hudson JI, Hiripi E, Pope HG Jr, Kessler RC. The prevalence and correlates of eating disorders in the National Comorbidity Survey Replication. Biol Psychiatry. 2007;61(3): 348–58.

183. Huhmann K. Menses requires energy: a review of how disordered eating, excessive exercise, and high stress lead to menstrual irregularities. Clin Ther. 2020;42(3):401–7.

184. Sundgot-Borgen J, Torstveit MK. Prevalence of eating disorders in elite athletes is higher than in the general population. Clin J Sport Med. 2004;14(1):25–32.

185. Liechty JM, Lee MJ. Longitudinal predictors of dieting and disordered eating among young adults in the U.S. Int J Eat Disord. 2013;46:790–800.

186. Loucks AB. The response of luteinizing hormone pulsatility to 5 days of low energy availability disappears by 14 years of gynecological age. J Clin Endocrinol Metab. 2006;91(8):3158–64.

187. Arcelus J, Mitchell AJ, Wales J, Nielsen S. Mortality rates in patients with anorexia nervosa and other eating disorders. A meta-analysis of 36 studies. Arch Gen Psychiatry. 2011;68(7):724–31.

188. Roberts CJ, Gill ND, Beaven CM, Posthumus LR, Sims ST. Application of a nutrition support protocol to encourage optimization of nutrient intake in provincial academy rugby union athletes in New Zealand: practical considerations and challenges from a team-based case study. Int J Sports Sci. 2022;18(6):174795412211241.

189. Joy E, Kussman A, Nattiv A. 2016 update on eating disorders in athletes: a comprehensive narrative review with a focus on clinical assessment and management. Br J Sports Med. 2016;50:154–62.

190. American Psychiatric Association. Diagnostic and statistical manual of mental disorders. 5th ed. Arlington (VA): American Psychiatric Publishing; 2013.

191. Fichter MM, Quadflieg N. Mortality in eating disorders—results of a large prospective clinical longitudinal study. Int J Eat Disord. 2016;49(4):391–401.

192. National Eating Disorders Association. Anorexia nervosa [Internet]. Accessed 2024 May 23. Available from: https://www.nationaleatingdisorders.org/anorexia-nervosa/

193. National Eating Disorders Association. Bulimia nervosa [Internet]. Accessed 2016 January 2. Available from: https://www.nationaleatingdisorders.org/learn/by-eating-disorder/bulimia

194. Rosen JC, Leitenberg H, Fisher C, Khazam C. Binge-eating episodes in bulimia nervosa: the amount and type of food consumed. Int J of Eat Disord. 1986;5(2):255–67.

195. Wilson GT, Sysko R. Frequency of binge eating episodes in bulimia nervosa and binge eating disorder: diagnostic considerations. Int J Eat Disord. 2009;42:603–10.

196. Crow SJ, Swanson SA, le Grange D, Feig EH, Merikangas KR. Suicidal behavior in adolescents and adults with bulimia nervosa. Compr Psychiatry. 2014;55(7):1534–9.

197. Rosling AM, Sparén P, Norring C, von Knorring A-L. Mortality of eating disorders: a follow-up study of treatment in a specialist unit 1974–2000. Int J Eat Disord. 2011;44:304–10.

198. National Eating Disorders Association. Binge eating disorder [Internet]. Accessed 2016 January 2. Available from: https://www.nationaleatingdisorders.org/binge-eating-disorder

199. Fairburn CG, Bohn K. Eating disorder NOS(EDNOS): an example of the troublesome "not otherwise specified" (NOS) category in DSM-IV. Behav Res Ther. 2005;43(6):691–701.

200. Stellingwerff T, Peeling P, Garvican-Lewis LA, Hall R, Koivisto AE, Heikura IA, and Burke LM. Nutrition and altitude: strategies to enhance adaptation, improve performance and maintain health: a narrative review. Sports Med. 2019;49(Suppl 2):169–84.

201. Roberts D, Smith DJ. Erythropoietin concentration and arterial hemoglobin saturation with supramaximal exercise. J Sports Sci. 1999;17(6):485–93.

202. Puype J, Ramaekers M, Van Thienen R, Deldicque L, Hespel P. No effect of dietary nitrate supplementation on endurance training in hypoxia. Scand J Med Sci Sports. 2015;25(2):234–41.

Diet Planning for Optimal Performance

CHAPTER OBJECTIVES

- Discuss energy metabolic systems and how different energy demands of different sports use each of these systems.
- Identify the different muscle fiber types, how they are different, and how different sports emphasize the usage of different types.
- Recognize anabolic and catabolic hormones and how these are used in normal metabolic reactions.
- Demonstrate an understanding of different energy stores in humans and how athletes

utilize these stores in different types of physical activity.
- Determine the factors that are necessary to successfully build muscle mass.
- Identify the nutritionally relevant factors for specific power sports.
- Recognize the nutritionally relevant factors for specific endurance sports.
- Explain how athletes involved in different sports require different eating plans to satisfy their energy requirements.

Case Study

Joanne was a bright, straight 15-year-old high school swimmer who was showing a great deal of promise. Her high school coach suggested to her parents that Joanne join a local (nonschool) swim club to help her excel. They and Joanne agreed to give it a try. The first swim practice would take place at 5:30 AM before school, followed by a quick drive home for some food and a quick change, and then off to school to be there from 8:30 AM to 3:00 PM. That would be followed by school team swim practice that ended at 5:00 PM, then a quick drive to the swim club for final practice from 6:00 PM to 7:00 PM, and a 10-minute drive home. Dinner was at 7:30 PM, homework until 10:00 PM, and repeat 5 days/week. On weekends, Saturday practice was from 10:00 AM to 2:00 PM, and there was no Sunday practice. Sounds tough, but Joanne loved it! She loved her coaches, and she was making some great swimming buddies at the local swim club—girls from other schools that she would not have met were it not for the club. After several weeks, Joanne was clearly beginning to drag and, to make matters worse, her algebra grade went from an A+ to a C. When her parents

got the report card, they did not say anything because they were sure it was because of Joanne's new algebra teacher and not Joanne. Without saying anything to Joanne, her dad went to the school at about 10:00 AM to talk with the principal about the new algebra teacher. This was the same time that Joanne was taking her algebra class, and when he entered the school and walked toward the principal's office, he walked past Joanne's classroom. He looked in the window and saw something he could not believe. Joanne was sitting at her desk with her head bobbing from exhaustion while her algebra teacher was lecturing. Joanne was trying hard to keep her eyes open, but just could not do it. That moment struck Joanne's dad hard, as he realized clearly what had happened. Joanne was doing triple the physical activity she was doing before, depleting her carbohydrate stores, but her eating pattern had not changed to ensure adequate glycogen recovery and stable blood sugar (important for brain function). She was still trying to satisfy all of her needs with breakfast, lunch, and dinner, and it was clear now that this strategy was not working.

So, Joanne's dad continued to the principal's office, but now with an entirely new discussion focus: He wanted to ask the principal if Joanne could bring some snacks to school with her that she could eat mid-morning and before her school swim practice. The principal understood completely and to her credit agreed that the snacks were a good idea. Joanne would just have to find a way to eat the snacks between classes so as not to disturb the other students/teachers. Joanne started having the snacks and in just a week her entire demeanor went from exhausted to enthusiastically energetic. To make matters even better, her 10-week report card returned to straight A's again, including in algebra. The human fuel tank can only receive so much energy at a time, particularly for carbohydrate, and if you let it get to empty and stay there, bad things happen.

CASE STUDY
DISCUSSION QUESTIONS

Maintaining a reasonably good energy balance (energy availability) of a good distribution of macronutrients through-out the day is important for ensuring the maintenance of normal blood sugar and carbohydrate stores. Failure to sustain normal blood sugar results in gluconeogenesis, often with muscle tissue catabolized to provide the liver with amino acids that can be converted to glucose, resulting in improved attention and lower mental fatigue. Mental fatigue can result in muscular fatigue, even if the muscles have adequate energy to continue functioning (1,2).

1. It is important to sustain real-time energy balance to avoid issues associated with Relative Energy Deficiency in Sport (RED-S). To do this for your own real-time energy balance, create a spreadsheet to assess your hourly energy balance for each hour of the day, by predicting the energy expended for each hour and by assessing the energy intake of the foods and beverages you consume each hour of the day (follow the procedure described in earlier chapters). Carry over the ending energy balance of each hour to begin the energy balance of the next hour. To do this, you will need the following:
   a. Obtain an estimate of your basal (resting) energy expenditure (REE) for 24 hours, divided by 24 so you have *hourly* energy expenditure. Use the Harris–Benedict equation revised by Mifflin et al. (3):
   Male REE = (10 × weight in kg) + (6.25 × height in cm) − (5 × age in years) + 5
   Female REE = (10 × weight in kg) + (6.25 × height in cm) − (5 × age in years) − 161

   b. Obtain an estimate of your average hourly energy expenditure using the following MET value scale with this as an example: If you slept from midnight to 6 AM (6 hours), each of these hours would represent your predicted REE. If you did an average of *very light* activity from 6 AM to 7 AM, this hour would represent your REE × 2. Follow this procedure for each hour of the day.

Factor Descriptions (4)

1.0 Resting, reclining: Sleeping, reclining, relaxing
1.5 Rest +: Normal, average sitting, standing daytime activity
2.0 Very light: More movement, mainly with upper body; equivalent to tying shoes, typing, brushing teeth
2.5 Very light +: Working harder than 2.0
3.0 Light: Movement with upper and lower body; equivalent to household chores
3.5 Light +: Working harder than 3.0; heart rate faster, but can do this all day without difficulty
4.0 Moderate: Walking briskly, etc.; heart rate faster, sweating lightly, etc., but comfortable
4.5 Moderate +: Working harder than 4.0; heart rate noticeably faster, breathing faster
5.0 Vigorous: Breathing clearly faster and deeper, heart rate faster, must take occasional deep breaths during sentence to carry on conversation
5.5 Vigorous +: Working harder than 5.0; breathing noticeably faster and deeper and must breathe deeply more often to carry on conversation
6.0 Heavy: You can still talk, but breathing is so hard and deep you would prefer not to; sweating profusely; heart rate very high
6.5 Heavy +: Working harder than 6.0; you can barely talk but would prefer not to. This is about as hard as you can go, but not for long
7.0 Exhaustive: Cannot continue this intensity long, as you are on the verge of collapse and are gasping for air. Heart rate is pounding

2. For those periods of the day with wide shifts in energy balance that exceed ±400 calories, add foods and beverages at different times of the day to see what it would take to correct the severe energy balance deficits and surpluses (5,6).

3. If you have control over your eating pattern and food/beverage availability, try eating in the corrected food pattern to see how you feel.

INTRODUCTION

Specific sporting activities place different demands on energy/metabolic systems. Power and speed activities typically require that the athlete have the explosive capacity to move quickly, jump high, or move a heavy weight. The greater the athlete's ability to perform sport-specific tasks, the more successful they will be. The power and speed training athletes perform must have the appropriate nutritional support. **Team sport** athletes require a combination of power and endurance (stamina) to perform well during competition. For example, soccer players must not only have the stamina (endurance) to jog for the entire match but also require quick bursts of speed to sprint toward a ball when necessary. Basketball players must not only have the capacity to jog the length of the court during the game but also have the explosive power to block a shot, to sprint for a shot, or to jump for a rebound. *Endurance athletes* must have a high level of oxidative competence to enable the capacity to burn a fuel, fat, that humans have a large supply of and minimize the utilization of limited carbohydrate stores. Because of the long duration of endurance events, successful athletes have pre-event strategies for optimizing glycogen stores and hydration state, and during-event strategies for avoiding dehydration, maintaining blood volume to ensure continued cooling capacity, and maintaining carbohydrate stores to enable the complete oxidation of fats and the capacity to go faster (*i.e.*, when passing a competitor) when necessary (Table 15.1). This chapter reviews the specific nutritional requirements for each type of activity, includes a practical guide on the basic elements of assessing athlete readiness, and provides sport-specific nutritional issues that should be considered.

Team Sport

Team sports, or stop-and-go sports, require a combination of fast bursts of speed (sprints) interspersed with periods of slower, predominantly aerobic motion or with temporary cessation of activity. Examples of team sports include basketball, soccer, and hockey, but similar energy requirements are seen in tennis and other sports with stop-and-go activity.

ENERGY METABOLIC SYSTEMS

In brief, the energy systems work as follows (7,8).

High-power/high-intensity exercise of short duration creates a high demand for adenosine triphosphate (ATP) because of the large volume of power required by hard-working muscles per unit of time. At the initiation of

Table 15.1	Energy Metabolic Systems	
System	**Characteristics**	**Duration**
Phosphocreatine (PCr) system	Anaerobic production of ATP from stored PCr.	Used for maximal intensity activities lasting no more than 9 s.
Anaerobic glycolysis (lactic acid system)	Anaerobic production of ATP from the breakdown of glycogen. By-product of this system is the production of lactic acid.	Used for extremely high-intensity activities that exceed the athlete's capacity to bring in sufficient oxygen. Can continue producing ATP with this system no more than 30 s.
Oxygen system (aerobic metabolism)	Aerobic production of ATP from the breakdown of carbohydrates and fats. ■ Aerobic metabolism of fats referred to as "β-oxidation." ■ Aerobic metabolism of glucose referred to as "aerobic glycolysis." ■ Aerobic metabolism of glycogen referred to as "aerobic glycogenolysis." **Note:** The common generic term for the aerobic metabolism of carbohydrate is *aerobic glycolysis.*	Aerobic metabolism of fats (β-oxidation) used for lower intensity activities of long duration that can produce a substantial volume of ATP, but without the production of system-limiting by-products. Aerobic metabolism of carbohydrates (aerobic glycolysis and glycogenolysis) used for high-intensity activities that require a large volume of ATP, but that are within the athlete's capacity to bring sufficient oxygen into the system. This system can produce ATP for up to 2 min.

ATP, adenosine triphosphate.

these high-intensity activities, the *phosphocreatine (PCr) metabolic system* becomes the predominant source of energy. Although the PCr system is capable of providing the greatest production of ATP per unit of time, there is only sufficient preformed PCr to provide energy for up to ~8 seconds, at which time the muscles must rely on other energy sources that cannot produce as great a volume of ATP per unit of time. The result is that the athlete must, at this point, slow down (lower exercise intensity) because of the lower level of ATP production.

The PCr system is followed by the *anaerobic glycolysis system* as the system with the second greatest capacity to produce ATP per unit of time. This system relies on carbohydrate/glycogen as a fuel and can provide energy for up to and an additional 10–30 seconds (depending on power production) before a buildup of **lactic acid** that the muscle cannot adequately clear. At the point of lactic acid buildup, the muscle experiences a loss of power and fatigue.

🗐 Lactic Acid

Lactic acid (lactate) is produced constantly from pyruvate during normal energy metabolism. It can be reconverted to pyruvate and used to create ATP energy. When the energy requirement exceeds the oxidative capacity of tissues, lactic acid builds up in the tissues and is released into the blood to avoid excess acid buildup in the tissues. However, blood lactate can only build up until it affects blood pH, at which point the tissue lactic acid builds up, causing a cessation of tissue (muscle) function.

The anaerobic glycolysis system is followed by the *aerobic glycolysis system* with the third greatest capacity to produce ATP per unit of time and is also reliant on carbohydrate/glycogen as a fuel. Although producing less ATP per unit of time than anaerobic glycolysis, and therefore has a lower power potential, this system has the capacity to provide energy longer to the working muscle. Aerobic glycolysis can produce ATP for ~1–2 minutes, depending on muscle power production, before the muscle experiences a loss of power and fatigue.

The aerobic glycolysis system is followed by the *aerobic energy system* (also referred to as β-oxidation, as two carbon atoms in a fatty acid molecule are oxidatively metabolized at a time). Although this system produces the lowest volume of ATP per unit of time (and therefore has the lowest power potential), it has the capacity to sustain the production of ATP for the longest period of time (typically more than 2 hours). This system relies predominantly on fats as a source of energy, but is also capable of metabolizing other energy substrates including blood glucose. This aerobic energy system uses Krebs cycle (citric acid cycle) and the electron transport system for the production of ATP.

It is important to consider that, under normal circumstances, *all* energy systems function simultaneously, but the amount of muscle power required influences which energy system becomes the predominant system in the production of ATP.

Muscle Fibers: Converting Chemical Energy into Mechanical Energy

Power and speed activities are highly reliant on fast-twitch, primarily anaerobic, **muscle fibers**. Also referred to as *type IIB* fibers, these fibers primarily store glycogen, but low levels of fat (triglycerides). Glycogen can be quickly metabolized as a fuel without oxygen (anaerobically), enabling these fibers to produce a high level of power so long as the glycogen does not run out. The intermediate fast-twitch muscle fibers, *type IIA*, also produce a tremendous amount of power, but these muscle fibers can be trained to behave more like the *type I slow-twitch fibers* that are characteristic of fibers used by endurance athletes (9). The type of training that is done is important, therefore, because it can influence the behavior of the *type IIA* muscle fibers (10) (Figure 15.1, Table 15.2).

🗐 Muscle Fibers

Muscles have different types of fibers with different energy metabolic potentials. Type I fibers (slow-twitch) are highly aerobic with the capacity to use oxygen well and burn fat to produce ATP and have high endurance. Type IIA fibers are highly anaerobic at their genetic baseline, but can be trained to improve oxidative capacity. Type IIB fibers are primarily anaerobic fibers that can produce a great deal of ATP in a short period, but have low endurance.

Because muscle fibers, particularly the *type IIA* fibers, are adaptable to the kinds of activities commonly practiced by individuals, the type of training pursued should closely mimic the type of sporting activity the athlete is involved in (9). For instance, pure power athletes require all of the power fibers capable of producing high power to be fully engaged as power fibers, but if the athlete undergoes significant aerobic/endurance training, the *type IIA* fibers will adapt by becoming more aerobically capable and lose some of their anaerobic power potential (Figure 15.1). It is not uncommon for power athletes to include a significant component of endurance exercise in the training protocol as part of a strategy to lower the

Characteristic	Red Fiber Type I	White Fiber Type II
Speed of contraction	Slow twitch	Fast twitch
Myoglobin content*	High	Low
Generation of ATP	Aerobic glycolysis† Oxidative phosphorylation	Anaerobic glycolysis‡
Number of mitochondria	Many	Few
Glycogen content	Low	High
Succinate dehydrogenase NADH dehydrogenase	High	Low
Glycolytic enzymes	Low	High

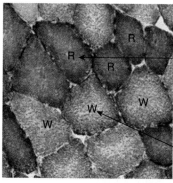

"R" fibers (Type I) are darker red because they have more mitochondria for oxidative metabolism.

"W" fibers (Type II) are lighter because they have fewer mitochondria.

FIGURE 15.1: Characteristics of different muscle fiber types. Type I fibers are referred to as endurance fibers; type II fibers are referred to as power fibers; and type IIA intermediate fibers (not pictured) produce more power than type I fibers, but less power than type II fibers. ATP, adenosine triphosphate; NADH, nicotinamide adenine dinucleotide. (From Dudek RW. High-yield histopathology. 2nd ed. Philadelphia [PA]: LWW [PE]; 2011.)

Table 15.2 Muscle Fiber Types

Fiber Type	Characteristics
Type I	Also referred to as *slow-twitch fibers*, these fibers have many mitochondria with a high level of oxidative enzymes that enable aerobic (*i.e.*, oxidative) metabolism. Speed of contraction is low. The high level of triglyceride (fat) storage in these muscles enables muscle contraction over a long period of time before reaching fatigue. However, the low level of glycogen (carbohydrate) storage in these muscle fibers lowers power potential, but the high level of blood supply enables refueling and fatigue resistance. These are the primary fibers used in aerobic, endurance-type activity, including events such as marathon running, triathlons, and cycling.
Type IIA	Also referred to as *intermediate fast-twitch fibers*, at their genetic baseline behave like *fast-twitch fibers* (type IIB), with high glycogen (carbohydrate) storage and low triglyceride (fat) storage. Speed of contraction is fast. They can produce a high level of power anaerobically, but achieve fatigue relatively quickly as glycogen stores become depleted (9). An interesting characteristic of these fibers is that endurance training helps to make these fibers more oxidatively capable, with increases in oxidative enzymes and triglycerides stores. However, cessation of aerobic training causes these fibers to revert to their genetic baseline as mainly power fibers.
Type IIB	Also referred to as *pure fast-twitch fibers*, they produce a high level of power anaerobically with fast muscle contraction. The primary fuel stored in these fibers is glycogen, and when glycogen is depleted the muscle fiber becomes fatigued. The relatively low level of blood supply also contributes to poor refueling and early fatigue, best suited for events such as sprinting, weight lifting, football linemen, and high-jumping/pole-vault.
Smooth	Smooth muscle is also referred to as *involuntary muscle*, because it is capable of contracting without conscious control. Most blood vessels and the walls of internal organs, including the heart, are composed of smooth muscle. Although the heart controls its own activity, it is also affected by other factors, including the hormonal and neural effects of exercise.

The characteristics listed are those that are generally observed. However, it has become increasingly clear that exercise training can have an impact on the primary characteristics of each of these fiber types. For instance, chronic pure power training will somewhat alter the power potential of the type I fibers, whereas chronic pure endurance training will somewhat alter the endurance potential of type IIB fibers.

Sources: Billeter R, Weber H, Lutz H, Howald H, Eppenberger HM, Jenny E. Myosin types in human skeletal muscle fibers. Histochemistry. 1980;65(3):249–259; Kenney WL, Murray R. Exercise physiology. In: Maughan R, editor. Sports nutrition: the encyclopaedia of sports medicine, an IOC Medical Commission Publication. London (England): Wiley Blackwell; 2014. p. 20–58; Schiaffino S, Reggiani C. Fiber types in mammalian skeletal muscles. Physiol Rev. 2011;91(4):1447–1531; Tesch PA, Karlsson J. Muscle fiber types and size in trained and untrained muscles of elite athletes. J Appl Physiol. 1985;59(6):1716–1720.

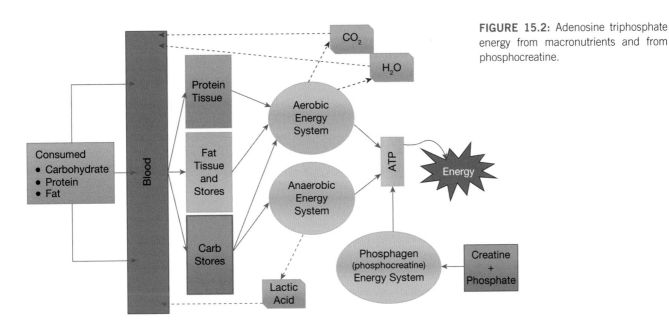

FIGURE 15.2: Adenosine triphosphate energy from macronutrients and from phosphocreatine.

body fat level. However, because fibers exhibit a degree of placidity in response to exercise training, doing so may compromise the total power capacity (9).

Short-duration activities, such as the 100-m sprint and the vault in gymnastics, demand instantly available fuel that can be quickly utilized by muscles. This fuel, PCr, can quickly supply large amounts of ATP energy to muscles, but the available storage of PCr is limited (Figure 15.2 shows how we derive ATP energy).

POWER AND STRENGTH IN THE ENERGY METABOLIC SYSTEMS

In well-nourished athletes, ATP production via PCr lasting no more than 5 and 9 seconds in sudden-onset, high-intensity activities. This is not sufficient energy availability for most activities, as even the Olympic time

for the 100 m sprint is ~10 seconds (11,12). As a result, muscle obtains the additional required energy anaerobically, mainly from stored muscle glycogen. It should be noted that children appear to have a PCr advantage over adults performing similar activities, as a greater proportion of oxidative ATP is formed in child versus adult muscle, enabling children to lower total PCr utilization and, therefore, begin subsequent activities with higher PCr concentrations (13). Anaerobic metabolism, however, causes the buildup of lactic acid, which limits the time an athlete can exercise intensely while in a predominantly anaerobic state. Most scientists believe that the *anaerobic threshold* (*i.e.*, the point at which the rate of blood lactate increase exceeds the rate of blood lactate removal) is ~1.5 minutes for someone working at maximal intensity (14). It is at this point that the athlete would need to reduce exercise intensity or stop exercising altogether (Table 15.3).

Table 15.3	Rate of Metabolism of Fat, Blood Glucose, Aerobic and Anaerobic Glycolysis, and Phosphocreatine	
System	Maximum Production of ATP (mmol/kg of dry mass/s)	Delay Time to Achieve Maximal ATP Production
Phosphocreatine (anaerobic)	9.0	Instantaneous
Glycolysis (anaerobic)	4.5	5–10 s
Glycolysis (aerobic)	2.8	More than 1 min
Blood glucose (aerobic)	1.0	1.5 h
Fat (aerobic)	1.0	More than 2 h

ATP, adenosine triphosphate.

Source: Maughan RJ, ed. Olympic encyclopaedia of sports medicine—An IOC Medical Commission Publication, nutrition in sport. London (England): Wiley Blackwell; 2000.

Aerobic metabolism refers to the metabolism of fuel *with* oxygen and, because it does not produce lactic acid, can continue much longer than anaerobic metabolic processes, provided the fuels and nutrients needed for metabolism are available. A lower amount of ATP energy per unit of time can be produced aerobically than the ATP produced anaerobically, resulting in lower power production/lower exercise intensity for predominantly aerobic activities when compared with predominantly anaerobic activities. However, there is far more fuel available for aerobic metabolism than for anaerobic metabolism, allowing for longer exercise times.

Important Factors to Consider

- Athletes who work hard and burn more fuel per unit of time require more oxygen to burn this fuel.
- When the amount of energy burned per unit of time exceeds the athlete's capacity to provide sufficient oxygen to metabolically active cells, fuel is burned that does not require oxygen (*i.e.*, burned anaerobically).
- With greater levels of anaerobic metabolism, the volume of lactic acid that is produced increases.
- If the threshold for removing cellular lactic acid is reached, the lactic acid builds up, resulting in the necessity to either exercise less intensely to produce less lactic acid or to stop exercising.

Well-conditioned athletes have better oxygen delivery to working muscles, enabling them to maintain oxidative metabolism at a faster rate and to go faster, longer before reaching fatigue. Imagine the speed of elite-level marathon runners, who now complete the 26.2-mile marathon distance at an average speed of ~4 minutes, 30 seconds per mile or less, achieved primarily through aerobic metabolism.

Having the right fuels available is critically important, because poor fuel availability will inhibit energy metabolism. Fat storage is rarely an issue, as even the leanest athletes have ample stores of fat that can be used to supply energy aerobically. However, a failure to also have sufficient carbohydrate stores results in the production of **ketones** (incompletely metabolized fats) that are acidic and result in premature muscular fatigue (15–17). Unlike fat, carbohydrate stores are limited and, therefore, an appropriate dietary plan that ensures adequate carbohydrate availability is required for the planned exercise. Protein is also a potential fuel source, but as we have no

storage depot for protein to metabolize for energy, the protein metabolized for energy is derived from the catabolism of lean mass (18). Because a primary purpose of exercise is intended to improve lean mass, the athlete should have a strategy that optimizes oxygen utilization and maximizes carbohydrate stores to limit the catabolism of protein as a source of energy.

Ketones

In humans, ketones are three water-soluble molecules that include acetoacetate, β-hydroxybutyrate, and acetone and are produced as a result of gluconeogenesis (production of glucose from noncarbohydrates) by the liver as a result of poor carbohydrate availability. Elevated blood ketones, therefore, represent a good indication of poor carbohydrate status. Most commonly, ketosis occurs during periods of fasting/starvation, ketogenic (carbohydrate-restrictive) diets, poor control of diabetes, and prolonged high-intensity exercise that is carbohydrate depleting. Acetone is the most common ketone as it is the product of the spontaneous metabolism of the other two ketones (acetoacetate and β-hydroxybutyrate). Ketones, which smell like nail polish remover (acetone), can be detected on a person's breath. A review of the impact of ketogenic diets in endurance athletes found no clear benefit when compared to a high carbohydrate diet (19). Athletes considering adopting a ketogenic diet should understand the risk of impaired performance in the higher-intensity aspects of competition, and the likelihood of early depletion of glycogen stores (20).

The energy stored in ATP and PCr (**energy stores**) provides sufficient energy, produced anaerobically, for up to ~9 seconds. This phosphagen system depends on PCr to quickly provide a high-energy phosphate molecule to form ATP. The theory behind creatine monohydrate supplements is that greater creatine tissue availability enables more efficient formation of PCr, which is then available to form ATP (see Chapter 13). The greater capacity to form PCr enables more ATP, allowing for more high-intensity anaerobic work.

A number of sports are highly dependent on the phosphagen system, including shot put, long jump, triple jump, discus throwers, gymnastics vault, and short sprints. In addition, other sports that have quick bursts of activity, such as football, volleyball, and hockey, also have a dependence on this energy pathway. In some of these sports, the capacity to perform repeated high-intensity actions may determine the winner. The high jumper, long jumper, and pole-vaulter all need two or three stellar efforts with the hope that one of them will be good enough to win, and the forward on a basketball team would like to have the capacity to jump as high in the last quarter as in the first to capture a rebound.

Energy Stores

Body energy stores are made of PCr, muscle glycogen, liver glycogen, blood glucose, fat, and muscle/organ tissue (protein). Of these, we store the most potential energy as fat, followed by protein (muscle/organ, and not intended to be burned as fuel), muscle glycogen, liver glycogen, and blood sugar.

Minimizing the utilization of protein to satisfy the athlete's energy requirements and to, therefore, have less available protein for the synthesis of creatine, consumption of both adequate protein and energy is required to ensure satisfactory synthesis of the creatine needed for multiple quick bursts of high-intensity activity (21,22). To improve the storage of ATP-PCr in the muscles, athletes must practice activities that focus on this system (*i.e.*, activities that are at maximal intensity for 8 seconds and that are repeated multiple times during an exercise session) (23). This type of training, by itself, is not sufficient to improve short-duration, high-intensity performance. Consumption of sufficient energy and protein, by itself, also is not sufficient to improve short-duration, high-intensity performance. However, when both proper training and nutritional strategies are combined, athletes can experience very real gains in short-duration, high-intensity performance.

It should be noted that, even with higher creatine storage, the maximum preformed PCr is sufficient to last up to only 8 seconds of hard physical work (11,12). There is wide variability between athletes in the regeneration of PCr, but athletes performing maximal exercise for up to 8 seconds typically allow 2–4 minutes for PCr regeneration before undertaking another maximal bout of exercise (6,24). It is here that proper nutrition management is important, as athletes with both sufficient substrates and training are capable of reforming PCr more efficiently and also can make the transfer to anaerobic glycolysis more efficiently. A 100-m sprinter accelerates over the first 8 seconds of the race, but during this 8 seconds when PCr runs low, anaerobic glycolysis is synthesizing a significant proportion of the required ATP. However, because anaerobic glycolysis does not produce as much ATP per unit of time as PCr, the winner of the 100-m dash is typically the person who slows down the least during the last 2 seconds of the race (Table 15.4).

With intense exercise, the primary fuel becomes stored muscle glycogen (the storage form of glucose/carbohydrate). When the stored glycogen becomes depleted, the athlete performing high-intensity activity fatigues quickly and the exercise stops (25,26). Although anaerobic metabolism typically provides only a small proportion of the total energy used by muscles, it is important because it can provide energy quickly and helps to fill the energy gap between the initiation of exercise (PCr) and the time it takes for aerobic energy metabolism to begin producing sufficient ATP. Maintenance of high-intensity (*i.e.*, anaerobic) activity is limited by glycogen storage, which is typically depleted within 1.5 minutes of high-intensity activity. Purely high-intensity sports are often intentionally limited to 1.5 minutes because of the realization that humans cannot perform continuous high-intensity activity for a longer period of time. For example, the floor routine in gymnastics is up to a 1.5-minute

Table 15.4	Energy Stores in a 70-kg (154-lb) Relatively Lean (10% Body Fat) Male Athlete		
Energy Source	**Mass (kg) [lb]**	**Energy (kJ) [kcal]**	**Theoretical Maximal Exercise Time (min)**[a]
Liver glycogen	(0.08) [0.176]	(1,280) [307]	16
Muscle glycogen	(0.40) [0.88]	(6,400) [1,530]	80
Blood glucose	(0.01) [0.022]	(160) [38]	2
Fat	(7.0) [15.4]	(260,000) [62,142]	3,250
Protein[b]	(13.0) [28.6]	(220,000) [52,581]	2,750

[a]Maximal exercise time is theoretical and assumes sole use of indicated energy source.

[b]Protein, although available as an energy source, is not intended to be a primary source of energy. Not more than a very small part (<1%) of the total protein is available for use during exercise.

Source: Gleeson M. Biochemistry of exercise. In: Maughan RJ, editor. Sports nutrition—The encyclopedia of sports medicine: An IOC Medical Commission Publication. London (England): Wiley Blackwell; 2014.

Table 15.5	Percent Contribution of Different Energy Systems in a Sample of Different Sports		
Sport	Phosphocreatine and Anaerobic Glycolysis	Anaerobic Glycolysis and Aerobic Glycolysis	Aerobic (β-Oxidation of Fats)
Distance running	10	20	70
Rowing	20	30	50
Soccer	50	20	30
Basketball	60	20	20
Tennis	70	20	10
Volleyball	80	5	15
Gymnastics	80	15	5
Sprints	90	10	0

Source: Fox EL, Foss ML, Keteyian SJ. Fox's physiological basis for exercise and sport. 6th ed. Madison (WI): William C Brown; 1998.

routine, as are Olympic boxing rounds. Sports with a higher aerobic/lower anaerobic component take longer to deplete muscle glycogen. In a 75-km cycling time trial lasting ~168 minutes, it was found that the cyclists experienced a 77% decrease in muscle glycogen (27). It has been found that in someone exercising at maximal intensity for 30 seconds, the rate of ATP resynthesis from PCr metabolism is highest in the first few seconds of exercise, but falls to almost zero after 20 seconds. The rate of ATP resynthesis from glycolysis peaks after about 5 seconds and is maintained for 15 seconds, but falls in the last 10 seconds of exercise (28).

Some sports are predominantly aerobic with a heavy reliance on fat metabolism, but may also have some reliance on anaerobic glycolysis during the competition. The long-distance runner who has managed most of the distance while preserving some muscle glycogen still has the glycogen energy reserves to finish the race with a strong (anaerobic) "kick," enabling him or her to pass runners at critical points during the end of the race (29). For runners in short-distance races, for swimmers in short races, and for hockey players skating at full bore at the end of a game to go for a winning score, the anaerobic pathway is the primary metabolic pathway, and having sufficient stored muscle glycogen is important for the athlete to continue exercising at a high intensity. Middle-distance runners experience extreme race intensity, with 800-m to 5,000-m racers experiencing VO2max levels of between 95% and 130% (30). The reliance on both anaerobic and aerobic metabolism in middle-distance athletes demands satisfying glycogen storage total energy requirements through appropriate dietary strategies.

The fact that power athletes utilize a high degree of PCr and glycogen via anaerobic glycolysis helps to explain the types of foods that power athletes should consume. The limited storage of fats in fast-twitch muscle fibers is a clear indication that the metabolism of fats is relatively limited when compared with the predominantly high–fat-storing slow-twitch fibers used by endurance athletes. Relatively high carbohydrate intakes have been found to enable better carbohydrate (i.e., glycogen) storage (31). Therefore, although power athletes often focus on consumption of high-protein diets, the energy metabolic systems they use suggests that they would do well to consider consuming relatively high-carbohydrate diets (31,32). It should be made clear that power athletes are breathing and bringing oxygen into the system, which supports the oxidative metabolism of fat. The high-intensity activity they do, however, is proportionately more reliant on anaerobic metabolism (Table 15.5).

In-season exercise patterns of power athletes help them metabolize consumed energy, but maintaining these patterns off-season is difficult and often associated with an enlargement of the body fat mass (33). There is also evidence that the weight cycling often experienced by power athletes increases obesity risk after they retire from the sport, and the associated weight fluctuations are associated with more frequent illnesses and earlier mortality (34,35).

Building Lean (Muscle) Mass

Power athletes look for nutrition strategies to enlarge muscle mass because more muscle per unit weight increases the potential for improving the strength-to-weight ratio and power production. There are many techniques employed for increasing muscle mass, including resistance training, consumption of more energy and protein at different points in the exercise day, and the consumption of products claiming to enhance muscle development (36–39). Some of these strategies have been shown to work well, whereas others do not. Athletes and those who work with them should carefully evaluate the adequacy of their diets before embarking on a regimen of costly and unproven supplements that are meant to enhance muscular development, muscular strength, or both.

It is generally recommended that competitive power athletes should consume ~1.7 g protein/kg mass (31,32). Surveys, however, suggest that the protein intake of some power athletes is often greater than 3 g/kg of body weight (40–42). Protein consumption that exceeds the individual's anabolic maximum, particularly if not well distributed throughout the day, is not likely to enhance the protein mass and will merely be used to satisfy the energy requirement or stored as fat (43). Whether this excess protein is stored or metabolized as energy, there is an increased need to excrete the nitrogen associated with protein, forcing greater urinary output that can result in dehydration. In fact, many athletes claim they lose weight on a high protein intake, but this may be due to the high level of body water that is lost rather than from the loss of fat (44). This may also be due to an increase in ketones from insufficient carbohydrate availability that results in incompletely burned fat, which causes nausea and reduces appetite (45). Athletes may also distribute the protein they consume wrongly, with the majority of protein intake coming at dinner (*i.e.*, the end of the day). There is increasingly clear evidence that protein is best utilized to improve muscle protein synthesis if it is evenly distributed throughout the day, with no more than ~30 g provided in any single meal (31). A simple guide for calculating protein intake and eating frequency is shown in Example 15.1.

Example 15.1: Calculating Protein Eating Frequency

170 lb male athlete requiring 1.5 g/kg protein per day[a]

1. Calculate weight in kg (170/2.2 = 77.3 kg)
2. Calculate total protein requirement (77.3 × 1.5 = 116 g protein)
3. Calculate the number of protein eating opportunities: (116 g/25[b] = 4.64)
4. This athlete should consume ~25 g of protein that is evenly distributed 4–5 times per day (*e.g.*, breakfast, lunch, mid-afternoon snack, dinner, and evening snack).

[a]The current recommended range of protein intake is 1.2–2.0 g/kg/day
[b]Maximal muscle protein synthesis occurs with a protein consumption of ~20–25 g of protein per meal. This example is using 25 g/meal.

Nutrients That Control Muscle Development

Muscle development occurs best in conjunction with a well-planned resistance program, a sustained energy and nutrient balance, and normal levels of human growth hormone (HGH), insulin, testosterone, and other **anabolic hormones** including insulin-like growth factor-1 (IGF-1) (46–49). **Catabolic hormones** are hormones that are involved in tissue breakdown and include cortisol, thyroxine, and epinephrine.

There is every reason to believe that an athlete who is in good energy and nutrient balance is already producing appropriate amounts of the anabolic hormones, so arbitrarily increasing protein intake is not likely to initiate an even greater muscle protein synthesis (43). (Remember: More than enough is not better than enough.)

📄 **Anabolic Hormones**

Hormones that are involved in building tissues such as muscle, including HGH, anabolic steroids such as testosterone, IGF-1, and insulin.

📄 **Catabolic Hormones**

Hormones that are involved in breaking down tissues, typically to make energy available to tissues, such as cortisol, glucagon, thyroxine, and epinephrine (adrenalin).

Individual amino acids have been widely tested to determine if their intake might change the production of HGH in athletes. It is important to note that amino acid mixtures are the largest category of supplements used by bodybuilders (50). Studies have shown that increasing the consumption (via supplement) of the amino acid ornithine may in some circumstances increase HGH production, but there is even more evidence that there is *no* significant increase in HGH from taking, either individually or in various combinations, the amino acids arginine, lysine, ornithine, and tyrosine (51–57). There is also evidence that taking a broad-range supplement containing all 20 amino acids has no effect on either HGH or testosterone production (58). Nutrient supplement companies often use studies to claim that specific amino acids stimulate HGH and increase muscle mass (59). However, they often fail to quote other studies that have better statistical procedures and demonstrate that supplementation with these amino acids has no significant impact on strength or endurance (60).

There is evidence to support protein consumption that is about double that for nonathletes (0.8 vs. 1.7 g/kg/day).

The higher requirement is because athletes have more muscle to support, experience an exercise-associated increase in muscle damage, and have relatively small but important protein losses in urine (40,31). Although the protein requirement for athletes is higher than for nonathletes, athlete total protein intakes are often higher than the recommended intake level (43). A possible exception to this is found in vegetarian athletes, who tend to satisfy the protein level recommended for nonathletes, but often consume below the recommended protein intake for athletes (61).

There are several concerns associated with excess protein consumption when excess levels are consumed per meal or per day. Excess protein consumption results in a portion of the protein to be used to satisfy the energy requirement or to be stored as fat. In either case, nitrogen must be removed from the amino acid molecules, and the nitrogenous wastes that are created result in increased urinary output and greater urinary calcium loss, which increases the risk of dehydration and may be associated with lower bone mineral density (62–64). There is also some limited evidence that chronic excess protein consumption may increase the risk of kidney disease (65). Because kidney disease often occurs gradually and its presence is often unknown, Friedman (65) suggests that individuals should test for normal kidney function before pursuing a high protein intake. However, most recommendations for limiting protein consumption are commonly based on the fact that individuals suffering from kidney failure benefit from reduced protein consumption. There is little evidence, however, to suggest that chronically high protein intakes of up to 2.8 g/kg/day are associated with increased kidney disease in individuals with normally functioning and healthy kidneys (43,66).

Athletes often take multivitamin and multimineral supplements with the belief that this will enhance the athletic endeavor, but evidence is largely lacking that these supplements enhance performance in sports that require power (64,67,68). Despite the lack of scientific evidence to support taking supplemental doses of vitamins, and some evidence that they inhibit performance, there is a common belief among power athletes that a number of these vitamins enhance strength (69). The consumption of dietary supplements in a group of surveyed Olympic athletes ($N = 372$) ranged from 52% to 92%, with 83% of surveyed speed and power athletes using dietary supplements (70). The authors of this study suggest that, because supplement purity cannot be assured, athletes should seek professional nutrition counseling to avoid potentially unsafe use of dietary supplements.

Power and Strength Summary

Power and strength are critical components for athletes doing quick, short-duration, high-intensity activities. Although also important for athletes involved in longer-duration activities, they are not the issue of central importance. A key nutritional element in building and maintaining muscle mass is the acquisition of sufficient energy. Although consuming large amounts of protein can help to satisfy the energy requirement, consumption of additional carbohydrate is less expensive and more effective. Power athletes are even more dependent on carbohydrates than endurance athletes because the muscle fibers they use do not have the capacity to burn fats effectively. Power athletes often make the mistake of thinking that protein is the key to their success, but high-protein consumption may limit the consumption of other essential nutrients, including carbohydrate, which is needed to optimize glycogen storage for anaerobic high-intensity activity. Similarly, the consumption of dietary supplements has not been found to improve the athletic endeavor in athletes consuming adequate diets, but their consumption may lead the athlete to believe that they need not be as diligent in the consumption of good foods (71). This problem is compounded by the fact that some supplements targeting athletes contain banned substances not listed on the label (72). Supplementation of vitamins, minerals, protein products, and fat analogs has not been found to be successful in improving power, muscle mass, or athletic performance in power athletes. Although the risk of taking these products is likely to be low, there are no data to know if these products are safe when consumed in the amounts and duration prescribed by the manufacturers of these products. A more sensible approach is to consume a balanced and varied diet that is high in carbohydrates (5.0–8.0 g/kg/day), moderate in protein (1.2–1.7 g/kg/day), and sufficient fat to satisfy the energy requirement (<30% of total energy consumed). Provided the food consumed comes from a variety of foods, this intake has the benefit of exposing tissues to required minerals and vitamins. As carbohydrates are metabolized cleanly (*i.e.*, no nitrogenous waste; only carbon dioxide and water), there is no question about the safety of consuming a varied diet high in good-quality carbohydrate-containing foods (Table 15.6 shows energy sources of different **power sports**).

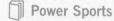 **Power Sports**

Power sports are considered to be those that require a great deal of energy over a relatively short period of time and include sports such as sprinting, gymnastics, and weight-lifting.

Table 15.6	Energy Sources of Different Sports				
				% Energy Contribution	
Event Time (min)	**Sample Event**	**VO$_{2max}$ (approx)**	**Phosphocreatine**	**Glycolysis (Anaerobic)**	**Aerobic Metabolism (Oxidative)**
0.5–1	400-m running; individual cycling time trial (500 m or 1 km); 100-m swimming	~150	~10	~47–60	~30–43
1.5–2	800-m running; 200-m swimming; 500-m canoe/kayak	113–130	~5	~29–45	~50–66
3–5	1,500-m running; cycling pursuit; 400-m swimming; 100-m canoe/kayak	103–115	~2	~14–28	~70–84
5–8	3,000-m running; 2,000-m rowing	98–102	<1	~10–12	~88–90

Note that longer durations involve relatively higher aerobic metabolism; shorter durations relatively higher anaerobic metabolism.

Source: Stellingwerff T, Maughan RJ, Burke LM. Nutrition for power sports: middle-distance running, track cycling, rowing, canoeing/kayaking, and swimming. J Sports Sci. 2011;29(S1):S79–S89.

ENDURANCE IN THE ENERGY METABOLIC SYSTEMS

Endurance athletes perform in events that have continuous movement for 20 minutes or longer, with many **endurance sports** requiring continuous movement over long distances or time periods (marathon, cross-country skiing, triathlon, etc.). There is a premium on supplying sufficient energy and fluid to ensure that the athlete does not become exhausted from the activity or overheated from the continuous energy metabolism. Failing to supply sufficient energy of the right type will result in early fatigue and poor athletic performance. Athletes taking supplements may have a false sense that nutrient needs are satisfied, but if the supplement consumption reduces energy intake from food, then this is counterproductive. There is also evidence that excess intake of certain common supplements may create difficulties in performance. In a study assessing both rats and humans, it has been found that vitamin C supplemental intake (1 g/day in humans; 0.24 mg/cm^2/day in rats) significantly hampered training-induced cellular adaptations to endurance activity [69]. The goal for the endurance athlete is, therefore, to establish a workable strategy for supplying sufficient nutrients, energy, and fluids before training/competition to begin the training session/competition with optimal glycogen stores and in a euhydrated state so as to enable sustained muscular work for a long duration and at the highest possible intensity. It is also an important goal for the endurance athlete to *plan* for a suitable recovery strategy that provides for easy and fast availability of fluids, carbohydrates, and protein [31].

Endurance Sports

Endurance sports are considered to be those that require a relatively low amount of energy per unit of time, but over long periods of time, and include sports such as distance running (marathon, ultra-endurance running, etc.), swimming, distance cycling, and triathlon.

The majority of endurance activity occurs at intensities that enable fats to contribute a high proportion of the fuel for muscular work. Because fat is amply available in even the leanest athlete, supplying fats before and during physical activity is not a concern and should not be a goal [73]. However, carbohydrate is involved in the complete combustion of fats, and because the storage capacity for carbohydrates is relatively low and easily depleted, the goal for endurance athletes is to find a way to supply enough carbohydrates before training/competition to optimize glycogen stores and to have a carbohydrate-containing beverage to consume during exercise to sustain blood sugar and buffer glycogen utilization [31]. Such a carbohydrate strategy will help to minimize the risk for premature fatigue. Ultimately, endurance athletes must consume sufficient total energy, a significant portion of which is carbohydrate, to enable muscular work over long time periods, and must have a strategy for supporting carbohydrate requirements during physical activity to help sustain the complete oxidation of fats.

Aerobic metabolism is the energy system of greatest importance for endurance athletes. In this energy pathway, oxygen is used to help transfer phosphorus into new ATP molecules. Unlike anaerobic metabolism, this energy pathway can use protein, fat, and carbohydrate for fuel by converting pieces of these energy substrates into acetyl coenzyme A (acetyl CoA), the intermediary compound in metabolism (74). Glucose is converted to pyruvic acid (an anaerobic, energy-releasing process), which can be converted either into acetyl CoA with the help of oxygen or to the energy storage product *lactic acid*. Excess production of lactic acid results in muscular fatigue, causing activity to stop. However, the lactic acid can be reconverted to pyruvic acid to be used as a fuel aerobically. Aerobic metabolism occurs in the mitochondria of cells, where the vast majority of all ATP is produced from the entering acetyl CoA. Fats can be converted to acetyl CoA through a process called the *β-oxidative metabolic pathway* (8). This pathway is oxygen dependent, which means that fats can only be burned aerobically.

The ability of an athlete to achieve a steady state of oxygen uptake into the cells is a function of how well an athlete is aerobically conditioned. Maximal oxygen uptake in males and females involved in different sports can be viewed in Chapter 11, Table 11.6. An athlete who frequently trains aerobically is likely to reach a steady state faster than one who does not train aerobically. For a well-conditioned person, it can take 5 minutes before enough oxygen is in the system to support aerobic metabolism at a steady state. The first 5 minutes of activity is supported by a combination of anaerobic and aerobic metabolism. Achievement of a fast steady state is therefore important because that diminishes the amount of time an athlete is obtaining energy via anaerobic pathways. This places a heavy burden on the most limited fuel—carbohydrates. In theory, once an athlete reaches a level of oxygen uptake that matches the oxygen requirement for the given level of exertion, the exercise could go on for as long as the body's carbohydrate level and fluids do not reach a critical state. For instance, a long-distance runner who is in a steady state could continue running provided the runner replaced the carbohydrates and fluids that are used in the activity. Therefore, endurance is enhanced with a periodic intake of carbohydrate and fluid during the activity.

Athletes in aerobic sports have an enhanced capacity to use oxygen than do athletes in power sports. Because even the leanest athletes have a great deal of energy stored as fat, this increased ability to burn fat dramatically improves endurance. However, as carbohydrate is needed for the complete combustion of fat, carbohydrate is still the limiting energy source for endurance work because athletes have relatively low carbohydrate stores. This is clearly demonstrated by findings that athletes consuming high-fat, low-carbohydrate diets have lower performance outcomes than those consuming low-fat, high-carbohydrate diets (73,75).

Athletes with different levels of conditioning are likely to achieve steady state at different levels of exercise intensity. A well-conditioned athlete may be capable of maintaining a steady state at a high enough level of exercise intensity to easily win a race. At the 1996 Olympic Games in Atlanta, Georgia, the winner of the marathon ran over 26 miles at a speed that averaged just over a 5-minute-per-mile pace. In the 2012 London Olympic Games, the pace was even faster, at about 4 minutes 50 seconds per mile (Table 15.7). However, an athlete with poor aerobic conditioning may only be able to run at a 10-minutes-per-mile pace and maintain a steady state. Each person has his or her own pace that allows maintenance of a steady state. Exceeding that pace causes a greater proportion of the muscular work to rely on anaerobic metabolism, with an associated increase in the reliance on carbohydrate fuel. Because of the limited storage of carbohydrate fuel, glycogen is depleted more quickly and the person becomes exhausted.

Endurance events, including marathon, ultraendurance running, triathlon, road cycling, and distance swimming, require a high level of aerobic fitness but also require periods of anaerobic power for bursts of speed at critical junctures in a race. The winning times of the men's Olympic marathon have gradually become faster (see Table 15.8). (Note that variations in speed between Olympic marathons may be due to differences in marathon course difficulty.)

The primary energy system for endurance sports is oxidative (aerobic), which represents a work intensity below maximal, allowing for sufficient oxygen to be brought into the system and delivered to cells. Although endurance athletes are unable to move as quickly as sprinters, they can continue activity for much longer distances because the oxidative system provides energy with limited production of lactate and uses a fuel (fat) that is in high supply. Factors that affect maximal oxygen uptake include (76):

- *Pulmonary diffusing capacity* (i.e., the ability to "grab" oxygen from air in the lungs and transfer it to red blood cells [RBCs])
- *Cardiac output* (i.e., the capacity of the heart to pump blood through the body to deliver oxygen to tissues)

Table 15.7	Winning Men's and Women's Marathon Times From the First Modern Olympic Games in 1896 to the Present			
Year	Men's Marathon	Time	Women's Marathon	Time
1896	Spiridon Lewis	2:58:50		
1900	Michel Théato	2:59:45		
1904	Thomas Hicks	3:28:53		
1906	William Sherring	2:51:23.6		
1908	John Hayes	2:55:18.4		
1912	Kenneth McArthur	2:36:54.8		
1920	Hannes Kolehmainen	2:32:35.8		
1924	Albin Stenroos	2:41:22.6		
1932	Juan Carlos Zabala	2:31:36.0		
1936	Kee-Chung Sohn	2:29:19.2		
1948	Delfo Cabrera	2:34:51.6		
1952	Emil Zátopek	2:23:02.2		
1956	Alain Mimoun	2:25:03.2		
1960	Abebe Bikila	2:15:16.2		
1964	Abebe Bikila	2:12:11.2		
1968	Mamo Wolde	2:20:26.4		
1972	Frank Shorter	2:12:19.8		
1976	Waldemar Cierpinski	2:09:55		
1980	Waldemar Cierpinski	2:11:03		
1984	Carlos Lopes	2:09:21	Joan Benoit	2:24:52
1988	Gelindo Bordin	2:10:32	Rosa Mota	2:25:40
1992	Hwang Yeong-Jo	2:13:23	Valentina Yegorova	2:32:41
1996	Josia Thugwane	2:12:36	Fatuma Roba	2:26:05
2000	Gazehegne Abera	2:10:11	Naoko Takahashi	2:23:14
2004	Stefano Baldini	2:10:55	Mizuki Noguchi	2:26:20
2008	*Samuel Wanjiru*[a]	*2:06:32*	Constantina Tomescu	2:26:44
2012	Stephen Kiprotich	2:08:01	*Tiki Gelana*[a]	*2:23:07*
2016	Eliud Kipchoge	2:08:44	Jemina Sumgong	2:24:04

First Women's Olympic Marathon was in 1984.
[a]Runner (in *italics*) = Olympic Record.

- *Oxygen-carrying capacity* (*i.e.*, the concentration of normal, healthy RBCs)
- *Skeletal muscles* (*i.e.*, the capacity of the muscle to take oxygen from the blood and transfer the oxygen into mitochondria for oxidative metabolism)

Training has the effect of increasing the capacity to deliver oxygen to cells, primarily as the result of an increase in maximal cardiac output (77). Studies assessing blood lactate concentration have found that trained athletes are far more capable of tolerating high levels of blood lactate than untrained subjects doing the same intensity of work, likely because of a larger blood volume (a common adaptation to training) that allows for improved lactate dilution and lesser pH impact (78,79). (Larger blood volumes are an adaptive benefit of aerobic fitness.) Even lean athletes have ample stored energy as fat, and improving oxygen delivery to tissues enhances fat metabolism while lowering the need to obtain fuel anaerobically. It is still important to consider, however, that fat requires carbohydrate for complete fat metabolism and the avoidance of ketone creation. Therefore,

Table 15.8	Nutritional Recommendations for Athletes Who Wish to Decrease, Maintain, or Increase Body Mass		
	Decreasing Body Mass	**Maintaining Body Mass**	**Increasing Body Mass**
Decreased training volume	Decreased calorie intake sufficient to lose ~0.25%–0.75% of body mass per week (larger caloric decrease to reflect decreased training volume) Minimum EA, 30 kca·kg^{-1} FFM CHO, 4–5 g·kg body mass^{-1} PRO, 1.6–2.4 g·kg body mass^{-1}	Slight decrease in caloric intake to reflect decreased training volume CHO, 4–7 g·kg body mass^{-1} PRO, 1.2–1.8 g·kg body mass^{-1}	Not recommended (not ideal for skeletal muscle hypertrophy and/or increased risk of fact accumulation)
No change in training volume	Decreased caloric intake sufficient to lose ~0.25%–0.75% of body mass per week Minimum EA, 30 kca·kg^{-1} FFM CHO, 4–5 g·kg body mass^{-1} PRO, 1.6–2.4 g·kg body mass^{-1}	No change in calorie intake CHO, 4–7 g/kg body mass^{-1} PRO, 1.2–1.8 g·kg body mass^{-1}	Increased calorie intake to increase body mass 0.1%–0.25% per week CHO, 6–7 g·kg body mass^{-1} PRO, 1.2–1.8 g·kg body mass^{-1}
Increased training volume	Not recommended (increased risk of overtraining or injury)	Slight increase in caloric intake to reflect increase in volume CHO, 4–7 g·kg body mass^{-1} PRO, 1.2–1.8 g·kg body mass^{-1}	Increased calorie intake to increase body mas 0.1%–0.25% per week (larger caloric increase to reflect increase in training volume) CHO, 6–7 g·kg body mass^{-1} PRO, 1.2–1.8 g·kg body mass^{-1}

Source: Reprinted from: Mota JA, Nuckols G, Smith-Ryan AE. Nutritional periodization: Applications for the strength athlete. Strength Cond J. 2019;41(5):69–78.

even athletes with a high capacity to metabolize fat may be compromised if they fail to store/supply sufficient carbohydrates during periods of predominantly oxidative metabolism. This is clearly demonstrated by studies finding that athletes who consume high-fat diets have maximal endurance time of ~57 minutes; those who consume a normal mixed diet experience an increase in endurance times to ~114 minutes; and those on high-carbohydrate diets have an increase in maximal endurance times to ~167 minutes (80). Distance athletes often have possibilities of in-race nutrition. For instance, marathoners have fluid stations available every 5 kilometers, with personal containers available at each station. It is important for these athletes to fully understand what works best for them, regarding carbohydrate volume and type and electrolyte concentration of the fluids consumed. It is also important for these athletes to understand when and if caffeine and/or nitrate should be consumed prior to or during competition (81).

Ultra-endurance athletes have extremely high nutrient/ fluid requirements, as these competitions typically last for at least 4 hours, with some lasting more than 10 hours. The current recommendations for ultraendurance athletes include a carbohydrate intake of 3–12 g/kg/day or 30–110 g of carbohydrate/hr (82). This high amount can result in GI symptoms if not consumed in a way that the athlete has become well adapted to. A unique study that analyzed the food and fluid intake of elite ultraendurance runners during a 24-hour world championship found that the majority (not all) of these runners surpassed nutritional recommendations and did not experience nutritionally related adverse effects (83). Those who failed to follow nutritional recommendations mainly had difficulties consuming sufficient energy and/or fluids to satisfy needs, often because of GI symptoms.

Vegetarianism has increased in popularity among athletes, and they may offer some advantages for endurance sports, as they are high in carbohydrate (better glycogen stores), tend to lower body fat (better strength: weight ratio), and high in naturally occurring nitrate (vasodilation/better oxygen deliver to cells with lower blood pressure) (84). It is clear that multiple factors influence the dietary choice of athletes, including social, psychological, economic, physiologic, biologic, lifestyle, beliefs, and knowledge (85). Teammates have an important influence on eating behaviors of athletes, suggesting the importance of working with teams and the athlete environment to more effectively improve the nutrient intake of individuals on the team, rather than only working with individual athletes (86). The effectiveness of vegetarian and other popular diets, including, ketogenic, intermittent fasting, gluten-free, and low FODMAP, have been assessed on endurance athletes, and all have potential benefits and problems associated with them. These include (87):

Vegan/Vegetarian Diet:
- Potential Positive Effects
  - Maintenance or improvement of aerobic capacity
  - No negative change in endurance performance
  - Lower inflammation and improved immune response
  - Lower exercise-associated oxidative stress
  - Enhance cardiovascular function
- Potential Negative Effects
  - Lower energy availability
  - Lower serum testosterone
  - Increased risk of micronutrient deficiency
  - Lower protein quality and quantity

Intermittent Fasting Diet:
- Potential Positive Effects
  - Elevated fat/ketone usage
  - Elevated metabolic, inflammatory, hormonal responses
- Potential Negative Effects
  - Lower endurance performance
  - Increase in delayed muscle soreness
  - Altered sleep pattern
  - Increased risk of dehydration

High-Fat Diet:
- Potential Positive Effects
  - Elevated use of fats and ketones
  - No change in aerobic capacity
  - No negative impact on muscle glycogen stores
- Potential Negative Effects
  - Reduced running economy
  - Lower appetite
  - Elevated oxygen cost
  - Reduced bone health

- Increased GI symptoms
- Increased fatigue

Gluten-Free Diet:
- Potential Positive Effects
  - Fewer exercise-induced GI symptoms
- Potential Negative Effects
  - Low energy availability
  - Lower macronutrient intake
  - Lower fiber intake

Low-FODMAP Diet:
- Potential Positive Effects
  - Fewer exercise-induced GI symptoms
- Potential Negative Effects
  - Negative impact on gut microbiome
  - Difficulty finding foods to consume
  - Lower fiber intake

GENERAL NUTRITION CONCERNS AND STRATEGIES FOR ATHLETES IN ALL SPORTS

Regardless of the athletic endeavor or sport, athletes must be mindful of some issues that could compromise their capacity to benefit from training. These include overtraining, overuse injury, poor fluid intake, and poor energy availability.

Overtraining

Overtraining is a stress-related condition that has a negative impact on the normal beneficial adaptation to training, impairs normal psychological well-being, and creates immune system problems that are manifested with increased illness frequency (88). Some well-established warning signs include:

- increased muscle soreness
- delayed muscle recovery
- inability to perform at the previous training load
- poor sleep
- decreased vigor
- swelling of lymph nodes
- high frequency of illness
- loss of appetite (89)

Many of these signs are a result of working at a level harder than the body's capacity to recover from it. Overtraining commonly results in poor performance because of the increased risk that the athlete will become sick or injured. It is a problem for an estimated 10%–20% of all athletes with intensive training and is commonly observed in endurance athletes. Importantly, poor intake of carbohydrates and fluids is commonly observed in athletes with overtraining syndrome (90). According to a joint consensus statement of the European College of Sport Science and the American College of Sports Medicine, overtraining syndrome can be effectively eliminated through a logical training program that allows for adequate rest and recovery with proper nutrition and hydration (90).

Overuse Injury

Overuse injuries occur when an athlete repeats the same physical task, causing repetitive stress to bone and muscles at a rate greater than the tissues can be repaired (91). A blister that results from the rubbing of a running shoe, a mild form of overuse injury, and the repeated stress on a bone from constant repeated pounding may result in a more serious form of overuse injury such as a stress fracture. Endurance athletes spend many hours in training involving repetitive motion, making overuse injury a concern for this group (92). Muscle tissue breakdown occurs as a common and natural component of physical activity, but trained athletes who are accustomed to the duration and intensity of the activity should have good muscle recovery without overuse injury, provided appropriate nutritional strategies (*e.g.,* consumption of good-quality protein, carbohydrate, and beverages soon after the end of training) are followed (93). Well-nourished athletes are better able to heal minor tissue damage that occurs during normal training and competition.

Poor Fluid Intake

Physical activity results in an inevitable loss of sweat-related body water loss to dissipate the heat associated with exercise-associated energy metabolism. There is a wide range of sweat loss, depending on the endurance sport, the environmental temperature, and humidity, with observed ranges from 4.9 to 12.7 L lost and 2.1 to 10.5 L ingested (94). There is evidence that the prevalence of poor hydration status at the initiation of training is high in both young and adult athletes, which has the effect of compromising the potential benefits that can and should be derived as a result of the training (95). Despite the high rates of sweat losses experienced by athletes, most athletes replace only a fraction of the body water loss, even when fluids are readily available to consume (96). The resulting dehydration, when associated with >2%

lowering of body weight, is associated with poor athletic performance (97,98). Importantly, using thirst as a guideline for when to consume fluids is not appropriate, as a high level of body water has already been lost, with a potentially negative impact on performance, before the thirst sensation occurs (99).

Poor Energy Availability

The energy demands of endurance athletes are extremely high, with estimates that cross-country skiers metabolize ~4,000 calories during a 50-km race, and metabolize even more energy during intensive training (100). It is generally recommended that endurance athletes should consume a minimum of 45 kcal/kg/day when daily training has a duration of 1.5 hours or more (101). It has been estimated that a 25-year-old 125-lb female marathoner who runs 10 miles in the morning and 8 miles in the afternoon would require ~4,331 kcal to satisfy the combined needs of activity and REE (102). Athletes with poor energy availability are at increased risk for both disease and injury (22). The long duration of endurance training places a high demand on energy stores, and without good planning the endurance athlete is at high risk of injury that results from insufficient energy (103). The higher risk of injury includes a wide array of problems, including higher risk of stress fractures and poor muscle recovery. The athlete with poor energy availability is also at high risk of psychological, metabolic, endocrine, and immunologic problems. Importantly, it is hard to imagine how an endurance athlete could properly benefit from endurance training without sufficient energy to optimally support the training. Female endurance athletes who fail to consume sufficient energy are at high risk of menstrual dysfunction, which is also associated with poor bone health (104,105). It is important to help athletes understand that, regardless of their age or sex, they should be encouraged to satisfy their nutrient requirements through consumption of whole foods rather than supplement intake (106).

General Nutrition Strategies That Are Important for All Athletes to Follow

1. Physical activity results in greater energy expenditure, and therefore requires more energy and nutrients to be consumed.
    a. It is important for athletes to satisfy the elevated energy expenditure through greater eating frequency rather than by increasing the caloric/nutrient load of the traditional 3 meals/day.

b. This requires meal and snack planning, as most athletes should try to satisfy their energy requirement by eating something approximately every 3 hours during the day. This eating frequency helps to sustain blood sugar, which diminishes the chance that cortisol (a catabolic hormone) will be produced. Elevated cortisol has a negative impact on bone and muscle mass, which is precisely what athletes do not want to happen.

c. Greater eating frequency also helps to assure that glycogen stores are sustained, which is an important factor in athletic performance.

2. The eating frequency should be dynamically planned with the physical activity in mind.

a. An example eating strategy would be breakfast, mid-morning snack, lunch, mid-afternoon snack, dinner, evening snack, and snack before bedtime. These meals and snacks should *all* contribute to both energy and nutrient requirements. This is best done by eating a wide variety of well-tolerated foods, avoiding highly processed foods, and making sure that the foods consumed don't interfere with physical activity by creating GI distress.

b. Athletes should have something available to eat (*e.g.,* Banana, Orange, Apple, etc.) soon after they wake up, as blood sugar is likely to be low. It is not desirable for athletes to wake up, shower, get dressed, and go to a cafeteria to eat breakfast 1 hour after they wake up. Have a little bit right away, then go have breakfast.

3. The foods that are consumed is important. Variety is key, as monotonous intakes are associated with malnutrition and poor athletic performance.

a. Consumption of fresh fruits, whole grain breads, and vegetables are beneficial in many ways: They are all a good source of carbohydrates, which is the fuel most likely to run out in physically active people; They provide a wide variety of nutrients necessary for staying healthy and keeping muscles functioning at their conditioned capacity.

b. Different foods have different nutrients, even if they have the same name. For instance, grapes come in different colors, and each color is associated with different phytonutrients, vitamins, and minerals. Using food "color" as a strategy for assuring food variety is an excellent strategy. For instance, if you ate something red for dinner last night, have something green for dinner tonight.

c. While there are many easily available and convenient foods/snacks, athletes should try to limit the intake of highly process foods, such as highly processed cereals and cookies, as these often fail to provide the nutrients athletes need and, because they are highly processed, they may be absorbed too quickly and result in a high insulin production. Elevated insulin results in too much energy entering cells too quickly. The cells can't process all this energy in real time, so the energy is converted to fat and stored. Athletes typically don't want high body fat levels, as this negatively impact the strength:weight ratio.

4. Athletes have an elevated protein intake requirement, at a level that is typically double the requirement for nonathletes (*i.e.,* 1.6 g/kg vs. 0.8 g/kg).

a. Increasing the per-meal protein intake to satisfy the protein requirement is not desirable, as the maximum amount of protein that most athletes can consume in a single meal/snack is approximately 30 g. This is one of the major reasons that eating frequency in athletes should be increased, so that the required protein can be delivered in amounts that the body can process as protein.

b. Having too much protein in a single meal has undesirable outcomes, including much of the protein being denitrogenated so the remaining carbon chains can be stored as fat. In addition, excessively high protein intakes in a single meal may expose tissues to too much leucine. The leucine delivered in good quality food that provides 30–40 g of protein functions as a muscle protein synthesis stimulator (good), but too much leucine at once has the opposite effect, by reducing muscle protein synthesis (bad).

c. The elevated blood urea nitrogen that results from excess protein being consumed at once must be excreted. This results in higher urinary nitrogen excretion that can result in dehydration, compromising athletic performance. In addition, urea is acidic, so the kidneys retain ionized calcium from the blood to neutralize the acidity. However, since this calcium is important for sustaining blood pH, the blood takes calcium from bones to replace the calcium retained by the kidneys, resulting in low bone mineral density.

d. There are many foods that are good sources of protein, but far too often athletes consume high-fat protein foods (*e.g.,* hamburger, fried chicken, etc.) that provides inflammatory fats, which is not desirable. Athletes should try to select low-fat protein foods (*i.e.,* boiled eggs vs. fried eggs, chicken breast without skin vs. fried chicken breast with skin, etc.), and also learn to eat more plant-based protein by combining foods that elevates the essential amino acid ratio (*i.e.*, beans with rice, oatmeal with nuts, etc.)

5. Athletes should substitute noninflammatory fats with inflammatory fats, but the total intake of these healthier fats should not increase fat intake above the generally expected maximum of approximately 30% of total calories.

   a. Fat intake is important for many reasons including delivering the fat-soluble vitamins (vitamins A, D, E, and K), and helping to satisfy the elevated energy requirement of athletes.

   b. Generally, nonhydrogenated fats are better to consume than hydrogenated fats. For instance, corn oil is a better choice than corn oil margarine, because the process of hydrogenating the fat to make it more solid increases the transfat content, which is inflammatory. When possible, it's desirable to have the oil rather than the tub or stick margarine made from the oil.

   c. Some foods, such as cold-water fish, have an elevated omega-3 fatty acid content, which are anti-inflammatory. By contrast, fatty and processed meats have more saturated fatty acids that are likely to be more inflammatory.

   d. Ideally, athletes should learn to satisfy their fat intake through the consumption of vegetable oils, cold water fish, seeds, and nuts.

6. Iron deficiency and iron deficiency anemia are common occurrences in athletes. Iron is a critically important component of compounds (*i.e.*, hemoglobin and myoglobin) involved in delivering oxygen to cells. Poor oxygen delivery results in a higher heart rate and early exhaustion, and a reduction in oxidative capacity, which also results in early exhaustion. Regular consumption of foods that are good sources of iron helps to diminish iron deficiency risk.

   a. Athletes have a faster breakdown and loss of RBCs than nonathletes, requiring a regular dietary intake of foods that are good sources of iron. Females of childbearing age have a higher requirement for iron than equivalently aged men because of the regular monthly menstrual loss of iron. While both male and female athletes have a relatively high risk of iron deficiency, this places female athletes at a higher risk.

   b. Heme iron is well absorbed and is provided by foods of animal origin.

   c. Nonheme iron is not as well absorbed as heme iron and is provided by vegetable sources, including leafy greens, whole grain cereals, dried beans, peas, nuts, seeds, and nuts. The preparation of foods containing nonheme iron sources is an important factor in the net absorption of iron from these foods. The two primary factors include reducing the content of oxalic acid, which binds iron and makes it unavailable for absorption, and increasing the proportionate content on heme iron in the foods. Oxalic acid is highly water soluble, so blanching vegetables such a spinach for a short time in a pot of boiling water leaches out the oxalic acid and improves iron availability. The conversion of nonheme to heme iron can be made by adding a source of vitamin C (*e.g.*, lemon juice) to the vegetable. Vitamin C is a reducing agent that reduces nonheme iron to its more elemental and better absorbed form, heme iron.

   d. Ideally, it is better to *not* have a high amount of iron at once, as typically provided by supplements, with meals. Iron is a divalent mineral that is competitively absorbed with other divalent minerals, including zinc, magnesium, and calcium. If a high amount of iron is consumed with to a meal, the iron is likely to take up a large proportion of the absorption site, resulting in limited absorption of the other divalent minerals. If this is done regularly, a deficiency of zinc, magnesium, and calcium may occur.

   e. Because iron is so critical for the athlete's oxygen carrying capacity, it is recommended that athletes have iron status tested on a regular basis. This test should be performed at least annually to evaluate hemoglobin, hematocrit, and ferritin. Higher-risk athletes should have a regular iron status exam biannually.

7. Vitamin D status is critically important for support of the immune system, healthy bones, and healthy muscles.

   a. Athletes involved in indoor sports may be at risk of vitamin D deficiency because of an inadequate time spent obtaining UV-B irradiation from sunlight. When skin is exposed to sunlight, the cholesterol contained in the subcutaneous fat is converted to 1-hydroxy vitamin D, the inactive form of vitamin D, which becomes available for activation by the liver and kidneys as needed.

   b. Even athletes who spend a great deal of time outdoors may be at risk for vitamin D deficiency because the clothing worn inhibits UV-B irradiation by the sun. As an example, football players often practice and play outdoors, but the clothing worn makes skin exposure to sunlight difficult.

  c. Because of the multiple important functions of vitamin D to health and the athletic endeavor, athletes should have serum vitamin D tested on a regular basis (*i.e.*, yearly), with a physician-recommended dose of vitamin D supplement taken if prescribed.

8. Athletes who fail to consume a wide variety of foods may compromise their immune system, placing them at increased risk of poor health and injury.

  a. Ideally, athletes will consume a wide variety of fresh fruits, vegetables, and whole grains to satisfy the needs for antioxidants, symbiotics, and zinc.

  b. Antioxidants help to protect cells from reactive oxygen species, which can damage cells and increase muscle soreness and risk of disease. There are a number of antioxidant nutrients that are best provided through the consumption of a wide variety of foods, included green-, yellow- and orange-colored fruits and vegetables, nuts and oils, and fresh fruits.

  c. Symbiotics (a combination of prebiotics and pro-biotics) help the body sustain a healthy gut microbiome, which is important for health. Food sources include foods that have been fermented (*i.e.*, yogurt, kefir, kombucha), and several other foods including green tea and garlic.

  d. Zinc is easily obtained from foods of animal origin (*e.g.*, red meat, poultry, fish), but there are also good vegetable sources of zinc, such as pumpkin seeds.

9. Athletes should develop strategies to *stay well hydrated*, rather than having a strategy to recover from a dehydrated state.

  a. Athletes should not begin a training session or a competition in a poorly hydrated state, as once the physical activity begins, they are likely to be able to lose body water at a rate faster than they can drink and absorb it. A good strategy is to drink ample amounts of water with meals, and to check urine color prior to exercise. A dark urine color is a sign that the kidneys are forced to concentrate urine because of a less than optimal hydration state. Dark urine should be a red flag that more fluid should be consumed prior to the initiation of exercise.

  b. When athletes exercise, blood sugar is used at a faster rate, sodium loss occurs at a faster rate because of the sodium content of sweat, and water is lost via sweat. The hotter the environment, the greater the sweat loss to sustain body temperature. The more humid the environment, the greater the sweat loss to sustain body temperature. Put simply, as three things (water, salt, and blood sugar) are being rapidly reduced with exercise, athletes should drink an appropriate constituted sports beverage that replaces these things. Water alone is insufficient.

  c. Because sweat is being lost as such a fast rate, athletes should not wait for thirst as an indicator of when to drink, as thirst should be considered an emergency sensation because it only occurs when the athlete has already lost ~1.5 L of water, and blood volume is significantly lower. Therefore, athlete should develop a drinking/sipping strategy that attempts to sustain the hydration state and not wait for thirst to drink.

SPECIFIC NUTRITION STRATEGIES FOR PRE-, DURING-, AND POSTCOMPETITION/PRACTICE

Pre-competition/Practice

It has become increasingly clear that when endurance athletes compete, carbohydrate availability is the limiting energy substrate for performance (107). Pre-exercise carbohydrate consumption, regardless of glycemic index, is associated with improved performance, with a general recommendation for 800–1,200 kcal be consumed between 2 and 3 hours prior to practice or competition (108–110). Ideally, this pre-exercise meal should also provide sufficient fluid to allow initiation of exercise in a well-hydrated state and should be moderate in protein and relatively low in fat and fiber to ensure efficient gastric emptying (31). The composition of what is consumed prior to exercise is an important factor, even if the relative content of carbohydrate, protein, and fat is the same. A study has found that a low glycemic index sports bar resulted in a performance benefit over a similarly constituted high glycemic index sports bar (111). There are also beginning data to suggest that other foods or food components may be useful in improving performance when consumed pre-exercise: caffeine, at a level ~10 mcg/mL but below 15 mcg/mL, may reduce the perception of fatigue, potentially allowing exercise to continue longer; nitrate (as commonly obtained from

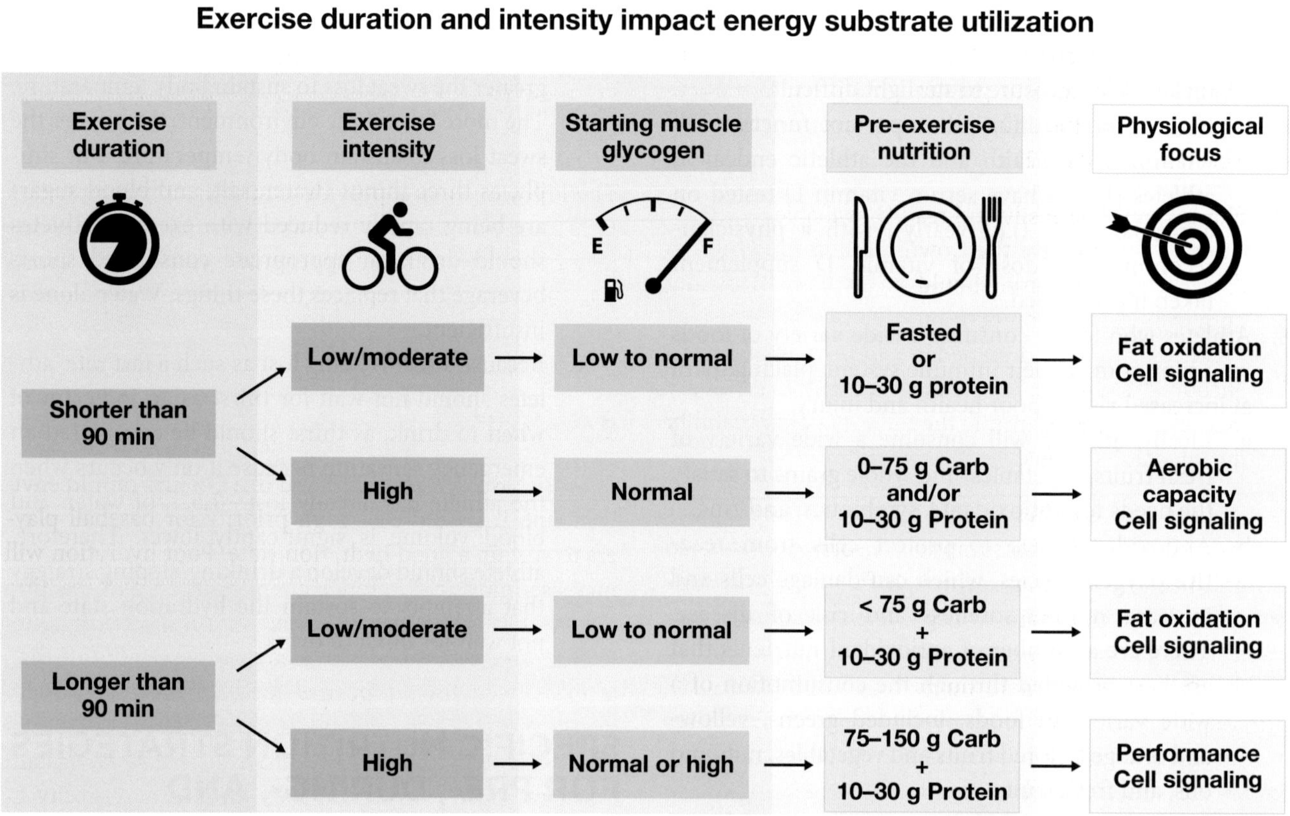

Exercise duration and intensity impact energy substrate utilization

Exercise duration	Exercise intensity	Starting muscle glycogen	Pre-exercise nutrition	Physiological focus
Shorter than 90 min	Low/moderate	Low to normal	Fasted or 10–30 g protein	Fat oxidation Cell signaling
	High	Normal	0–75 g Carb and/or 10–30 g Protein	Aerobic capacity Cell signaling
Longer than 90 min	Low/moderate	Low to normal	< 75 g Carb + 10–30 g Protein	Fat oxidation Cell signaling
	High	Normal or high	75–150 g Carb + 10–30 g Protein	Performance Cell signaling

FIGURE 15.3: Pre-exercise nutrition considerations for protein and carbohydrate intake. (Reprinted from figure 9 of Rothschild JA, Kilding AE, Plus DJ. What should I eat before exercise? Pre-exercise nutrition and the response to endurance exercise: Current prospective and future directions. Nutrients. 2020;12:3473.)

beetroot juice) increases nitric oxide availability with the effect of lowering the oxygen cost of exercise, thereby improving exercise performance (112–116). The recommended food consumed prior to exercise has much to do with exercise intensity and duration, and the athlete's state of glycogen stores. Figure 15.3 illustrates the variability in the recommended carbohydrate and protein consumption prior to exercise for athletes involved in different activities.

Consumption of fluids before exercise/competition is also important to ensure effective glycogen storage, which is stored with water, and to begin the exercise/competition in a well-hydrated state. There is also evidence that consumption of cold fluids or ice slurry before exercise on a hot day may be an effective strategy of precooling core temperature, which can improve endurance performance (117,118). It is common for athletes to consume fluids only when thirsty, so a planned effort should be made to encourage fluid consumption prior to exercise/competition to a point where urine color is clear (119). Consumption of sports beverages prior to exercise is useful because they provide the two things athletes require: carbohydrates and fluids. The American College of Sports Medicine position on fluids states that (120):

- the fluid consumed should be flavored and sweetened to encourage fluid intake;
- to help maintain training intensity, the fluid should contain carbohydrate; and
- to stimulate rapid and complete rehydration, the beverage should contain sodium chloride (salt).

Sports beverages that meet these criteria are particularly useful in helping to deliver both carbohydrates and fluids to athletes.

During Competition/Practice

Fluids are available at fixed 5 km intervals in organized 10-km races and marathons, and athletes should be encouraged to take advantage of each fluid station and consume fluids. However, to be ensured that the athlete can tolerate fluid consumption at this interval, they should practice consuming fluids at the same intervals during training sessions. This will have the advantage of helping the athlete adapt to the fluid consumed and will also improve tolerance to greater fluid consumption to better offset sweat loss. The following recommendations have been suggested (121):

- Fluids should be easily and readily available.
- Athletes should have their own bottle from which to drink, and this bottle should be with them during both training and competition.
- Practices should be designed in a way that enables and encourages athletes to drink frequently, with every possible attempt to mimic the fluid intake availability during competitions.

Athletes and coaches should know that sweat rates can far exceed fluid consumption/absorption rates, so diminishing this difference through frequent fluid consumption is an important strategy. There is concern that some athletes may consume excess fluids, resulting in weight increase (*i.e.*, more fluids consumed than lost). Although a rare occurrence, overconsumption of fluids is a potential cause of hyponatremia (*i.e.*, blood sodium below 125 mmol/L), which can result in bloating, vomiting, confusion, respiratory distress, and possible death that may result from brain edema (120,122,123). Other causes of hyponatremia include excess sodium loss in sweat and consumption of beverages that fail to supply sufficient sodium (31).

Postcompetition/Practice

Carbohydrate consumption immediately postexercise is useful because it maximizes the availability of glycogen synthetase to optimize glycogen resynthesis and storage (124). Even delaying carbohydrate consumption for as little as 2 hours reduces glycogen synthesis (125). There is also strong evidence suggesting that skeletal muscle breakdown increases with endurance training and/or with a single endurance exercise bout, and athletes who consume foods immediately following endurance activity have improved muscle protein synthesis and recovery (126). Providing a combination of good-quality protein and carbohydrate 1 hour postexercise resulted in three times greater muscle protein synthesis than when the same foods are provided 3 hours postexercise (127). While many athletes focus on protein supplementation as an ideal recovery nutrient, a good recovery strategy should simultaneously satisfy the needs related to carbohydrate refueling, rehydration, and the protein requirement for muscle repair (128,129).

NUTRITION ISSUES FOR SELECTED SPORTS WITH A HIGH POWER COMPONENT

The following sports provide examples of how nutrition influences power and speed activities. The list of sports is not intended to be comprehensive. Rather, the sports provide the reader with ideas for how to apply the science to athletes involved in different activities.

Baseball

Because baseball is often played in a hot and humid environment, it should be a high priority for baseball players to sustain a good hydration state. Poor hydration will increase injury risk, reduce attention span and reaction time, result in early fatigue, and diminish coordination (130,131). Fitness is also a factor, as it was found that, at exercise intensities normal for baseball, players with greater fitness sustained body temperature better than less fit players because of improved capacity to sustain sweat rates and cooling capacity (132). The capacity to sustain blood flow to the pitching arm is a factor in performance that is also related to hydration state. It has been found that blood flow increased with up to 40 pitches but steadily declined after that, and by the 100th pitch blood flow to the pitching arm was 30% below baseline (133). It is likely that the reduction in pitching arm blood flow is associated with hydration state. Taken together, these studies suggest that baseball players should make efforts to sustain hydration state using strategies described in Chapter 7.

Baseball players play many games over the course of any in-season week or month, predisposing them to overuse injuries if they fail to get adequate rest, fluids, and energy. Preventing low energy availability has been found to be an important factor in sustaining throwing capacity and avoiding increased injury and health risks (134). Pitchers, in particular, may be at high risk of overuse injury (135,136). The reduced throwing power observed over the course of the season may be due to a combination of overuse injury and reduced leg strength, both of which would affect the throwing motion (137). Catchers work hard and carry more equipment weight, so they are likely to need more sports beverages than other players. They should take every advantage of dugout time when on offense to consume fluids that help to satisfy both carbohydrate and hydration requirements. Both reduced muscular strength and lower muscular strength could be associated with poor hydration and poor energy availability (22,130). Baseball requires power and speed with a high reliance on PCr and carbohydrate for muscular fuel. Although PCr is synthesized from three amino acids, requiring an adequate protein consumption, humans have an energy-first system mandating that energy consumption is also adequate to ensure the consumed protein can be used to manufacture needed substances (including PCr) rather than contributing to the requirement for energy. Put simply, baseball players who focus excessively on protein consumption but who fail to meet total energy needs are at risk of poor performance. Because normal blood sugar is typically maintained for only a short period of 1 to less than 3 hours, and baseball games typically last for ~3 hours, baseball players should consume a carbohydrate-containing sports beverage between innings. The amounts consumed should be related to sweat rates, with the goal of maintaining postgame weights that are within 2% of pregame weights (31). Failure to maintain blood sugar will result in a loss of concentration, poor reaction time, and mental and muscular fatigue.

Bodybuilding

To achieve a high level of muscle mass, bodybuilders place a high level of repetitive stress (typically via free weights and muscle resistance equipment) on each muscle group with high-intensity repetitions that rarely last longer than 30 seconds per muscle group and never last longer than 1.5 minutes (138). In preparation for competition, bodybuilders combine this hard muscle training with the consumption of extra energy, often composed of high-protein foods coupled with nutrient supplements, to enlarge the muscle mass. Because a single training session may result in an up to 40% drop in muscle glycogen stores, it is possible that glycogen depletion may result in impaired training (139). Although bodybuilders have protein requirements at the upper end of the recommended range (~1.7 g/kg/day), typical protein consumption is well above this level at the expense of carbohydrate, which should be in the range of 4–7 g/kg/day (138). Note also that it was found that there was no scientific evidence for 42% of the products for which beneficial nutritional claims were made in bodybuilding magazines, with 32% of the products having misleading information (59). Bodybuilders may restrict fluids and salt to enhance the appearance of being "cut" but fluid restriction has been found to be dangerous, particularly in younger bodybuilders, who are predisposed to developing hypokalemia (low potassium that predisposes the athlete to fatigue,

weakness, and cramping), hypophosphatemia (low phosphorus that predisposes the athlete to muscle dysfunction and weakness, and irritability), rhabdomyolysis (refers to damaged muscle that is associated with muscle pain and weakness), and flaccid tetraparesis (refers to muscle weakness affecting all four limbs) with fluid restriction (140). It has been reported that the majority of bodybuilders follow regimens that result in severe dehydration associated with glycogen depletion (141,142). There is also evidence that the energy (calorie) restriction common in the period immediately prior to competition results in a loss of lean mass, suggesting that the energy restriction is excessive (143). There are different nutritional recommendations for athletes who wish to decrease, maintain, or increase body mass that should be considered (Table 15.8).

Bodybuilders have repetitive patterns of weight gain and weight loss to try to enlarge muscle while reducing body fat. Typical weight loss during the competitive season alternatingly decreases (~6.8 kg; 15 lb) and increases (~6.2 kg; 14 lb). This dieting pattern results in food preoccupation that leads to both binge eating and psychological stress following competitions (144). Importantly, bodybuilders should be made aware of the increased risk of developing eating disorders that may result from the repetitive pattern of weight adjustments (145). A more appropriate strategy is to follow a pattern that sustains energy balance by dynamically matching intake with energy expenditure and provides sufficient carbohydrate and protein to satisfy both glycogen and muscle protein needs. This would simultaneously optimize musculature while minimizing fat tissue acquisition (146). Athletes in weight category sports attempt to gain an advantage by competing in a weight category that is below their regular weight by attempting weight loss strategies that are likely to be dangerous. It has been recommended that the competition weight should be based on preseason weight and body composition, combined with a prohibition of unhealthy weight loss strategies (147). In addition, these athletes should be guided by certified sports nutritionists to develop a healthy eating and exercise pattern for optimal performance.

Diving

Diving requires a combination of power, body control, and flexibility, which all require sustaining good energy and hydration needs (148). The training regimen for divers is similar to that of gymnastics that emphasizes dry-land fitness and focuses on tumbling and water entry. Dietary restriction is often used as a strategy to achieve the desirable muscular and lean physique in divers (149). There is strong evidence that the common strategy of dietary restriction has a negative impact on both health and performance, with greater disease risk from an impaired immune system, dizziness and weakness, and low bone mineral density (150–153). In addition, there is evidence that restrictive eating results in higher body fat percent and greater risk of menstrual disorder (151,154). For the pretraining or precompetition period divers should have a planned meal and/or snack ~1–4 hours prior to exercise that is relatively high in carbohydrate and low in fats (31). This intake should help the diver practice/perform with both normal muscle/liver glycogen and blood sugar, thereby diminishing the risk of mental disorientation and premature muscular fatigue. Training far exceeds energy and hydration needs than divers experience during competition (148). As a result, divers should plan to have multiple opportunities during training to consume small quantities of carbohydrate so as to ensure normal blood sugar and muscle carbohydrate availability (155). During the postcompetition and posttraining period, divers should consume sufficient fluids, electrolytes, and energy to recover glycogen stores and to enhance muscle recovery and muscle protein synthesis (156). Ideally, divers should consume foods and beverages soon after training/competition to optimize the benefit (148). There is evidence that, particularly postcompetition, alcohol is commonly consumed (157). However, alcohol consumption interferes with nutrient and hydration recovery and also has a negative multiday effect that can interfere with both training and competition (158). As a result, alcohol should be avoided.

Football (United States)

American football is highly anaerobic, with plays rarely exceeding 15 seconds, followed by a period of rest/recovery after each play. Football players are getting bigger and stronger each year and have a relatively positive body image when compared with other male athletes (159). Players carry the extra burden of heavy equipment, which adds to the energy requirement. Because the primary fuels used in this activity are PCr and muscle glycogen, it is doubtful that the traditional "steak and potatoes" pregame meal, which overemphasizes protein and underemphasizes carbohydrate, will optimize glycogen storage. Studies of athletes, including football players, have found that a wide range of dietary supplement consumption is common and, although there is no firm indication that

this supplementation negatively influences health, there are also no data confirming that such supplementation improves performance (68). Studies of collegiate football players have found that the rate of vitamin and mineral supplements ranges from 23% to 50% (160,161).

The stop-and-go nature of football is also associated with a high level of body water loss, which can affect the ability to concentrate and perform (162). Maintenance of plasma volume is strongly associated with athletic performance, which should encourage football players to consume a well-designed sports beverage to maintain endurance and performance (163). A recent assessment of National Collegiate Athletic Association Division 1 football players suggested that there should be significant efforts made to improve hydration awareness among football teams to avoid serious health consequences (including possible hydration-associated fatalities) that could occur, especially among higher weight players (i.e., linemen) (164).

The higher weight of current football players compared with the weight of past players is, by itself, not necessarily a good thing. It was found that football linemen with higher body fat percentages and higher body mass indexes had higher rates of lower extremity injuries, and players with higher body fat levels had a 2.5 times greater relative risk of injury than those with lower body fat (165,166). These findings strongly imply that weight per se is the wrong metric for football players. Instead, any increase in weight should be accompanied with relative enlargement of the lean mass to minimize injury risk. This can only be accomplished with a dynamic interplay between appropriate training and eating, with well-distributed energy and protein and avoidance of relative energy deficiency (22). A recent study found that players who ingest protein in a relatively good energy-balanced state had higher lean mass and lower fat mass, and those consuming an appropriate level of protein (1.2–2.0 g/kg/day) while not in a state of negative energy balance had even higher lean mass and lower fat mass (167). Importantly, it has been determined that the dietary intakes of team-sport athletes, both professional and semiprofessional, fail to meet current recommendations from the International Olympic Committee, and the American College of Sports Medicine, resulting in underconsumption of both total energy and carbohydrate (168). It has also been found that nutrition education focused on team sport athletes is an effective strategy for improving eating habits, resulting in improved body composition and performance (169).

Gymnastics

Artistic gymnasts are small, and there is a high level of pressure to keep both stature and weight low (170). As a result, gymnasts are considered to be at high risk of eating disorders and disordered eating, which can increase risks for poor health and also lower athletic performance (151,171,172). Even in men's gymnastics, it is suggested that controlling energy intake to achieve lower weight is an appropriate and desired approach if a gymnast is to achieve success (173). Although lowering mass may lower the risk of traumatic injuries to joints in gymnastics, achieving lower mass through inappropriate means places the gymnast at higher skeletal injury risk (22, 174).

As with other predominantly anaerobic athletes, gymnasts have a heavy reliance on type IIB (pure fast-twitch) and type IIA (intermediate fast-twitch) muscle fibers (175). As a result, gymnastic activity is heavily dependent on PCr and carbohydrate (both blood glucose and muscle and liver glycogen) to fuel activity. This reliance suggests that gymnasts should consume a diet that provides ample carbohydrate to optimize glycogen storage, with a distribution of energy and protein to ensure optimal muscle protein synthesis and muscle recovery. A number of studies have evaluated the nutrient intake of elite gymnasts. In general, these studies demonstrate an inadequacy in the intake of total energy, iron, and calcium (171,176,177). Inadequate calcium, coupled with the fact that virtually all gymnastic training is indoors, increasing risk for poor vitamin D status, suggests that gymnasts may be at high risk for stress fracture. Poor iron intake is associated with anemia, which is a risk factor in the development of amenorrhea (178). Gymnasts have delayed menarche, often past the age of 15, which may play a role in bone health (170). The possible causes of either primary amenorrhea (never having experienced a period; delayed menarche) or secondary amenorrhea (no period for the past 3 months) include the following (22):

- relative energy deficiency
- poor iron status
- high physical stress
- high psychological stress
- high cortisol level, which interferes with the production of estrogen (often the result of relative energy deficiency; low blood sugar).

Competitive gymnasts often reach their competitive peak between the ages of 16 and 18 (170). As adolescents, they have the combined nutritional requirements to satisfy growth and development and the physical demands of sport. Satisfying these high nutritional needs is difficult without appropriate planning. Ideally, this should be done in cooperation with the training facility to ensure availability of foods and beverages.

Hockey

For both men and women, hockey is a high-speed, full-effort sport. With frequent substitutions that allow hockey skaters to perform continuously at high intensity, it is rare for a skater to be on the ice for more than 1.5 minutes before being replaced. This high-intensity effort focuses on PCr and carbohydrate (glycogen and glucose). Although nutrition knowledge of hockey players appears to be poor, there is good indication that hockey players and team management are open to making appropriate nutritional changes (179,180).

A study of elite Swedish hockey players found that skating performance (speed, distance skated, number of shifts, amount of time per shift) improved with carbohydrate loading (181). It was also found that ~60% of quadriceps glycogen is metabolized during a single game (182). It is conceivable that successive game days and/or successive days of practice (both common in hockey) could contribute to glycogen depletion and performance reduction. Although data suggest that players commonly consume a high-protein diet, the heavy reliance on glycogen suggests that hockey players should consume a diet relatively high in carbohydrate (182). Because high-protein diets are also often higher fat diets, players appropriately changing to a high-carbohydrate diet should be aware that the lower energy concentration may result in an inadequate total energy consumption (183). Switching to foods that are lower in fat and higher in carbohydrate, while maintaining the same eating frequency, may result in a negative energy balance that is likely to increase health risks and also be detrimental to performance (184,185).

The high-intensity activity common in hockey results in high sweat rates, suggesting that players should strategize for how to sustain hydration state during a game and should arrive at the game in a well-hydrated state. It has been found that 1% body weight loss is common in hockey players, suggesting that a conscious strategy of frequent sports beverage consumption is necessary (186).

Power/Speed Track and Field Events

Track and field competition includes a number of high-intensity, short-duration events that are primarily anaerobic. These include sprints, short distance hurdles, jumping (long jump, high jump, and pole-vault), and throwing (javelin, shot put, and discus). All of these events are highly reliant on PCr and glycogen (carbohydrate) to satisfy energy needs (187). A study assessing different levels of carbohydrate consumption found that high carbohydrate intakes (~75% of total calories) produced better sprint performance than lower intakes (<45% of total calories) of carbohydrate (188). It is now well established that sprint performance is regulated by the content of skeletal muscle glycogen, which is largely influenced by carbohydrate ingestion. Higher carbohydrate intakes of ~70% of total calories result in higher glycogen storage levels (31,189–191).

The combination of carbohydrate (25 g) and caffeine (100 mg) has been found to improve intermittent sprint performance when ingested 1 hour before exercise (192). This study found higher glucose levels during the final states of exercise, a finding that could be important for competitive field events where several tries/rounds (i.e., long-jump, pole-vault) are necessary to determine the winner.

Pure sprinters should consider carefully whether carbohydrate supercompensation (*i.e.*, maximizing glycogen storage through reduced glycogen utilization through avoidance of higher intensity activity, and higher glycogen formation through high carbohydrate intake) is necessary, because glycogen is stored with water (1 g glycogen to 3–4 g water) (193). Having a level of glycogen storage that exceeds the requirement of a single competitive performance may add unnecessary (water) weight, thereby putting the sprinter at a disadvantage. Sprinters should sustain relatively high carbohydrate intakes but make a performance-related self-determination regarding whether following a carbohydrate supercompensation strategy is warranted.

Swimming (100–400 m)

Swimmers spend a great deal of time in water training to practice techniques that help to overcome drag. Typical energy expenditures of swimmers range between 3,600 and 4,800 kcal/day for males and 1,900 and 2,600 kcal/day for females (194). During competitions, the shorter (sprint) distances derive most of the required energy anaerobically from PCr and glycogen (see Table 15.5). Studies have found a large between-swimmer variation in energy intakes, with male swimmers more likely to satisfy energy needs than female swimmers (195,196). This finding suggests that a large proportion of swimmers have dietary habits that fail to optimally support training and competition needs.

The need for carbohydrate is estimated to be in the range of 3–10 g/kg, depending on training demands (197). Protein requirements, which are in the range of 1.2–1.6 g/kg/day, appear to be met, but many swimmers often fail to optimally time protein consumption to optimize muscle recovery and muscle protein synthesis (198,199). Ideally, high-quality protein should be consumed in 20–25 g amounts evenly distributed over 4–5 meals/snacks during the day (199).

Competitive training for swimmers often begins at a young age, with many of them in junior high school and high school. Training often occurs before school begins in the early morning and often continues immediately after school. This schedule, particularly for adolescent swimmers experiencing a growth spurt, requires a high-energy intake that must be planned for to ensure normal growth and development and no additional health risks. Relative energy deficiency in this young group of athletes could have both negative performance effects (i.e., reduced performance, increased injury risk, decreased coordination) and long-term health implications (i.e., poor bone health, poor growth and development, poor menstrual function in female athletes) (22,194).

Sprinting times that exceed 2 minutes should be followed with a recovery time of at least 4 minutes to regenerate PCr. Without an appropriate recovery period, swimmers will be forced to train shorter durations at lower intensities, which could negatively affect competition (164,194,200).

It may appear odd that swimmers may suffer from poor hydration because they train in a water environment, but it has been found that poor hydration is prevalent in swimmers (201). Although the level of dehydration is mild, swimmers should take steps to sustain normal hydration by having readily available sports beverages during training and competition.

Wrestling

Surveys of wrestling coaches assessing nutrition knowledge suggest that a high proportion of the coaches have a less-than-adequate knowledge base to be guiding young athletes in these areas (202). The American College of Sports Medicine position on weight loss in wrestlers states (203):

> Despite a growing body of evidence admonishing the behavior, weight cutting (rapid weight reduction) remains prevalent among wrestlers. Weight cutting has significant adverse consequences that may affect competitive performance, physical

health, and normal growth and development. To enhance the education experience and reduce the health risks for the participants, the ACSM recommends measures to educate coaches and wrestlers toward sound nutrition and weight control behaviors, to curtail "weight cutting," and to enact rules that limit weight loss.

The general goal of this weight-loss strategy is to qualify for a weight class during a weigh-in on the night before a match, and to gain as much weight as possible between the weigh-in and the match on the next day. Sadly, there is evidence that wrestling at a weight below the predicted minimum wrestling weight appears to be associated with greater wrestling success (204). There is also good evidence that successful weight gain during this short period is important for success. In one study evaluating the relative weight gains of wrestlers, the heavier wrestler was successful 57% of the time (205).

There is concern on many levels about the weight-loss techniques commonly practiced by wrestlers. There is some evidence that undernutrition may lead to altered growth hormone production in wrestlers that, if present over several seasons, could lead to growth impairment (206). In another study, it was determined that dietary restriction reduced protein nutrition to an average of 0.9 g/kg/day, which is below recommended levels, and also lowered muscular performance (207). These data are confirmed by findings indicating that weight loss by energy restriction significantly reduced anaerobic performance of wrestlers. Those on a high-carbohydrate refeeding diet tended to recover their performance, whereas those with lower intakes of carbohydrate did not (208). Besides the obvious physiologic changes that occur from rapid weight loss, there is good evidence that rapid weight loss in collegiate wrestlers causes an impairment of short-term memory, a fact that could have an impact on scholastic achievement in these student athletes (209).

"Making weight" is a hazard to both performance and health. There is ample evidence to suggest that the weight cycling associated with making weight (*i.e.*, weight loss to make weight followed by weight recovery for performance) is dangerous and can lead to glycogen depletion, a lower muscle mass, a lower REE, and an increase in body fat (34). Should this occur with frequency, it is likely that the reduction in REE could make it more difficult for dietary restriction to achieve the desired weight, leading the wrestler to take more draconian (and more dangerous) measures to achieve the desired weight outcome. Wrestlers and coaches should follow a reasonable model for achieving desired weight, such as that offered

by the Wisconsin Interscholastic Athletic Association, to avoid health and performance difficulties (210). This program develops reasonable goals for weight and provides nutrition education information to help wrestlers achieve desired weight reasonably and to understand the implications of improper weight-loss methods. The basic message of these weight-achievement guidelines is that a cap is placed on the maximum amount of weight change that can occur during the course of a season, and a monitoring system has been added to ensure that sudden and dramatic weight change does not occur at any point in the season.

NUTRITION ISSUES FOR SELECTED SPORTS WITH A HIGH ENDURANCE COMPONENT

The following sports provide examples of how nutrition influences endurance activities. The list of sports is not intended to be comprehensive. Rather, the sports provide the reader with ideas for how to apply the science to athletes involved in different activities.

Distance Running

Distance running involving distances of 10,000 m (6.2 miles) or longer places a high reliance on aerobic metabolism, with only 2%–7% of the total energy obtained derived anaerobically (138). Despite this relatively low reliance on glycogen, the fact that distance runners have continuous activity far longer than power athletes places a high demand for glycogen. Put simply, although the proportion of glycogen utilized is relatively low, the volume of glycogen used is high because of the long time spent in the activity (211). As a result, high muscle and liver glycogen stores prior to the run and carbohydrate delivery during the run are important factors for runners to consider.

Gastrointestinal (GI) issues occur with high frequency in long-distance runners, often the result of the consumption of fluids that are hyperosmolar, with excessive concentrations of carbohydrate (>8% carbohydrate solution), electrolytes (>200 mg sodium/250 mL), or both (212). It is important for individual runners to know their tolerance for the beverages they consume during the run, as higher carbohydrate concentrations are typically associated with improved performance, but may also be associated with higher levels of GI distress. These symptoms include nausea, abdominal cramping, vomiting, and diarrhea (213).

Box 15.1   How to Calculate the Percent of Carbohydrate in a Sports Drink

1. Convert the serving size from fluid ounces (oz) or milliliters (mL) to grams (g).
   a. Fluid ounces (oz): Divide the total ounces by 0.03527 for grams
      i. Example: 16 oz/0.03526 = 453.77 g
   b. Milliliters (mL): Divide the amount in mL by 1
      i. Example: 500 mL/1 = 500 g

2. Calculate the carbohydrate percent in a serving size by dividing the carbohydrate amount in 100 g and then multiply by 100.
   a. A drink containing 6 g of carbohydrate per 100 mL (or 100 g) = 6/100 = 0.06
   b. 0.06 × 100 = 6% carbohydrate solution

More serious problems can include blood loss in the feces as a result of damage to the intestines (211). Distance runners train for long hours with repeated motion, which may increase the risk of stress fractures (214). Stress fractures occur more frequently in women runners than in male runners, particularly if the female runner is amenorrheic (215). There is a clear relationship between amenorrhea and lower bone density, so amenorrheic runners should seek the advice of a physician to determine if there are reasonable steps that can be taken, including running "softer" through stride modifications and runner surface changes, to reduce the risk of stress fractures (22,215,216). A review of stress fractures in runners found that being female and a prior history of stress fractures were predictive of future fractures (217). Sufficient energy and consumption of calcium and vitamin D are important to ensure normal bone development. Although vitamin D is likely to be adequate, particularly for runners who train during the day and have ample sun exposure, runners must be purposeful in consuming diets that provide sufficient energy and calcium (218). Inadequate energy intake is a red flag that nutrient intake may also be low (food is the carrier of both nutrients *and* energy) and that the runner is at high risk for both disease and reduced performance (22). The nonmenstruating female runners had lower intakes of fat, and higher fat intakes were associated with more adequate total energy consumption (219). These findings suggest that high-carbohydrate diets, which are preferred for optimal performance, may make it more difficult to consume the high level of needed energy because carbohydrates have a lower caloric density than high-fat foods.

Surveys of distance runners confirm that total energy intake is below recommended levels, suggesting that runners must make a concerted effort to consume the recommended amounts before, during, and after exercise (220).

Runners should learn to manage hydration state by taking pre- and posttraining weight in different environmental conditions. This strategy will help them understand the degree to which they are satisfying body fluid needs (31). Studies of distance runners suggest a range of weight loss averaging ~3%, with individual ranges from 0.8% to 5.0% (221). Surveys of runners have found that, despite knowing that hydration is important, a large proportion of runners (41%–54.4%) have poor hydration habits, particularly during training, and that 35.4% of runners consumed sports drinks, whereas nearly 4% never consumed fluids of any kind in training (222). Studies strongly suggest that 7% carbohydrate solutions with electrolytes are effective as both fluid and energy replacement beverages (31,223). Long-distance runners should develop the habit of frequent fluid consumption to maintain body water status, whether they are thirsty or not. See Box 15.1 for the calculation of the percent of carbohydrate in a sports drink.

Triathlon

The Olympic-Distance Triathlon consists of a 1.5-km swim, a 40-km cycle, and a 10-km run. The most well-known IRONMAN competition in Hawaii (Kona) includes a 2.4-mile swim, a 112-mile bike run, and a 26-mile, 385-yard run. A survey of triathletes found that the average weekly training distances were: swimming 8.8 km (5.47 miles); cycling 270 km (167.77 miles), and running 58.2 km (36.16 miles) (224). Interestingly, there appears to be a high level of overtraining, as a study found statistically significant performance improvements when triathletes reduced the total time spent during training prior to a competition (225). The improvement is likely due to improvement in net glycogen storage associated with a reduction in intense activity that is coupled with a relatively high carbohydrate intake (31).

Different sporting activities may influence athletes to consume different foods and to consume different supplements, resulting in different nutrient exposure (226). In an athlete survey it was found that calcium intake was lower in triathletes than in athletes participating in team sports, including volleyball and basketball, with more pronounced lower intakes in female triathletes (227). Consumption of sufficient calcium is an important component of reducing stress fracture risk.

Maintenance of normal hydration is important to sustain sweat rates and blood volume. There are indications that triathletes may not consume sufficient fluids, which would affect performance and increase risk for heat stress. One study found that pre- and postevent weight declined significantly, whereas urine osmolarity increased significantly, both signs of underhydration (228). Triathletes appear to have difficulty sustaining good hydration during a competition, with body weight loss that commonly exceeds 4% (229). Particularly when competing in warm climates, triathletes should develop well-practiced fluid consumption behaviors to minimize dehydration risk. It is important to note that consumption of ice slurry is useful for cooling core temperature in triathletes when they compete or train in hot environments, resulting in improved performance (117,118).

The majority of Olympic-distance triathletes appear to consume sufficient carbohydrate to satisfy prerace guidelines, but carbohydrate consumption during the race varies widely between athletes, with a large proportion of them failing to satisfy recommended carbohydrate intake levels (230). This is significant, as the carbohydrate demands in the triathlete are greater than the capacity of the athlete to store it (231). Therefore, it is important for triathletes to have a strategy for adequate carbohydrate intake during competition, which should be in the range of 1.0–1.5 g/kg/hr (31). Nutrition interventions encouraging the consumption of more fluid and carbohydrates by triathletes have been successful, with triathletes consuming a level of energy closer to the requirement than before the intervention, which was associated with improved performance (232).

Long-Distance Swimming

Distance swimmers must spend a great deal of time training in water to achieve incrementally small improvements in time and performance (194). Swimming performance is based on a swimmer's ability to create forward propulsion while minimizing the drag created as he or she moves through water, a task that is better enabled with a relatively lean physique (200). Achieving this level of endurance and body composition requires avoidance of relative energy deficiency, which could compromise lean mass and diminish necessary glycogen stores (233). Ideally, needed energy should be provided before, during, and after training to optimize the training benefit. Male and female swimmers report energy intakes of up to 4,800 kcal/day and 2,600 kcal/day, respectively (194).

When compared with other athletes, swimmers often have higher upper body strength but lower bone mineral densities (234,235). There are likely to be three reasons for this, including inadequate energy availability, poor vitamin D status associated with many hours training in an indoor pool without exposure to sunlight, and less physiologic stress being placed on bone because swimmers train in water, which is essentially a gravity-free environment (236). This latter reason suggests that at least a portion of the training by swimmers, particularly young adolescent swimmers who are undergoing the adolescent growth spurt and large changes in bone development, should place resistance on both the upper and lower body.

The volume of training by distance swimmers will deplete muscle glycogen stores, indicating a high need for carbohydrate replacement strategies (197). Consuming fluids during training that are carbohydrate containing would serve to satisfy both carbohydrate and fluid requirements (199).

Cycling

The Tour de France cycle race has extreme endurance demands on participating athletes, with a distance of 4,000 km traveled in just over 3 weeks with only a single day of rest. The energy expended is the highest values ever reported for athletes over a period longer than 7 days (237). Consumption patterns indicate a high carbohydrate diet (62% carbohydrate; 15% protein; 23% fat), with ~50% of total consumed energy between standard meals, and about 30% of energy is consumed as a carbohydrate-containing sports beverage (238).

Asthma prevalence in elite cyclists appears to be approximately twice that of the general population (239). As a result, it may be prudent to make careful allergy inquiries before making recommendations on food and beverage consumption so as to avoid triggering an allergic response.

Cyclists can easily carry fluids and foods on the bike frame or in jersey pockets, and because there is less jarring motion in cycling than in running, cyclists can consume some solid foods without experiencing GI distress. Cyclists should take advantage of this on long rides by bringing along sport beverages to drink and some crackers, bananas, carbohydrate gel, or bread to consume, but whatever is consumed should be known to be well tolerated. Although the need for carbohydrate is highest, many cyclists believe that higher protein foods are beneficial for performance. However, there is no indication that protein foods consumed during cycling enhance performance, and because these foods detract from the consumption of carbohydrate foods they may be performance reducing (240).

GENERAL ATHLETE ASSESSMENT STRATEGIES TO ENSURE NUTRITIONAL READINESS

The assessment and status of an athlete's health typically include health/medical history, body composition, and food intake and energy balance.

Health/Medical History

Health/medical history is typically obtained via an in-depth athlete interview and includes a discussion of:

- medical history that provides information on prescribed and nonprescribed (over-the-counter) drug usage;
- alcohol consumption;
- typical eating environment (*i.e.*, university cafeteria; cooks for self in apartment);
- chronic disease state (*e.g.*, diabetes, amenorrhea);
- relevant acute conditions (*e.g.*, broken bones, muscle strains);
- allergies (food and nonfood), food intolerances, and food sensitivities;
- understanding of changes that may have occurred in appetite;
- if athlete has self-initiated or been placed on a special diet that may put the athlete at nutritional risk;
- family history of disease states (*e.g.*, cardiovascular disease; kidney disease)
- results of any past blood tests indicating normal or abnormal values (*e.g.*, serum iron test for diagnosis of anemia); and
- recommendations for biologic tests (*e.g.*, blood tests, urine tests) where risk of disease/condition is

suggested by health history results (*e.g.*, athlete is considered to be at risk of anemia because of food avoidance pattern).

Body Composition Assessment

Body composition assessment is a multicomponent analysis, involving:

- measurement of height, weight, body fat percent, lean mass percent;
- comparison of these values with sport-specific norms;
- trend analysis to assess how body composition values have changed. Note: it is important to use the same validated measurement strategies for this purpose; and
- Z-score analysis to assess how athlete body composition values differ from position-specific team values.

Food Intake and Energy Balance Assessment

Food intake and energy balance assessment involves the following:

- computerized food intake analysis to include assessment of micronutrient and macronutrient intakes compared with age/gender-specific dietary reference intakes;
- understanding of food avoidance/food preference patterns;
- review of any possible disease states and clinical conditions with associated drug intake that could affect nutrient needs;
- prediction of energy balance values to assess within-day relative energy availability and 24-hour energy balance, for typical training and nontraining days;
- gain an understanding of possible cultural, religious, and/or cultural-associated food intake patterns that may influence macro- and micronutrient intake; and
- under some circumstances, measuring hydration state via assessment of urine-specific gravity.

See online Appendix A for sample athlete health history, nutritional status, and body composition questionnaire and online Appendix B for three examples of dietary intake analysis and eating plans. Please note that Nutri-Timing, which accesses the United States Department of Agriculture nutrient database and the Harris–Benedict equation for predicting REE, was used to create the food plans in online Appendix B.

SUMMARY

- The type of activity performed impacts the type of energy metabolized, but this difference does not necessarily have an impact on the types and frequency of foods/beverages that should be consumed. Although high-intensity power activities (*e.g.*, sprinting) are highly reliant on glycogen as a source of fuel and low-intensity endurance activities (*e.g.*, marathon) are highly reliant on fat as a source of fuel, glycogen storage is the limiting substrate for both types of activities because of the high duration of endurance activities. Therefore, regular dietary sources of carbohydrates should be consumed by all types of athletes to ensure optimal glycogen storage (31).

- Because power athletes are heavily reliant on glycogen stores to fuel the activity, a practice lasting several hours will require regular consumption of carbohydrate to avoid glycogen depletion and a reduction in performance.

- Although endurance athletes are heavily reliant on fat stores to fuel the activity, glycogen is still being used over the long duration of training and competition. Therefore, a regular intake of carbohydrate during training and competition is needed to avoid glycogen depletion and a reduction in performance.

- Different types of muscle fibers have different power potential, with type II fibers producing more power than type I fibers. The type IIA intermediate fibers behave more like power fibers than endurance fibers, but the type of chronic activity that is performed can change the behavior of these fibers. For instance, an athlete who does more endurance activity will modify their type IIA fibers to develop more mitochondria and oxidative capacity, so they begin to look more like type I fibers.

- Well-conditioned athletes have a better capacity to deliver and use oxygen in working muscles, enabling better performance and a longer time before reaching fatigue. Because even the leanest of athletes have ample body fat stores that can be called upon for fuel but glycogen storage is relatively limited in all athletes, a greater capacity to use fat as a fuel (the result of better oxygen utilization), the less likely that glycogen will become depleted.

- Carbohydrate insufficiency during exercise will increase ketone production from gluconeogenesis (*i.e.*, the creation of carbohydrate from noncarbohydrate sources).

- PCr, a source of instantaneous ATP, storage is limited to ~9 seconds of high-intensity activity. Assuming sufficient availability of creatine (likely with sufficient intake of energy/protein), depleted PCr stores can be regenerated with 2–4 minutes of rest.

- Consumption of more protein, by itself, will not result in an increased muscle mass. Increasing muscle mass is multifactorial, requiring a reasonably good sustained energy and nutritional balance, resistance training, and a timing and quality of food intake that can take advantage of muscle protein synthesis potential.

- Although the recommended protein intake for athletes is approximately double that of nonathletes, most athletes appear to consume sufficient amounts of protein from foods alone. A possible exception is vegetarian athletes who do not as consistently obtain sufficient protein.

- Anabolic hormones are involved in tissue building and include testosterone, insulin, HGH, and IGF-1.

- Catabolic hormones are involved in tissue breakdown and include cortisol, thyroxine, and epinephrine.

- There is limited evidence that dietary supplements are useful in improving athletic performance. Ideally, athletes should take a "food-first" approach to meeting nutritional needs.

- Sustaining a good hydration state is important for *all* athletes, regardless of the sport. One of the adaptations to physical activity is to enlarge the blood volume, enabling a better sustained state of hydration if the athletes follow a hydration protocol that maintains both blood volume and fluid balance between the extracellular (blood) and intracellular (tissues) environments. As little as a 2% drop in body weight, resulting from more body water lost than replaced, can have a significant impact on athletic performance.

- Overtraining is associated with multiple problems that is likely to reduce athletic performance, including high muscle soreness and delayed muscle recovery. Athletes should have a training play that incorporates an adequate diet to meet energy/nutrient needs and sufficient rest to recover from training.

- Optimal nutritional/hydration preparation for practice/competition cannot occur in the meal just before physical activity. Athletes require a consistent daily plan for ensuring adequate energy, protein, carbohydrate, fluids, and nutrients to ensure that nutrition is positive factor in athletic performance.

- Excess fluid consumption resulting in weight gain increases the risk of hyponatremia, which can result in bloating, respiratory distress, and brain edema with a potentially fatal outcome.

- Blood sugar typically remains in the normal range for ~3 hours when performing normal daily activity. However, physical activity increases the rate at which brain and muscle tissues utilize blood sugar, dramatically reducing the length of time that blood sugar stays in the normal range. As a result, athletes should have a strategy of carbohydrate consumption, typically by consuming a carbohydrate-containing beverage, during physical activity that helps to sustain normal blood sugar.

- Much of the information that athletes receive about nutrition comes from false nutritional claims in magazine advertisements and stories that target athletes. A significant proportion of the "evidence" presented in these magazines is false.

- Alcohol consumption can negatively impact athletic performance, with even a single serving (*i.e.*, one beer, one glass of wine) affecting reaction time for multiple days. If an athlete consumes alcohol, they should be aware of the performance sequelae of doing so.

- Athletes are at high risk of iron deficiency for multiple reasons, including faster breakdown of RBCs, poor dietary intake, and increased urinary and fecal loses of iron. It is not possible for an athlete with iron deficiency or iron deficiency anemia to perform up to their conditioned capacity.

- Athletes in sports where "making weight" (*e.g.*, wrestling) or sports where appearance (*e.g.*, figure skating, gymnastics) is a factor in scoring are at risk for following dietary patterns that will hinder performance. Relative energy deficiency in sport is now documented to cause numerous performance and health problems that may prematurely cause an athlete to fail athletically and leave the sport prematurely.

- Athletes who train indoors (*i.e.*, basketball, gymnastics, figure skating) are at risk of vitamin D deficiency because of a failure to receive adequate ultraviolet B radiation from the sun. Vitamin D deficiency has multiple negative health and performance outcomes, including low bone density, increased illness frequency, and poor muscle recovery.

- Preparticipation evaluations that include a health/medical history are important and should be performed annually in all athletes to identify health and nutritional risks.

- Body composition assessment is an important component of the nutritional assessment to ensure that the athlete is eating in a way to achieve body composition goals. However, care must be taken to use body composition results in a way that will result in positive outcomes. As an example, the risk that an athlete will follow a low-calorie diet that fails to provide sufficient energy is greater if told that their body fat percent is too high, than if they are told that lean body mass percent is too low.

Practical Application Activity

Imagine two young adults, age 23, of the same sex, height, weight, and body composition. Person A has spent the last 5 years running long distances of ~5 miles (8 km) every other day, and he has participated in several half-marathon races. Person B is a talented tennis player who has been playing competitive tennis for the past 5 years. Both are healthy and fit. Now imagine that Persons A and B have met at a party, and Person A invites Person B to go for a long morning run. They agree, and go for a morning run. After about 1 mile, Person A is carrying on a conversation with Person B, but Person B is starting to get short of breath and cannot participate in the conversation without taking frequent gasps for air. In addition, Person A is running faster but with greater ease than Person B, who is now struggling to keep up. Explain what is happening:

1. Is there a difference in the trained metabolic systems that could be the cause of this difference in comfort level while running?

2. How do training differences impact muscle fibers, and could this difference help to explain why Person A and Person B are responding differently to this morning run?

3. Who (Person A or B) is likely to more efficiently burn fat as an energy substrate, and how would this difference impact time to fatigue?

4. If the tables were turned, and Person B asked Person A to participate in stop-and-go activity such as tennis, would Person A now become fatigued more quickly? If so, what is the metabolic explanation for this?

5. If you were making dietary recommendations to both Person A and Person B, would these recommendations differ? If so, in what ways would they be different?

CHAPTER QUESTIONS

1. Of the following, which energy metabolic system is used for high-intensity activities that require a large volume of ATP, but that are within the athlete's capacity to bring sufficient oxygen into the system?
   a. PCr system
   b. Anaerobic glycolysis
   c. Aerobic glycolysis
   d. Aerobic metabolism
   e. b and c
   f. c and d

2. Of the following muscle fibers, which stores a high level of glycogen and remain primarily anaerobic regardless of conditioning protocol?
   a. Type I
   b. Type IIA
   c. Type IIB
   d. Type III

3. Preformed PCr has sufficient energy to supply an athlete with up to _____ seconds of sudden-onset, high-intensity activity.
   a. 3
   b. 9
   c. 20
   d. 60

4. The delay time to achieve maximal ATP production with aerobic glycolysis is approximately:
   a. 0–1 seconds (instantaneous)
   b. 5–10 seconds
   c. More than 60 seconds
   d. More than 20 minutes

5. Well-conditioned athletes have better oxygen delivery to working muscles, enabling them to maintain oxidative metabolism at a faster rate and to go faster longer before reaching fatigue.
   a. True
   b. False

6. A relatively lean male athlete weighing 154 lb will store ~_____ calories as fat?
   a. 500
   b. 1,000
   c. 50,000
   d. 90,000

7. The percent contribution of aerobic β-oxidation to total energy needs in distance running is approximately:
   a. 30%
   b. 50%
   c. 70%
   d. 90%

8. The percent contribution of aerobic β-oxidation to total energy needs in gymnastics is approximately:
   a. 5%
   b. 20%
   c. 40%
   d. 60%

9. Of the following hormones, which is not anabolic to muscle mass development?
   a. Insulin
   b. Creatine
   c. Growth hormone
   d. Testosterone

10. The eating pattern of bodybuilders leading in weight loss and weight gain over a competitive season increases preoccupation with food that may result in both binge eating and psychological stress following competitions.
    a. True
    b. False

ANSWERS TO CHAPTER QUESTIONS

1. c
2. c
3. b
4. c
5. a

6. d
7. c
8. a
9. b
10. a

REFERENCES

1. Enoka RM, Duchateau J. Muscle fatigue: what, why and how it influences muscle function. J Physiol. 2008;586(1):11–23.
2. Marcora SM, Staiano W, Manning V. Mental fatigue impairs physical performance in humans. J Appl Physiol. 2009;106(3):857–64.
3. Mifflin MD, St Jeor ST, Hill LA, Scott BJ, Daugherty SA, Koh YO. A new predictive equation for resting energy expenditure in health individuals. Am J Clin Nutr. 1990;51(2):241–7.
4. National Research Council. Recommended dietary allowances. 10th ed. Washington (DC): The National Academies Press; 1989. Accessed 2018 May 23. Available from: https://doi.org/10.17226/13286.
5. Fahrenholtz IL, Sjödin A, Benardot D, Tornberg ÅB, Skouby S, Faber J, Sundgot-Borgen JK, Melin AK. Within-day energy deficiency and reproductive function in female endurance athletes. Scand J Med Sci Sports. 2018:1–8.
6. Torstveit MK, Fahrenholtz I, Stenqvist TB, Sylta Ø, Melin A. Within-day energy deficiency and metabolic perturbation in male endurance athletes. Int J Sport Nutr Exerc Metab. 2018: 1–8.
7. Kenney WL, Wilmore J, Costill D. Fuel for exercise. In: Physiology of sport and exercise. 6th ed. Champaign (IL): Human Kinetics; 2015.
8. McArdle WD, Katch FI, Katch VL. Exercise physiology: nutrition, energy, and human performance. Baltimore (MD): Lippincott Williams & Wilkins; 2010.
9. Ingalls CP. Nature vs. nurture: can exercise really alter fiber type composition in human skeletal muscle? J Appl Physiol. 2004;97(5):1591–2.
10. Schiaffino S, Reggiani C. Fiber types in mammalian skeletal muscles. Physiol Rev. 2011;91(4):1447–531.
11. Hirvonen J, Nummela A, Rusko H, Rehunen S, Härkönen M. Fatigue and changes of ATP, creatine phosphate, and lactate during the 400-m sprint. Can J Sport Sci. 1992;17(2):141–4.
12. Hirvonen J, Rehunen S, Rusko H, Härkönen M. Breakdown of high-energy phosphate compounds and lactate accumulation during short supramaximal exercise. Eur J Appl Physiol Occup Physiol. 1987;56(3):253–9.
13. Kappenstein J, Ferrauti A, Runkel B, Fernandez-Fernandez J, Müller K, Zange J. Changes in phosphocreatine concentration of skeletal muscle during high-intensity intermittent exercise in children and adults. Eur J Appl Physiol. 2013;113(11):2769–79.
14. Ghosh AK. Anaerobic threshold: its concept and role in endurance sport. Malays J Med Sci. 2004;11(1):24–36.
15. Probart CK, Bird PK, Parker KA. Diet and athletic performance. Med Clin North Am. 1993;77(4):757–72.
16. Weibel J, Glonek T. Ketone production in ultra marathon runners. J Sports Med Phys Fitness. 2007;47(4):491–5.
17. White AM, Johnston CS, Swan PD, Tjonn SL, Sears B. Blood ketones are directly related to fatigue and perceived effort during exercise in overweight adults adhering to low-carbohydrate diets for weight loss: a pilot study. J Am Diet Assoc. 2007;107(10):1792–6.
18. Campbell B, Kreider RB, Ziegenfuss T, La Bounty P, Roberts M, Burke D, Landis J, Lopez H, Antonio J. International Society of Sports Nutrition Position Stand: protein and exercise. J Int Soc Sports Nutr. 2007;4(8):1–7.
19. Bailey CP, Hennessy E. A review of the ketogenic diet for endurance athletes: performance enhancer or placebo effect? J Int Soc Sports Nutr. 2020; 17:33.
20. Burke LM. Ketogenic low-CHO, high-fat diet: the future of elite endurance sport? J Physiol. 2021;599(3):819–43.
21. Koenig CA, Benardot D, Cody M, Thompson W. Comparison of creatine monohydrate and carbohydrate supplementation on repeated jump height performance. J Strength Cond Res. 2008;22(4):1081–6.
22. Mountjoy M, Sudgot-Borgen J, Burke L, Carter S, Constantini N, Lebrun C, Meyer N, Sherman R, Steffen K, Budgett R, Ljungqvist A. The IOC consensus statement: beyond the Female Athlete Triad—Relative Energy Deficiency in Sport (RED-S). Br J Sports Med. 2014;48(7):491–7.
23. Marocolo M, Willardson JM, Marocolo IC, da Mota GR, Simão R, Maior AS. Ischemic preconditioning and placebo intervention improves resistance exercise performance. J Strength Cond Res. 2016;30(5):1462–9.
24. Arnold DL, Matthews PM, Radda GK. Metabolic recovery after exercise and the assessment of mitochondrial function *in vivo* in human skeletal muscle by means of ^{31}P NMR. Magn Reson Med. 1984;1(3):307–15.
25. Hesse E, Renaud J-M. Modulation of skeletal muscle fatigue kinetics by extracellular glucose and glycogen content. FASEB J. 2015;29(1 Suppl):824.10.
26. Ørtenblad N, Westerblad H, Nielsen J. Muscle glycogen stores and fatigue. J Physiol. 2013;591(18):4405–13.
27. Nieman DC, Shanely RA, Zwetsloot KA, Meaney MP, Farris GE. Ultrasonic assessment of exercise-induced change in skeletal muscle glycogen content. BMC Sports Sci Med Rehabil. 2015;7:9.
28. Maughan RJ, Greenhaff PL, Leiper JB, Ball D, Lambert CP, Gleeson M. Diet composition and the performance of high-intensity exercise. J Sports Sci. 1997;15(3):265–75.
29. Fogelholm M, Tikkanen H, Naveri H, Harkonen M. High-carbohydrate diet for long distance runners: a practical viewpoint. Br J Sports Med. 1989;23(2):94–6.
30. Stellingwerff T, Bovim IM, Whitfield J. Contemporary nutrition interventions to optimize performance in middle-distance runners. Int J Sport Nutr Exerc Metab. 2019;29:106–16.
31. Thomas DT, Erdman KA, Burke LM, MacKillop M. American College of Sports Medicine Joint Position Statement. Nutrition and athletic performance. Med Sci Sports Exerc. 2016;48(3):543–68.
32. Hoffman JR, Ratamess NA, Kang J, Falvo MJ, Faigenbaum AD. Effect of protein intake on strength, body composition and endocrine changes in strength/power athletes. J Int Soc Sports Nutr. 2006;3(2):12–8.
33. Binkley TL, Daughters SW, Weidauer LA, Vukovich MD. Changes in body composition in division I football players over a competitive season and recovery in off-season. J Strength Cond Res. 2015;29(9):2503–12.
34. Horswill CA. Weight loss and weight cycling in amateur wrestlers: Implications for performance and resting metabolic rate. Int J Sport Nutr. 1993;3(3):245–60.
35. Strauss RH, Lanese RR, Leizman DJ. Illness and absence among wrestlers, swimmers, and gymnasts at a large university. Am J Sports Med. 1988;16(6):653–5.

36. Cook CJ, Kilduff LP, Beaven CM. Improving strength and power in trained athletes with 3 weeks of occlusion training. Int J Sports Physiol Perform. 2013;9(1):166–72.

37. Holway FE, Spriet LL. Sport-specific nutrition: practical strategies for team sports. J Sports Sci. 2011;29 Suppl 1):S115–25.

38. Moore DR, Camera DM, Areta JL, Hawley JA. Beyond muscle hypertrophy: why dietary protein is important for endurance athletes. Appl Physiol Nutr Metab. 2014;39(9):987–97.

39. Pasiakos SM, Lieberman HR, McLellan TM. Effects of protein supplements on muscle damage, soreness and recovery of muscle function and physical performance: a systematic review. Sports Med. 2014;44(5):655–70.

40. Fox EA, McDaniel JL, Preitbach AP, Weiss EP. Perceived protein needs and measured protein intake in collegiate male athletes: an observational study. J Int Soc Sports Nutr. 2011; 8(9): http://www.jissn.com/content/8/1/9

41. Gillen JB, Trommelen J, Wardenaar FC, Brinkmans NY, Versteegen JJ, Jonvik KL, Kapp C, de Vries J, van den Borne JJ, Gibala MJ, van Loon LJC. Dietary protein intake and distribution patterns of well-trained Dutch athletes. Int J Sport Nutr Exerc Metab. 2017;25(2):105–14.

42. Van Erp-Baart AM, Saris WHM, Binkhorst RA, Vos JA, Elvers JWH. Nationwide survey on nutritional habits in elite athletes: part 1-Energy, carbohydrate, protein, and fat intake. Int J Sports Med. 1989;10:S3–10.

43. Phillips SM. A brief review of higher dietary protein diets in weight loss: a focus on athletes. Sports Med. 2014;44(Suppl 2): S149–53.

44. Bhasin B, Velez JCQ. Evaluation of polyuria: the roles of solute loading and water diuresis. Am J Kidney Dis. 2016;67(3):507–11.

45. Ortinau LC, Hoertel HA, Douglas SM, Leidy HJ. Effects of high-protein vs. high-fat snacks on appetite control, satiety, and eating imitation in healthy women. Nutr J. 2014;13:97.

46. Binnerts A, Swart G, Wilson J, Hoogerbrugge N, Pols HA, Birkenhager JC, Lamberts SW. The effect of growth hormone administration in growth hormone deficient adults on bone, protein, carbohydrate, and lipid homeostasis, as well as on body composition. Clin Endocrinol. 1992;37(1):79–87.

47. Deyssig R, Frisch H, Blum W, Waldhor T. Effect of growth hormone treatment on hormonal parameters, body composition, and strength in athletes. Acta Endorinol. 1993;128:313–8.

48. Gregory J, Greene S, Thompson J, Scrimgeour C, Rennie M. Effects of oral testosterone undecanoate on growth, body composition, strength and energy expenditure of adolescent boys. Clin Endocrinol. 1992;37(3):207–13.

49. Yarasheki K, Campbell, J, Smith, K, Rennie MJ, Holloszy J, Bier DM. Effect of growth hormone and resistance exercise on muscle growth in young men. Am J Physiol. 1992;262(3):E261–7.

50. Chromiak JA, Antonio J. Use of amino acids as growth hormone-releasing agents by athletes. Nutrition. 2002;18(7–8):657–61.

51. Bucci L, Hickson J, Pivarnik J, Wolinsky I, McMahon J, Turner S. Ornithine ingestion and growth hormone release in bodybuilders. Nutr Res. 1990;10(3):239–45.

52. Bucci L, Hickson J, Wolinksy I, Pivarnik J. Ornithine supplementation and insulin release in bodybuilders. Int J Sport Nutr. 1992;2(3):287–91.

53. Elam R. Morphological changes in adult males from resistance exercise and amino acid supplementation. J Sports Med Phys Fitness. 1988;28(1):35–9.

54. Elam R, Hardin D, Sutton R, Hagen L. Effects of arginine and ornithine on strength, lean body mass, and urinary hydroxyproline in adult males. J Sports Med Phys Fitness. 1989;29(1): 52–6.

55. Lambert GP, Bleiler TL, Change RT, Johnson AK, Gisolfi CV. Effects of carbonated and noncarbonated beverages at specific intervals during treadmill running in the heat. Int J Sport Nutr. 1993;3(2):177–93.

56. Pasiakos SM, McLellan TM, Lieberman HR. The effects of protein supplements on muscle mass, strength, and aerobic and anaerobic power in healthy adults: a systematic review. Sports Med. 2015;45(1):111–31.

57. Suminski, RR, Robertson RJ, Goss FL, Robinson AG, DaSilva SG, Kang J, Utter AC, Metz KF. The effect of amino acid ingestion and resistance exercise on growth hormone responses in young males. Med Sci Sports Exerc. 1993;25(5):S77.

58. Fry A, Kraemer W, Stone M, Warren BJ, Kearney JT, Maresh CM, Weseman CA, Fleck SJ. Endocrine and performance responses to high volume training and amino acid supplementation in elite junior weightlifters. Int J Sport Nutr. 1993; 3(3):306–22.

59. Barron RL, Vanscoy GJ. Natural products and the athlete: facts and folklore. Ann Pharmacother. 1993;27(5):607–15.

60. Hawkins CE, Walberg-Rankin J, Sebolt DR. Oral arginine does not affect body composition or muscle function in male weightlifters. Med Sci Sports Exerc. 1991;23:S15.

61. Geil PB, Anderson JW. Nutrition and health implications of dry beans: a review. J Am Coll Nutr. 1994;13(6):549–58.

62. Mares-Perlman JA, Subar AF, Block G, Greger JL, Luby MH. Zinc intake and sources in the U.S. adult population: 1976–1980. J Am Coll Nutr. 1995;14:349–57.

63. Pate RR, Miller BJ, Davis JM, Slentz CA, Klingshirn LA. Iron status of female runners. Int J Sport Nutr. 1993;3(2): 222–31.

64. Telford R, Catchpole E, Deakin V, Hahn A, Plank A. The effect of 7 to 8 months of vitamin/mineral supplementation on athletic performance. Int J Sport Nutr. 1992;2(2):135–53.

65. Friedman AN. High-protein diets: potential effects on the kidney in renal health and disease. Am J Kidney Dis. 2004; 44(6):950–62.

66. Brandle E, Sieberth HG, Hautmann RE. Effect of chronic dietary protein intake on the renal function in healthy subjects. Eur J Clin Nutr. 1996;50(11):734–40.

67. Maughan RJ, Burke LM, Dvorak J, Larson-Meyer DE, Peeling P, Phillips SM, Rawson ES, Walsh NP, Garthe I, Geyer H, Meeusen R, van Loon LJC, Shirreffs SM, Spriet LL, Stuart M, Vernec A, Currell K, Ali VM, Budgett RG, Ljungqvist A, Mountjoy M, Pitsiladis YP, Soligard T, Erdener U, Engebretsen L. IOC consensus statement: dietary supplements and the high-performance athlete. Br J Sports Med. 2018;52(7):439–55.

68. Sinnott RA, Maddela RL, Bae S, Best T. The effect of dietary supplements on the quality of life of retired professional football players. Glob J Health Sci. 2012;5(2):13–26.

69. Gomez-Cabrera M-C, Domenech E, Romagnoli M, Arduini A, Borras C, Pallardo FV, Sastre J, Viña J. Oral administration of vitamin C decreases muscle mitochondrial biogenesis an hampers training-induced adaptations in endurance performance. Am J Clin Nutr. 2008;87(1):142–9.

70. Heikkinen A, Alaranta A, Helenius I, Vasankari T. Use of dietary supplements in Olympic athletes is decreasing: a follow-up study between 2002 and 2009. J Int Soc Sports Nutr. 2011;8:1–8. Accessed May 23, 2018. Available from: http://www.jissn.com/content/8/1/1

71. Lukaski HC. Vitamin and mineral status: effects on physical performance. Nutrition. 2004;20(7–8):632–44.

72. Maughan RJ, King DS, Lea T. Dietary supplements. J Sports Sci. 2004;22(1):95–113.

73. Burke LM. Re-examining high-fat diets for sports performance: did we call the "nail in the coffin" too soon? Sports Med. 2015;45(Suppl. 1):S33–49.

74. Chance B, Leigh JS, Clark BJ Jr, Maris J, Kent J, Nioka S, Smith D. Control of oxidative metabolism and oxygen delivery in human skeletal muscle: a steady-state analysis of the work/energy cost transfer function. Proc Natl Acad Sci U S A. 1985; 82(24):8384–8.

75. Burke LM, Ross ML, Garvican-Lewis LA, Welvaert M, Heikura IA, Forbes SG, Mirtschin JG, Cato LE, Strobel N, Sharma AP, Hawley JA. Low carbohydrate, high fat diet impairs exercise economy and negates the performance benefit from intensified training in elite race walkers. J Physiol. 2017;595(9):2785–807.

76. Bassett DR, Howley ET. Limiting factors for maximum oxygen uptake and determinants of endurance performance. Med Sci Sports Exerc. 2000;32(1):70–84.

77. Ekblom B, Åstrand PO, Saltin B, Stenberg J, Wallstrom B. Effect of training on circulatory response to exercise. J Appl Physiol. 1968;24(4):518–28.

78. Åstrand PO, Rodahl K. Textbook of work physiology. New York (NY): McGraw-Hill; 1970. p. 279–430.

79. Heinonen I, Koga S, Kalliokoski KK, Musch TI, Poole DC. Herterogeneity of muscle blood flow and metabolism: influence of exercise, aging and disease states. Exerc Sport Sci Rev. 2015;43(3):117–24.

80. Sizer F, Whitney E. Nutrition: concepts and controversies. 7th ed. Albany (NY): West/Wadsworth; 1997. p. 383.

81. Burke LM, Jeukendrup AE, Jones AM, Mooses M. Contemporary nutrition strategies to optimize performance in distance runners and race walkers. Int J Sport Nutr Exerc Metab. 2019;29:117–29.

82. Costa RJS, Hoffman MD, Stellingwerff T. Considerations for ultra-endurance activities: part 1-nutrition. Research in Sports Medicine. 2019;37(2):166–81.

83. Lavoué C, Siracusa J, Chalchat É, Bourrilhon C, Charlotte K. Analysis of food and fluid intake in elite ultra-endurance runners during a 24-hour world championship. J Int Soc Sports Nutr. 2020;17:36.

84. Barnard ND, Goldman DM, Loomis JF, Kahleova H, Levin SM, Neabore S, Batts TC. Plant-based diets for cardiovascular safety and performance in endurance sports. Nutrients. 2019;11:130.

85. Malsagova KA, Kopylov AT, Siitsyna AA, Stepanov AA, Izotov AA, Butkova TV, Chingin K, Klyuchnikov MS, Kaysheva AL. Sports nutrition: diets, selection factors, recommendations. Nutrients. 22021;13:3771.

86. Scott CL, Haycraft E, Plateau CR. Teammate influences on the eating attitudes and behaviors of athletes: a systematic review. Psychol Sport Exerc. 2019;43:183–94.

87. Devrim-Lanpir A, Hill L, Knechtle B. Efficacy of popular diets applied by endurance athletes on sports performance: beneficial or detrimental? A narrative review. Nutrients. 2021;13:491.

88. Angeli A, Minetto M, Dovio A, Paccotti P. The overtraining syndrome in athletes: a stress-related disorder. J Endocrinol Invest. 2004;27(6):603–12.

89. Budgett R. Fatigue and underperformance in athletes: the overtraining syndrome. Br J Sports Med. 1998;32(2):107–10.

90. Meeusen R, Duclos M, Foster C, Meeusen R, Duclos M, Foster C, Fry A, Gleeson M, Nieman D, Raglin J, Rietjens G, Steinacker J, Urhausen A; European College of Sport Science; American College of Sports Medicine. Prevention, diagnosis and treatment of the overtraining syndrome: joint consensus statement of the European College of Sport Science and the American College of Sports Medicine. Med Sci Sports Exerc. 2013;45(1):186–205.

91. Krivickas LS. Anatomical factors associated with overuse sports injuries. Sports Med. 1997;24(2):132–46.

92. Wen DY. Risk factors for overuse injuries in runners. Curr Sports Med Rep. 2007;6(5):307–13.

93. Dressendorfer RH, Wade CE. Effects of a 15-d race on plasma steroid levels and leg muscle fitness in runners. Med Sci Sports Exerc. 1991;23(8):954–8.

94. Armstrong LE, Johnson EC, McKenzie AL, Ellis LA, Williamson KH. Ultraendurance cycling in a hot environment: thirst, fluid consumption, and water balance. J Strength Cond Res. 2015;29(4):869–76.

95. Arnaoutis G, Kavouras SA, Angelopoulou A, Skoulariki C, Bismpikou S, Mourtakos S, Sidossis LS. Fluid balance during training in elite young athletes of different sports. J Strength Cond Res. 2015;29(12):3447–52.

96. Hargreaves M, Dillo P, Angus D, Febbraio M. Effect of fluid ingestion on muscle metabolism during prolonged exercise. J Appl Physiol. 1996;80(1):363–6.

97. Armstrong LE, Costill DL, Fink WJ. Influence of diuretic-induced dehydration on competitive running performance. Med Sci Sports Exerc. 1985;17(4):456–61.

98. Walsh RM, Noakes TD, Hawley JA, Dennis SC. Impaired high-intensity cycling performance time at low levels of dehydration. Int J Sport Nutr. 1994;15(7):392–8.

99. Armstrong LE, Johnson EC, Bergeron MF. Counterview: is drinking to thirst adequate to appropriately maintain hydration status during prolonged endurance exercise? No. Wilderness Environ Med. 2016;27(2):195–8.

100. Ekblom B, Bergh U. Physiology and nutrition for cross-country skiing. In: Lamb D, Knuttgen K, Murray R, editors. Perspectives in exercise science and sports medicine: physiology and nutrition for competitive sport. Indianapolis (IN): Benchmark Press; 1996.

101. Economos CD, Bortz SS, Nelson ME. Nutritional practices of elite athletes. Sports Med. 1993;16(6):381–99.

102. Murray R, Horswill CA. Nutrient requirements for competitive sports. In: Wolinsky I, editor. Nutrition in exercise and sport. 3rd ed. Boca Raton (FL): CRC Press; 1998. p. 521–58.

103. Fontana L, Klein S, Holloszy JO. Effects of long-term caloric restriction and endurance exercise on glucose tolerance, insulin action, and adipokine production. Age. 2010;32(1):97–108.

104. Nattiv A. Stress fractures and bone health in track and field athletes. J Sci Med Sport. 2000;3(3):268–79.

105. Schnackenburg KE, Macdonald HM, Ferber R, Wiley JP, Boyd SK. Bone quality and muscle strength in female athletes with lower limb stress fractures. Med Sci Sports Exerc. 2011;43(11):2110–9.

106. Desbrow B, Burd NA, Tarnopolski M, Moore DR. Nutrition for special populations: young, female, and maters athletes. Int J Sport Nutr Exerc Metab. 2019;29:220–7.

107. Hawley JA, Leckey JJ. Carbohydrate dependence during prolonged, intense endurance exercise. Sports Med. 2015;45(Suppl 1):5–12.

108. Burdon CA, Spronk I, Cheng HL, O'Connor HT. Effect of glycemic index of a pre-exercise meal on endurance exercise performance: a systematic review and meta-analysis. Sports Med. 2016;47(6):1087–101.

109. Coggan AR, Swanson SC. Nutritional manipulations before and during endurance exercise: effects on performance. Med Sci Sports Exerc. 1992;24(9 Suppl):S331–5.

110. Sherman WM. Metabolism of sugars and physical performance. Am J Clin Nutr. 1995;62(1):228S–41S.

111. Kaviani M, Chilibeck PD, Gall S, Joachim J, Zello GA. The effects of low- and high-glycemic index sports nutrition bars on metabolism and performance in recreational soccer players. Nutrients. 2020;12:982.

112. Astorino TA, Roberson DW. Efficacy of acute caffeine ingestion for short-term high-intensity exercise performance: a systematic review. J Strength Cond Res. 2010;24(1):257–65.

113. Burke L, Desbrow B, Spriet L. Caffeine for sports performance. Champaign (IL): Human Kinetics; 2013.

114. Jones AM. Influence of dietary nitrate on the physiological determinants of exercise performance: a critical review. Appl Physiol Nutr Metab. 2014;39(9):1019–28.

115. Ormsbee MJ, Bach CW, Baur DA. Pre-exercise nutrition: the role of macronutrients, modified starches and supplements on metabolism and endurance performance. Nutrients. 2014;6(5):1782–808.

116. Tarnopolsky MA. Caffeine and creatine use in sport. Ann Nutr Metab. 2010;57(Suppl 2):1–8.

117. Stevens CJ, Dascombe B, Boyko A, Sculley D, Callister R. Ice slurry ingestion during cycling improves Olympic distance triathlon performance in the heat. J Sports Sci. 2013;31(12):1271–9.

118. Tan PMS, Lee JKW. The role of fluid temperature and form on endurance performance in the heat. Scand J Med Sci Sports. 2015;25(Suppl 1):39–51.

119. Havemann L, Goedecke JH. Nutritional practices of male cyclists before and during an ultraendurance event. Int J Sport Nutr Exerc Metab. 2008;18(6):551–66.

120. Sawka MN, Burke LM, Eichner ER, Maughan RJ, Montain SJ, Stachenfield NS; American College of Sports Medicine. American College of Sports Medicine Position Stand: exercise and fluid replacement. Med Sci Sports Exerc. 2007;39(2):377–90.

121. Broad EM, Burke LM, Cox GR, Heeley P, Riley M. Body weight changes and voluntary fluid intakes during training and competition sessions in team sports. Int J Sport Nutr. 1996;6(3):307–20.

122. Armstrong LE, Casa DJ, Millard-Stafford M, Moran DS, Pyne SW, Roberts WO; American College of Sports Medicine. American College of Sports Medicine Position Stand: exertional heat illness during training and competition. Med Sci Sports Exerc. 2007;39(3):556–72.

123. Hew-Butler T, Rosner MH, Fowkes-Godek S, Dugas JP, Hoffman MD, Lewis DP, Maughan RJ, Miller KC, Montain SJ, Rehrer NJ, Roberts WO, Rogers IR, Siegel AJ, Stuempfle KJ, Winger JM, Verbalis JG. Statement of the Third International Exercise-Associated Hyponatremia Consensus Development Conference, Carlsbad, California, 2015. Clin J Sport Med. 2015;25(4):303–20.

124. Beck KL, Thomson JS, Swift RJ, von Hurst PR. Role of nutrition in performance enhancement and postexercise recovery. Open Access J Sports Med. 2015;6:259–67.

125. Ivy JL, Katz AL, Cutler CL, Sherman WM, Coyle EF. Muscle glycogen synthesis after exercise: effect of time of carbohydrate ingestion. J Appl Physiol. 1985;64(4):1480–5.

126. Rodriguez NR, Vislocky LM, Courtney GP. Dietary protein, endurance exercise, and human skeletal-muscle protein turnover. Curr Opin Clin Nutr Metab Care. 2007;10(1):40–5.

127. Levenhagen DK, Gresham JD, Carlson MG, Maron DJ, Borel MJ, Flakoll PJ. Postexercise nutrient intake timing in humans is critical to recovery of leg glucose and protein homeostasis. Am J Physiol Endocrinol Metab. 2001;280(6):E982–93.

128. Kim J, Kim E-K. Nutritional strategies to optimize performance and recovery in rowing athletes. Nutrients. 2020;12:1685.

129. Polios A, Georgakouli K, Draganidis D, Deli CK, Tsimeas PD, Chatzinikolaou A, Papanikolaou K, Batrakoulis A, Mohr M, Jamurtas AZ, Fatouros IG. Protein-based supplementation to enhance recovery in team sports: what is the evidence? J Sports Sci Med. 2019;18:523–36.

130. Herring SA, Putukian M, Kibler WB, LeClere L, Boyajian-O'Neill L, Day MA, Franks RR, Indelicato P, Matuszak J, Miller TL, O'Connor F. Team Physician Consensus Statement: Return to Sport/Return to Play and the Team Physician: A Team Physician Consensus Statement—2023 Update. Curr Sports Med Rep. 2024;23(5):183-91.

131. Murray R. Dehydration, hyperthermia, and athletes: science and practice. J Athl Train. 1996;31(3):248–52.

132. Yoshida T, Nakai S, Yorimoto A, Kawabata T, Morimoto T. Effect of aerobic capacity on sweat rate and fluid intake during outdoor exercise in the heat. Eur J Appl Physiol Occup Physiol. 1995;71(2–3):235–9.

133. Bast SC, Perry JR, Poppiti R, Vangsness CT, Weaver FA. Upper extremity blood flow in collegiate and high school baseball pitchers: a preliminary report. Am J Sports Med. 1996;24(6):847–51.

134. Sygo J, Glass AK, Killer SC, Stellingwerff T. Fueling for the field: Nutrition for jumps, throws, and combined events. Int J Sport Nutr Exerc Metab. 2019;29:95–105.

135. Whitley JD, Terrio T. Changes in peak torque arm-shoulder strength of high school baseball pitchers during the season. Percept Mot Skills. 1998;86(3 suppl):1361–2.

136. Yang J, Mann BJ, Guettler JH, Dugas JR, Irrgang JJ, Fleisig GS, Albright JP. Risk-prone pitching activities and injuries in youth baseball: findings from a national sample. Am J Sports Med. 2014;42(6):1456–63.

137. MacWilliams BA, Choi T, Perezous MK, Chao EY, McFarland EG. Characteristic ground-reaction forces in baseball pitching. Am J Sports Med. 1998;26(1):66–71.

138. Sloniger MA, Cureton KJ, O'Bannon PJ. One-mile run-walk performance in young men and women: role of anaerobic metabolism. Med Sci Sports Exerc. 1997;22(4):337–50.

139. Koopman R, Manders RJ, Jonkers RA, Hul GB, Kuipers H, van Loon, LJ. Intramyocellular lipid and glycogen content are reduced following resistance exercise in untrained healthy males. Eur J Appl Physiol. 2006;96(5):525–34.

140. Britschgi F, Zünd G. Bodybuilding: hypokalemia and hypophosphatemia. Schweiz Med Wochenschr. 1991;21(33):1163–5.

141. di Corcia M, Tartaglia N, Polito R, Ambrosi A, Messina G, Francavilla VC, Cincione RI, della Malva A, Ciliberti MG, Sevi A, Messina G, Albenzio M. Functional Properties of Meat in Athletes' Performance and Recovery. Int. J. Environ. Res. Public Health. 2022, 19,5145. https://doi.org/10.3390/ijerph19095145

142. Slater G, Phillips SM. Nutrition guidelines for strength sports: sprinting, weightlifting, throwing events, and bodybuilding. J Sports Sci. 2011;29(S1):S67–77.

143. Hickson JF, Johnson TE, Lee W, Sidor RJ. Nutrition and the precontent preparations of a male bodybuilder. J Am Diet Assoc. 1990;90(2):264–7.

144. Andersen RE, Barlett SJ, Morgan GD, Brownell KD. Weight loss, psychological, and nutritional patterns in competitive male body builders. Int J Eat Disord. 1995;181(1):49–57.

145. Helms ER, Aragon AA, Fitschen PJ. Evidence-based recommendations for natural bodybuilding contest preparation: nutrition and supplementation. J Int Soc Sports Nutr. 2014;11:20.

146. Benardot D. Timing of energy and fluid intake: new concepts for weight control and hydration. ACSMs Health Fit J. 2007;11(4):13–9.

147. Burke LM, Slater GJ, Matthews JJ, Langan-Evans C, Horswill CA. ACSM Expert Consensus Statement on Weight Loss in Weight-Category Sports. Current Sports Medicine Reports. 2021;20(4):199–217. ISSN 1537–890X

148. Benardot D, Zimmermann W, Cox GR, Marks S. Nutritional recommendations for divers. Int J Sport Nutr Exerc Metab. 2014;24(2):392–403.

149. Loucks AB, Kiens B, Wright HH. Energy availability in athletes. J Sports Sci. 2011;29(Suppl 1):S7–15.

150. Barrack MT, Rauth MJ, Barkai H-S, Nichols JF. Dietary restraint and low bone mass in female adolescent endurance runners. Am J Clin Nutr. 2008;87:36–43.

151. Deutz B, Benardot D, Martin D, Cody MM. Relationship between energy deficits and body composition in elite female gymnasts and runners. Med Sci Sports Exerc. 2000;32(3):659–68.

152. Ersoy, G. Dietary status and anthropometric assessment of child gymnasts. J Sports Med Phys Fitness. 1991;31(4):577–80.

153. Nova E, Montero A, López-Varela S, Marcos A. Are elite gymnasts really malnourished? Evaluation of diet, anthropometry and immunocompetence. Nutr Res. 2001;21(1–2):15–29.

154. Sundgot-Borgen J. Risk and trigger factors for the development of eating disorders in female elite athletes. Med Sci Sports Exerc. 1994;26(4):414–9.

155. Burke LM, Hawley JA, Wong SH, Jeukendrup AE. Carbohydrates for training and competition. J Sports Sci. 2011;29(Suppl 1):S17–27.

156. Millard-Stafford M, Childers WL, Conger SA, Kampfer AJ, Rahnert JA. Recovery nutrition: timing and composition after endurance exercise. Curr Sports Med Rep. 2008;7(4):193–201.

157. Yusko DA, Buckman JF, White HR, Pandina RJ. Alcohol, tobacco, illicit drugs, and performance enhancers: a comparison of use by college student athletes and nonathletes. J Am Coll Health. 2008;57(3):281–90.

158. Shirreffs SM, Maughan RJ. The effect of alcohol on athletic performance. Curr Sports Med Rep. 2006;5(4):192–6.

159. Parks PS, Read MH. Adolescent male athletes: body image, diet, and exercise. Adolescence. 1997;32(127):593–602.

160. Jonnalagadda SS, Rosenbloom CA, Skinner R. Dietary practices, attitudes, and physiological status of collegiate freshman football players. J Strength Cond Res. 2001;15(4):507–13.

161. Short SH, Short WR. Four year study of university athletes' dietary intake. J Am Diet Assoc. 1983;82(6):632–45.

162. Burke LM, Hawley JA. Fluid balance in team sports: guidelines for optimal practices. Sports Med. 1997;24(1):38–54.

163. Criswell D, Powers D, Lawler J, Tew J, Dodd S, Iryiboz Y, Tulley R, Wheeler K. Influence of a carbohydrate-electrolyte beverage on performance and blood homeostasis during recovery from football. Int J Sport Nutr. 1991;1(2):178–91.

164. Judge LW, Kumley RF, Bellar DM, Pike KL, Pierson EE, Weidner T, Pearson D, Friesen CA. Hydration and fluid replacement knowledge, attitudes, barriers, and behaviors of NCAA Division 1 American football players. J Strength Cond Res. 2016;30(11):2972–8.

165. Gomez JE, Ross SK, Calmbach WL, Kimmel RB, Schmidt DR, Dhanda R. Body fatness and increased injury rates in high school football linemen. Clin J Sport Med. 1998;8(2):115–20.

166. Kaplan TA, Digel SL, Scavo VA, Arellana SB. Effect of obesity on injury risk in high school football players. Clin J Sport Med. 1995;5(1):43–7.

167. Garber L, Benardot D, Thompson WR, Wanders D. The Relationships Between Energy Balance, Timing and Quantity of Protein Consumption, and Body Composition in Collegiate Football Players. Thesis, Georgia State University, 2016. Accessed May 22, 2018. Available from: http://scholarworks.gsu.edu/nutrition_theses/79

168. Jenner SL, Buckley GL, Belski R, Devlin BL, Forsyth AK. Dietary intakes of professional and semi-professional team sport athletes do no meet sports nutrition recommendations – A systematic literature review. Nutrients. 2019;11:1160.

169. Sánchez-Díaz S, Yanci J, Castillo D, Scanlan AT, Raya-González J. Effects of nutrition education interventions in team sport players. A systematic review. Nutrients. 2020;12:3664.

170. Georgopoulos NA, Markou KB, Theodoropoulou A, Benardot D, Leglise M, Vagenakis AG. Growth retardation in artistic compared with rhythmic elite female gymnasts. J Clin Endocrinol Metab. 2002;87(7):3169–73.

171. Benardot D, Czerwinski C. Selected body composition and growth measures of junior elite gymnasts. J Am Diet Assoc. 1991;91(1):29–33.

172. Jonnalagadda SS, Benardot D, Nelson M. Energy and nutrient intakes of the United States national women's artistic gymnastics team. Int J Sport Nutr Exerc Metab. 1998;8(4):331–44.

173. Maddux GT. Men's gymnastics. Pacific Palisades (CA): Goodyear Publishing; 1970. p. 9.

174. Houtkooper LB, Going SB. Body composition: how should it be measured? Does it affect sport performance? Sports Sci Exch. 1994;52(5s):7.

175. Bortz S, Schoonen JC, Kanter M, Kosharek S, Benardot D. Physiology of anaerobic and aerobic exercise. In: Benardot D, editor. Sports nutrition: a guide for the professional working with active people. Chicago (IL): American Dietetic Association; 1993. p. 2–10.

176. Benardot D. Working with young athletes: views of a nutritionist on the Sports Medicine team. Int J Sport Nutr. 1996; 6(2):110–20.

177. Benardot D, Schwarz M, Heller DW. Nutrient intake in young, highly competitive gymnasts. J Am Diet Assoc. 1989; 89(3):401–3.

178. Loosli AR. Reversing sports-related iron and zinc deficiencies. Phys Sportsmed. 1993;21(6):70–8.

179. Burns J, Dugan L. Working with professional athletes in the rink: the evolution of a nutrition program for an NHL team. Int J Sport Nutr. 1994;4(2):132–4.

180. Reading KJ, McCargar LJ, Marriage BJ. Adolescent and young adult male hockey players: Nutrition knowledge and education. Can J Diet Pract Res. 1999;60(3):166–9.

181. Akermark C, Jacobs I, Rasmussen M, Karlsson J. Diet and muscle glycogen concentration in relation to physical performance in Swedish elite ice hockey players. Int J Sport Nutr. 1996;6(3):272–84.

182. Houston ME. Nutrition and ice hockey performance. Can J Appl Sport Sci. 1979;4(1):98–9.

183. Tegelman R, Aberg T, Pousette, A, Carlstrom K. Effects of a diet regimen on pituitary and steroid hormones in male ice hockey players. Int J Sports Med. 1992;13(5):424–30.

184. Benardot D. Energy thermodynamics revisited: energy intake strategies for optimizing athlete body composition and performance. J Exerc Sci Health (Revista de Ciencias del Ejercicio y la Salud). 2013;11(2):1–13.

185. Horswill CA, Hickner RC, Scott JR, Costill DL, Gould D. Weight loss, dietary carbohydrate modifications, and high intensity, physical performance. Med Sci Sports Exerc. 1990; 22(4):470–6.

186. Palmer MS, Spriet LL. Sweat rate, salt loss, and fluid intake during an intense on-ice practice in elite Canadian male junior hockey players. Appl Physiol Nutr Metab. 2008;33(2):263–71.

187. Kreider RB, Ferreira M, Wilson M, Grindstaff P, Plisk S, Reinardy J, Cantler E, Almada AL. Effects of creatine supplementation on body composition, strength, and sprint performance. Med Sci Sports Exerc. 1998;30(1):73–82.

188. Nevill ME, Williams C, Roper D, Slater C, Nevill AM. Effect of diet on performance during recovery from intermittent sprint exercise. J Sports Sci. 1993;11(2):119–26.

189. Balsom PD, Gaitanos GC, Söderlund K, Ekblom B. High-intensity exercise and muscle glycogen availability in humans. Acta Physiol Scand. 1999;165(4):337–45.

190. Couto PG, Bertuzzi R, de Souza CC, Lima HM, Kiss MA, de-Oliveira FR, Lima-Silva AE. High carbohydrate diet induces faster final sprint and overall 10,000 m times of young runners. Pediatr Exerc Sci. 2015;27(3):355–63.

191. Skein M, Duffield R, Kelly BT, Marino FE. The effects of carbohydrate intake and muscle glycogen content on self-paced intermittent-sprint exercise despite no knowledge of carbohydrate manipulation. Eur J Appl Physiol. 2012;112: 2859–70.

192. Cooper R, Naclerio F, Allgrove J, Larumbe-Zabala E. Effects of a carbohydrate and caffeine gel on intermittent sprint performance in recreationally trained males. Eur J Sport Sci. 2014;14(4):353–61.

193. Olsson K-E, Saltin B. Variation in total body water with muscle glycogen changes in man. Acta Physiol Scand. 1970; 80(1):11–8.

194. Shaw G, Boyd KT, Burke LM, Kovisto A. Nutrition for swimming. Int J Sport Nutr Exerc Metab. 2014;24(4):360–72.

195. Berning JR, Troup JP, VanHandel PJ, Daniels J, Daniels N. The nutritional habits of young adolescent swimmers. Int J Sport Nutr. 1991;1(3):240–8.

196. Kabasakalis A, Kalitsis K, Tsalis G, Mougios V. Imbalanced nutrition of top-level swimmers. Int J Sports Med. 2007;28:1–7.

197. Shaw G, Koivisto A, Gerrard D, Burke LM. Nutrition considerations for open-water swimming. Int J Sport Nutr Exerc Metab. 2014;24(4):373–81.

198. Areta JL, Burke LM, Ross ML, Camera DM, West DW, Broad EM, Jeacocke NA, Moore DR, Stellingwerff T, Phillips SM, Hawley JA, Coffey VG. Timing and distribution of protein ingestion during prolonged recovery from resistance exercise alters myofibrillar protein synthesis. J Physiol. 2013;591(9):2319–31.

199. Burke LM, Mujika I. Nutrition recovery in aquatic sports. Int J Sport Nutr Exerc Metab. 2014;24(4):425–36.

200. Pyne D, Sharp RL. Physical and energy requirements of competitive swimming events. Int J Sport Nutr Exerc Metab. 2014;24(4):351–9.

201. Robillard JI, Adams JD, Johnson EC, Bardis CN, Summers LG, Huffman A, Vidal T, Hammer ML, Kavouras SA. Fluid balance of adolescent swimmers during training. Int J Exerc Sci. 2014;11(2). Accessed May 23, 2018. Available from: http://digitalcommons.wku.edu/ijesab/vol11/iss2/48.

202. Sossin K, Gizis F, Marquart, LF, Sobal J. Nutrition beliefs, attitudes, and resource use of high school wrestling coaches. Int J Sport Nutr. 1997;7(3):219–28.

203. Oppliger RA, Case HS, Horswill CA, Landry GL, Shelter AC. American College of Sports Medicine position stand: weight loss in wrestlers. Med Sci Sports Exerc. 1996;28(6):ix–xii.

204. Wroble RR, Moxley DP. Weight loss patterns and success rates in high school wrestlers. Med Sci Sports Exerc. 1998;30(4): 625–8.

205. Wroble RR, Moxley DP. Acute weight gain and its relationship to success in high school wrestlers. Med Sci Sports Exerc. 1998;30(6):949–51.

206. Roemmich JN, Sinning WE. Weight loss and wrestling training: effects on growth-related hormones. J Appl Physiol. 1997;82(6):1760–4.

207. Roemmich JN, Sinning WE. Weight loss and wrestling training: effects on nutrition, growth, maturation, body composition, and strength. J Appl Physiol. 1997;2(6):1751–9.

208. Rankin JW, Ocel JV, Craft LL. Effect of weight loss and refeeding diet composition on anaerobic performance in wrestlers. Med Sci Sports Exerc. 1996;28(10):1292–9.

209. Choma CW, Sforzo GA, Keller BA. Impact of rapid weight loss on cognitive function in collegiate wrestlers. Med Sci Sports Exerc. 1998;30(5):746–9.

210. Oppliger RA, Harms RD, Herrmann DE, Streich CM, Clark RR. The Wisconsin wrestling minimum weight project: a model for weight control among high school wrestlers. Med Sci Sports Exerc. 1995;27(8):1220–4.

211. Jeukendrup AE. Nutrition for endurance sports: marathon, triathlon, and road cycling. J Sports Sci. 2011;29(S1):S91–9.

212. Pfeiffer B, Stellingwerff T, Hodgson AB, Randell R, Pöttgen K, Res P, Jeukendrup AE. Nutritional intake and gastrointestinal problems during competitive endurance events. Med Sci Sports Exerc. 2012;44(2):344–51.

213. Rehrer, NJ, van Kemenade M, Meester W, Brouns F, Saris WH. Gastrointestinal complaints in relation to dietary intake in triathletes. Int J Sport Nutr. 1992;2(1):48–59.

214. Penn IW, Wan ZM, Buhl KM, Allison DB, Burastero SE, Heymsfield SB. Body composition and two-compartment model assumptions in male long-distance runners. Med Sci Sports Exerc. 1994;26(3):392–7.

215. Warden SJ, Davis IS, Fredericson MD. Management and prevention of bone stress injuries in long-distance runners. J Orthop Sports Phys Ther. 2014;44(10):749–65.

216. Reeder MT, Dick BH, Atkins JK, Pribis AB, Martinez JM. Stress fractures: current concepts of diagnosis and treatment. Sports Med. 1996;22(3):198–212.

217. Wright AA, Taylor JB, Ford KR, Siska L, Smoliga JM. Risk factors associated with lower extremity stress fractures in runners: a systematic review with meta-analysis. Br J Sports Med. 2015;49(23):1517–23.

218. Wentz LM, Liu P-Y, Ilich JZ, Haymes EM. Female distance runners training in southeastern United States have adequate vitamin D status. Int J Sport Nutr Exerc Metab. 2016;26(5):397–403.

219. Deuster PA, Kyle SB, Moser PB, Vigersky RA, Singh A, Schoomaker EB. Nutritional intakes and status of highly trained amenorrheic and eumenorrheic women runners. Fertil Steril. 1986;46(4):636–43.

220. Beidleman BA, Puhl JL, DeSouza MJ. Energy balance in female distance runners. Am J Clin Nutr. 1995;61(2):303–11.

221. Del Coso J, Fernández D, Albián-Vicen J, Salinero JJ, González-Millán C, Areces F, Ruiz D, Gallo C, Calleja-González J, Pérez-González B. Running pace decrease during marathon is positively related to blood markers of muscle damage. PLoS One. 2013;8(2):e57602.

222. Geralda Ferreira F, Gonçalves Pereira L, Rodrigues Xavier WD, Ana Paula MG, Ângela Maria CS, Neuza Maria BC, João Carlos BM. Hydration practices of runners during training vs competition. Arch Med Deporte. 2016; 33(171):11–7.

223. Millard-Stafford ML, Sparling PB, Rosskopf LB, DiCarlo LJ. Carbohydrate-electrolyte replacement improves distance running performance in the heat. Med Sci Sports Exerc. 1992;24(8):934–40.

224. Gulbin JP, Gaffney PT. Ultraendurance triathlon participation: typical race preparation of lower-level triathletes. J Sports Med Phys Fitness. 1999;39(1):12–5.

225. Banister EW, Carter JB, Zarkadas PC. Training theory and taper: validation in triathlon athletes. Eur J Appl Physiol. 1999;79(2):182–91.

226. Giannopoulou I, Noutsos K, Apostolidis N, Baylos I, Nassis GP. Performance level affects the dietary supplement intake of both individual and team sports athletes. J Sports Sci Med. 2013;12(1):190–6.

227. Guezennec CY, Chalabi H, Bernard J, Fardellone P, Krentowski R, Zerath E, Meunier PJ. Is there a relationship between physical activity and dietary calcium intake? A survey in 10,373 young French subjects. Med Sci Sports Exerc. 1998;30(5):732–9.

228. Baillot M, Hue O. Hydration and thermoregulation during a half-ironman performed in tropical climate. J Sports Sci Med. 2015;14(2):263–8.

229. Rogers G, Goodman C, Rosen C. Water budget during ultra-endurance exercise. Med Sci Sports Exerc. 1997;29(11):1477–81.

230. Cox GR, Snow RJ, Burke LM. Race-day carbohydrate intakes of elite triathletes contesting Olympic-distance triathlon events. Int J Sport Nutr Exerc Metab. 2010;20(4):299–306.

231. Robins A. Nutritional recommendations for competing in the ironman triathlon. Curr Sports Med Rep. 2007;6(4):241–8.

232. Frentsos JA, Baer JT. Increased energy and nutrient intake during training and competition improves elite triathletes' endurance performance. Int J Sport Nutr. 1997;7(1):61–71.

233. Melin A, Torstveit MK, Burke LM, Marks S, Sundgot-Borgen J. Disordered eating and eating disorders in aquatic sports. Int J Sport Nutr Exerc Metab. 2014;24(4):450–9.

234. Bentley DJ, Wilson GJ, Davie AJ, Zhou S. Correlations between peak power output, muscular strength, and cycle time trial performance in triathletes. J Sports Med Phys Fitness. 1998;38(3):201–7.

235. Lee EJ, Long KA, Risser WL, Poindexter HB, Gibbons WE, Goldzieher J. Variations in bone status of contralateral and regional sites in young athletic women. Med Sci Sports Exerc. 1995;27(10):1354–61.

236. Manolagas SC, O'Brien CA, Almeida M. The role of estrogen and androgen receptors in bone health and disease. Nat Rev Endocrinol. 2013;9:699–712.

237. Saris WH, Schrijver J, van Erp Baart MA, Brouns F. Adequacy of vitamin supply under maximal sustained workloads: The Tour de France. Int J Vitam Nutr Res Suppl. 1989;30(Suppl):205–12.

238. Brouns F, Saris WH, Stroecken J, Beckers E, Thijssen R, Rehrer JN, ten Hoor F. Eating, drinking, and cycling: a controlled Tour de France simulation study, Part II. Effect of diet manipulation. Int J Sports Med. 1989;10(S1):S41–8.

239. Weiler JM, Layton T, Hunt M. Asthma in United States Olympic athletes who participated in the 1996 Summer Games. J Allergy Clin Immunol. 1998;102(5):722–6.

240. Hansen M, Bangsbo J, Jensen J, Krause-Jensen M, Bibby BM, Sollie O, Hall UA, Madsen K. Protein intake during training sessions has no effect on performance and recovery during a strenuous training camp for elite cyclists. J Int Soc Sports Nutr. 2016;13(9):9.

Index

Note: Page numbers followed by *f* and *t* indicate figures and tables, respectively.

A